FIRST AID FOR THE®

USMLE STEP 1 2015

TAO LE, MD, MHS
Associate Clinical Professor
Chief, Section of Allergy and Immunology
Department of Medicine
University of Louisville

VIKAS BHUSHAN, MD
Diagnostic Radiologist
Los Angeles

MATTHEW SOCHAT, MD
Resident, Department of Neurology
New York University School of Medicine

PATRICK SYLVESTER
The Ohio State University College of Medicine
Class of 2015

MICHAEL MEHLMAN
University of Queensland, Australia
Class of 2015

KIMBERLY KALLIANOS, MD
Resident, Department of Radiology and Biomedical Imaging
University of California, San Francisco

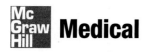 **Medical**

New York / Chicago / San Francisco / Lisbon / London / Madrid / Mexico City
Milan / New Delhi / San Juan / Seoul / Singapore / Sydney / Toronto

First Aid for the® USMLE Step 1 2015: A Student-to-Student Guide

Previous editions copyright © 1991 through 2014 by Vikas Bhushan and Tao Le. First edition copyright © 1990, 1989 by Vikas Bhushan, Jeffrey Hansen, and Edward Hon.

Photo and line art credits for this book begin on page 669 and are considered an extension of this copyright page. Portions of this book identified with the symbol ℞ are copyright © USMLE-Rx.com (MedIQ Learning, LLC). Portions of this book identified with the symbol RU are copyright © Dr. Richard Usatine. Portions of this book identified with the symbol ✴ are under license from other third parties. Please refer to page 669 for a complete list of those image source attribution notices.

First Aid for the® is a registered trademark of McGraw-Hill Education.

1 2 3 4 5 6 7 8 9 0 RMN/RMN 15 14

ISBN 978-0-07-184006-4
MHID 0-07-184006-0
ISSN 1532-6020

Notice

Medicine is an ever-changing science. As new research and clinical experience broaden our knowledge, changes in treatment and drug therapy are required. The authors and the publisher of this work have checked with sources believed to be reliable in their efforts to provide information that is complete and generally in accord with the standards accepted at the time of publication. However, in view of the possibility of human error or changes in medical sciences, neither the authors nor the publisher nor any other party who has been involved in the preparation or publication of this work warrants that the information contained herein is in every respect accurate or complete, and they disclaim all responsibility for any errors or omissions or for the results obtained from use of the information contained in this work. Readers are encouraged to confirm the information contained herein with other sources. For example and in particular, readers are advised to check the product information sheet included in the package of each drug they plan to administer to be certain that the information contained in this work is accurate and that changes have not been made in the recommended dose or in the contraindications for administration. This recommendation is of particular importance in connection with new or infrequently used drugs.

This book was set in Electra LT Std by Rainbow Graphics.
The editors were Catherine A. Johnson and Peter J. Boyle.
Project management was provided by Rainbow Graphics.
The production supervisor was Jeffrey Herzich.
RR Donnelley was printer and binder.

This book is printed on acid-free paper.

McGraw-Hill Education books are available at special quantity discounts to use as premiums and sales promotions, or for use in corporate training programs. To contact a representative please visit the Contact Us pages at www.mhprofessional.com.

Dedication

To the contributors to this and past editions, who took time to share their knowledge, insight, and humor for the benefit of students.

Contents

▶ SECTION I — GUIDE TO EFFICIENT EXAM PREPARATION — 1

▶ SECTION I SUPPLEMENT — SPECIAL SITUATIONS — 23

▶ SECTION II — HIGH-YIELD GENERAL PRINCIPLES — 43

Contributing Authors

DANIEL AARONSON
Sackler School of Medicine
Class of 2016

MARK D. ARD, MA
Editor, firstaidteam.com
Loma Linda University School of Medicine
Class of 2016

YASH CHAVDA
NYIT College of Osteopathic Medicine
Class of 2015

FRANCIS DENG
Washington University School of Medicine in St. Louis
Class of 2016

NATHANIEL R. GREENBAUM
Sackler School of Medicine
Class of 2016

ANN R. HUA
University of Texas Health Science Center at San Antonio
Class of 2017

JACK HUA
University of Texas Health Science Center at San Antonio
Class of 2015

JOUZIF IBRAHIM, MD
Resident, Department of Anesthesiology
New York State University at Buffalo School of Medicine

MEHBOOB KALANI
University of St. Eustatius School of Medicine
Class of 2015

M. SCOTT MOORE, DO
Resident, Department of Pathology
University of Arizona School of Medicine

JUDITH RAMEL, MD
American University of the Caribbean
Class of 2014

NINO SIKHARULIDZE, MD
Department of Endocrinology
Tbilisi State Medical University

JARED A. WHITE, MS
University of Mississippi School of Medicine
Class of 2016

IMAGE AND ILLUSTRATION TEAM

PRAMOD THEETHA KARIYANNA, MD
Resident, Department of Internal Medicine
Brookdale University Hospital and Medical Center

RICHARD P. USATINE, MD
Professor, Dermatology and Cutaneous Surgery
Professor, Family and Community Medicine
University of Texas Health Science Center San Antonio

Associate Authors

JESSIE DHALIWAL
Western University of Health Sciences College of Osteopathic Medicine
Class of 2016

ASHWANI GORE
St. George's University School of Medicine
Class of 2015

JAN ANDRE GRAUMAN, MA
San Juan Bautista School of Medicine
Class of 2016

ERIC DAEHO KIM
Western University of Health Sciences College of Osteopathic Medicine
Class of 2016

RYAN K. MEYER
Rutgers New Jersey Medical School
Class of 2016

SATYAJIT REDDY
Alpert Medical School of Brown University
Class of 2015

IMAGE AND ILLUSTRATION TEAM

WENDY E. ABBOTT
Kentucky College of Osteopathic Medicine
Class of 2015

KEVIN AU
Albany Medical College
Class of 2015

JOCELYN T. COMPTON
Columbia University College of Physicians and Surgeons
Class of 2015

JULIA KING
New York University School of Medicine
MD/PhD Candidate

Faculty Reviewers

MARIA ANTONELLI, MD

Rheumatology Fellow, Department of Medicine
Case Western Reserve University School of Medicine

BRIAN S. APPLEBY, MD

Associate Professor, Department of Neurology
Case Western Reserve University School of Medicine

HERMAN BAGGA, MD

Fellow, Department of Urology
Cleveland Clinic

ADITYA BARDIA, MBBS, MPH

Attending Physician, Massachusetts General Hospital
Harvard Medical School

JOHN BARONE, MD

Anatomic and Surgical Pathology
BaroneRocks.com

BROOKS D. CASH, MD

Professor of Medicine, Division of Gastroenterology
University of South Alabama School of Medicine

LINDA S. COSTANZO, PhD

Professor of Physiology & Biophysics
Virginia Commonwealth University School of Medicine

ANTHONY L. DeFRANCO, PhD

Professor of Microbiology and Immunology
University of California, San Francisco School of Medicine

CHARLES S. DELA CRUZ, MD, PhD

Assistant Professor, Department of Pulmonary and Critical Care Medicine
Yale School of Medicine

CONRAD FISCHER, MD

Residency Program Director, Brookdale University Hospital
Brooklyn, New York
Associate Professor of Medicine, Physiology, and Pharmacology
Touro College of Medicine

STUART D. FLYNN, MD

Dean, College of Medicine
University of Arizona College of Medicine, Phoenix

JEFFREY J. GOLD, MD

Associate Professor, Department of Neurology
University of California, San Diego School of Medicine

WHITNEY GREEN, MD

Resident, Department of Pathology
Johns Hopkins Hospital

RYAN C. W. HALL, MD

Assistant Professor, Department of Psychiatry
University of South Florida

MARGARET HAYES, MD

Pulmonary and Critical Care Fellow
Johns Hopkins Hospital

JEFFREY W. HOFMANN, PhD

The Warren Alpert Medical School of Brown University
MD Candidate

DEEPALI JAIN, MD

Assistant Professor, Department of Pathology
All India Institute of Medical Sciences

BRIAN C. JENSEN, MD

Assistant Professor of Medicine and Pharmacology
University of North Carolina McAllister Heart Institute

JENNIFER LE, MD

Associate Professor, Division of Child and Adolescent Psychiatry
University of Louisville School of Medicine

GERALD LEE, MD

Assistant Professor, Department of Pediatrics
University of Louisville School of Medicine

KACHIU LEE, MD, MPH

Department of Dermatology
Harvard Medical School

WARREN LEVINSON, MD, PhD

Professor, Department of Microbiology & Immunology
University of California, San Francisco School of Medicine

NICHOLAS MAHONEY, MD
Assistant Professor of Ophthalmology
Wilmer Eye Institute/Johns Hopkins Hospital

PETER MARKS, MD, PhD
Associate Professor, Department of Internal Medicine
Yale School of Medicine

J. RYAN MARTIN, MD
Assistant Professor of Obstetrics, Gynecology, and Reproductive Sciences
Yale University School of Medicine

JEANNINE RAHIMIAN, MD, MBA
Associate Professor of Obstetrics and Gynecology
David Geffen School of Medicine at UCLA

SOROUSH RAIS-BAHRAMI, MD
Assistant Professor of Urology and Radiology
The University of Alabama at Birmingham School of Medicine

SASAN SAKIANI, MD
Fellow, Division of Gastroenterology and Hepatology
Case Western Reserve University School of Medicine

JOSEPH L. SCHINDLER, MD
Assistant Professor of Neurology and Neurosurgery
Yale School of Medicine

NATHAN W. SKELLEY, MD
Resident, Department of Orthopaedic Surgery
Washington University School of Medicine in St. Louis

HOWARD M. STEINMAN, PhD
Assistant Dean of Biomedical Science Education
Professor, Department of Biochemistry
Albert Einstein College of Medicine

STEPHEN F. THUNG, MD
Associate Professor, Department of Obstetrics and Gynecology
Ohio State University College of Medicine

HILARY J. VERNON, MD, PhD
Assistant Professor, McKusick Nathans Institute of Genetic Medicine
Johns Hopkins University

ADAM WEINSTEIN, MD
Assistant Professor, Section of Pediatric Nephrology
Geisel School of Medicine at Dartmonth

Twenty-Fifth Anniversary Foreword

Our exam experiences remain vivid in our minds to this day as we reflect on 25 years of *First Aid*. In 1989, our big idea was to cobble together a "quick and dirty" study guide so that we would never again have to deal with the USMLE Step 1. We passed, but in a Faustian twist, we now relive the exam yearly while preparing each new edition.

Like all students before us, we noticed that certain topics tended to appear frequently on examinations. So we compulsively bought and rated review books and pored through a mind-numbing number of "recall" questions, distilling each into short facts. We had a love-hate relationship with mnemonics. They went against our purist desires for conceptual knowledge, but remained the best way to absorb the vocabulary and near-random associations that unlocked questions and eponyms.

To pull it all together, we used a then–"state-of-the-art" computer database (Paradox/MS DOS 4) that fortuitously limited our entries to 256 characters. That single constraint mandated brevity, while the three-column layout created structure—and this was the blueprint upon which *First Aid* was founded.

The printed, three-column database was first distributed in 1989 at the University of California, San Francisco. The next year, the official first edition was self-published under the title *High-Yield Basic Science Boards Review: A Student-to-Student Guide*. The following year, our new publisher dismissed the *High-Yield* title as too confusing and came up with *First Aid for the Boards*. We thought the name was a bit cheesy, but it proved memorable. Interestingly, our "High-Yield" name resurfaced years later as the title of a competing board review series.

We lived in San Francisco and Los Angeles during medical school and residency. It was before the Web, and before med students could afford cell phones and laptops, so we relied on AOL e-mail and bulky desktops. One of us would drive down to the other person's place for multiple weekends of frenetic revisions fueled by triple-Swiss white chocolate lattes from the Coffee Bean & Tea Leaf, with R.E.M. and the Nusrat Fateh Ali Khan playing in the background. Everything was marked up on 11- by 17-inch "tearsheets," and at the end of the marathon weekend we would converge at the local 24-hour Kinko's followed by the FedEx box near LAX (10 years before these two great institutions merged). These days we work with our online collaborative platform A.nnotate, GoToMeeting, and ubiquitous broadband Internet, and sadly, we rarely get to see each other.

What hasn't changed, however, is the collaborative nature of the book. Thousands of authors, editors, and contributors have enriched our lives and made this book possible. Most helped for a year or two and moved on, but a few, like Ted Hon, Chirag Amin, and Andi Fellows, made lasting contributions. Like the very first edition, the team is always led by student authors who live and breathe (and fear) the exam, not professors years away from that reality.

We're proud of the precedent that *First Aid* set for the many excellent student-to-student publications that followed. More importantly, *First Aid* itself owes its success to the global community of medical students and international medical graduates (IMGs) who each year contribute ideas, suggestions, and new content. In the early days, we used book coupons and tear-out business reply mail forms. These days, we get more than 20,000 comments and suggestions each year via our blog FirstAidTeam.com and A.nnotate.

At the end of the day, we don't take any of this for granted. There are big changes in store for the USMLE, and a bigger job ahead of us to try to keep *First Aid* indispensable to students and IMGs. We want and need your participation in the *First Aid* community. (See How to Contribute, p. xix.) With your help, we hope editing *First Aid* for the next 25 years will be just as fun and rewarding as the past 25 years have been.

Louisville   Tao Le

Los Angeles   Vikas Bhushan

First Aid for the USMLE Step 1 Through the Years

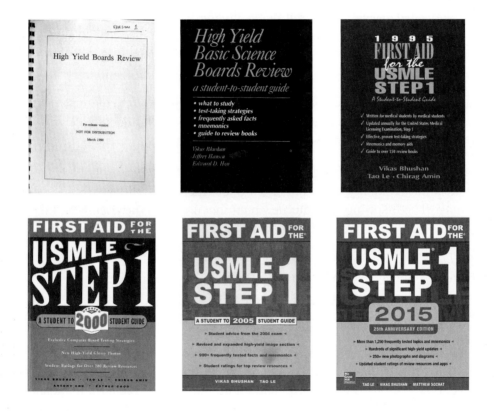

Preface

With the 25th anniversary edition of *First Aid for the USMLE Step 1,* we continue our commitment to providing students with the most useful and up-to-date preparation guide for the USMLE Step 1. This edition represents an outstanding revision in many ways, including:

- Dozens of entirely new facts and hundreds of major fact updates culled from more than 20,000 comments and suggestions.

- Extensive text revisions, new mnemonics, clarifications, and corrections curated by a team of 25 student authors who excelled on their Step 1 examinations and verified by a team of expert faculty and nationally recognized USMLE instructors.

- Updated with more than 250 new full-color images to help visualize various disorders, descriptive findings, and basic science concepts. Labeled and captioned photographs have been selected to aid retention by engaging visual memory in a manner complementary to mnemonics.

- Updated with dozens of new and revised diagrams. We continue to expand our collaboration with USMLE-Rx (MedIQ Learning, LLC) to develop and enhance illustrations with improved information design to help students integrate pathophysiology, therapeutics, and diseases into memorable frameworks for annotation and personalization.

- A revised exam preparation guide with updated data from the NBME and NRMP. The guide also features new high-yield techniques for efficient and effective test preparation.

- An updated summary guide to student-recommended USMLE Step 1 review resources, including mobile apps for iOS and Android. The full resource guide with detailed descriptions can be found at our blog, **www.firstaidteam.com**.

- Real-time Step 1 updates and corrections can also be found exclusively on our blog.

We invite students and faculty to share their thoughts and ideas to help us continually improve *First Aid for the USMLE Step 1* through our blog and collaborative editorial platform. (See How to Contribute, p. xix.)

Louisville	Tao Le
Los Angeles	Vikas Bhushan
New York City	Matthew Sochat
Queensland	Michael Mehlman
Athens, Ohio	Patrick Sylvester
San Francisco	Kimberly Kallianos

Special Acknowledgments

This has been a collaborative project from the start. We gratefully acknowledge the thousands of thoughtful comments, corrections, and advice of the many medical students, international medical graduates, and faculty who have supported the authors in our continuing development of *First Aid for the USMLE Step 1*.

We provide special acknowledgment and thanks to the following students who made exemplary contributions to this edition through our voting, proofreading, and crowdsourcing platform: Ram Baboo, Kash Badar, Maria Bakkal, Gauri Barlingay, Jorge Martinez Bencosme, Kenneth Max Brock, Anup Chalise, Ujval Choksi, Jensyn Cone, Eliana Costantino, Andrew Crisologo, John Cummins, Solomon Dawson, Kathryn Demitruk, Isaac M. Dodd, Daniel Franco, Jared Gans, Okubit Gebreyonas, Alejandro Gener, Maikel Ragaei Ramzi Fahmi Gerges, Jacqueline Hairston, Joyce Ho, M. Ho, Sakshi Jain, Benjamin Hans Jeuk, Shirley Ju, Suthasenthuran Kanagalingam, Tamer Khashab, Mariah Kirsch, Vladimer Kitiashvili, Mary Lan, Yedda Li, Matthew Lippmann, Robert McKenna, Nicolaus Mephis, Caroline Murrell, Natia Murvelashvili, Shehni Nadeem, Yeon-Kyeong Noh, Vanessa Pascoe, Iqra Patoli, Arun Rajaratnam, Josean Ramos, Huma Rasheed, Dolly Sharma, Jared Shenson, Yue Shi, Huijuan Song, Justin Sysol, and Sandra Tomlinson-Hansen.

For help on the Web, thanks to Mark Ard, Edison Cano, Tim Durso, Ryan Nguyen, and Joe Savarese. For support and encouragement throughout the process, we are grateful to Thao Pham and Jonathan Kirsch, Esq. Thanks to Louise Petersen for organizing and supporting the project. Thanks to our publisher, McGraw-Hill, for the valuable assistance of its staff, including Midge Haramis and Jeffrey Herzich. For enthusiasm, support, and commitment for this ongoing and ever-challenging project, thanks to our editor, Catherine Johnson.

We are also very grateful to Dr. Fred Howell and Dr. Robert Cannon of Textensor Ltd for providing us extensive customization and support for their powerful A.nnotate collaborative editing platform, which allows us to efficiently manage thousands of contributions. Many thanks to Dr. Richard Usatine for his outstanding dermatologic and clinical image contributions. Thanks also to Jean-Christophe Fournet (*www.humpath.com*), Dr. Ed Uthman, and Dr. Frank Gaillard (*www.radiopaedia.org*) for generously allowing us to access some of their striking photographs.

For exceptional editorial support, enormous thanks to our tireless senior editor, Emma D. Underdown, and her team of editors, Christine Diedrich, Linda Davoli, Janene Matragrano, Isabel Nogueira, and Rebecca Stigall. Many thanks to Tara Price for page design and all-around InDesign expertise. Special thanks to Jan Bednarczuk for a greatly improved index. We are also grateful to our medical illustrators, Andrea Charest, Justin Klein, Karina Metcalf, and Hans Neuhart, for their creative work on the new and updated illustrations. Lastly, tremendous thanks to Rainbow Graphics, especially David Hommel and Donna Campbell, for remarkable ongoing editorial and production support under time pressure.

Louisville	Tao Le
Los Angeles	Vikas Bhushan
New York City	Matthew Sochat
Queensland	Michael Mehlman
Athens, Ohio	Patrick Sylvester
San Francisco	Kimberly Kallianos

General Acknowledgments

This year, we were fortunate to receive the input of thousands of medical students and graduates who provided new material, clarifications, and potential corrections through our Web site and our collaborative editing platform. This has been a tremendous help in clarifying difficult concepts, correcting errata from the previous edition, and minimizing new errata during the revision of the current edition. This reflects our long-standing vision of a true, student-to-student publication. We have done our best to thank each person individually below, but we recognize that errors and omissions are likely. Therefore, we will post an updated list of acknowledgements at our Web site, www.firstaidteam.com/. We will gladly make corrections if they are brought to our attention.

Special thanks to our mnemonics contest contributors: Dr. Cheryl Bernstein, Jonathan Berkman, Thomas Campi Jr., François-Xavier Crahay, Ryan Austin Denu, Rajkumar Doshi, Ethan Fram, Marcel T. Ghanim, Jessica Glatz, Alan Groves, Raven G. Harris, Ali Khan, Jacob T. Luty, Ryan Makipour, Alireza Mofid, Daniel Razzano, Paul T. Rutkowski, Kate Ryan, Yoni Samocha, Shan Siddiqi, Christopher Steele, James West, and Dane Yomtov.

For submitting contributions and corrections, many thanks to Mohamed Abou-Kassem, Nauri Abreu, Amin Abu Khatir, Budri Abubaker-Sharif, Omar Abudayyeh, Mishuka Adhikary, Cameron Adler, Arsalan Aftab, Azka Afzal, Anuj Agarwal, Abhi Aggarwal, Joshua Agranat, Gaby Aguilera Nunez, Anosh Ahmed, Muhammad Ahsan Ahsan, Lisa Akiyama, Riad Akkari, Ameen Al-Aghil, Mohammad Alam, Suliaman Alaqeel, Waseem Albasha, Lauren Albers, Lourdes Alberty, Majed Alfi, Muhammad Ali, Andrei Stephan Allicock, Salvador Alonso Martinez, Netanel Alper, Mohammad Jamal Al-Tibi, Muqaddam Ahmed Salim Al-Yafai, Mesfer Alyami, Abhimanyu Amarnani, Andrew Ames, Shannon Amirie, Zhibo An, Sewak Anand, Jen Anderson, Laura Andreias, Kevin Andres, Jonathan Angel, Iffat Anindo, Saeed Arefanian, Miguel Arribas, Seyed Arshia Arshad, Praag Arya, Hosam Asal, Syed Ashraf, Junaid Aslam, Andrew Athanassiou, Jeremiah Au, Jasmine Aulakh, Katherine Austin, John C. Axley, Ibrahim Azar, Alexander Babazadeh, Bradley Baker, David Ballard, Pavan Bang, Raksha Bangalore, Hamza Mohammad Bani Younis, Faustino Banuelos, Perel Baral, Carlos Barbosa, Ayse Dalsu Baris, Luis Barraza, Josh Barrick, Patrick Bartholomew Jr., Matthew Bartow, Eric Basler, Elizabeth Bast, James Bates, Dick Batka, Priya Batta, Mahmoud Bayoumi, Austin Beck, Sabrina Bedell, Alexis Begezda, Juliana Belen-Rodriguez, Peter Belin, Philip Bell, Ryan Bentley, Daniel Benzo, Alexandra Berger, Jonathan Berkman, Bjorn Bernhardsen, Corbett Berry, Rayyan Bhuiyan, Shea Bielby, Jordan Bilezikian, Ryan Birdsall, Brian Birnbaum, Kendra Black, Aaron Blackshaw, Casi Blanton, Ryan Bober, Valentina Bonev, Peter Boulos, Abdelhak Boumenir, Amanda Bowers, Daniel Bradley, Hannes Brandt, Brian Mayrsohn, Kelly Brown, Sareena Brown, Alejandro Bugarini, Abraham Burshan, Saad R. Butt, Matthew Cable-Fabiszak, Ming Cai, Katharine Caldwell, Thomas R. Campi Jr., Stephanie Cantu, Jessica Cao, Justin Cappuzzo, Daniel Carlyle, Blaise Carney, Timothy Carswell, Martin Castaneda, Kenan Celtik, Nikhita Ch., Aron Chacko, Japjot Chahal, Garvin Chan, Arjun Chandrasekaran, Jenny Chen, Jin Chen, Lilyanne Chen, Simon Chen, Wendy Chen, Nancy Cheng, Habib Chera, Hymie Chera, Karan Chhabra, Richa Chhibba, Priyanka Chilakamarri, Shahzad Chindhy, Dheeraj Chinnam, David Chitty, Joshua Cho, Shua Cho, Tony Choi, William Chong, Manita Choudhary, Yun Chu, Alice Chuang, Donald Chuang, Andrew Cibulas, Devin Clark, Beth Clymer, Elizabeth Coffee, Matt Cohn, Lauren Coleman, William Coleman, Joseb A. Colón, Michael Connor, Laura Coonfield, Jared Cooper, Amarilis Cornejo, Matthew Correia, ChenChen Costelloe, Alina Cote, Francesca Cottini, Rachel Courtney, Blake Cross, Jennifer Cushman, Alexander Dabrowiecki, Joseph Daibes, Amulya Dakka, Hiren Darji, Nishedh Dave, Abel David, Michael Davidson, Carine Davila, Brian Dawes, Charles De Jesus, Carlo De la Sancha, Colette DeJong, Ann Ann Delacruz, Lei Deng, Ryan Denu, Henry Derbes III, Yaanik Desai, Asela Dharmadasa, Joseph

Diaz, Peter Dietrich, Cheri Dijamco, Om Parkash Dinani, Corina Din-Lovinescu, Tim Dino, Bill Diplas, Gregory Dorilus, Milap Dubal, James Dui, Robert Duprey, Amer Durrani, Tim Durso, Marco Duverseau, Andrew Dym, Angel Eads, Ryan Eaton, Pasquale Eckert, Mitchell Edwards, Carl Engelke, Nicolas Enriquez, Emmanuel Fadiora, Giselle Falconi, Joseph Farahany, David Farchadi, Tooba Farooqui, Benjamin Feibel, Calvin Feng, Valerie Fernandez, Nicholas Field, Andrew Figoni, Marielys Figueroa Sierra, Matthew Fishman, Trenden Flanigan, Robert Flick, Sara Fondriest, Cody Fowers, Ethan B. Fram, Elizabeth Watts Freeman, Gabrielle Fridman, Brian Fromm, Chuck Fryberger, Debbie Fubara, James Gabriel, Mairre James Gaddi, Abdulaziz Galadari, Vincent Galdi, Michael Gallo, Himali Gandhi, Oliver Gantz, Joseph Garcia, Norberto Garcia, Russell Garcia, Eric Garfinkel, Amanda Garlish, Colby Genrich, Nicholas George, Alex Germano, Lindsey Gerngross, Asem Ghanim, Marcel Ghanim, Zane Giffen, Kurren Gill, Zachary Gillooly, Christin Giordano, Jessica Glatz, Stephanie Gleicher, Ezequiel Gleichgerrcht, Naomi Goldstein, Jolana Gollero, Dibson Gondim, Jessica Gonzalez, Shawn Greenan, Justin Greene, David Greenky, Michael J. E. Greff, Fiorella Grillon Garelli, Ashley Griswold, Allison Grossman, Astrid Grouls, Adam Grumke, Russ Guin, Angad Guliani, Landon Guntman, Nita Gupta, Daniel Gutierrez, Olga Guzovsky, Ryan Hadden, Sam Haider, Mohammad Halaibeh, Jillian Halper, Brittney Hanerhoff, Katelyn Harris, Raven Harris, Rebecca Hartog, William Harvey, Hunaid Hasan, Muhammad Hassan, Sean Healton, Aryles Hedjar, Richard Hickman, Timothy Hicks, Baker Hillawy, Johnson Ho, Keren Ho, Aaron Hodes, Dana Holiday, David Hopkins, Hehua Huang, Jiancheng Huang, Julio Huapaya, Meredith Hubbard, I-Chun Hung, Jenny Huo, Zachary Huttinger, Oluyinka Igberase, Imoh Ikpot, Brian Imada, Joseph Imbus, Brandon Imp, Ameen Iqbal, Amrin Islam, Yehuda Isseroff, Mangala Iyengar, Seema Jaga, Brian James, Marlene Jean, Nathalie Jean-Noel, Salman Ali Jehangir, Krishan Jethwa, Benjamin Jeuk, Jerry John, Jocelyn John, Charlie Jones, Collin Juergens, John Jung, Danielle Kacen, Nashreen Kadri, Michael Kagan, Casey Kaisi, Takayoshi Kakiuchi, Shana Kalaria, Julia Kang, David Kapp, Yvonne Kaptein, Andrew Karas, Nabin Raj Karki, Jay Karri, Ibrahim Kashoor, Sameena Kaur, Billy Kennedy, Marriam Khan, Saber Khan, Yousuf Khan, Zara Khan, Chirag Kher, Edwina Khneisser, Arshia Khorasani-Zadeh, Elias Khorasni-zadeh, Rohan Khurana, Charles Kim, David Kim, Rachel Kim, Youn Kim, Nikhar Kinger, Kathryn Kinser, Sakal Kiv, Catherine Koertje, Monique Konstantinovic, Yelen Korotkaya, Kathleen Kramer, Srikanth Krishnan, Sabin Kshattry, Sudhir Kunchala, Monika Kusuma-Pringle, Maryana Kutuzova, Marcin Kuzma, Alyssa Kwok, Joel Labha, Curtis Lacy, Isabella Lai, Sarah Langdon, Michael Lanni, Thomas Larrew, Michael Larson, Grace Lassiter, Jake Laun, Dimitri Laurent, Stephenie Le, Edward Lee, Joseph Lee, Paul Lee, Susan Lee, Woojin Lee, Claudia Leung, David Levine, Rebecca Levin-Epstein, Bradford Levison, Edgar Miles Leviste, Jack Li, Jun Lim, Franck Lin, Jillian Liu, Christian Lobo, Ben Longwell, Melissa Lopez, Lyz Annette Lopez Perez, Laura Lopez-Roca, Alnardo Lora, Alina Lou, Kein Lowder, Nicholas Lowe, Carlos Loya-Valencia, Kevin Lu, Raulee Lucero, Ternce Lynn, Sean Mackman, Ashwini Mahadev, Lauren Mahale, Lubna Mahmoud, Leann Mainis, Ojas Mainkar, Ryan Makipour, Nicholas Mangnitz, Ninad Maniar, Mahmoud Mansour, Mohamed B. Mansour, Benoit Mapa, Lila Martin, Jorge Martínez, Deborah Martins, Shehryar Masood, Blaine Massey, Michelle Matzko, Mark Mayeda, Sandy Mazzoni, Dustin McCurry, Melissa Meghpara, Drew Mehta, Dillon Meier, Yuzhong Meng, Pranav Merchant, Michael Kingberg, Jonathan Michaels, Patrick Michelier, Sarah Michelson, Alyssa Mierjeski, Lauren Miller, Wesley Miller, Muhammad Minhaj, Dennis Miraglia, Lucas Miranda, Mitch Mitchell, Takudzwa Mkorombindo, Alireza Mofid, Maryam Mohammed, Hassan Reyad Mohsen, Shahir Monsuruddin, Tatsuno Moorhouse, Jarrad Morgan, Marie Morris, Sohrab Mosaddad, Shawn Moshrefi, Giorgio Mottola, Mayssan Muftah, Shawn Munafo, Amir Munir, Tina Munjal, Annamalai Nadarajan, Daniel Naftalovich, Menachem Nagar, Anna Nanigian, Warren Naselsky, Brenton Nash, Iraj Nasrabadi, Rodda Naveen, Shariq Nawab, Nijas Nazar, Derek Nelsen, Bryan Nevil, Jun Yen Ng, Julius Ngu, Cang Nguyen, Mai-Trang Nguyen, Michael Nguyen, Joseph Nicolazzi, Thomas Nienaber, Frank Noto, Vanessa Obas, Ololade Ogunsuyi, Anderson Okafor, Okwudili Okpaleke, Gebreyonas Okubit, Fatai Oluyadi, Owen Ortmayer, Thomas Osinski, Giulia M. Ottaviani, Jordan Owens, Amisha Oza, Denizhan Ozdemir, Samuel Pabon, Monica Pajdak, Kristen Palis, James Palmer, Jason Pan, Khang Wen Pang, Scott Pangonis, Robert Papas, Abhishek Parikh, Ishan Patel, Jay Patel, Kishan Patel, Krishna Patel, Kunal Patel, Pratik Patel, Saikrishna Patibandla, Ricardo Patron Madge, Eric Pease, Rafael De Jesus Perez Rodriguez, Matthew Peters, Pete Peterson, Noona Peto, Jimmy Tam Huy Pham, Allen L. Pimienta, Keyhan Piran, Peter Plumeri, Jayce Porter, Arun Prashar, Vishnu Prathap, Preston Pugh, Audrey Pulitzer, Nisha Punatar, Steven Punzell, Anthony Purgianto, Matthew Purkey, Muhammad Sher Khoh Qaisrani, Muhammad Sohaib Qamar, Xiaoming Qi, Xiaoliang Qiu, Javier Quintero, Elisa Quiroz, Sara Radmard, Ambreen Rafiq, Jonathan Ragheb, Saad Rahmat, Milap Raikundalia, Michael Rains, Vinaya Rajan, Robert Rakowczyk, Priya Ramaswamy, Dhakshitha Rao, Ethan Rault, Amruta Ravan, Mohsin Raza, Tong Ren, David Retamar, Meredith Rideout, Miriam Rivera-Mendoza,

Leah Roberts, Moshe Roberts, Juliana D. Rodriguez, Daniel Rodriguez Benzo, Tova Rogers, Melissa Rojas, Yoram Andres Roman Casul, Mattan Rozenek, Julietta Rubin, Jose Ruiz, Barry Rush, Brian Russ, James Russell, Nicholas Russo, Paul Rutkowski, Muhammad Saad Mostafa, Shoaib Saadat, James Sacca, Mahniya Sadiq, Yelena Safarpour, Glorimar Salcedo, Mohamad Saleh, Ahmed Salem, Sumeet Salhotra, Jorge Salim, Jordan Salmon, Tareq Salous, Linsen Samuel, Yair Saperstein, Sapna Tandon, Sasmit Sarangi, Naveed Sarmast, Ryan Sarver, Mostafa Sarya, Neha Satyanarayana, Frank Scali, Kevin Schafer, Stephen Schale, Michael Schmid, Caroline Schrodt, Christine Schultheiss, Justin Schultz, Nicholas Schwartz, Anthony Scott, Eric Seachrist, Simone Sealey-David, Allen Seba, Serin Seckin, Lara Seiden, Ashley Self, Anna Sevilla, Anand Sewak, Lorenzo Sewanan, Anna Shah, Harsh Shah, Jarna Shah, Bryan Shapiro, Zan Shareef, Amir Sharim, Ahmed Sheikh, Tarick Sheikh, Dhara Sheth, Jia Shi, Muhammad Shuaib, Vincent Sicari, Virinder Sidhu, Brittany Simpson, Vikal Singh, Vishavpreet Singh, Donald Skenandore, Jeremy Slosberg, Matthew Snyder, Peter Sohn, Jun Song, Wilbur Song, Gayathry Sooriyakumar, Mihir Soparkar, Vlasios Sotirchos, Joshua Speirs, John Squiers, Nandita Sriram, Priya Srivastava, Tansha Srivastava, Amelia St. Ange, Cara Staszewski, Yizhen Su, Alisha Subervi-Vázquez, Matthew Sugimoto, Sunam Sujanani, Rafia Sultan, James Sun, Kevin Sun, Feba Sunny, Kriti Suwal, Gorica Svalina, Sujan Swearingen, Rumman Syed, Josh Symes, David Szafron, Janeta Szczepanik, Daniel Tabari, Daniel Tahsoh, Benjamin Tan, Sapna Tandon, Huasong Tang, Andrew Tarr, Sammy Tayiem, David Taylor, Steven Taylor, Jason Teach, Shahrzad Tehranian, Zi Yi Tew, Jessica M. Thomas, Adam Tiagonce, Gloria Tran, Tri Trang, Stefan Trela, Janson Trieu, Michael Troy, Adam Truong, Gavin Tucker, Harika Reddy Tula, Christine Tung, James Tunovic, Alex Turin, Nkechi Ukeekwe, Mark Unger, Sana Usman, Akash Vadhavana, Joseph Valentin, Olivier Van Houtte, Leah Vance, Arden Vanderwall, Fernando Vazquez de Lara, Erick Candido Velasquez Centellas, Hampton Vernon, Charles Vu, Nicholas Vu, Swetha Vuyyuru, Shaan Wadhawan, Yangyang Waiwai, Jordan Walker, Emily Walzer, Ezekiel Wang, Kaiser Wang, Leo Wang, Sophie Wang, Wei Wang, Yolanda Wang, Connor Wann, Itaat Wasty, Joseph Waters, Shawna Watson, Jer Weekes, Adam Weiner, Robert Weir, Tristan Weir, Robert Welborn, Lindsey Welch, David Weltman, Gong Weng, Wells Weymouth, Rand Wilcox Vanden Berg, James Wilhite, Mark Winter, Emily Wirtz, Sunnie Wong, John Worth, James Wrubel, Tianyi Wu, Rong Xia, David Xu, Owais Yahya, Yakov Yakubov, Rian Yalamanchili, Jason Yan, Xiaofeng Yan, Daniel Yang, George Yang, William Yang, Vadim Yerokhin, James Yoon, Christopher Young, Eric Young, Andrew Yousef, Shahrukh A. Yousfi, Ibbad Yousuf, Amy Yu, Guo Yu, Sezzy Yun, Syed Tabish A. Zaidi, Sabina Zawadzka, Antonia Zecevic, Lichuan Zeng, Henry Zhan, Han Zhang, Jessica Zhang, Xueqing Zhang, Jennifer Zhao, Xiao Zheng, Joseph Zilisch, Morgan Zingsheim, Patrick Zito, Isabelle Zuchelkowski, Kathleen Zuniga, and Andrew Zureick.

How to Contribute

This version of *First Aid for the USMLE Step 1* incorporates hundreds of contributions and improvements suggested by student and faculty reviewers. We invite you to participate in this process. Please send us your suggestions for:

- Study and test-taking strategies for the USMLE Step 1

- New facts, mnemonics, diagrams, and clinical images

- High-yield topics that may appear on future Step 1 exams

- Personal ratings and comments on review books, question banks, apps, videos, and courses

For each new entry incorporated into the next edition, you will receive up to a **$20 Amazon.com gift card** as well as personal acknowledgment in the next edition. Significant contributions will be compensated at the discretion of the authors. Also, let us know about material in this edition that you feel is low yield and should be deleted.

All submissions including potential errata should ideally be supported with hyperlinks to two current references:

- A dynamically updated Web resource such as *Wikipedia, eMedicine,* or *UpToDate*; and

- A link to an authoritative specialty textbook (search the "topic + *Inkling*" in Google and link to the courtesy pages available from a wide variety of major medical textbooks)

We welcome potential errata on grammar and style if the change improves readability. Please note that *First Aid* style is somewhat unique; for example, we have fully adopted the *AMA Manual of Style* recommendations on eponyms: "We recommend that the possessive form be omitted in eponymous terms."

The preferred way to submit new entries, clarifications, mnemonics, or potential corrections with a valid, authoritative reference is via our Web site: **www.firstaidteam.com**.

This Web site will be continuously updated with validated errata, new high-yield content, and a new online platform to contribute suggestions, mnemonics, diagrams, clinical images, and potential errata.

Alternatively, you can email us at: **firstaidteam@yahoo.com**.

Contributions submitted by **May 15, 2015**, receive priority consideration for the 2016 edition of *First Aid for the USMLE Step 1*. We thank you for taking the time to share your experience and apologize in advance that we cannot individually respond to all contributors as we receive thousands of contributions each year.

▶ NOTE TO CONTRIBUTORS

All contributions become property of the authors and are subject to editing and reviewing. Please verify all data and spellings carefully. Contributions should be supported by at least two high-quality references.

Please include supporting hyperlinks on all content and errata suggestions. Check our Web site first to avoid duplicate submissions. In the event that similar or duplicate entries are received, only the first complete entry received with a valid, authoritative reference will be credited. Please follow the style, punctuation, and format of this edition as much as possible.

▶ JOIN THE FIRST AID TEAM

The *First Aid* author team is pleased to offer part-time and full-time paid internships in medical education and publishing to motivated medical students and physicians. Internships range from a few months (e.g., a summer) up to a full year. Participants will have an opportunity to author, edit, and earn academic credit on a wide variety of projects, including the popular *First Aid* series.

For 2015, we are actively seeking passionate medical students and graduates with a specific interest in improving our medical illustrations, expanding our database of medical photographs, and developing the software that supports our crowdsourcing platform. We welcome people with prior experience and talent in these areas. Relevant skills include clinical imaging, digital photography, digital asset management, information design, medical illustration, graphic design, and software development.

Please email us at **firstaidteam@yahoo.com** with a CV and summary of your interest or sample work.

How to Use This Book

Medical students who have used previous editions of this guide have given us feedback on how best to make use of the book.

START EARLY: Use this book as early as possible while learning the basic medical sciences. The first semester of your first year is not too early! Devise a study plan by reading Section I: Guide to Efficient Exam Preparation, and make an early decision on resources to use by reading Section IV: Top-Rated Review Resources.

LET FIRST AID BE YOUR GUIDE: Annotate material from other resources such as class notes or comprehensive textbooks into your copy of *First Aid*. Use it as a framework for distinguishing between high-yield and low-yield material. Note that *First Aid* is neither a textbook nor a comprehensive review book, and it is not a panacea for inadequate preparation during the first two years of medical school. We strongly recommend that you invest in the latest edition of at least one or two top-rated review resources on each subject to ensure that you learn the material thoroughly.

CONSOLIDATE THE MATERIAL: As you study new material, use the corresponding high-yield facts in *First Aid for the USMLE Step 1* as a means of consolidating knowledge. Make high-yield connections between different organ systems and general principles and focus on material that is most likely to be tested.

INTEGRATE STUDY WITH CASES AND QUESTIONS: To broaden your learning strategy, consider integrating your *First Aid* study with case-based reviews (e.g., *First Aid Cases for the USMLE Step 1*) and practice questions (e.g., *First Aid Q&A for the USMLE Step 1* or the USMLE-Rx Qmax Step 1 question bank). After reviewing a discipline or organ system chapter within *First Aid*, review cases on the same topics and test your knowledge with relevant practice questions. Maintain access to more comprehensive resources (e.g., *First Aid for the Basic Sciences: General Principles* and *Organ Systems*, *First Aid Express* and the *Ultimate* video courses) for deeper review as needed.

PRIME YOUR MEMORY: Return to your annotated Sections II and III several days before taking the USMLE Step 1. The book can serve as a useful way of retaining key associations and keeping high-yield facts fresh in your memory just prior to the exam. The Rapid Review section includes high-yield topics to help guide your studying.

CONTRIBUTE TO FIRST AID: Reviewing the book immediately after your exam can help us improve the next edition. Decide what was truly high and low yield and send us your comments. Feel free to send us scanned images from your annotated *First Aid* book as additional support. Of course, always remember that all examinees are under agreement with the NBME to not disclose the specific details of copyrighted test material.

Common USMLE Laboratory Values

* = Included in the Biochemical Profile (SMA-12)

Blood, Plasma, Serum	Reference Range	SI Reference Intervals
*Alanine aminotransferase (ALT, GPT at 30°C)	8–20 U/L	8–20 U/L
Amylase, serum	25–125 U/L	25–125 U/L
*Aspartate aminotransferase (AST, GOT at 30°C)	8–20 U/L	8–20 U/L
Bilirubin, serum (adult)		
Total // Direct	0.1–1.0 mg/dL // 0.0–0.3 mg/dL	2–17 μmol/L // 0–5 μmol/L
*Calcium, serum (Total)	8.4–10.2 mg/dL	2.1–2.8 mmol/L
*Cholesterol, serum (Total)	140–200 mg/dL	3.6–6.5 mmol/L
*Creatinine, serum (Total)	0.6–1.2 mg/dL	53–106 μmol/L
Electrolytes, serum		
Sodium	135–147 mEq/L	135–147 mmol/L
Chloride	95–105 mEq/L	95–105 mmol/L
* Potassium	3.5–5.0 mEq/L	3.5–5.0 mmol/L
Bicarbonate	22–28 mEq/L	22–28 mmol/L
Gases, arterial blood (room air)		
P_{O_2}	75–105 mmHg	10.0–14.0 kPa
P_{CO_2}	33–44 mmHg	4.4–5.9 kPa
pH	7.35–7.45	[H^+] 36–44 nmol/L
*Glucose, serum	Fasting: 70–110 mg/dL	3.8–6.1 mmol/L
	2-h postprandial: < 120 mg/dL	< 6.6 mmol/L
Growth hormone – arginine stimulation	Fasting: < 5 ng/mL	< 5 μg/L
	provocative stimuli: > 7 ng/mL	> 7 μg/L
Osmolality, serum	275–295 mOsm/kg	275–295 mOsm/kg
*Phosphatase (alkaline), serum (p-NPP at 30°C)	20–70 U/L	20–70 U/L
*Phosphorus (inorganic), serum	3.0–4.5 mg/dL	1.0–1.5 mmol/L
*Proteins, serum		
Total (recumbent)	6.0–7.8 g/dL	60–78 g/L
Albumin	3.5–5.5 g/dL	35–55 g/L
Globulins	2.3–3.5 g/dL	23–35 g/L
*Urea nitrogen, serum (BUN)	7–18 mg/dL	1.2–3.0 mmol/L
*Uric acid, serum	3.0–8.2 mg/dL	0.18–0.48 mmol/L
Cerebrospinal Fluid		
Glucose	40–70 mg/dL	2.2–3.9 mmol/L

(continues)

Hematologic

Erythrocyte count	Male: 4.3–5.9 million/mm^3	$4.3–5.9 \times 10^{12}$/L
	Female: 3.5–5.5 million/mm^3	$3.5–5.5 \times 10^{12}$/L
Hematocrit	Male: 41–53%	0.41–0.53
	Female: 36–46%	0.36–0.46
Hemoglobin, blood	Male: 13.5–17.5 g/dL	2.09–2.71 mmol/L
	Female: 12.0–16.0 g/dL	1.86–2.48 mmol/L
Reticulocyte count	0.5–1.5% of red cells	0.005–0.015
Hemoglobin, plasma	1–4 mg/dL	0.16–0.62 μmol/L
Leukocyte count and differential		
Leukocyte count	4500–11,000/mm^3	$4.5–11.0 \times 10^9$/L
Segmented neutrophils	54–62%	0.54–0.62
Band forms	3–5%	0.03–0.05
Eosinophils	1–3%	0.01–0.03
Basophils	0–0.75%	0–0.0075
Lymphocytes	25–33%	0.25–0.33
Monocytes	3–7%	0.03–0.07
Mean corpuscular hemoglobin	25.4–34.6 pg/cell	0.39–0.54 fmol/cell
Mean corpuscular volume	80–100 μm^3	80–100 fL
Platelet count	150,000–400,000/mm^3	$150–400 \times 10^9$/L
Prothrombin time	11–15 seconds	11–15 seconds
Activated partial thromboplastin time	25–40 seconds	25–40 seconds
Sedimentation rate, erythrocyte (Westergren)	Male: 0–15 mm/h	0–15 mm/h
	Female: 0–20 mm/h	0–20 mm/h
Proteins in urine, total	< 150 mg/24 h	< 0.15 g/24 h

First Aid Checklist for the USMLE Step 1

This is an example of how you might use the information in Section I to prepare for the USMLE Step 1. Refer to corresponding topics in Section I for more details.

Years Prior
☐ Select top-rated review resources as study guides for first-year medical school courses.
☐ Ask for advice from those who have recently taken the USMLE Step 1.

Months Prior
☐ Review computer test format and registration information.
☐ Register six months in advance. Carefully verify name and address printed on scheduling permit. Call Prometric or go online for test date ASAP.
☐ Define goals for the USMLE Step 1 (e.g., comfortably pass, beat the mean, ace the test).
☐ Set up a realistic timeline for study. Cover less crammable subjects first. Review subject-by-subject emphasis and clinical vignette format.
☐ Simulate the USMLE Step 1 to pinpoint strengths and weaknesses in knowledge and test-taking skills.
☐ Evaluate and choose study methods and materials (e.g., review books, question banks).

Weeks Prior
☐ Simulate the USMLE Step 1 again. Assess how close you are to your goal.
☐ Pinpoint remaining weaknesses. Stay healthy (exercise, sleep).
☐ Verify information on admission ticket (e.g., location, date).

One Week Prior
☐ Remember comfort measures (loose clothing, earplugs, etc.).
☐ Work out test site logistics such as location, transportation, parking, and lunch.
☐ Call Prometric and confirm your exam appointment.

One Day Prior
☐ Relax.
☐ Lightly review short-term material if necessary. Skim high-yield facts.
☐ Get a good night's sleep.
☐ Make sure the name printed on your photo ID appears EXACTLY the same as the name printed on your scheduling permit.

Day of Exam
☐ Relax. Eat breakfast. Minimize bathroom breaks during the exam by avoiding excessive morning caffeine.
☐ Analyze and make adjustments in test-taking technique. You are allowed to review notes/study material during breaks on exam day.

After the Exam
☐ Celebrate, regardless.
☐ Send feedback to us on our Web site at **www.firstaidteam.com.**

Guide to Efficient Exam Preparation

"A mind of moderate capacity which closely pursues one study must infallibly arrive at great proficiency in that study."

—Mary Shelley, *Frankenstein*

"Finally, from so little sleeping and so much reading, his brain dried up and he went completely out of his mind."

—Miguel de Cervantes Saavedra, *Don Quixote*

▶ INTRODUCTION

Relax.

This section is intended to make your exam preparation easier, not harder. Our goal is to reduce your level of anxiety and help you make the most of your efforts by helping you understand more about the United States Medical Licensing Examination, Step 1 (USMLE Step 1). As a medical student, you are no doubt familiar with taking standardized examinations and quickly absorbing large amounts of material. When you first confront the USMLE Step 1, however, you may find it all too easy to become sidetracked from your goal of studying with maximal effectiveness. Common mistakes that students make when studying for Step 1 include the following:

- Not understanding how scoring is performed or what the score means
- Starting to study (including *First Aid*) too late
- Starting to study intensely too early and burning out
- Starting to prepare for boards before creating a knowledge foundation
- Using inefficient or inappropriate study methods
- Buying the wrong books or buying more books than you can ever use
- Buying only one publisher's review series for all subjects
- Not using practice examinations to maximum benefit
- Not using review books along with your classes
- Not analyzing and improving your test-taking strategies
- Getting bogged down by reviewing difficult topics excessively
- Studying material that is rarely tested on the USMLE Step 1
- Failing to master certain high-yield subjects owing to overconfidence
- Using *First Aid* as your sole study resource
- Trying to do it all alone

> ▶ *The test at a glance:*
> - *8-hour exam*
> - *Total of 322 multiple choice items*
> - *7 test blocks (60 min/block)*
> - *46 test items per block*
> - *45 minutes of break time, plus another 15 if you skip the tutorial*

In this section, we offer advice to help you avoid these pitfalls and be more productive in your studies.

▶ USMLE STEP 1—THE BASICS

The USMLE Step 1 is the first of three examinations that you must pass in order to become a licensed physician in the United States. The USMLE is a joint endeavor of the National Board of Medical Examiners (NBME) and the Federation of State Medical Boards (FSMB). The USMLE serves as the single examination system for U.S. medical students and international medical graduates (IMGs) seeking medical licensure in the United States.

The Step 1 exam includes test items drawn from the following content areas[1]:
- Anatomy
- Behavioral sciences
- Biochemistry
- Microbiology

- Pathology
- Pharmacology
- Physiology
- Interdisciplinary topics, such as nutrition, genetics, and aging

How Is the Computer-Based Test (CBT) Structured?

The CBT Step 1 exam consists of one "optional" tutorial/simulation block and seven "real" question blocks of 46 questions each (see Figure 1) for a total of 322 questions, timed at 60 minutes per block. A short 11-question survey follows the last question block. The computer begins the survey with a prompt to proceed to the next block of questions.

Once an examinee finishes a particular question block on the CBT, he or she must click on a screen icon to continue to the next block. Examinees **cannot** go back and change their answers to questions from any previously completed block. However, changing answers is allowed **within** a block of questions as long as the block has not been ended and if time permits—**unless** the questions are part of a sequential item test set (see p. 4).

What Is the CBT Like?

Given the unique environment of the CBT, it's important that you become familiar ahead of time with what your test-day conditions will be like. In fact, you can easily add 15 minutes to your break time! This is because the 15-minute tutorial offered on exam day may be skipped if you are already familiar with the exam procedures and the testing interface. The 15 minutes is then added to your allotted break time of 45 minutes for a total of 1 hour of potential break time. You can download the tutorial from the USMLE Web site and do it before test day. This tutorial is the exact same interface you will use in the exam; learn it now and you can skip taking it during the exam, giving you 15 extra minutes of break time. You can also gain experience with the CBT format by taking the 150 practice questions available online or by signing up for a practice session at a test center.

> ▶ If you know the format, you can skip the tutorial and add 15 minutes to your break time!

FIGURE 1. Schematic of CBT Exam.

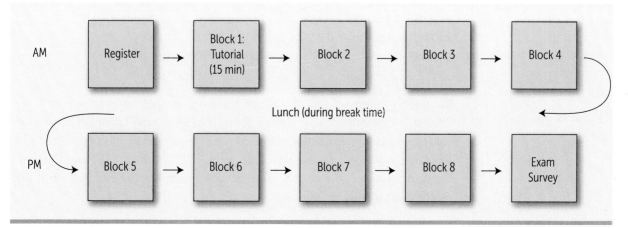

For security reasons, examinees are not allowed to bring any personal electronic equipment into the testing area. This includes both digital and analog watches, iPods, tablets, calculators, cellular telephones, and electronic paging devices. Examinees are also prohibited from carrying in their books, notes, pens/pencils, and scratch paper. Food and beverages are also prohibited in the testing area. The testing centers are monitored by audio and video surveillance equipment. However, most testing centers allot each examinee a small locker outside the testing area in which he or she can store snacks, beverages, and personal items.

> ▶ Keyboard shortcuts:
> - A, B, etc.—letter choices
> - Enter or spacebar—move to next question
> - Esc—exit pop-up Lab and Exhibit windows
> - Alt-T—countdown timers for current session and overall test

The typical question screen in the CBT consists of a question followed by a number of choices on which an examinee can click, together with several navigational buttons on the top of the screen. There is a countdown timer on the lower left corner of the screen as well. There is also a button that allows the examinee to mark a question for review. If a given question happens to be longer than the screen (which occurs very rarely), a scroll bar will appear on the right, allowing the examinee to see the rest of the question. Regardless of whether the examinee clicks on an answer choice or leaves it blank, he or she must click the "Next" button to advance to the next question.

The USMLE features a small number of media clips in the form of audio and/or video. There may even be a question with a multimedia heart sound simulation. In these questions, a digital image of a torso appears on the screen, and the examinee directs a digital stethoscope to various auscultation points to listen for heart and breath sounds. The USMLE orientation materials include several practice questions in these formats. During the exam tutorial, examinees are given an opportunity to ensure that both the audio headphones and the volume are functioning properly. If you are already familiar with the tutorial and planning on skipping it, first skip ahead to the section where you can test your headphones. After you are sure the headphones are working properly, proceed to the exam.

> ▶ Heart sounds are tested via media questions. Make sure you know how different heart diseases sound on auscultation.

The USMLE also has a sequential item test format. These questions are grouped together in the list of questions on the left side of the screen and must be completed in order. After an examinee answers the first question, he or she will be given the option to proceed to the next item but will be warned that the answer to the first question will be locked. **After proceeding, examinees will not be able to change the answer selected for that question.** The question stem and the answer chosen will be available to the examinee as he or she answers the next question(s) in the sequence.

> ▶ Test illustrations include:
> - Gross photos
> - Histology slides
> - Radiographs
> - Electron micrographs
> - Line drawings

The examinee can call up a window displaying normal laboratory values. In order to do so, he or she must click the "Lab" icon on the top part of the screen. Afterward, the examinee will have the option to choose between "Blood," "Cerebrospinal," "Hematologic," or "Sweat and Urine." The normal-values screen may obscure the question if it is expanded. The examinee may have to scroll down to search for the needed lab values. You might want to memorize some common lab values so you spend less time on questions that require you to analyze these.

> ▶ Familiarize yourself with the commonly tested lab values.

The CBT interface provides a running list of questions on the left part of the screen at all times. The software also permits examinees to highlight or cross out information by using their mouse. Finally, there is a "Notes" icon on the top part of the screen that allows students to write notes to themselves for review at a later time. Being familiar with these features can save time and may help you better organize the information you need to answer a question.

> ▶ Ctrl-Alt-Delete are the keys of death during the exam. Don't touch them!

For those who feel they might benefit, the USMLE offers an opportunity to take a simulated test, or "CBT Practice Session at a Prometric center." Students are eligible to register for this three-and-one-half-hour practice session after they have received their scheduling permit.

The same USMLE Step 1 sample test items (150 questions) available on the USMLE Web site, www.usmle.org, are used at these sessions. **No new items will be presented.** The session is divided into a short tutorial and three 1-hour blocks of 50 test items each at a cost of about $75, if your testing region is in the United States or Canada. Students receive a printed percent-correct score after completing the session. **No explanations of questions are provided.**

> ▶ You can take a shortened CBT practice test at a Prometric center.

You may register for a practice session online at www.usmle.org. A separate scheduling permit is issued for the practice session. Students should allow two weeks for receipt of this permit.

How Do I Register to Take the Exam?

Prometric test centers offer Step 1 on a year-round basis, except for the first two weeks in January and major holidays. The exam is given every day except Sunday at most centers. Some schools administer the exam on their own campuses. Check with the test center you want to use before making your exam plans.

> ▶ The Prometric Web site will display a calendar with open test dates.

U.S. students can apply to take Step 1 at the NBME Web site. This application allows you to select one of 12 overlapping three-month blocks in which to be tested (e.g., April–May–June, June–July–August). Choose your three-month eligibility period wisely. If you need to reschedule outside your initial three-month period, you can request a one-time extension of eligibility for the next contiguous three-month period, and pay a rescheduling fee. The application also includes a photo ID form that must be certified by an official at your medical school to verify your enrollment. After the NBME processes your application, it will send you a scheduling permit.

The scheduling permit you receive from the NBME will contain your USMLE identification number, the eligibility period in which you may take the exam, and two additional numbers. The first of these is known as your "scheduling number." You must have this number in order to make your exam appointment with Prometric. The second number is known as the "candidate identification number," or CIN. Examinees must enter their CINs at the Prometric workstation in order to access their exams. Prometric has no access to the codes. **Do not lose your permit!** You will not be allowed to take the exam unless you present this permit along with an unexpired, government-

▶ *The confirmation emails that Prometric and NBME send are not the same as the scheduling permit.*

issued photo ID that includes your signature (such as a driver's license or passport). Make sure the name on your photo ID exactly matches the name that appears on your scheduling permit.

Once you receive your scheduling permit, you may access the Prometric Web site or call Prometric's toll-free number to arrange a time to take the exam. You may contact Prometric two weeks before the test date if you want to confirm identification requirements. Although requests for taking the exam may be completed more than six months before the test date, examinees will not receive their scheduling permits earlier than six months before the eligibility period. The eligibility period is the three-month period you have chosen to take the exam. Most medical students choose the April–June or June–August period. Because exams are scheduled on a "first-come, first-served" basis, it is recommended that you contact Prometric as soon as you receive your permit. After you've scheduled your exam, it's a good idea to confirm your exam appointment with Prometric at least one week before your test date. Prometric will provide appointment confirmation on a print-out and by email. Be sure to read the *2015 USMLE Bulletin of Information* for further details.

▶ *Test scheduling is done on a "first-come, first-served" basis. It's important to call and schedule an exam date as soon as you receive your scheduling permit.*

What If I Need to Reschedule the Exam?

You can change your test date and/or center by contacting Prometric at 1-800-MED-EXAM (1-800-633-3926) or www.prometric.com. Make sure to have your CIN when rescheduling. If you are rescheduling by phone, you must speak with a Prometric representative; leaving a voice-mail message will not suffice. To avoid a rescheduling fee, you will need to request a change at least 31 calendar days before your appointment. Please note that your rescheduled test date must fall within your assigned three-month eligibility period.

▶ *Register six months in advance for seating and scheduling preference.*

When Should I Register for the Exam?

Although there are no deadlines for registering for Step 1, you should plan to register at least six months ahead of your desired test date. This will guarantee that you will get either your test center of choice or one within a 50-mile radius of your first choice. For most U.S. medical students, the desired testing window is in June, since most medical school curricula for the second year end in May or June. Thus, U.S. medical students should plan to register before January in anticipation of a June test date. The timing of the exam is more flexible for IMGs, as it is related only to when they finish exam preparation. Talk with upperclassmen who have already taken the test so you have real-life experience from students who went through a similar curriculum, then formulate your own strategy.

Where Can I Take the Exam?

Your testing location is arranged with Prometric when you call for your test date (after you receive your scheduling permit). For a list of Prometric locations nearest you, visit www.prometric.com.

How Long Will I Have to Wait Before I Get My Scores?

The USMLE reports scores in three to four weeks, unless there are delays in score processing. Examinees will be notified via email when their scores are available. By following the online instructions, examinees will be able to view, download, and print their score report. Additional information about score timetables and accessibility is available on the official USMLE Web site.

What About Time?

Time is of special interest on the CBT exam. Here's a breakdown of the exam schedule:

15 minutes	Tutorial (skip if familiar with test format and features)
7 hours	Seven 60-minute question blocks
45 minutes	Break time (includes time for lunch)

> ▶ Gain extra break time by skipping the tutorial or finishing a block early.

The computer will keep track of how much time has elapsed on the exam. However, the computer will show you only how much time you have remaining in a given block. Therefore, it is up to you to determine if you are pacing yourself properly (at a rate of approximately one question per 78 seconds).

The computer will not warn you if you are spending more than your allotted time for a break. You should therefore budget your time so that you can take a short break when you need one and have time to eat. You must be especially careful not to spend too much time in between blocks (you should keep track of how much time elapses from the time you finish a block of questions to the time you start the next block). After you finish one question block, you'll need to click on a button to proceed to the next block of questions. If you do not click to proceed to the next question block, you will automatically be entered into a break period.

Forty-five minutes is the minimum break time for the day, but you are not required to use all of it, nor are you required to use any of it. You can gain extra break time (but not time for the question blocks) by skipping the tutorial or by finishing a block ahead of the allotted time. Any time remaining on the clock when you finish a block gets added to your remaining break time. Once a new question block has been started, you may not take a break until you have reached the end of that block. If you do so, this will be recorded as an "unauthorized break" and will be reported on your final score report.

> ▶ Be careful to watch the clock on your break time.

Finally, be aware that it may take a few minutes of your break time to "check out" of the secure resting room and then "check in" again to resume testing, so plan accordingly. The "check-in" process may include fingerprints and pocket checks. Some students recommend pocketless clothing on exam day to streamline the process.

If I Freak Out and Leave, What Happens to My Score?

Your scheduling permit shows a CIN that you will enter onto your computer screen to start your exam. Entering the CIN is the same as breaking the seal on a test book, and you are considered to have started the exam when you do so. However, no score will be reported if you do not complete the exam. In fact, if you leave at any time from the start of the test to the last block, no score will be reported. The fact that you started but did not complete the exam, however, will appear on your USMLE score transcript. Even though a score is not posted for incomplete tests, examinees may still get an option to request that their scores be calculated and reported if they desire; unanswered questions will be scored as incorrect.

The exam ends when all question blocks have been completed or when their time has expired. As you leave the testing center, you will receive a printed test-completion notice to document your completion of the exam. To receive an official score, you must finish the entire exam.

What Types of Questions Are Asked?

▶ *Nearly three fourths of Step 1 questions begin with a description of a patient.*

One-best-answer multiple choice items (either singly or as part of a sequential item set) are the only question type on the exam. Most questions consist of a clinical scenario or a direct question followed by a list of five or more options. You are required to select the single best answer among the options given. There are no "except," "not," or matching questions on the exam. A number of options may be partially correct, in which case you must select the option that best answers the question or completes the statement. Additionally, keep in mind that experimental questions may appear on the exam, which do not affect your score.

How Is the Test Scored?

Each Step 1 examinee receives an electronic score report that includes the examinee's pass/fail status, a three-digit test score, and a graphic depiction of the examinee's performance by discipline and organ system or subject area. The actual organ system profiles reported may depend on the statistical characteristics of a given administration of the examination.

▶ *The mean Step 1 score for U.S. medical students continues to rise, from 200 in 1991 to 228 in 2013.*

The NBME provides a three-digit test score based on the total number of items answered correctly on the examination (see Figure 2). Since some questions may be experimental and are not counted, it is possible to get different scores for the same number of correct answers. The most recent mean score was 228 with a standard deviation of approximately 21.

FIGURE 2. Scoring Scale for the USMLE Step 1.

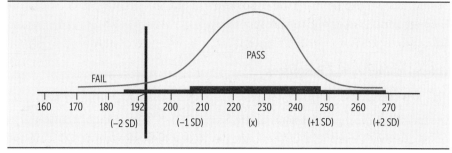

A score of **192** or higher is required to pass Step 1. The NBME does not report the minimum number of correct responses needed to pass, but estimates that it is roughly 60–70%. The NBME may adjust the minimum passing score in the future, so please check the USMLE Web site or www.firstaidteam.com for updates.

According to the USMLE, medical schools receive a listing of total scores and pass/fail results plus group summaries by discipline and organ system. Students can withhold their scores from their medical school if they wish. Official USMLE transcripts, which can be sent on request to residency programs, include only total scores, not performance profiles.

Consult the USMLE Web site or your medical school for the most current and accurate information regarding the examination.

What Does My Score Mean?

The most important point with the Step 1 score is passing versus failing. Passing essentially means, "Hey, you're on your way to becoming a fully licensed doc." As Table 1 shows, the majority of students pass the exam, so remember, we told you to relax.

TABLE 1. Passing Rates for the 2012–2013 USMLE Step 1.

	2012		2013	
	No. Tested	% Passing	No. Tested	% Passing
Allopathic 1st takers	18,723	96%	19,108	97%
Repeaters	1,133	68%	915	72%
Allopathic total	19,856	94%	20,023	95%
Osteopathic 1st takers	2,496	92%	2,680	94%
Repeaters	68	68%	46	74%
Osteopathic total	2,564	91%	2,726	94%
Total U.S./Canadian	22,420	94%	22,749	95%
IMG 1st takers	14,201	76%	14,649	79%
Repeaters	4,261	40%	3,772	44%
IMG total	18,462	68%	18,421	72%
Total Step 1 examinees	40,882	82%	41,170	85%

TABLE 2. CBSE to USMLE Score Prediction.

CBSE Score	Step 1 Equivalent
≥ 94	≥ 260
92	255
90	250
88	245
86	240
84	235
82	230
80	225
78	220
76	215
74	210
72	205
70	200
68	195
66	190
64	185
62	180
60	175
58	170
56	165
54	160
52	155
50	150
48	145
46	140
≤ 44	≤ 135

▶ Practice questions may be easier than the actual exam.

Beyond that, the main point of having a quantitative score is to give you a sense of how well you've done on the exam and to help schools and residencies rank their students and applicants, respectively.

Official NBME/USMLE Resources

The NBME offers a Comprehensive Basic Science Examination (CBSE) for practice that is a shorter version of the Step 1. The CBSE contains four blocks of 50 questions each and covers material that is typically learned during the basic science years. Scores range from 45 to 95 and correlate with a Step 1 equivalent (see Table 2). The standard error of measurement is approximately 3 points, meaning a score of 80 would estimate the student's proficiency is somewhere between 77 and 83. In other words, the actual Step 1 score could be predicted to be between 218 and 232. Of course, these values do not correlate exactly, and they do not reflect different test preparation methods. Many schools use this test to gauge whether a student is expected to pass Step 1. If this test is offered, it is usually conducted at the end of regular didactic time before any dedicated Step 1 preparation. Use the information to help set realistic goals and timetables for your success.

The NBME also offers the Comprehensive Basic Science Self-Assessment (CBSSA). Students who prepared for the exam using this Web-based tool reported that they found the format and content highly indicative of questions tested on the actual exam. In addition, the CBSSA is a fair predictor of USMLE performance (see Table 3).

The CBSSA exists in two forms: a standard-paced and a self-paced format, both of which consist of four sections of 50 questions each (for a total of 200 multiple choice items). The standard-paced format allows the user up to 65 minutes to complete each section, reflecting time limits similar to the actual exam. By contrast, the self-paced format places a 4:20 time limit on answering all multiple choice questions.

Keep in mind that this bank of questions is available only on the Web. The NBME requires that users log on, register, and start the test within 30 days of registration. Once the assessment has begun, users are required to complete the sections within 20 days. Following completion of the questions, the CBSSA provides a performance profile indicating the user's relative strengths and weaknesses, much like the report profile for the USMLE Step 1 exam. The profile is scaled with an average score of 500 and a standard deviation of 100. Please note that the CBSSAs do not list the correct answers to the questions at the end of the session. However, some forms can be purchased with an extended feedback option; these tests show you which questions you answered incorrectly, but do not show you the correct answer or explain why your choice was wrong. Feedback from the self-assessment takes the form of a performance profile and nothing more. The NBME charges $50 for assessments without feedback and $60 for assessments with expanded feedback. The fees are payable by credit card or money order. For more information regarding the CBSE and the CBSSA, visit the NBME's Web site at www.nbme.org.

The NBME scoring system is weighted for each assessment exam. While some exams seem more difficult than others, the score reported takes into account these inter-test differences when predicting Step 1 performance. Also, while many students report seeing Step 1 questions "word-for-word" out of the assessments, the NBME makes special note that no live USMLE questions are shown on any NBME assessment.

Lastly, the International Foundations of Medicine (IFOM) offers a Basic Science Examination (BSE) practice exam at participating Prometric test centers for $200. Students may also take the self-assessment test online for $35 through the NBME's Web site. The IFOM BSE is intended to determine an examinee's relative areas of strength and weakness in general areas of basic science—not to predict performance on the USMLE Step 1 exam—and the content covered by the two examinations is somewhat different. However, because there is substantial overlap in content coverage and many IFOM items were previously used on the USMLE Step 1, it is possible to roughly project IFOM performance onto the USMLE Step 1 score scale. More information is available at http://www.nbme.org/ifom/.

TABLE 3. CBSSA to USMLE Score Prediction.

CBSSA Score	Approximate USMLE Step 1 Score
200	164
250	175
300	185
350	196
400	207
450	217
500	228
550	239
600	249
650	260
700	271
750	281
800	292

▶ DEFINING YOUR GOAL

It is useful to define your own personal performance goal when approaching the USMLE Step 1. Your style and intensity of preparation can then be matched to your goal. Furthermore, your goal may depend on your school's requirements, your specialty choice, your grades to date, and your personal assessment of the test's importance. Do your best to define your goals early so that you can prepare accordingly.

Certain highly competitive residency programs, such as those in plastic surgery and orthopedic surgery, have acknowledged their use of Step 1 scores in the selection process. In such residency programs, greater emphasis may be placed on attaining a high score, so students who seek to enter these programs may wish to consider aiming for a very high score on the Step 1 exam (see Figure 3). At the same time, your Step 1 score is only one of a number of factors that are assessed when you apply for residency. In fact, many residency programs value other criteria such as letters of recommendation, third-year clerkship grades, honors, and research experience more than a high score on Step 1. Fourth-year medical students who have recently completed the residency application process can be a valuable resource in this regard.

▶ *Fourth-year medical students have the best feel for how Step 1 scores factor into the residency application process.*

▶ *Some competitive residency programs place more weight on Step 1 scores in their selection process.*

FIGURE 3. Median USMLE Step 1 Score by Specialty for Matched U.S. Seniors.[a]

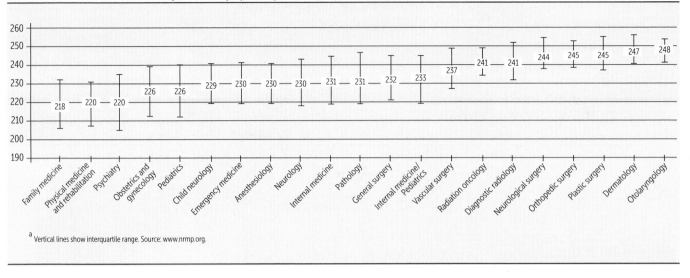

[a] Vertical lines show interquartile range. Source: www.nrmp.org.

▶ EXCELLING IN THE PRECLINICAL YEARS

Many students feel overwhelmed during the first few weeks of medical school and struggle to find a workable system. Strategies that worked during your undergraduate years may or may not work as you prepare for the USMLE Step 1. Below are three study methods to use during the preclinical years and their effectiveness for Step 1 preparation. Regardless of your choice, the foundation of knowledge you build during your basic science years is the most important resource for success on the USMLE Step 1.

Highlight, Read, and Reread

The most passive of the three methods, this generally consists of sitting through lectures and highlighting relevant material (sometimes in an assortment of colors). Notes are jotted in the margins, but the general bulk of information is in the same order presented by the various lecturers. Students then go home and reread the notes, focusing on the highlights. It is difficult to test integration of concepts. These notes (usually in the thousands of pages) are almost useless for Step 1 preparation.

Flash cards

There is no shortage of flash card applications, from make-your-own cards to purchasable premade decks. Self-made flash cards, if done correctly, offer the ability to objectively test necessary facts. Written in an open-ended format and coupled with spaced repetition, they train both recognition and recall. Apps exist for various smartphones and tablets, so the flash cards are always accessible. However, the speed of creating digital cards and sharing can lead to flash card overload (it is unsustainable to make 50 flash cards per lecture!). Even at a modest pace, the thousands upon thousands of cards are too many for Step 1 preparation. Unless you have specified high-yield cards

▶ *Watch out for flash card overload!*

(and checked the content with high-yield resources), stick to premade cards by reputable sources that curate the vast amount of knowledge for you.

Differential Tables and Summaries

This is the most active (and time intensive) form of learning. It consists of integrating the pertinent information from paragraphs on each subject into tables that cut across topics within the same category. The key is to synthesize the sequentially presented material. Sensitive and specific findings should be highlighted. This material is also the easiest to share and can complement other methods. While many review sources offer this material in various styles and formats, your own notes may in fact be concise enough to use as an adjunct for Step 1 preparation, and they have the added benefit of being organized to your liking.

▶ TIMELINE FOR STUDY

Before Starting

Your preparation for the USMLE Step 1 began when you entered medical school. Organize and commit to studying from the beginning so that when the time comes to prepare for the USMLE, you will be ready with a strong foundation.

Make a Schedule

After you have defined your goals, map out a study schedule that is consistent with your objectives, your vacation time, the difficulty of your ongoing coursework, and your family and social commitments (see Figure 4). Determine whether you want to spread out your study time or concentrate it into 14-hour study days in the final weeks. Then factor in your own history in preparing for standardized examinations (e.g., SAT, MCAT). Talk to students at your school who have recently taken Step 1. Ask them for their study schedules, especially those who have study habits and goals similar to yours.

▶ *Customize your schedule. Tackle your weakest section first.*

Typically, U.S. medical students allot between five and seven weeks for dedicated preparation for Step 1. The time you dedicate to exam preparation will depend on your target score as well as your success in preparing yourself during the first two years of medical school. Some students reserve about a week at the end of their study period for final review; others save just a few days. When you have scheduled your exam date, do your best to adhere to it. Studies show that a later testing date does not translate into a higher score, so avoid pushing back your test date without good reason.[2]

Make your schedule realistic, and set achievable goals. Many students make the mistake of studying at a level of detail that requires too much time for a comprehensive review—reading *Gray's Anatomy* in a couple of days is not a realistic goal! Have one catch-up day per week of studying. No matter how

▶ *"Crammable" subjects should be covered later and less crammable subjects earlier.*

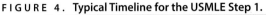

FIGURE 4. Typical Timeline for the USMLE Step 1.

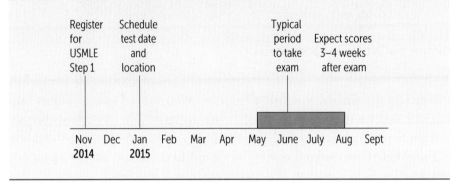

well you stick to your schedule, unexpected events happen. But don't let yourself procrastinate because you have catch-up days; stick to your schedule as closely as possible and revise it regularly on the basis of your actual progress. Be careful not to lose focus. Beware of feelings of inadequacy when comparing study schedules and progress with your peers. **Avoid others who stress you out.** Focus on a few top-rated resources that suit your learning style—not on some obscure books your friends may pass down to you. Accept the fact that you cannot learn it all.

You will need time for uninterrupted and focused study. Plan your personal affairs to minimize crisis situations near the date of the test. Allot an adequate number of breaks in your study schedule to avoid burnout. Maintain a healthy lifestyle with proper diet, exercise, and sleep.

▶ *Avoid burnout. Maintain proper diet, exercise, and sleep habits.*

Another important aspect of your preparation is your studying environment. **Study where you have always been comfortable studying.** Be sure to include everything you need close by (review books, notes, coffee, snacks, etc.). If you're the kind of person who cannot study alone, form a study group with other students taking the exam. The main point here is to create a comfortable environment with minimal distractions.

Year(s) Prior

The knowledge you gained during your first two years of medical school and even during your undergraduate years should provide the groundwork on which to base your test preparation. Student scores on NBME subject tests (commonly known as "shelf exams") have been shown to be highly correlated with subsequent Step 1 scores.[3] Moreover, undergraduate science GPAs as well as MCAT scores are strong predictors of performance on the Step 1 exam.[4]

▶ *Buy review books early (first year) and use while studying for courses.*

We also recommend that you buy highly rated review books early in your first year of medical school and use them as you study throughout the two years. When Step 1 comes along, these books will be familiar and personalized to the way in which you learn. It is risky and intimidating to use unfamiliar review books in the final two or three weeks preceding the exam. Some students find it helpful to personalize and annotate *First Aid* throughout the curriculum.

Months Prior

Review test dates and the application procedure. Testing for the USMLE Step 1 is done on a year-round basis. If you have disabilities or special circumstances, contact the NBME as early as possible to discuss test accommodations (see First Aid for the Student with a Disability, p. 41).

Use this time to finalize your ideal schedule. Consider upcoming breaks and whether you want to relax or study. Work backward from your test date to make sure you finish at least one question bank. Also add time to redo missed or flagged questions (which may be half the bank). This is the time to build a structured plan with enough flexibility for the realities of life.

Begin doing blocks of questions from reputable question banks under "real" conditions. Don't use tutor mode until you're sure you can finish blocks in the allotted time. It is important to continue balancing success in your normal studies with the Step 1 test preparation process.

> ▶ Simulate the USMLE Step 1 under "real" conditions before beginning your studies.

Weeks Prior (Dedicated Preparation)

Your dedicated prep time may be one week or two months. You should have a working plan as you go into this period. Finish your school work strong, take a day off, and then get to work. Start by simulating a full-length USMLE Step 1 if you haven't yet done so. Consider doing one NBME CBSSA and the 150 free questions from the NBME Web site. Alternatively, you could choose 7 blocks of randomized questions from a commercial question bank. Make sure you get feedback on your strengths and weaknesses and adjust your studying accordingly. Many students study from review sources or comprehensive programs for part of the day, then do question blocks. Also, keep in mind that reviewing 46 questions can take upward of two hours. Feedback from CBSSA exams and question banks will help you focus on your weaknesses.

> ▶ In the final two weeks, focus on review, practice questions, and endurance. Stay confident!

One Week Prior

Make sure you have your CIN (found on your scheduling permit) as well as other items necessary for the day of the examination, including a current driver's license or another form of photo ID with your signature (make sure the name on your **ID exactly** matches that on your scheduling permit). Confirm the Prometric testing center location and test time. Work out how you will get to the testing center and what parking and traffic problems you might encounter. Drive separately from other students taking the test on the same day, and exchange cell phone numbers in case of emergencies. If possible, visit the testing site to get a better idea of the testing conditions you will face. Determine what you will do for lunch. Make sure you have everything you need to ensure that you will be comfortable and alert at the test site. It may be beneficial to adjust your schedule to start waking up at the same time that you will on your test day. And of course, make sure to maintain a healthy lifestyle and get enough sleep.

> ▶ One week before the test:
> ▪ Sleep according to the same schedule you'll use on test day
> ▪ Review the CBT tutorial one last time
> ▪ Call Prometric to confirm test date and time

One Day Prior

Try your best to relax and rest the night before the test. Double-check your admissions and test-taking materials as well as the comfort measures discussed earlier so that you will not have to deal with such details on the morning of the exam. At this point it will be more effective to review short-term memory material that you're already familiar with than to try to learn new material. The Rapid Review section at the end of this book is high yield for last-minute studying. Remember that regardless of how hard you have studied, you cannot know everything. There will be things on the exam that you have never even seen before, so do not panic. Do not underestimate your abilities.

Many students report difficulty sleeping the night prior to the exam. This is often exacerbated by going to bed much earlier than usual. Do whatever it takes to ensure a good night's sleep (e.g., massage, exercise, warm milk, no back-lit screens at night). Do not change your daily routine prior to the exam. Exam day is not the day for a caffeine-withdrawal headache.

▶ No notes, books, calculators, pagers, cell phones, recording devices, or watches of any kind are allowed in the testing area, but they are allowed in lockers.

Morning of the Exam

On the morning of the Step 1 exam, wake up at your regular time and eat a normal breakfast. If you think it will help you, have a close friend or family member check to make sure you get out of bed. Make sure you have your scheduling permit admission ticket, test-taking materials, and comfort measures as discussed earlier. Wear loose, comfortable clothing. Plan for a variable temperature in the testing center. Arrive at the test site 30 minutes before the time designated on the admission ticket; however, do not come too early, as doing so may intensify your anxiety. When you arrive at the test site, the proctor should give you a USMLE information sheet that will explain critical factors such as the proper use of break time. Seating may be assigned, but ask to be reseated if necessary; you need to be seated in an area that will allow you to remain comfortable and to concentrate. Get to know your testing station, especially if you have never been in a Prometric testing center before. Listen to your proctors regarding any changes in instructions or testing procedures that may apply to your test site.

▶ Arrive at the testing center 30 minutes before your scheduled exam time. If you arrive more than half an hour late, you will not be allowed to take the test.

Finally, remember that it is natural (and even beneficial) to be a little nervous. Focus on being mentally clear and alert. Avoid panic. When you are asked to begin the exam, take a deep breath, focus on the screen, and then begin. Keep an eye on the timer. Take advantage of breaks between blocks to stretch, maybe do some jumping jacks, and relax for a moment with deep breathing or stretching.

After the Test

After you have completed the exam, be sure to have fun and relax regardless of how you may feel. Taking the test is an achievement in itself. Remember, you are much more likely to have passed than not. Enjoy the free time you have before your clerkships. Expect to experience some "reentry" phenomena as you try to regain a real life. Once you have recovered sufficiently from the test (or from partying), we invite you to send us your feedback, corrections, and suggestions for entries, facts, mnemonics, strategies, resource ratings, and the like (see p. xix, How to Contribute). Sharing your experience will benefit fellow medical students and IMGs.

▶ STUDY MATERIALS

Quality and Cost Considerations

Although an ever-increasing number of review books and software are now available on the market, the quality of such material is highly variable. Some common problems are as follows:

- Certain review books are too detailed to allow for review in a reasonable amount of time or cover subtopics that are not emphasized on the exam.
- Many sample question books were originally written years ago and have not been adequately updated to reflect recent trends.
- Some question banks test to a level of detail that you will not find on the exam.

Review Books

In selecting review books, be sure to weigh different opinions against each other, read the reviews and ratings in Section IV of this guide, examine the books closely in the bookstore, and choose carefully. You are investing not only money but also your limited study time. Do not worry about finding the "perfect" book, as many subjects simply do not have one, and different students prefer different formats. Supplement your chosen books with personal notes from other sources, including what you learn from question banks.

> ▶ If a given review book is not working for you, stop using it no matter how highly rated it may be or how much it costs.

There are two types of review books: those that are stand-alone titles and those that are part of a series. Books in a series generally have the same style, and you must decide if that style works for you. However, a given style is not optimal for every subject.

You should also find out which books are up to date. Some recent editions reflect major improvements, whereas others contain only cursory changes. Take into consideration how a book reflects the format of the USMLE Step 1.

> ▶ Charts and diagrams may be the best approach for physiology and biochemistry, whereas tables and outlines may be preferable for microbiology.

Practice Tests

Taking practice tests provides valuable information about potential strengths and weaknesses in your fund of knowledge and test-taking skills. Some students use practice examinations simply as a means of breaking up the monotony of studying and adding variety to their study schedule, whereas other students rely almost solely on practice. You should also subscribe to one

▶ *Most practice exams are shorter and less clinical than the real thing.*

or more high-quality question banks. In addition, students report that many current practice-exam books have questions that are, on average, shorter and less clinically oriented than those on the current USMLE Step 1.

After taking a practice test, spend time on each question and each answer choice whether you were right or wrong. There are important teaching points in each explanation. Knowing why a wrong answer choice is incorrect is just as important as knowing why the right answer is correct. Do not panic if your practice scores are low as many questions try to trick or distract you to highlight a certain point. Use the questions you missed or were unsure about to develop focused plans during your scheduled catch-up time.

▶ *Use practice tests to identify concepts and areas of weakness, not just facts that you missed.*

Clinical Review Books

Keep your eye out for more clinically oriented review books; purchase them early and begin to use them. A number of students are turning to Step 2 CK books, pathophysiology books, and case-based reviews to prepare for the clinical vignettes. Examples of such books include:

- *First Aid Cases for the USMLE Step 1* (McGraw-Hill)
- *First Aid for the Wards* (McGraw-Hill)
- *First Aid Clerkship* series (McGraw-Hill)
- *Blueprints* clinical series (Lippincott Williams & Wilkins)
- *PreTest Physical Diagnosis* (McGraw-Hill)
- *Washington Manual* (Lippincott Williams & Wilkins)

Texts, Syllabi, and Notes

Limit your use of textbooks and course syllabi for Step 1 review. Many textbooks are too detailed for high-yield review and include material that is generally not tested on the USMLE Step 1 (e.g., drug dosages, complex chemical structures). Syllabi, although familiar, are inconsistent across medical schools and frequently reflect the emphasis of individual faculty, which often does not correspond to that of the USMLE Step 1. Syllabi also tend to be less organized than top-rated books and generally contain fewer diagrams and study questions.

▶ TEST-TAKING STRATEGIES

▶ *Practice! Develop your test-taking skills and strategies well before the test date.*

Your test performance will be influenced by both your knowledge and your test-taking skills. You can strengthen your performance by considering each of these factors. Test-taking skills and strategies should be developed and perfected well in advance of the test date so that you can concentrate on the test itself. We suggest that you try the following strategies to see if they might work for you.

Pacing

You have seven hours to complete 322 questions. Note that each one-hour block contains 46 questions. This works out to about 78 seconds per question. If you find yourself spending too much time on a question, mark the question, make an educated guess, and move on. If time permits, come back to the question later. Remember that some questions may be experimental and do not count for points (and reassure yourself that these experimental questions are the ones that are stumping you). In the past, pacing errors have been detrimental to the performance of even highly prepared examinees. The bottom line is to keep one eye on the clock at all times!

▶ *Time management is an important skill for exam success.*

Dealing with Each Question

There are several established techniques for efficiently approaching multiple choice questions; find what works for you. One technique begins with identifying each question as easy, workable, or impossible. Your goal should be to answer all easy questions, resolve all workable questions in a reasonable amount of time, and make quick and intelligent guesses on all impossible questions. Most students read the stem, think of the answer, and turn immediately to the choices. A second technique is to first skim the answer choices to get a context, then read the last sentence of the question (the lead-in), and then read through the passage quickly, extracting only information relevant to answering the question. Try a variety of techniques on practice exams and see what works best for you. If you get overwhelmed, remember that a 30-second time out to refocus may get you back on track.

Guessing

There is **no penalty** for wrong answers. Thus, **no test block should be left with unanswered questions.** A hunch is probably better than a random guess. If you have to guess, we suggest selecting an answer you recognize over one with which you are totally unfamiliar.

Changing Your Answer

The conventional wisdom is not to change answers that you have already marked unless there is a convincing and logical reason to do so—in other words, go with your "first hunch." Many question banks tell you how many questions you changed from right to wrong, wrong to wrong, and wrong to right. Use this feedback to judge how good a second-guesser you are. If you have extra time, reread the question stem and make sure you didn't misinterpret the question.

▶ *Go with your first hunch, unless you are certain that you are a good second-guesser.*

▶ CLINICAL VIGNETTE STRATEGIES

> ▶ *Be prepared to read fast and think on your feet!*

In recent years, the USMLE Step 1 has become increasingly clinically oriented. This change mirrors the trend in medical education toward introducing students to clinical problem solving during the basic science years. The increasing clinical emphasis on Step 1 may be challenging to those students who attend schools with a more traditional curriculum.

What Is a Clinical Vignette?

A clinical vignette is a short (usually paragraph-long) description of a patient, including demographics, presenting symptoms, signs, and other information concerning the patient. Sometimes this paragraph is followed by a brief listing of important physical findings and/or laboratory results. The task of assimilating all this information and answering the associated question in the span of one minute can be intimidating. So be prepared to read quickly and think on your feet. Remember that the question is often indirectly asking something you already know.

> ▶ *Practice questions that include case histories or descriptive vignettes are critical for Step 1 preparation.*

Strategy

Remember that Step 1 vignettes usually describe diseases or disorders in their most classic presentation. So look for cardinal signs (e.g., malar rash for SLE or nuchal rigidity for meningitis) in the narrative history. Be aware that the question will contain classic signs and symptoms instead of buzzwords. Sometimes the data from labs and the physical exam will help you confirm or reject possible diagnoses, thereby helping you rule answer choices in or out. In some cases, they will be a dead giveaway for the diagnosis.

> ▶ *Step 1 vignettes usually describe diseases or disorders in their most classic presentation.*

Making a diagnosis from the history and data is often not the final answer. Not infrequently, the diagnosis is divulged at the end of the vignette, after you have just struggled through the narrative to come up with a diagnosis of your own. The question might then ask about a related aspect of the diagnosed disease. Consider skimming the answer choices and lead-in before diving into a long stem. However, be careful with skimming the answer choices; going too fast may warp your perception of what the vignette is asking.

▶ IF YOU THINK YOU FAILED

After the test, many examinees feel that they have failed, and most are at the very least unsure of their pass/fail status. There are several sensible steps you can take to plan for the future in the event that you do not achieve a passing score. First, save and organize all your study materials, including review books, practice tests, and notes. Familiarize yourself with the reapplication procedures for Step 1, including application deadlines and upcoming test dates.

Make sure you know both your school's and the NBME's policies regarding retakes. The NBME allows a maximum of six attempts to pass each Step examination.[5] You may take Step 1 no more than three times within a 12-month period. Your fourth and subsequent attempts must be at least 12 months after your first attempt at that exam and at least six months after your most recent attempt at that exam.

> ▶ *If you pass Step 1, you are not allowed to retake the exam.*

The performance profiles on the back of the USMLE Step 1 score report provide valuable feedback concerning your relative strengths and weaknesses. Study these profiles closely. Set up a study timeline to strengthen gaps in your knowledge as well as to maintain and improve what you already know. Do not neglect high-yield subjects. It is normal to feel somewhat anxious about retaking the test, but if anxiety becomes a problem, seek appropriate counseling.

▶ IF YOU FAILED

Even if you came out of the exam room feeling that you failed, seeing that failing grade can be traumatic, and it is natural to feel upset. Different people react in different ways: For some it is a stimulus to buckle down and study harder; for others it may "take the wind out of their sails" for a few days; and it may even lead to a reassessment of individual goals and abilities. In some instances, however, failure may trigger weeks or months of sadness, feelings of hopelessness, social withdrawal, and inability to concentrate—in other words, true clinical depression. If you think you are depressed, please seek help.

▶ TESTING AGENCIES

- **National Board of Medical Examiners (NBME)**
  Department of Licensing Examination Services
  3750 Market Street
  Philadelphia, PA 19104-3102
  (215) 590-9500
  Fax: (215) 590-9457
  Email: webmail@nbme.org
  www.nbme.org

- **Educational Commission for Foreign Medical Graduates (ECFMG)**
  3624 Market Street
  Philadelphia, PA 19104-2685
  (215) 386-5900
  Fax: (215) 386-9196
  Email: info@ecfmg.org
  www.ecfmg.org

- **Federation of State Medical Boards (FSMB)**
  400 Fuller Wiser Road, Suite 300
  Euless, TX 76039-3856
  (817) 868-4041
  Fax: (817) 868-4098
  Email: usmle@fsmb.org
  www.fsmb.org

- **USMLE Secretariat**
  3750 Market Street
  Philadelphia, PA 19104-3102
  (215) 590-9700
  Fax: (215) 590-9457
  Email: webmail@nbme.org
  www.usmle.org

▶ REFERENCES

1. United States Medical Licensing Examination. Available at: http://www.usmle.org/bulletin/exam-content/#step1. Accessed October 20, 2014.
2. Pohl, Charles A., Robeson, Mary R., Hojat, Mohammadreza, and Veloski, J. Jon, "Sooner or Later? USMLE Step 1 Performance and Test Administration Date at the End of the Second Year," *Academic Medicine*, 2002, Vol. 77, No. 10, pp. S17–S19.
3. Holtman, Matthew C., Swanson, David B., Ripkey, Douglas R., and Case, Susan M., "Using Basic Science Subject Tests to Identify Students at Risk for Failing Step 1," *Academic Medicine*, 2001, Vol. 76, No. 10, pp. S48–S51.
4. Basco, William T., Jr., Way, David P., Gilbert, Gregory E., and Hudson, Andy, "Undergraduate Institutional MCAT Scores as Predictors of USMLE Step 1 Performance," *Academic Medicine*, 2002, Vol. 77, No. 10, pp. S13–S16.
5. United States Medical Licensing Examination. 2014 USMLE Bulletin of Information. http://www.usmle.org/pdfs/bulletin/2014bulletin.pdf. Accessed September 26, 2014.

Special Situations

▶ FIRST AID FOR THE INTERNATIONAL MEDICAL GRADUATE

"International medical graduate" (IMG) is the accepted term now used to describe any student or graduate of a non-U.S., non-Canadian, non–Puerto Rican medical school, regardless of whether he or she is a U.S. citizen or resident. Technically the term IMG encompasses FMGs (foreign medical graduates; i.e., medical graduates from medical schools outside the United States who are not residents of the United States—that is, U.S. citizens or green-card holders), although the terms IMG and FMG are often used interchangeably.

▶ *IMGs make up approximately 25% of the U.S. physician population.*

IMG's Steps to Licensure in the United States

To be eligible to take the USMLE Steps, you (the applicant) must be officially enrolled in a medical school located outside the United States and Canada that is listed in the International Medical Education Directory (IMED; http://www.faimer.org/resources/imed.html), both at the time you apply for examination and on your test day. In addition, your "Graduation Year" must be listed as "Current" at the time you apply and on your test day.

▶ *More detailed information can be found in the ECFMG Information Booklet, available at www.ecfmg.org/pubshome.html.*

If you are an IMG, you must go through the following steps (not necessarily in this order) to apply for residency programs and become licensed to practice in the United States. You must complete these steps even if you are already a practicing physician and have completed a residency program in your own country.

▶ *Applicants may apply online for USMLE Step 1, Step 2 CK, or Step 2 CS at www.ecfmg.org.*

- Pass USMLE Step 1, Step 2 CK, and Step 2 CS, as well as obtain a medical school diploma (not necessarily in this order). All three exams can be taken during medical school. If you have already graduated prior to taking any of the Steps, then you will need to verify your academic credentials (confirmation of enrollment and medical degree) prior to applying for any Step exam.
- You will be certified electronically by the Educational Commission for Foreign Medical Graduates (ECFMG) after above steps are successfully completed. You should receive your formal ECFMG certificate in the mail within the next 1–2 weeks. The ECFMG will not issue a certificate (even if all the USMLE scores are submitted) until it verifies your medical diploma with your medical school.
- You must have a valid ECFMG certificate before entering an accredited residency program in the United States, although you can begin the Electronic Residency Application Service (ERAS) application and interviews before you receive the certificate. However, many programs prefer to interview IMGs who have an ECFMG certificate, so obtaining it by the time you submit your ERAS application is ideal.
- Apply for residency positions in your fields of interest, either directly or through the ERAS and the National Residency Matching Program (NRMP), otherwise known as "the Match." To be entered into the Match, you need to have passed all the examinations necessary for ECFMG

certification (i.e., Step 1, Step 2 CK, and Step 2 CS) by the rank order list deadline (usually in late February before the Match). If you do not pass these exams by the deadline, you will be withdrawn from the Match.

- If you are not a U.S. citizen or green-card holder (permanent resident), obtain a visa that will allow you to enter and work in the United States.
- Sign up to receive the ECFMG and ERAS email newsletter to keep up to date with their most current policies and deadlines.
- If required by the state in which your residency program is located, obtain an educational/training/limited medical license. Your residency program may assist you with this application. Note that medical licensing is the prerogative of each individual state, not of the federal government, and that states vary with respect to their laws about licensing.
- Once you have the ECFMG certification, take the USMLE Step 3 during your residency, and then obtain a full medical license. Once you have a state-issued license, you are permitted to practice in federal institutions such as Veterans Affairs (VA) hospitals and Indian Health Service facilities in any state. This can open the door to "moonlighting" opportunities and possibilities for an H1B visa application if relevant. For details on individual state rules, write to the licensing board in the state in question or contact the Federation of State Medical Boards (FSMB). If you need to apply for an H1B visa for starting residency, you will need to take and pass the USMLE Step 3 exam, preferably before you Match.
- Complete your residency and then take the appropriate specialty board exams if you wish to become board certified (e.g., in internal medicine or surgery). If you already have a specialty certification in another country, some specialty boards may grant you six months' or one year's credit toward your total residency time.
- Currently, most residency programs are accepting applications through ERAS. For more information, see *First Aid for the Match* or contact:

> **ECFMG/ERAS Program**
> 3624 Market Street
> Philadelphia, PA 19104-2685 USA
> (215) 386-5900
> Email: eras-support@ecfmg.org
> www.ecfmg.org/eras

- For detailed information on the USMLE Steps, visit the USMLE Web site at http://www.usmle.org.

▶ Keep informed by signing up for the ECFMG email newsletter at www.ecfmg.org/resources.

The USMLE and the IMG

The USMLE is a series of standardized exams that give IMGs and U.S. medical graduates a level playing field. The passing marks for IMGs for Step 1, Step 2 CK, and Step 2 CS are determined by a statistical distribution that is based on the scores of U.S. medical school students. For example, to pass Step 1, you will probably have to score higher than the bottom 8–10% of U.S. and Canadian graduates.

> ▶ *IMGs have a maximum of six attempts to pass any USMLE Step, and must pass the USMLE Steps required for ECFMG certification within a seven-year period.*

Under USMLE program rules, a maximum of six attempts will be permitted to pass any USMLE Step or component exam. There is a limit of three attempts within a 12-month period for any of the USMLE Steps.

Timing of the USMLE

For an IMG, the timing of a complete application is critical. It is extremely important that you send in your application early if you are to obtain the maximum number of interviews. Complete all exam requirements by August of the year in which you wish to apply. Check the ECFMG Web site for deadlines to take and pass the various Step exams to be eligible for the NRMP Match.

IMG applicants must pass the USMLE Steps required for ECFMG certification within a seven-year period. The USMLE program recommends, although not all jurisdictions impose, a seven-year limit for completion of the three-step USMLE program.

In terms of USMLE exam order, arguments can be made for taking the Step 1 or the Step 2 CK exam first. For example, you may consider taking the Step 2 CK exam first if you have just graduated from medical school and the clinical topics are still fresh in your mind. However, keep in mind that there is substantial overlap between Step 1 and Step 2 CK topics in areas such as pharmacology, pathophysiology, and biostatistics. You might therefore consider taking the Step 1 and Step 2 CK exams close together to take advantage of this overlap in your test preparation.

USMLE Step 1 and the IMG

Significance of the Test. Step 1 is one of the three exams required for the ECFMG certification. Since most U.S. graduates apply to residency with their Step 1 scores only, it may be the only objective tool available with which to compare IMGs with U.S. graduates.

Eligibility Period. A three-month period of your choice.

Fee. The fee for Step 1 is $850 plus an international test delivery surcharge (if you choose a testing region other than the United States or Canada).

Statistics. In 2013–2014, 79% of IMG examinees passed Step 1 on their first attempt, compared with 97% of MD degree examinees from the United States and Canada.

> ▶ *A higher Step 1 score will improve your chances of getting into a highly competitive specialty.*

Tips. Although few if any students feel totally prepared to take Step 1, IMGs in particular require serious study and preparation in order to reach their full potential on this exam. It is also imperative that IMGs do their best on Step 1, as a poor score on Step 1 is a distinct disadvantage in applying for most residencies. Remember that if you pass Step 1, you cannot retake it in an attempt to improve your score. Your goal should thus be to beat the mean, because you can then assert with confidence that you have done better than average for U.S. students (see Table 4). Higher Step 1 scores will also lend credibility to your residency application and help you get into highly competitive specialties such as radiology, orthopedics, and dermatology.

Commercial Review Courses. Do commercial review courses help improve your scores? Reports vary, and such courses can be expensive. For some students these programs can provide a more structured learning environment with professional support. However, review courses consume a significant chunk of time away from independent study. Many IMGs participate in review courses as they typically need higher scores to compete effectively with U.S. and Canadian candidates for residency positions. (For more information on review courses, see Section IV.)

USMLE Step 2 CK and the IMG

What Is the Step 2 CK? It is a computerized test of the clinical sciences consisting of up to 355 multiple-choice questions divided into eight blocks. It can be taken at Prometric centers in the United States and several other countries.

Content. The Step 2 CK includes test items in the following content areas:

- Internal medicine
- Obstetrics and gynecology-

> ▶ The areas tested on the Step 2 CK relate to the clerkships provided at U.S. medical schools.

TABLE 4. USMLE Step 1 Mean Score of Matched Applicants in 2014.

Specialty	U.S. Graduates	U.S. IMGs	Non-U.S. IMGs
All specialties	230	217	227
Anesthesiology	230	234	226
Dermatology[a]	247	—	—
Emergency medicine	230	225	226
Family medicine	218	206	213
Internal medicine	231	221	231
Neurology	230	216	230
Obstetrics and gynecology	226	221	226
Pathology	231	224	226
Pediatrics	226	216	223
Physical medicine and rehabilitation	220	223	220
Psychiatry	220	205	214
Diagnostic radiology	241	237	232
General surgery	232	227	233

[a]No PGY-1 positions were filled by IMGs. Fourteen PGY-2 positions were filled by IMGs. Source: www.nrmp.org.

- Pediatrics
- Preventive medicine
- Psychiatry
- Surgery
- Other areas relevant to the provision of care under supervision

Significance of the Test. The Step 2 CK is required for the ECFMG certificate. It reflects the level of clinical knowledge of the applicant. It tests clinical subjects, primarily internal medicine. Other areas tested are orthopedics, ENT, ophthalmology, safety science, epidemiology, professionalism, and ethics.

Eligibility. Students and graduates from medical schools that are listed in IMED are eligible to take the Step 2 CK. Students must have completed at least two years of medical school. This means that students must have completed the basic medical science component of the medical school curriculum by the beginning of the eligibility period selected.

Eligibility Period. A three-month period of your choice.

Fee. The fee for the Step 2 CK is $850 plus an international test delivery surcharge (if you choose a testing region other than the United States or Canada).

Statistics. In 2012–2013, 84% of ECFMG candidates passed the Step 2 CK on their first attempt, compared with 98% of MD degree examinees from U.S. and Canadian schools.

> ▶ Be familiar with topics that are heavily emphasized in U.S. medicine, such as cholesterol screening.

Tips. It's better to take the Step 2 CK after your internal medicine rotation because most of the questions on the exam give clinical scenarios and ask you to make medical diagnoses and clinical decisions. In addition, because this is a clinical sciences exam, cultural and geographic considerations play a greater role than is the case with Step 1. For example, if your medical education gave you ample exposure to malaria, brucellosis, and malnutrition but little to alcohol withdrawal, child abuse, and cholesterol screening, you must work to familiarize yourself with topics that are more heavily emphasized in U.S. medicine. You must also have a basic understanding of the legal and social aspects of U.S. medicine, because you will be asked questions about communicating with and advising patients.

USMLE Step 2 CS and the IMG

What Is the Step 2 CS? The Step 2 CS is a test of clinical and communication skills administered as a one-day, eight-hour exam. It includes 10 to 12 encounters with standardized patients (15 minutes each, with 10 minutes to write a note after each encounter).

Content. The Step 2 CS tests the ability to communicate in English as well as interpersonal skills, data-gathering skills, the ability to perform a physical exam, and the ability to formulate a brief note, a differential diagnosis, and a list of diagnostic tests. The areas that are covered in the exam are as follows:

- Internal medicine
- Surgery
- Obstetrics and gynecology
- Pediatrics
- Psychiatry
- Family medicine

Unlike the USMLE Step 1, Step 2 CK, or Step 3, **there are no numerical grades for the Step 2 CS**—it's simply either a "pass" or a "fail." To pass, a candidate must attain a passing performance in **each** of the following three components:

▶ *The Step 2 CS is graded as pass/fail.*

- Integrated Clinical Encounter (ICE): includes Data Gathering, Physical Exam, and the Patient Note
- Spoken English Proficiency (SEP)
- Communication and Interpersonal Skills (CIS)

According to the NBME, the most commonly failed component for IMGs is the CIS.

Significance of the Test. The Step 2 CS assesses spoken English language proficiency and is required for the ECFMG certificate. The Test of English as a Foreign Language (TOEFL) is no longer required.

Eligibility. Students must have completed at least two years of medical school in order to take the test. That means students must have completed the basic medical science component of the medical school curriculum at the time they apply for the exam.

Fee. The fee for the Step 2 CS is $1480.

Scheduling. You must schedule the Step 2 CS within **four months** of the date indicated on your notification of registration. You must take the exam within 12 months of the date indicated on your notification of registration. It is generally advisable to take the Step 2 CS as soon as possible in the year before your Match, as often the results either come in late or arrive too late to allow you to retake the test and pass it before the Match.

▶ *Try to take the Step 2 CS the year before you plan to Match.*

Test Site Locations. The Step 2 CS is currently administered at the following five locations:

- Philadelphia, PA
- Atlanta, GA
- Los Angeles, CA
- Chicago, IL
- Houston, TX

For more information about the Step 2 CS exam, please refer to *First Aid for the Step 2 CS.*

USMLE Step 3 and the IMG

What Is the USMLE Step 3? It is a two-day computerized test in clinical medicine consisting of 454 multiple-choice questions and 13 computer-based case simulations (CCS). The exam aims to test your knowledge and its application to patient care and clinical decision making (i.e., this exam tests if you can safely practice medicine independently and without supervision). Please go to the USMLE Web site to learn more about recent changes to the exam.

Significance of the Test. Taking Step 3 before residency is critical for IMGs seeking an H1B visa and is also a bonus that can be added to the residency application. Step 3 is also required to obtain a full medical license in the United States and can be taken during residency for this purpose.

Fee. The fee for Step 3 is $815.

Eligibility. Examinees are no longer required to apply to the Step 3 exam under the eligibility requirements of a specific medical licensing authority. Those wishing to sit for the Step 3 exam, independent of the place of residence, must meet the following requirements:

- Have completed an MD or DO degree from an LCME- or AOA-accredited U.S. or Canadian medical school, or from a medical school outside the U.S. and Canada listed in the International Medical Education Directory.
- Have taken and passed the Step 1, Step 2 CK, and Step 2 CS exams.
- If an IMG: be certified by the ECFMG or have completed a Fifth Pathway program.

The Step 3 exam is not available outside the United States. Applications can be found online at www.fsmb.org and must be submitted to the FSMB.

Statistics. In 2013–2014, 87% of IMG candidates passed the Step 3 on their first attempt, compared with 96% of MD degree examinees from U.S. and Canadian schools.

> ▶ Complete the Step 3 exam before you apply for an H1B visa.

Residencies and the IMG

In the Match, the number of U.S.-citizen IMG applications has grown over the past few years, while the percentage accepted has remained constant (see Table 5). More information about residency programs can be obtained at www.ama-assn.org.

The Match and the IMG

Given the growing number of IMG candidates with strong applications, you should bear in mind that good USMLE scores are not the only way to gain a competitive edge. However, USMLE Step 1 and Step 2 CK scores continue to be used as the initial screening mechanism when candidates are being considered for interviews.

TABLE 5. IMGs in the Match.

Applicants	2012	2013	2014
U.S.-citizen IMGs	4,279	5,095	5,133
% U.S.-citizen IMGs accepted	49	53	53
Non-U.S.-citizen IMGs	6,828	7,568	7,334
% non-U.S.-citizen IMGs accepted	41	48	49.5
U.S. seniors (non-IMGs)	16,527	17,487	17,374
% U.S. seniors accepted	95	94	94

Source: www.nrmp.org.

Based on accumulated IMG Match experiences over recent years, here are a few pointers to help IMGs maximize their chances for a residency interview:

- **Apply early.** Programs offer a limited number of interviews and often select candidates on a first-come, first-served basis. Because of this, you should aim to complete the entire process of applying for the ERAS token, registering with the Association of American Medical Colleges (AAMC), mailing necessary documents to ERAS, and completing the ERAS application by mid-September (see Figure 5). Community programs usually send out interview offers earlier than do university and university-affiliated programs.

- **U.S. clinical experience helps.** Externships and observerships in a U.S. hospital setting have emerged as an important credential on an IMG application. Externships are like short-term medical school internships and offer hands-on clinical experience. Observerships, also called "shadowing," involve following a physician and observing how he or she manages patients. Some programs require students to have participated in an externship or observership before applying. It is best to gain such an experience before or at the time you apply to various programs so that you can mention it on your ERAS application. If such an experience or opportunity comes up after you apply, be sure to inform the programs accordingly.

> ▶ Most U.S. hospitals allow externship only when the applicant is actively enrolled in a medical school, so plan ahead.

- **Clinical research helps.** University programs are attracted to candidates who show a strong interest in clinical research and academics. They may even relax their application criteria for individuals with unique backgrounds and strong research experience. Publications in well-known journals are an added bonus.

- **Time the Step 2 CS well.** ECFMG has published the new Step 2 CS score-reporting schedule for 2014–2015 at http://www.ecfmg.org. Most program directors would like to see a passing score on the Step 1, Step 2 CK, and Step 2 CS exams before they rank an IMG on their rank order list in mid-February. There have been many instances in which candidates have lost a potential Match—either because of delayed CS results or because they have been unable to retake the exam on time

FIGURE 5. IMG Timeline for Application.

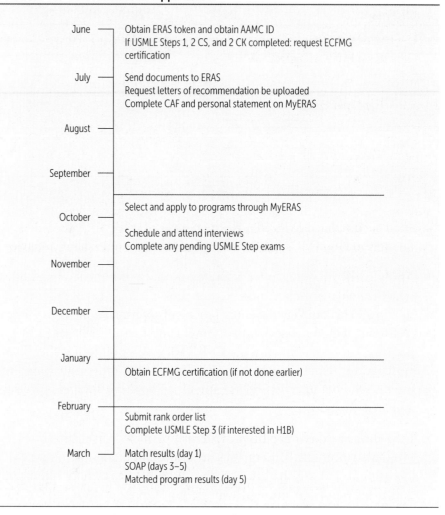

June	Obtain ERAS token and obtain AAMC ID If USMLE Steps 1, 2 CS, and 2 CK completed: request ECFMG certification
July	Send documents to ERAS Request letters of recommendation be uploaded Complete CAF and personal statement on MyERAS
August	
September	
October	Select and apply to programs through MyERAS Schedule and attend interviews Complete any pending USMLE Step exams
November	
December	
January	Obtain ECFMG certification (if not done earlier)
February	Submit rank order list Complete USMLE Step 3 (if interested in H1B)
March	Match results (day 1) SOAP (days 3–5) Matched program results (day 5)

following a failure. It is difficult to predict a result on the Step 2 CS, since the grading process is not very transparent. Therefore, it is advisable to take the Step 2 CS as early as possible in the application year.

- **U.S. letters of recommendation help.** Letters of recommendation from clinicians practicing in the United States carry more weight than recommendations from home countries.

- **Step up the Step 3.** If H1B visa sponsorship is desired, aim to have Step 3 results by January of the Match year. In addition to the visa advantage you will gain, an early and good Step 3 score may benefit IMGs who have been away from clinical medicine for a while as well as those who have low scores on Step 1 and the Step 2 CK.

- **Verify medical credentials in a timely manner.** Do not overlook the medical school credential verification process. The ECFMG certificate arrives only after credentials have been verified and after you have passed

▶ *A good score on the Step 3 may help offset poorer scores on the Step 1 or 2 CK exams.*

Step 1, the Step 2 CK, and the Step 2 CS, so you should keep track of the process and check with the ECFMG from time to time about your status.

- **Don't count on a pre-Match.** Programs participating in NRMP Match can no longer offer a pre-Match.

What if You Do Not Match?

For applicants who do not Match into a residency program, there's SOAP (Supplemental Offer and Acceptance Program). Under SOAP, unmatched applicants will have access to the list of unfilled programs at noon Eastern time on the Monday of Match week. The unfilled programs electing to participate in SOAP will offer positions to unmatched applicants through the Registration, Ranking, and Results (R3) system. A series of "rounds" will begin at noon Eastern time on Wednesday of Match week until 5:00 P.M. Eastern time on Friday of Match week. Detailed information about SOAP can be found at the NRMP Web site at http://www.nrmp.org.

▶ *The Scramble has been replaced by SOAP (Supplemental Offer and Acceptance Program).*

Resources for the IMG

- **ECFMG**
  3624 Market Street
  Philadelphia, PA 19104-2685
  (215) 386-5900
  Fax: (215) 386-9196
  www.ecfmg.org

  The ECFMG telephone number is answered only between 9:00 A.M.–5:00 P.M. Monday through Friday EST. The ECFMG often takes a long time to answer the phone, which is frequently busy at peak times of the year, and then gives you a long voice-mail message—so it is better to write or fax early than to rely on a last-minute phone call. Do not contact the NBME, as all IMG exam matters are conducted by the ECFMG. The ECFMG also publishes an information booklet on ECFMG certification and the USMLE program, which gives details on the dates and locations of forthcoming Step tests for IMGs together with application forms. It is free of charge and is also available from the public affairs offices of U.S. embassies and consulates worldwide as well as from Overseas Educational Advisory Centers. You may order single copies of the handbook by calling (215) 386-5900, preferably on weekends or between 6 P.M. and 6 A.M. Eastern time, or by faxing to (215) 386-9196. Requests for multiple copies must be made by fax or mail on organizational letterhead. The full text of the booklet is also available on the ECFMG's Web site at www.ecfmg.org.

- **FSMB**
  400 Fuller Wiser Road, Suite 300
  Euless, TX 76039
  (817) 868-4041
  Fax: (817) 868-4098
  Email: usmle@fsmb.org
  www.fsmb.org

The FSMB has a number of publications available, including free policy documents. To obtain these publications, print and mail the order form on the Web site listed above. Alternatively, write to Federation Publications at the above address. All orders must be prepaid with a personal check drawn on a U.S. bank, a cashier's check, or a money order payable to the FSMB. Foreign orders must be accompanied by an international money order or the equivalent, payable in U.S. dollars through a U.S. bank or a U.S. affiliate of a foreign bank. For Step 3 inquiries, the telephone number is (817) 868-4041.

The AMA has dedicated a portion of its Web site to information on IMG demographics, residencies, immigration, and the like. This information can be found at www.ama-assn.org.

Other resources that may be useful and of interest to IMGs include the following:

- *The International Medical Graduate's Guide to US Medicine and Residency Training*, by Patrick C. Alquire, Gerald P. Whelan, and Vijay Rajput (2009; ISBN 9781934465080).
- *The International Medical Graduate's Best Hope*, by Franck Belibi and Suzanne Belibi (2009; ISBN 9780979877308).

▶ FIRST AID FOR THE OSTEOPATHIC MEDICAL STUDENT

What Is the COMLEX-USA Level 1?

The National Board of Osteopathic Medical Examiners (NBOME) administers the Comprehensive Osteopathic Medical Licensing Examination, or COMLEX-USA. Like the USMLE, the COMLEX-USA is administered over three levels.

The COMLEX-USA series assesses osteopathic medical knowledge and clinical skills using clinical presentations and physician tasks. A description of the COMLEX-USA Written Examination Blueprints for each level, which outline the various clinical presentations and physician tasks that examinees will encounter, is given on the NBOME Web site. Another stated goal of the COMLEX-USA Level 1 is to create a more primary care–oriented exam that integrates osteopathic principles into clinical situations.

To be eligible to take the COMLEX-USA Level 1, you must have satisfactorily completed your first year in an American Osteopathic Association (AOA)–approved medical school. The office of the dean at each school informs the NBOME that a student has completed his or her first year of school and is in good standing. At this point, the NBOME sends out an email with detailed instructions on how to register for the exam.

For all three levels of the COMLEX-USA, raw scores are converted to a percentile score and a score ranging from 5 to 800. For Levels 1 and 2, a score of 400 is required to pass; for Level 3, a score of 350 is needed. COMLEX-USA scores are posted at the NBOME Web site 4–6 weeks after the test and usually mailed within 8 weeks after the test. The mean score is always 500.

If you pass a COMLEX-USA examination, you are not allowed to retake it to improve your grade. If you fail, there is no specific limit to the number of times you can retake it in order to pass. However, a student may not take the exam more than four times in one year. Levels 2 and 3 exams must be passed in sequential order within seven years of passing Level 1.

Note that effective July 1, 2016, candidates taking COMLEX-USA examinations will be limited to a total of six attempts for each examination.

What Is the Structure of the COMLEX-USA Level 1?

The COMLEX-USA Level 1 is a computer-based examination consisting of 400 questions over an eight-hour period in a single day (nine hours if you count breaks). Most of the questions are in one-best-answer format, but a small number are matching-type questions. Some one-best-answer questions are bundled together around a common question stem that usually takes the form of a clinical scenario. Every section of the COMLEX-USA Level 1 ends with either matching questions, multiple questions around a single stem, or both. New question formats may gradually be introduced, but candidates will be notified if this occurs. Multimedia questions are also included on the exam.

Questions are grouped into eight sections of 50 questions each in a manner similar to the USMLE. Reviewing and changing answers may be done only in the current section. A "review page" is presented for each block in order to advise test takers of questions completed, questions marked for further review, and incomplete questions for which no answer has been given.

Breaks are even more structured with COMLEX-USA than they are with the USMLE. Students are allowed to take a 10-minute break at the end of the second and sixth sections. Students who do not take these 10-minute breaks can apply the time toward their test time. After section 4, students are given a 40-minute lunch break. These are the only times a student is permitted a break. More information about the computer-based COMLEX-USA examinations can be obtained from www.nbome.org.

What Is the Difference Between the USMLE and the COMLEX-USA?

According to the NBOME, the COMLEX-USA Level 1 focuses broadly on the following categories, with osteopathic principles and practices integrated into each section:

- Health promotion and disease prevention
- The history and physical
- Diagnostic technologies
- Management
- Scientific understanding of mechanisms
- Health care delivery

> ▶ The test interface for the COMLEX-USA Level 1 is not the same as the USMLE Step 1 interface.

Although the COMLEX-USA and the USMLE are similar in scope, content, and emphasis, some differences are worth noting. For example, the interface is different; you cannot search for lab values. The expectation is that you can make a diagnosis without having performed testing. Fewer details are given about a patient's condition, so a savvy student needs to know how to differentiate between similar pathologies. Also, age, gender, and race are key factors for diagnosis on the COMLEX-USA. Images are embedded in the question stem and the examinee has to click an attachment button to see the image. If you don't read the question carefully, the attachment buttons are very easy to miss.

COMLEX-USA Level 1 tests osteopathic principles in addition to basic science materials but does not emphasize lab techniques. Although both exams often require that you apply and integrate knowledge over several areas of basic science to answer a given question, many students who took both tests reported that the questions differed somewhat in style. Students reported, for example, that USMLE questions generally required that the test taker reason and draw from the information given (often a two-step process), whereas those on the COMLEX-USA exam tended to be more straightforward. Furthermore, USMLE questions were on average found to be considerably longer than those on the COMLEX-USA.

COMLEX-USA test takers can expect to have only a few questions on biochemistry, molecular biology, or lab technique. On the other hand, microbiology is very heavily tested by clinical presentation and by lab identification. Another main difference is that the COMLEX-USA exam stresses osteopathic manipulative medicine. Therefore, question banks specific to the USMLE will not be adequate, and supplementation with a question bank specific to the COMLEX-USA is highly recommended.

Students also commented that the COMLEX-USA utilized "buzzwords," although limited in their use (e.g., "rose spots" in typhoid fever), whereas the USMLE avoided buzzwords in favor of descriptions of clinical findings or symptoms (e.g., rose-colored papules on the abdomen rather than rose spots). Finally, USMLE appeared to have more photographs than did the COMLEX-USA. In general, the overall impression was that the USMLE was a more "thought-provoking" exam, while the COMLEX-USA was more of a "knowledge-based" exam.

Who Should Take Both the USMLE and the COMLEX-USA?

Aside from facing the COMLEX-USA Level 1, you must decide if you will also take the USMLE Step 1. We recommend that you consider taking both the USMLE and the COMLEX-USA under the following circumstances:

- **If you are applying to allopathic residencies.** Although there is growing acceptance of COMLEX-USA certification on the part of allopathic residencies, some allopathic programs prefer or even require passage of the USMLE Step 1. These include many academic programs, programs in competitive specialties (e.g., orthopedics, ophthalmology, or dermatology), and programs in competitive geographic areas (e.g., Vermont, Utah, and California). Fourth-year doctor of osteopathy (DO) students who have already Matched may be a good source of information about which programs and specialties look for USMLE scores. It is also a good idea to contact program directors at the institutions you are interested in to ask about their policy regarding the COMLEX-USA versus the USMLE.

- **If you are unsure about your postgraduate training plans.** Successful passage of both the COMLEX-USA Level 1 and the USMLE Step 1 is certain to provide you with the greatest possible range of options when you are applying for internship and residency training.

> ▶ If you're not sure whether you need to take either the COMLEX-USA Level 1 or the USMLE Step 1, consider taking both to keep your Match options open.

In addition, the COMLEX-USA Level 1 has in recent years placed increasing emphasis on questions related to primary care medicine and prevention. Having a strong background in family or primary care medicine can help test takers when they face questions on prevention.

How Do I Prepare for the COMLEX-USA Level 1?

Student experience suggests that you should start studying for the COMLEX-USA four to six months before the test is given, as an early start will allow you to spend up to a month on each subject. The recommendations made in Section I regarding study and testing methods, strategies, and resources, as well as the books suggested in Section IV for the USMLE Step 1, hold true for the COMLEX-USA as well.

Another important source of information is in the *Examination Guidelines and Sample Exam*, a booklet that discusses the breakdown of each subject while also providing sample questions and corresponding answers. Many students, however, felt that this breakdown provided only a general guideline and was not representative of the level of difficulty of the actual COMLEX-USA. The sample questions did not provide examples of clinical vignettes, which made up approximately 25% of the exam. You will receive this publication with registration materials for the COMLEX-USA Level 1, but you can also receive a copy and additional information by writing:

NBOME
8765 W. Higgins Road, Suite 200
Chicago, IL 60631-4174
(773) 714-0622
Fax: (773) 714-0631
www.nbome.org

The NBOME developed the Comprehensive Osteopathic Medical Self-Assessment Examination (COMSAE) series to fill the need for self-assessment on the part of osteopathic medical students. Many students take the COMSAE exam before the COMLEX-USA in addition to using test-bank questions and board review books. Students can purchase a copy of this exam at www.nbome.org/comsae.asp.

In recent years, students have reported an emphasis in certain areas. For example:

- There was an increased emphasis on upper limb anatomy/brachial plexus.
- Specific topics were repeatedly tested on the exam. These included cardiovascular physiology and pathology, acid-base physiology, diabetes, benign prostatic hyperplasia, sexually transmitted diseases, measles, and rubella. Thyroid and adrenal function, neurology (head injury), specific drug treatments for bacterial infection, migraines/cluster headaches, and drug mechanisms also received heavy emphasis.
- Behavioral science questions were based on psychiatry.
- High-yield osteopathic manipulative technique (OMT) topics included an emphasis on the sympathetic and parasympathetic innervations of viscera and nerve roots, rib mechanics/diagnosis, and basic craniosacral theory. Students who spend time reviewing basic anatomy, studying nerve and dermatome innervations, and understanding how to perform basic OMT techniques (e.g., muscle energy or counterstrain) can improve their scores.

▶ *You must know the Chapman reflex points and the obscure names of physical exam signs.*

The COMLEX-USA Level 1 also includes multimedia-based questions. Such questions test the student's ability to perform a good physical exam and to elicit various physical diagnostic signs (e.g., Murphy sign).

Since topics that were repeatedly tested appeared in all four booklets, students found it useful to review them in between the two test days. It is important to understand that the topics emphasized on the current exam may not be stressed on future exams. However, some topics are heavily tested each year, so it may be beneficial to have a solid foundation in the above-mentioned topics.

▶ FIRST AID FOR THE PODIATRIC MEDICAL STUDENT

The National Board of Podiatric Medical Examiners (NBPME) offers the American Podiatric Medical Licensing Examinations (APMLE), which are designed to assess whether a candidate possesses the knowledge required to practice as a minimally competent entry-level podiatric surgeon. The APMLE is used as part of the licensing process governing the practice of podiatric medicine and surgery. The APMLE is recognized by all 50 states and the District of Columbia, the U.S. Army, the U.S. Navy, and the Canadian provinces of Alberta, British Columbia, and Ontario. Individual states use the examination scores differently; therefore, doctor of podiatric medicine (DPM) candidates should refer to the *APMLE Bulletin of Information: 2014 Examinations.*

The APMLE Part I is generally taken after the completion of the second year of podiatric medical education. Unlike the USMLE Step 1, there is no behavioral science section, nor is biomechanics tested. The exam samples seven basic science disciplines: general anatomy (13%); lower extremity anatomy (25%); biochemistry (7%); physiology (13%); microbiology and immunology (15%); pathology (12%); and pharmacology (15%). A detailed outline of topics and subtopics covered on the exam can be found in the *APMLE Bulletin of Information*, available at www.apmle.org.

▶ *Areas tested on the NBPME Part I:*
- *General anatomy*
- *Lower extremity anatomy*
- *Biochemistry*
- *Physiology*
- *Medical microbiology & immunology*
- *Pathology*
- *Pharmacology*

Your APMLE Appointment

In early spring, your college registrar will have you fill out an application for the APMLE Part I. New this year, applicants can register for the exam online at www.prometric.com/NBPME. The exam will be offered at an independent Prometric testing facility in each city with a podiatric medical school (New York, Philadelphia, Miami, Cleveland, Chicago, Des Moines, Phoenix, Pomona, and San Francisco), along with any other city Prometric deems necessary. Please contact Prometric for a full list of testing sites. You may take the exam at any of these locations regardless of which school you attend. However, you must designate on your application which testing location you desire. Specific instructions about exam dates and registration deadlines can be found in the *APMLE Bulletin.*

Exam Format

The APMLE Part I is a written exam consisting of 205 questions. The test consists of multiple choice questions that have one best answer or multiple "select all that apply" answers, as well as a drag-and-drop section. Examinees have four hours in which to complete the exam and are given scratch paper and a calculator, both of which must be turned in at the end of the exam. Some questions on the exam will be "trial questions." These questions are evaluated as future board questions but are not counted in your score.

Interpreting Your Score

Three to four weeks following the exam date, the dean's office at the student's respective school will receive scores. APMLE scores are reported as pass/fail, with a scaled score of at least 75 needed to pass. Historically, 85% of first-time test takers pass the APMLE Part I. Failing candidates receive a report with a score between 55 and 74 in addition to diagnostic messages intended to help identify strengths or weaknesses in specific content areas. If you fail the APMLE Part I, you must retake the entire examination at a later date. There is no limit to the number of times you can retake the exam.

Preparation for the APMLE Part I

Begin studying for the APMLE Part I at least three months prior to the test date. The suggestions made in Section I regarding study and testing methods for the USMLE Step 1 can be applied to the APMLE as well. This book should, however, be used as a supplement and not as the sole source of information. Neither you nor your school or future residency will ever see your actual passing numerical score. Competing with colleagues should not be an issue, and study groups are beneficial to many.

> ▶ *Know the anatomy of the lower extremity!*

A study method that helps many students is to copy the outline of the material to be tested from the *APMLE Bulletin*. Check off each topic during your study, because doing so will ensure that you have engaged each topic. If you are pressed for time, prioritize subjects on the basis of their weight on the exam. A full 25% of the APMLE Part I focuses on lower extremity anatomy. In this area, students should rely on the notes and material that they received from their class. Remember, lower extremity anatomy is the podiatric physician's specialty—so everything about it is important. Do not forget to study osteology. Keep your old tests and look through old lower extremity class exams, since each of the podiatric colleges submits questions from its faculty. This strategy will give you an understanding of the types of questions that may be asked. On the APMLE Part I, you will see some of the same classic lower extremity anatomy questions you were tested on in school.

The APMLE, like the USMLE, requires that you apply and integrate knowledge over several areas of basic science in order to answer exam questions. Students report that many questions emphasize clinical presentations; however, the facts in this book are very useful in helping students recall the various diseases and organisms. DPM candidates should expand on the high-yield pharmacology section and study antifungal drugs and treatments for *Pseudomonas*, methicillin-resistant *S. aureus*, candidiasis, and erythrasma. The high-yield section focusing on pathology is very useful; however, additional emphasis on diabetes mellitus and all its secondary manifestations, particularly peripheral neuropathy, should not be overlooked. Students should also focus on renal physiology and drug elimination, the biochemistry of gout, and neurophysiology, all of which have been noted to be important topics on the APMLE Part I exam.

A sample set of questions is found on the APMLE website www.apmle.org. These samples are somewhat similar in difficulty to actual board questions. If you have any questions regarding registration, fees, test centers, authorization forms, or score reports, please contact your college registrar or:

Prometric
Phone: 877-302-8952
Fax: 800-813-6670
Email: nbpmeinquiry@prometric.com
www.prometric.com

▶ FIRST AID FOR THE STUDENT WITH A DISABILITY

The USMLE provides accommodations for students with documented disabilities. The basis for such accommodations is the Americans with Disabilities Act (ADA) of 1990. The ADA defines a disability as "a significant limitation in one or more major life activities." This includes both "observable/physical" disabilities (e.g., blindness, hearing loss, narcolepsy) and "hidden/mental disabilities" (e.g., attention-deficit hyperactivity disorder, chronic fatigue syndrome, learning disabilities).

To provide appropriate support, the administrators of the USMLE must be informed of both the nature and the severity of an examinee's disability. Such documentation is required for an examinee to receive testing accommodations. Accommodations include extra time on tests, low-stimulation environments, extra or extended breaks, and zoom text.

> ▶ U.S. students seeking ADA-compliant accommodations must contact the NBME directly; IMGs, contact the ECFMG.

Who Can Apply for Accommodations?

Students or graduates of a school in the United States or Canada that is accredited by the Liaison Committee on Medical Education (LCME) or the AOA may apply for test accommodations directly from the NBME. Requests are granted only if they meet the ADA definition of a disability. If you are a disabled student or a disabled graduate of a foreign medical school, you must contact the ECFMG (see the following page).

Who Is Not Eligible for Accommodations?

Individuals who do not meet the ADA definition of disabled are not eligible for test accommodations. Difficulties not eligible for test accommodations include test anxiety, slow reading without an identified underlying cognitive deficit, English as a second language, and learning difficulties that have not been diagnosed as a medically recognized disability.

Understanding the Need for Documentation

Although most learning-disabled medical students are all too familiar with the often exhausting process of providing documentation of their disability, you should realize that **applying for USMLE accommodation is different from these previous experiences.** This is because the NBME determines whether an individual is disabled solely on the basis of the guidelines set by the ADA. **Previous accommodation does not in itself justify provision of an accommodation for the USMLE,** so be sure to review the NBME guidelines carefully.

Getting the Information

The first step in applying for USMLE special accommodations is to contact the NBME and obtain a guidelines and questionnaire booklet. For the Step 1, Step 2 CK, and Step 2 CS exams, this can be obtained by calling or writing to:

Disability Services
National Board of Medical Examiners
3750 Market Street
Philadelphia, PA 19104-3102
(215) 590-9509
Fax: (215) 590-9457
Email: disabilityservices@nbme.org
www.usmle.org/test-accommodations

Internet access to this information is also available at www.nbme.org. This information is also relevant for IMGs, since the information is the same as that sent by the ECFMG.

Foreign graduates should contact the ECFMG to obtain information on special accommodations by calling or writing to:

ECFMG
3624 Market Street
Philadelphia, PA 19104-2685
(215) 386-5900
www.ecfmg.org

When you get this information, take some time to read it carefully. The guidelines are clear and explicit about what you need to do to obtain accommodations.

SECTION II

High-Yield
General Principles

"There comes a time when for every addition of knowledge you forget something that you knew before. It is of the highest importance, therefore, not to have useless facts elbowing out the useful ones."
—Sir Arthur Conan Doyle, A *Study in Scarlet*

"Never regard study as a duty, but as the enviable opportunity to learn."
—Albert Einstein

"Live as if you were to die tomorrow. Learn as if you were to live forever."
—Gandhi

The 2015 edition of *First Aid for the USMLE Step 1* contains a revised and expanded database of basic science material that students, student authors, and faculty authors have identified as high yield for board review. The information is presented in a partially organ-based format. Hence, Section II is devoted to pathology and the foundational principles of behavioral science, biochemistry, microbiology, immunology, and pharmacology. Section III focuses on organ systems, with subsections covering the embryology, anatomy and histology, physiology, pathology, and pharmacology relevant to each. Each subsection is then divided into smaller topic areas containing related facts. Individual facts are generally presented in a three-column format, with the **Title** of the fact in the first column, the **Description** of the fact in the second column, and the **Mnemonic** or **Special Note** in the third column. Some facts do not have a mnemonic and are presented in a two-column format. Others are presented in list or tabular form in order to emphasize key associations.

The database structure used in Sections II and III is useful for reviewing material already learned. These sections are **not** ideal for learning complex or highly conceptual material for the first time.

The database of high-yield facts is not comprehensive. Use it to complement your core study material and not as your primary study source. The facts and notes have been condensed and edited to emphasize the essential material, and as a result, each entry is "incomplete" and arguably "over-simplified." Often, the more you research a topic, the more complex it becomes, with certain topics resisting simplification. Work with the material, add your own notes and mnemonics, and recognize that not all memory techniques work for all students.

We update the database of high-yield facts annually to keep current with new trends in boards emphasis, including clinical relevance. However, we must note that inevitably many other high-yield topics are not yet included in our database.

We actively encourage medical students and faculty to submit high-yield topics, well-written entries, diagrams, clinical images, and useful mnemonics so that we may enhance the database for future students. We also solicit recommendations of alternate tools for study that may be useful in preparing for the examination, such as charts, flash cards, apps, and online resources (see How to Contribute, p. xix).

Image Acknowledgments

All images and diagrams marked with ▣ are © USMLE-Rx.com (MedIQ Learning, LLC) and reproduced here by special permission. All images marked with ℞ are © Dr. Richard P. Usatine, author of *The Color Atlas of Family Medicine*, *The Color Atlas of Internal Medicine*, and *The Color Atlas of Pediatrics*, and are reproduced here by special permission (www.usatinemedia.com). Images and diagrams marked with ✳ are adapted or reproduced with permission of other sources as listed on page 669. Images and diagrams with no acknowledgment are part of this book.

Disclaimer

The entries in this section reflect student opinions of what is high yield. Because of the diverse sources of material, no attempt has been made to trace or reference the origins of entries individually. We have regarded mnemonics as essentially in the public domain. Errata will gladly be corrected if brought to the attention of the authors, either through our online errata submission form at www.firstaidteam.com or directly by email to firstaidteam@yahoo.com.

Behavioral Science

"It is a mathematical fact that fifty percent of all doctors graduate in the bottom half of their class."

—Author Unknown

"It's psychosomatic. You need a lobotomy. I'll get a saw."

—Calvin, "Calvin & Hobbes"

"There are two kinds of statistics: the kind you look up and the kind you make up."

—Rex Stout

"On a long enough time line, the survival rate for everyone drops to zero."

—Chuck Palahniuk

A heterogeneous mix of epidemiology, biostatistics, ethics, psychology, sociology, and more falls under the heading of behavioral science. Many medical students do not diligently study this discipline because the material is felt to be easy or a matter of common sense. In our opinion, this is a missed opportunity.

Behavioral science questions may seem less concrete than questions from other disciplines, as they require an awareness of the psychosocial aspects of medicine. For example, if a patient does or says something, what should you do or say in response? These so-called quote questions now constitute much of the behavioral science section. Medical ethics and medical law are also appearing with increasing frequency. In addition, the key aspects of the doctor-patient relationship (e.g., communication skills, open-ended questions, facilitation, silence) are high yield, as are biostatistics and epidemiology. Make sure you can apply biostatistical concepts such as sensitivity, specificity, and predictive values in a problem-solving format.

▶ BEHAVIORAL SCIENCE—EPIDEMIOLOGY/BIOSTATISTICS

Observational studies

STUDY TYPE	DESIGN	MEASURES/EXAMPLE
Cross-sectional study	Collects data from a group of people to assess frequency of disease (and related risk factors) at a particular point in time. Asks, "What is happening?"	Disease prevalence. Can show risk factor association with disease, but does not establish causality.
Case-control study Retrospective	Compares a group of people with disease to a group without disease. Looks for prior exposure or risk factor. Asks, "What happened?"	Odds ratio (OR). "Patients with COPD had higher odds of a history of smoking than those without COPD."
Cohort study Prospective or retrospective	Compares a group with a given exposure or risk factor to a group without such exposure. Looks to see if exposure ↑ the likelihood of disease. Can be prospective (asks, "Who will develop disease?") or retrospective (asks, "Who developed the disease [exposed vs. nonexposed]?").	Relative risk (RR). "Smokers had a higher risk of developing COPD than nonsmokers."
Twin concordance study	Compares the frequency with which both monozygotic twins or both dizygotic twins develop the same disease.	Measures heritability and influence of environmental factors ("nature vs. nurture").
Adoption study	Compares siblings raised by biological vs. adoptive parents.	Measures heritability and influence of environmental factors.

Clinical trial	Experimental study involving humans. Compares therapeutic benefits of 2 or more treatments, or of treatment and placebo. Study quality improves when study is randomized, controlled, and double-blinded (i.e., neither patient nor doctor knows whether the patient is in the treatment or control group). Triple-blind refers to the additional blinding of the researchers analyzing the data.

DRUG TRIALS	TYPICAL STUDY SAMPLE	PURPOSE
Phase I	Small number of healthy volunteers.	"Is it safe?" Assesses safety, toxicity, pharmacokinetics, and pharmacodynamics.
Phase II	Small number of patients with disease of interest.	"Does it work?" Assesses treatment efficacy, optimal dosing, and adverse effects.
Phase III	Large number of patients randomly assigned either to the treatment under investigation or to the best available treatment (or placebo).	"Is it as good or better?" Compares the new treatment to the current standard of care.
Phase IV	Postmarketing surveillance of patients after treatment is approved.	"Can it stay?" Detects rare or long-term adverse effects. Can result in treatment being withdrawn from market.

Evaluation of diagnostic tests	Uses 2×2 table comparing test results with the actual presence of disease. TP = true positive; FP = false positive; TN = true negative; FN = false negative. Sensitivity and specificity are fixed properties of a test. PPV and NPV vary depending on disease prevalence.	

Sensitivity (true-positive rate)	Proportion of all people with disease who test positive, or the probability that a test detects disease when disease is present. Value approaching 100% is desirable for **ruling out** disease and indicates a **low false-negative rate**. High sensitivity test used for screening in diseases with low prevalence.	$= TP / (TP + FN)$ $= 1 -$ false-negative rate **SN-N-OUT** = highly **SeN**sitive test, when **N**egative, rules **OUT** disease If sensitivity is 100%, $TP / (TP + FN) = 1$, $FN = 0$, and all negatives must be TNs
Specificity (true-negative rate)	Proportion of all people without disease who test negative, or the probability that a test indicates no disease when disease is absent. Value approaching 100% is desirable for **ruling in** disease and indicates a **low false-positive rate**. High specificity test used for confirmation after a positive screening test.	$= TN / (TN + FP)$ $= 1 -$ false-positive rate **SP-P-IN** = highly **SP**ecific test, when **P**ositive, rules **IN** disease If specificity is 100%, $TN / (TN + FP) = 1$, $FP = 0$, and all positives must be TPs
Positive predictive value (PPV)	Proportion of positive test results that are true positive. Probability that person actually has the disease given a positive test result.	$= TP / (TP + FP)$ PPV varies directly with prevalence or pretest probability: high pretest probability → high PPV
Negative predictive value (NPV)	Proportion of negative test results that are true negative. Probability that person actually is disease free given a negative test result.	$= TN / (TN + FN)$ NPV varies inversely with prevalence or pretest probability: high pretest probability → low NPV

POSSIBLE CUTOFF VALUES
A = 100% sensitivity cutoff value
B = practical compromise between specificity and sensitivity
C = 100% specificity cutoff value

Incidence vs. prevalence	Incidence rate $= \dfrac{\text{\# of new cases}}{\text{\# of people at risk}}$ (during a time period) Prevalence $= \dfrac{\text{\# of existing cases}}{\text{\# of people at risk}}$ (at a point in time) Prevalence ≈ incidence for short duration disease (e.g., common cold).	**Incidence** looks at new cases (**incidents**). Prevalence looks at **all** current cases. Prevalence ≈ pretest probability.

| **Quantifying risk** | Definitions and formulas are based on the classic 2×2 or contingency table. |

Disease

		⊕	⊖
Risk factor or intervention	⊕	a	b
	⊖	c	d

Odds ratio (OR)	Typically used in case-control studies. Odds that the group with the disease (cases) was exposed to a risk factor (a/c) divided by the odds that the group without the disease (controls) was exposed (b/d).	$OR = \dfrac{a/c}{b/d} = \dfrac{ad}{bc}$
Relative risk (RR)	Typically used in cohort studies. Risk of developing disease in the exposed group divided by risk in the unexposed group (e.g., if 21% of smokers develop lung cancer vs. 1% of nonsmokers, RR = 21/1 = 21). If prevalence is low, OR ≈ RR.	$RR = \dfrac{a/(a+b)}{c/(c+d)}$
Attributable risk (AR)	The difference in risk between exposed and unexposed groups, or the proportion of disease occurrences that are attributable to the exposure (e.g., if risk of lung cancer in smokers is 21% and risk in nonsmokers is 1%, then 20% of the lung cancer risk in smokers is attributable to smoking).	$AR = \dfrac{a}{a+b} - \dfrac{c}{c+d}$
Relative risk reduction (RRR)	The proportion of risk reduction attributable to the intervention as compared to a control (e.g., if 2% of patients who receive a flu shot develop the flu, while 8% of unvaccinated patients develop the flu, then RR = 2/8 = 0.25, and RRR = 0.75).	$RRR = 1 - RR$
Absolute risk reduction (ARR)	The difference in risk (not the proportion) attributable to the intervention as compared to a control (e.g., if 8% of people who receive a placebo vaccine develop the flu vs. 2% of people who receive a flu vaccine, then ARR = 8% − 2% = 6% = .06).	$ARR = \dfrac{c}{c+d} - \dfrac{a}{a+b}$
Number needed to treat (NNT)	Number of patients who need to be treated for 1 patient to benefit.	$NNT = 1/ARR$
Number needed to harm (NNH)	Number of patients who need to be exposed to a risk factor for 1 patient to be harmed.	$NNH = 1/AR$

Precision vs. accuracy

Precision	The consistency and reproducibility of a test (reliability).	Random error ↓ precision in a test.
	The absence of random variation in a test.	↑ precision → ↓ standard deviation.
		↑ precision → ↑ statistical power $(1 - \beta)$.
Accuracy	The trueness of test measurements (validity).	Systematic error ↓ accuracy in a test.
	The absence of systematic error or bias in a test.	

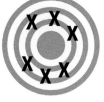
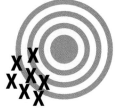

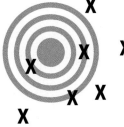
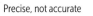

Accurate, not precise

Precise, not accurate

Accurate and precise

Not accurate, not precise

Bias and study errors

TYPE	DEFINITION	EXAMPLES	STRATEGY TO REDUCE BIAS
Recruiting participants			
Selection bias	Error in assigning subjects to a study group resulting in an unrepresentative sample. Most commonly a sampling bias.	Berkson bias—study population selected from hospital is less healthy than general population. Healthy worker effect—study population is healthier than the general population. Non-response bias— participating subjects differ from nonrespondents in meaningful ways	Randomization. Ensure the choice of the right comparison/reference group
Performing study			
Recall bias	Awareness of disorder alters recall by subjects; common in retrospective studies.	Patients with disease recall exposure after learning of similar cases	Decrease time from exposure to follow-up
Measurement bias	Information is gathered in a way that distorts it.	Miscalibrated scale consistently overstates weights of subjects	Use standardized method of data collection
Procedure bias	Subjects in different groups are not treated the same.	Patients in treatment group spend more time in highly specialized hospital units	Blinding and use of placebo reduce influence of participants and researchers on procedures and interpretation of outcomes as neither are aware of group allocation
Observer-expectancy bias	Researcher's belief in the efficacy of a treatment changes the outcome of that treatment (aka Pygmalion effect; self-fulfilling prophecy).	If observer expects treatment group to show signs of recovery, then he is more likely to document positive outcomes	
Interpreting results			
Confounding bias	When a factor is related to both the exposure and outcome, but not on the causal pathway → factor distorts or confuses effect of exposure on outcome.	Pulmonary disease is more common in coal workers than the general population; however, people who work in coal mines also smoke more frequently than the general population	Multiple/repeated studies. Crossover studies (subjects act as their own controls). Matching (patients with similar characteristics in both treatment and control groups)
Lead-time bias	Early detection is confused with ↑ survival.	Early detection makes it seem as though survival has increased, but the natural history of the disease has not changed	Measure "back-end" survival (adjust survival according to the severity of disease at the time of diagnosis)

Statistical distribution

Measures of central tendency	Mean = (sum of values)/(total number of values).	Most affected by outliers (extreme values).
	Median = middle value of a list of data sorted from least to greatest.	If there is an even number of values, the median will be the average of the middle two values.
	Mode = most common value.	Least affected by outliers.
Measures of dispersion	Standard deviation = how much variability exists from the mean in a set of values.	σ = SD; n = sample size.
	Standard error of the mean = an estimate of how much variability exists between the sample mean and the true population mean.	SEM = $\sigma/\sqrt{n}$. SEM ↓ as n ↑.
Normal distribution	Gaussian, also called bell-shaped. Mean = median = mode.	

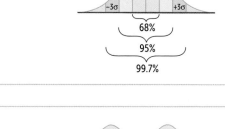

Nonnormal distributions

Bimodal	Suggests two different populations (e.g., metabolic polymorphism such as fast vs. slow acetylators; age at onset of Hodgkin lymphoma; suicide rate by age).	
Positive skew	Typically, mean > median > mode. Asymmetry with longer tail on right.	
Negative skew	Typically, mean < median < mode. Asymmetry with longer tail on left.	

Statistical hypotheses

Null (H_0)	Hypothesis of no difference or relationship (e.g., there is no association between the disease and the risk factor in the population).	
Alternative (H_1)	Hypothesis of some difference or relationship (e.g., there is some association between the disease and the risk factor in the population).	

	Reality	
	H_1	H_0
Study results — H_1	Power (1 − β)	α Type I error
Study results — H_0	β Type II error	Correct

Outcomes of statistical hypothesis testing

Correct result	Stating that there is an effect or difference when one exists (null hypothesis rejected in favor of alternative hypothesis). Stating that there is not an effect or difference when none exists (null hypothesis not rejected).	
Incorrect result		
Type I error (α)	Stating that there is an effect or difference when none exists (null hypothesis incorrectly rejected in favor of alternative hypothesis). α is the probability of making a type I error. p is judged against a preset α level of significance (usually $< .05$). If $p < 0.05$, then there is less than a 5% chance that the data will show something that is not really there.	Also known as false-positive error. α = you saw a difference that did not exist (e.g., convicting an innocent man).
Type II error (β)	Stating that there is not an effect or difference when one exists (null hypothesis is not rejected when it is in fact false). β is the probability of making a type II error. β is related to statistical power $(1 - \beta)$, which is the probability of rejecting the null hypothesis when it is false. ↑ power and ↓ β by: ▪ ↑ sample size ▪ ↑ expected effect size ▪ ↑ precision of measurement	Also known as false-negative error. β = you were blind to the truth (e.g., setting a guilty man free). If you ↑ sample size, you ↑ power. There is **power in numbers**.
Confidence interval	Range of values in which a specified probability of the means of repeated samples would be expected to fall. CI = mean ± Z(SEM). The 95% CI (corresponding to $p = .05$) is often used. For the 95% CI, Z = 1.96. For the 99% CI, Z = 2.58.	If the 95% CI for a mean difference between 2 variables includes 0, then there is no significant difference and H_0 is not rejected. If the 95% CI for odds ratio or relative risk includes 1, H_0 is not rejected. If the CIs between 2 groups do not overlap → statistically significant difference exists. If the CIs between 2 groups overlap → usually no significant difference exists.

Common statistical tests

t-test	Checks differences between **means** of **2** groups.	Tea is **meant** for **2**. Example: comparing the mean blood pressure between men and women.
ANOVA	Checks differences between means of **3** or more groups.	**3** words: **AN**alysis **O**f **VA**riance. Example: comparing the mean blood pressure between members of 3 different ethnic groups.
Chi-square (χ^2)	Checks differences between 2 or more percentages or proportions of **categorical** outcomes (not mean values).	Pronounce **Chi-tegorical**. Example: comparing the percentage of members of 3 different ethnic groups who have essential hypertension.

Pearson correlation coefficient (*r*)	*r* is always between −1 and +1. The closer the absolute value of *r* is to 1, the stronger the linear correlation between the 2 variables. Positive *r* value → positive correlation (as one variable ↑, the other variable ↑). Negative *r* value → negative correlation (as one variable ↑, the other variable ↓). Coefficient of determination = r^2 (value that is usually reported).

Disease prevention

Primary	Prevent disease occurrence (e.g., HPV vaccination)	PST: Prevent
Secondary	Screening early for disease (e.g., Pap smear)	Screen Treat
Tertiary	Treatment to reduce disability from disease (e.g., chemotherapy)	Quaternary—identifying patients at risk of unnecessary treatment, protecting from the harm of new interventions

Medicare and Medicaid	Medicare and Medicaid—federal programs that originated from amendments to the Social Security Act. Medicare is available to patients ≥ 65 years old, < 65 with certain disabilities, and those with end-stage renal disease. Medicaid is joint federal and state health assistance for people with very low income.	Medicar**E** is for **E**lderly. Medicai**D** is for **D**estitute. The 4 parts of Medicare: ▪ Part **A**: Hospital insurance ▪ Part **B**: Basic medical bills (e.g., doctor's fees, diagnostic testing) ▪ Part **C**: (Parts **A**+**B**) delivered by approved private companies ▪ Part **D**: Prescription drugs

▸ BEHAVIORAL SCIENCE—ETHICS

Core ethical principles

Autonomy	Obligation to respect patients as individuals (truth-telling, confidentiality), to create conditions necessary for autonomous choice (informed consent), and to honor their preference in accepting or not accepting medical care.
Beneficence	Physicians have a special ethical (fiduciary) duty to act in the patient's best interest. May conflict with autonomy (an informed patient has the right to decide) or what is best for society (traditionally patient interest supersedes).
Nonmaleficence	"Do no harm." Must be balanced against beneficence; if the benefits outweigh the risks, a patient may make an informed decision to proceed (most surgeries and medications fall into this category).
Justice	To treat persons fairly and equitably. This does not always imply equally (e.g., triage).

Informed consent	A process (not just a document/signature) that requires: ■ Disclosure: discussion of pertinent information ■ Understanding: ability to comprehend ■ Capacity: ability to reason and make one's own decisions (distinct from competence, a legal determination) ■ Voluntariness: freedom from coercion and manipulation Patients must have an intelligent understanding of their diagnosis and the risks/benefits of proposed treatment and alternative options, including no treatment. Patient must be informed that he or she can revoke written consent at any time, even orally.	Exceptions to informed consent: ■ Patient lacks decision-making capacity or is legally incompetent ■ Implied consent in an emergency ■ Therapeutic privilege—withholding information when disclosure would severely harm the patient or undermine informed decision-making capacity ■ Waiver—patient explicitly waives the right of informed consent
Consent for minors	A minor is generally any person < 18 years old. Parental consent laws in relation to health care vary by state. In general, parental consent should be obtained unless emergent treatment is required (e.g., blood transfusion) even if it opposes parental religious/cultural beliefs, or if a minor is legally emancipated (e.g., is married, is self supporting, or is in the military).	Situations in which parental consent is usually not required: ■ **Sex** (contraception, STIs, pregnancy) ■ **Drugs** (addiction) ■ **Rock and roll** (emergency/trauma) Physicians should always encourage healthy minor-guardian communication.

Decision-making capacity	Physician must determine whether the patient is psychologically and legally capable of making a particular health care decision. Components: ▪ Patient is ≥ 18 years old or otherwise legally emancipated ▪ Patient makes and communicates a choice ▪ Patient is informed (knows and understands) ▪ Decision remains stable over time ▪ Decision is consistent with patient's values and goals, not clouded by a mood disorder ▪ Decision is not a result of altered mental status (delusions, delirium, hallucinations)

Advance directives	Instructions given by a patient in anticipation of the need for a medical decision. Details vary per state law.
Oral advance directive	Incapacitated patient's prior oral statements commonly used as guide. Problems arise from variance in interpretation. If patient was informed, directive was specific, patient made a choice, and decision was repeated over time to multiple people, then the oral directive is more valid.
Living will (written advance directive)	Describes treatments the patient wishes to receive or not receive if he/she loses decision-making capacity. Usually, patient directs physician to withhold or withdraw life-sustaining treatment if he/she develops a terminal disease or enters a persistent vegetative state.
Medical power of attorney	Patient designates an agent to make medical decisions in the event that he/she loses decision-making capacity. Patient may also specify decisions in clinical situations. Can be revoked anytime patient wishes (regardless of competence). More flexible than a living will.

Surrogate decision-maker	If a patient loses decision-making capacity and has not prepared an advance directive, individuals (surrogates) who know the patient must determine what the patient would have done. Priority of surrogates: spouse > adult children > parents > adult siblings > other relatives.

Confidentiality	Confidentiality respects patient privacy and autonomy. If patient is not present or is incapacitated, disclosing information to family and friends should be guided by professional judgment of patient's best interest. The patient may voluntarily waive the right to confidentiality (e.g., insurance company request). General principles for exceptions to confidentiality: ▪ Potential physical harm to others is serious and imminent ▪ Likelihood of harm to self is great ▪ No alternative means exists to warn or to protect those at risk ▪ Physicians can take steps to prevent harm Examples of exceptions to patient confidentiality (many are state-specific) include: ▪ Reportable diseases (e.g., STIs, TB, hepatitis, food poisoning)—physicians may have a duty to warn public officials, who will then notify people at risk ▪ The Tarasoff decision—California Supreme Court decision requiring physician to directly inform and protect potential victim from harm ▪ Child and/or elder abuse ▪ Impaired automobile drivers (e.g., epileptics) ▪ Suicidal/homicidal patients

Ethical situations

SITUATION	APPROPRIATE RESPONSE
Patient is not adherent.	Attempt to identify the reason for nonadherence and determine his/her willingness to change; do not coerce the patient into adhering or refer him/her to another physician.
Patient desires an unnecessary procedure.	Attempt to understand why the patient wants the procedure and address underlying concerns. Do not refuse to see the patient or refer him/her to another physician. Avoid performing unnecessary procedures.
Patient has difficulty taking medications.	Provide written instructions; attempt to simplify treatment regimens; use teach-back method (ask patient to repeat medication regimen back to physician) to ensure patient comprehension.
Family members ask for information about patient's prognosis.	Avoid discussing issues with relatives without the patient's permission.
A patient's family member asks you not to disclose the results of a test if the prognosis is poor because the patient will be "unable to handle it."	Attempt to identify why the family member believes such information would be detrimental to the patient's condition. Explain that as long as the patient has decision-making capacity and does not indicate otherwise, communication of information concerning his/her care will not be withheld.
A child wishes to know more about his/her illness.	Ask what the parents have told the child about his/her illness. Parents of a child decide what information can be relayed about the illness.
A 17-year-old girl is pregnant and requests an abortion.	Many states require parental notification or consent for minors for an abortion. Unless there are specific medical risks associated with pregnancy, a physician should not attempt to sway the decision of the patient to have an elective abortion (regardless of maternal age or fetal condition).
A 15-year-old girl is pregnant and wants to keep the child. Her parents want you to tell her to give the child up for adoption.	The patient retains the right to make decisions regarding her child, even if her parents disagree. Provide information to the teenager about the practical issues of caring for a baby. Discuss the options, if requested. Encourage discussion between the teenager and her parents to reach the best decision.
A terminally ill patient requests physician assistance in ending his/her own life.	In the overwhelming majority of states, refuse involvement in any form of physician-assisted suicide. Physicians may, however, prescribe medically appropriate analgesics that coincidentally shorten the patient's life.
Patient is suicidal.	Assess the seriousness of the threat. If it is serious, suggest that the patient remain in the hospital voluntarily; patient can be hospitalized involuntarily if he/she refuses.
Patient states that he/she finds you attractive.	Ask direct, closed-ended questions and use a chaperone if necessary. Romantic relationships with patients are never appropriate. Never say, "There can be no relationship while you are a patient," because this implies that a relationship may be possible if the individual is no longer a patient.
A woman who had a mastectomy says she now feels "ugly."	Find out why the patient feels this way. Do not offer falsely reassuring statements (e.g., "You still look good").
Patient is angry about the amount of time he/she spent in the waiting room.	Acknowledge the patient's anger, but do not take a patient's anger personally. Apologize for any inconvenience. Stay away from efforts to explain the delay.
Patient is upset with the way he/she was treated by another doctor.	Suggest that the patient speak directly to that physician regarding his/her concerns. If the problem is with a member of the office staff, tell the patient you will speak to that person.
An invasive test is performed on the wrong patient.	Regardless of the outcome, a physician is ethically obligated to inform a patient that a mistake has been made.
A patient requires a treatment not covered by his/her insurance.	Never limit or deny care because of the expense in time or money. Discuss all treatment options with patients, even if some are not covered by their insurance companies.

Apgar score	Assessment of newborn vital signs following labor via a 10-point scale evaluated at 1 minute and 5 minutes. **Apgar** score is based on **A**ppearance, **P**ulse, **G**rimace, **A**ctivity, and **R**espiration (≥ 7 = good; 4–6 = assist and stimulate; < 4 = resuscitate). If Apgar score remains < 4 at later time points, there is ↑ risk that the child will develop long-term neurologic damage.

Low birth weight	Defined as < 2500 g. Caused by prematurity or intrauterine growth restriction (IUGR). Associated with ↑ risk of sudden infant death syndrome (SIDS) and with ↑ overall mortality. Other problems include impaired thermoregulation and immune function, hypoglycemia, polycythemia, and impaired neurocognitive/emotional development. Complications include infections, respiratory distress syndrome, necrotizing enterocolitis, intraventricular hemorrhage, and persistent fetal circulation.

Early developmental milestones

Milestone dates are ranges that have been approximated and vary by source. Children not meeting milestones may need assessment for potential developmental delay.

AGE	MOTOR	SOCIAL	VERBAL/COGNITIVE
Infant	**Parents**	**Start**	**Observing**
0–12 mo	Primitive reflexes disappear—Moro (by 3 mo), rooting (by 4 mo), palmar (by 6 mo), Babinski (by 12 mo) Posture—lifts head up prone (by 1 mo), rolls and sits (by 6 mo), crawls (by 8 mo), stands (by 10 mo), walks (by 12–18 mo) Picks—passes toys hand to hand (by 6 mo), Pincer grasp (by 10 mo) Points to objects (by 12 mo)	Social smile (by 2 mo) Stranger anxiety (by 6 mo) Separation anxiety (by 9 mo)	Orients—first to voice (by 4 mo), then to name and gestures (by 9 mo) Object permanence (by 9 mo) Oratory—says "mama" and "dada" (by 10 mo)
Toddler	**Child**	**Rearing**	**Working**
12–36 mo	Cruises, takes first steps (by 12 mo) Climbs stairs (by 18 mo) Cubes stacked—number = age (yr) × 3 Cultured—feeds self with fork and spoon (by 20 mo) Kicks ball (by 24 mo)	Recreation—parallel play (by 24–36 mo) Rapprochement—moves away from and returns to mother (by 24 mo) Realization—core gender identity formed (by 36 mo)	Words—200 words by age 2 (2 zeros), 2-word sentences
Preschool	**Don't**	**Forget, they're still**	**Learning!**
3–5 yr	Drive—tricycle (3 wheels at 3 yr) Drawings—copies line or circle, stick figure (by 4 yr) Dexterity—hops on one foot (by 4 yr), uses buttons or zippers, grooms self (by 5 yr)	Freedom—comfortably spends part of day away from mother (by 3 yr) Friends—cooperative play, has imaginary friends (by 4 yr)	Language—1000 words by age 3 (3 zeros), uses complete sentences and prepositions (by 4 yr) Legends—can tell detailed stories (by 4 yr)

Changes in the elderly

Sexual changes:
- Men—slower erection/ejaculation, longer refractory period
- Women—vaginal shortening, thinning, and dryness

Sleep patterns: ↓ REM and slow-wave sleep; ↑ sleep onset latency and ↑ early awakenings

↑ suicide rate

↓ vision, hearing, immune response, bladder control

↓ renal, pulmonary, GI function

↓ muscle mass, ↑ fat

Sexual interest does not decrease.
Intelligence does not decrease.

Presbycusis—sensorineural hearing loss (often of higher frequencies) due to destruction of hair cells at the cochlear base (preserved low-frequency hearing at apex).

Common causes of death (U.S.) by age

	<1 YR	1–14 YR	15–34 YR	35–44 YR	45–64 YR	65+ YR
#1	Congenital malformations	Unintentional injury	Unintentional injury	Unintentional injury	Cancer	Heart disease
#2	Preterm birth	Cancer	Suicide	Cancer	Heart disease	Cancer
#3	SIDS	Congenital malformations	Homicide	Heart disease	Unintentional injury	Chronic respiratory disease

Biochemistry

"Biochemistry is the study of carbon compounds that crawl."
—Mike Adams

"We think we have found the basic mechanism by which life comes from life."
—Francis H. C. Crick

This high-yield material includes molecular biology, genetics, cell biology, and principles of metabolism (especially vitamins, cofactors, minerals, and single-enzyme-deficiency diseases). When studying metabolic pathways, emphasize important regulatory steps and enzyme deficiencies that result in disease, as well as reactions targeted by pharmacologic interventions. For example, understanding the defect in Lesch-Nyhan syndrome and its clinical consequences is higher yield than memorizing every intermediate in the purine salvage pathway. Do not spend time on hard-core organic chemistry, mechanisms, or physical chemistry. Detailed chemical structures are infrequently tested; however, many structures have been included here to help students learn reactions and the important enzymes involved. Familiarity with the biochemical techniques that have medical relevance—such as ELISA, immunoelectrophoresis, Southern blotting, and PCR—is useful. Review the related biochemistry when studying pharmacology or genetic diseases as a way to reinforce and integrate the material.

▶ BIOCHEMISTRY—MOLECULAR

Chromatin structure

DNA double-helix

H1 histone (linker)

DNA

Nucleosome (H2A, H2B, H3, H4) ×2

Supercoiled structure

Metaphase chromosome

DNA exists in the condensed, chromatin form in order to fit into the nucleus. Negatively charged DNA loops twice around positively charged histone octamer to form nucleosome **"beads on a string."** Histones are rich in the amino acids lysine and arginine. H1 binds to the nucleosome and to "linker DNA," thereby stabilizing the chromatin fiber.

In mitosis, DNA condenses to form chromosomes. DNA and histone synthesis occur during S phase.

Heterochromatin	Condensed, appears darker on EM. Transcriptionally inactive, sterically inaccessible.	HeteroChromatin = Highly Condensed. Barr bodies (inactive X chromosomes) are heterochromatin.
Euchromatin	Less condensed, appears lighter on EM. Transcriptionally active, sterically accessible.	Eu = true, "truly transcribed."
DNA methylation	Template strand cytosine and adenine are methylated in DNA replication, which allows mismatch repair enzymes to distinguish between old and new strands in prokaryotes. DNA methylation at CpG islands represses transcription.	CpG Methylation Makes DNA Mute.
Histone methylation	Usually reversibly represses DNA transcription, but can activate it in some cases depending on methylation location.	Histone Methylation Mostly Makes DNA Mute. *(gene silencing)*
Histone acetylation	Relaxes DNA coiling, allowing for transcription.	Histone Acetylation makes DNA Active.

histones = positively charged d/+ basic aa & Mg^{2+}
· linker DNA = more prone to nuclease activity

SAM (S-adenosyl methionine) = methyl donor to histones

Nucleotides

PURines (**A, G**)—2 rings.
PYrimidines (**C, T, U**)—1 ring.
Thymine has a methyl.
Deamination of cytosine makes uracil.
Uracil found in RNA; thymine in DNA.
G-C bond (3 H bonds) stronger than A-T bond
(2 H bonds). ↑ G-C content → ↑ melting
temperature of DNA.

PUR**e A**s **G**old.
CUT the **PY** (pie).
Thymine has a me**thyl**.

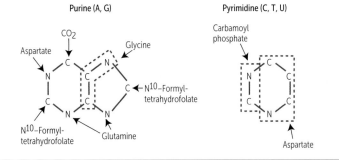

Purine (A, G)

Pyrimidine (C, T, U)

GAG—Amino acids necessary for purine
synthesis:
Glycine
Aspartate
Glutamine
NucleoSide = base + (deoxy)ribose (**S**ugar).
NucleoTide = base + (deoxy)ribose + phospha**Te**;
linked by 3′-5′ phosphodiester bond.

De novo pyrimidine and purine synthesis

Purines	Pyrimidines
	Make temporary base (orotic acid)
Start with sugar + phosphate (PRPP)	Add sugar + phosphate (PRPP)
Add base	Modify base

Ribonucleotides are synthesized first and
are converted to deoxyribonucleotides by
ribonucleotide reductase.
Carbamoyl phosphate is involved in 2 metabolic
pathways: de novo pyrimidine synthesis and the
urea cycle.

Various immunosuppressive, antineoplastic, and
antibiotic drugs function by interfering with
nucleotide synthesis:
- Leflunomide inhibits dihydroorotate
  dehydrogenase
- Mycophenolate and ribavirin inhibit IMP
  dehydrogenase
- Hydroxyurea inhibits ribonucleotide
  reductase
- 6-mercaptopurine (6-MP) and its prodrug
  azathioprine inhibit de novo purine synthesis
- 5-fluorouracil (5-FU) inhibits thymidylate
  synthase (↓ deoxythymidine monophosphate
  [dTMP])
- Methotrexate (MTX), trimethoprim (TMP),
  and pyrimethamine inhibit dihydrofolate
  reductase (↓ dTMP) in humans, bacteria, and
  protozoa, respectively

Pyrimidine base production
(requires aspartate)

Purine base production or
reuse from salvage pathway
*(de novo requires aspartate,
glycine, glutamine, and THF)*

Ribose 5-P

Glutamine + CO₂

2 ATP
2 ADP + Pᵢ + Glutamate

Carbamoyl phosphate synthetase II

PRPP (phosphoribosyl pyrophosphate) synthetase

Carbamoyl phosphate

Leflunomide ⊖

Aspartate

Orotic acid

PRPP

6-MP ⊖

Impaired in orotic aciduria

UMP

IMP ⊖ Mycophenolate, ribavirin

Hydroxyurea ⊖

UDP

AMP   GMP

Ribonucleotide reductase

dUDP   CTP

N⁵N¹⁰-methylene THF

dUMP

THF

DHF

Dihydrofolate reductase ⊖

Thymidylate synthase ⊖ 5-FU

dTMP

MTX, TMP, pyrimethamine

Purine salvage deficiencies

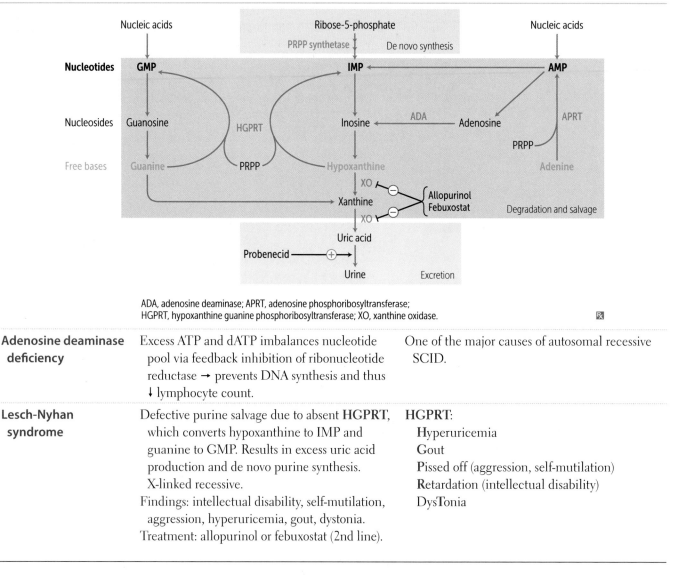

ADA, adenosine deaminase; APRT, adenosine phosphoribosyltransferase;
HGPRT, hypoxanthine guanine phosphoribosyltransferase; XO, xanthine oxidase.

Adenosine deaminase deficiency	Excess ATP and dATP imbalances nucleotide pool via feedback inhibition of ribonucleotide reductase → prevents DNA synthesis and thus ↓ lymphocyte count.	One of the major causes of autosomal recessive SCID.
Lesch-Nyhan syndrome	Defective purine salvage due to absent **HGPRT**, which converts hypoxanthine to IMP and guanine to GMP. Results in excess uric acid production and de novo purine synthesis. X-linked recessive. Findings: intellectual disability, self-mutilation, aggression, hyperuricemia, gout, dystonia. Treatment: allopurinol or febuxostat (2nd line).	**HGPRT:** **H**yperuricemia **G**out **P**issed off (aggression, self-mutilation) **R**etardation (intellectual disability) Dys**T**onia

Genetic code features

Unambiguous	Each codon specifies only 1 amino acid.	
Degenerate/ redundant	Most amino acids are coded by multiple codons.	Exceptions: methionine and tryptophan encoded by only 1 codon (AUG and UGG, respectively).
Commaless, nonoverlapping	Read from a fixed starting point as a continuous sequence of bases.	Exceptions: some viruses.
Universal	Genetic code is conserved throughout evolution.	Exception in humans: mitochondria.

DNA replication — Eukaryotic DNA replication is more complex than the prokaryotic process but uses many enzymes analogous to those listed below. In both prokaryotes and eukaryotes, DNA replication is semiconservative and involves both continuous and discontinuous (Okazaki fragment) synthesis.

A Origin of replication	Particular consensus sequence of base pairs in genome where DNA replication begins. May be single (prokaryotes) or multiple (eukaryotes).	
B Replication fork	Y-shaped region along DNA template where leading and lagging strands are synthesized.	
C Helicase	Unwinds DNA template at replication fork.	
D Single-stranded binding proteins	Prevent strands from reannealing.	
E DNA topoisomerases	Create a single- or double-stranded break in the helix to add or remove supercoils.	Fluoroquinolones—inhibit prokaryotic enzymes topoisomerase II (DNA gyrase) and topoisomerase IV.
F Primase	Makes an RNA primer on which DNA polymerase III can initiate replication.	
G DNA polymerase III	Prokaryotic only. Elongates leading strand by adding deoxynucleotides to the 3′ end. Elongates lagging strand until it reaches primer of preceding fragment. 3′ → 5′ exonuclease activity "proofreads" each added nucleotide.	DNA polymerase III has 5′ → 3′ synthesis and proofreads with 3′ → 5′ exonuclease.
H DNA polymerase I	Prokaryotic only. Degrades RNA primer; replaces it with DNA.	Has same functions as DNA polymerase III but also excises RNA primer with 5′ → 3′ exonuclease.
I DNA ligase	Catalyzes the formation of a phosphodiester bond within a strand of double-stranded DNA (i.e., joins Okazaki fragments).	Seals.
Telomerase	An RNA-dependent DNA polymerase that adds DNA to 3′ ends of chromosomes to avoid loss of genetic material with every duplication. Eukaryotes only.	

Mutations in DNA	Severity of damage: silent ≪ missense < nonsense < frameshift. For point (silent, missense, and nonsense) mutations: ▪ Transition—purine to purine (e.g., A to G) or pyrimidine to pyrimidine (e.g., C to T). ▪ Transversion—purine to pyrimidine (e.g., A to T) or pyrimidine to purine (e.g., C to G).	
Silent	Nucleotide substitution but codes for same (synonymous) amino acid; often base change in 3rd position of codon (tRNA wobble).	
Missense	Nucleotide substitution resulting in changed amino acid (called conservative if new amino acid is similar in chemical structure).	Sickle cell disease (substitution of glutamic acid with valine).
Nonsense	Nucleotide substitution resulting in early **stop** codon.	Stop the **nonsense**!
Frameshift	Deletion or insertion of a number of nucleotides not divisible by 3, resulting in misreading of all nucleotides downstream, usually resulting in a truncated, nonfunctional protein.	Duchenne muscular dystrophy

***Lac* operon**	Classic example of a genetic response to an environmental change. Glucose is the preferred metabolic substrate in *E. coli*, but when glucose is absent and lactose is available, the *lac* operon is activated to switch to lactose metabolism. Mechanism of shift: ▪ Low glucose → ↑ adenylyl cyclase activity → ↑ generation of cAMP from ATP → activation of catabolite activator protein (CAP) → ↑ transcription. ▪ High lactose → unbinds repressor protein from repressor/operator site → ↑ transcription.

DNA repair

Single strand

Nucleotide excision repair	Specific endonucleases release the oligonucleotides containing damaged bases; DNA polymerase and ligase fill and reseal the gap, respectively. Repairs bulky helix-distorting lesions. Occurs in G_1 phase of cell cycle.	Defective in xeroderma pigmentosum, which prevents repair of pyrimidine dimers because of ultraviolet light exposure.
Base excision repair	Base-specific glycosylase removes altered base and creates AP site (apurinic/apyrimidinic). One or more nucleotides are removed by AP-endonuclease, which cleaves the 5′ end. Lyase cleaves the 3′ end. DNA polymerase-β fills the gap and DNA ligase seals it. Occurs throughout cell cycle.	Important in repair of spontaneous/toxic deamination.
Mismatch repair	Newly synthesized strand is recognized, mismatched nucleotides are removed, and the gap is filled and resealed. Occurs predominantly in G_2 phase of cell cycle.	Defective in hereditary nonpolyposis colorectal cancer (HNPCC).

Double strand

Nonhomologous end joining	Brings together 2 ends of DNA fragments to repair double-stranded breaks. No requirement for homology. Some DNA may be lost.	Mutated in ataxia telangiectasia; Fanconi anemia.

DNA/RNA/protein synthesis direction	DNA and RNA are both synthesized 5′ → 3′. The 5′ end of the incoming nucleotide bears the triphosphate (energy source for bond). Protein synthesis is N-terminus to C-terminus.	mRNA is read 5′ to 3′. The triphosphate bond is the target of the 3′ hydroxyl attack. Drugs blocking DNA replication often have modified 3′ OH, preventing addition of the next nucleotide ("chain termination").

Start and stop codons

mRNA start codons	AUG (or rarely GUG).	AUG inAUGurates protein synthesis.
Eukaryotes	Codes for methionine, which may be removed before translation is completed.	
Prokaryotes	Codes for N-formylmethionine (fMet).	fMet stimulates neutrophil chemotaxis.
mRNA stop codons	UGA, UAA, UAG.	UGA = U Go Away. UAA = U Are Away. UAG = U Are Gone.

Functional organization of a eukaryotic gene

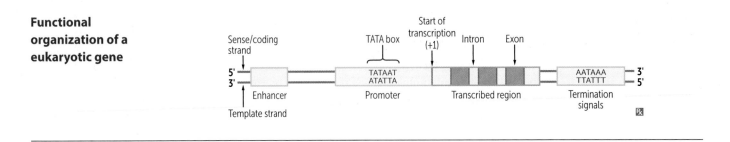

Regulation of gene expression

Promoter	Site where RNA polymerase II and multiple other transcription factors bind to DNA upstream from gene locus (AT-rich upstream sequence with TATA and CAAT boxes).	Promoter mutation commonly results in dramatic ↓ in level of gene transcription.
Enhancer	Stretch of DNA that alters gene expression by binding transcription factors.	Enhancers and silencers may be located close to, far from, or even within (in an intron) the gene whose expression it regulates.
Silencer	Site where negative regulators (repressors) bind.	

RNA polymerases

Eukaryotes	RNA polymerase I makes **r**RNA (most numerous RNA, **r**ampant). RNA polymerase II makes **m**RNA (largest RNA, **m**assive). RNA polymerase III makes **t**RNA (smallest RNA, **t**iny). No proofreading function, but can initiate chains. RNA polymerase II opens DNA at promoter site.	I, II, and III are numbered as their products are used in protein synthesis. α-amanitin, found in *Amanita phalloides* (death cap mushrooms), inhibits RNA polymerase II. Causes severe hepatotoxicity if ingested. Rifampin inhibits RNA polymerase in prokaryotes. Actinomycin D inhibits RNA polymerase in both prokaryotes and eukaryotes.
Prokaryotes	1 RNA polymerase (multisubunit complex) makes all 3 kinds of RNA.	

RNA processing (eukaryotes)

	Initial transcript is called heterogeneous nuclear RNA (hnRNA). hnRNA is then modified and becomes mRNA. The following processes occur in the nucleus following transcription: ▪ Capping of 5′ end (addition of 7-methylguanosine cap) ▪ Polyadenylation of 3′ end (≈ 200 A's) ▪ Splicing out of introns Capped, tailed, and spliced transcript is called mRNA.	mRNA is transported out of the nucleus into the cytosol, where it is translated. mRNA quality control occurs at cytoplasmic P-bodies, which contain exonucleases, decapping enzymes, and microRNAs; mRNAs may be stored in P-bodies for future translation. Poly-A polymerase does not require a template. AAUAAA = polyadenylation signal.

Splicing of pre-mRNA

❶ Primary transcript combines with small nuclear ribonucleoproteins (snRNPs) and other proteins to form spliceosome.

❷ Lariat-shaped (looped) intermediate is generated.

❸ Lariat is released to precisely remove intron and join 2 exons.

Antibodies to spliceosomal snRNPs (anti-Smith antibodies) are highly specific for SLE. Anti-U1 RNP antibodies are highly associated with mixed connective tissue disease (MCTD).

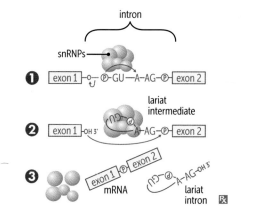

Introns vs. exons

Exons contain the actual genetic information coding for protein.

Introns are intervening noncoding segments of DNA.

Different exons are frequently combined by alternative splicing to produce a larger number of unique proteins.

Introns are intervening sequences and stay in the nucleus, whereas exons exit and are expressed.

Abnormal splicing variants are implicated in oncogenesis and many genetic disorders (e.g., β-thalassemia).

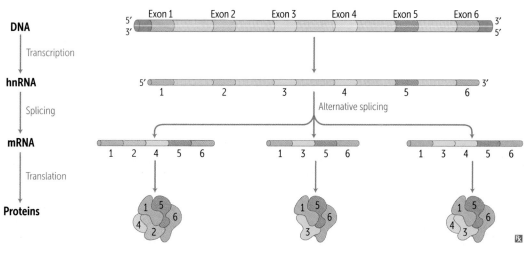

tRNA

Structure	75–90 nucleotides, 2° structure, cloverleaf form, anticodon end is opposite 3′ aminoacyl end. All tRNAs, both eukaryotic and prokaryotic, have CCA at 3′ end along with a high percentage of chemically modified bases. The amino acid is covalently bound to the 3′ end of the tRNA. **CCA** **C**an **C**arry **A**mino acids. T-arm: contains the TΨC (thymine, pseudouracil, cytosine) sequence necessary for tRNA-ribosome binding. D-arm: contains dihydrouracil residues necessary for tRNA recognition by the correct aminoacyl-tRNA synthetase. Acceptor stem: the 5′-CCA-3′ is the amino acid acceptor site.
Charging	Aminoacyl-tRNA synthetase (1 per amino acid; "matchmaker"; uses ATP) scrutinizes amino acid before and after it binds to tRNA. If incorrect, bond is hydrolyzed. The amino acid-tRNA bond has energy for formation of peptide bond. A mischarged tRNA reads usual codon but inserts wrong amino acid. Aminoacyl-tRNA synthetase and binding of charged tRNA to the codon are responsible for accuracy of amino acid selection.

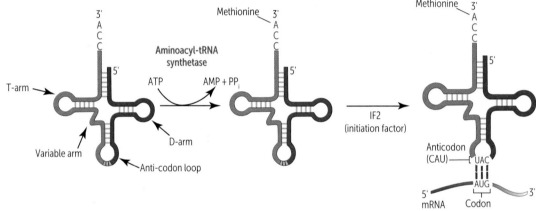

Wobble	Accurate base pairing is usually required only in the first 2 nucleotide positions of an mRNA codon, so codons differing in the 3rd "wobble" position may code for the same tRNA/amino acid (as a result of degeneracy of genetic code).

Protein synthesis

Initiation	Initiated by GTP hydrolysis; initiation factors (eukaryotic IFs) help assemble the 40S ribosomal subunit with the initiator tRNA and are released when the mRNA and the ribosomal 60S subunit assemble with the complex.	Eukaryotes: 40S + 60S → 80S (Even). PrOkaryotes: 30S + 50S → 70S (Odd). ATP—tRNA Activation (charging). GTP—tRNA Gripping and Going places (translocation).
Elongation	1. Aminoacyl-tRNA binds to A site (except for initiator methionine) 2. rRNA ("ribozyme") catalyzes peptide bond formation, transfers growing polypeptide to amino acid in A site 3. Ribosome advances 3 nucleotides toward 3′ end of mRNA, moving peptidyl tRNA to P site (translocation)	Think of "going **APE**": A site = incoming Aminoacyl-tRNA. P site = accommodates growing Peptide. E site = holds Empty tRNA as it Exits.
Termination	Stop codon is recognized by release factor, and completed polypeptide is released from ribosome.	

Posttranslational modifications

Trimming	Removal of N- or C-terminal propeptides from zymogen to generate mature protein (e.g., trypsinogen to trypsin).
Covalent alterations	Phosphorylation, glycosylation, hydroxylation, methylation, acetylation, and ubiquitination.

Chaperone protein	Intracellular protein involved in facilitating and/or maintaining protein folding. For example, in yeast, heat shock proteins (e.g., Hsp60) are expressed at high temperatures to prevent protein denaturing/misfolding.

▶ BIOCHEMISTRY—CELLULAR

Cell cycle phases	Checkpoints control transitions between phases of cell cycle. This process is regulated by cyclins, cyclin-dependent kinases (CDKs), and tumor suppressors. M phase (shortest phase of cell cycle) includes mitosis (prophase, prometaphase, metaphase, anaphase, telophase) and cytokinesis (cytoplasm splits in two). G_1 and G_0 are of variable duration.

REGULATION OF CELL CYCLE

CDKs	Constitutive and inactive.	
Cyclins	Regulatory proteins that control cell cycle events; phase specific; activate CDKs.	
Cyclin-CDK complexes	Phosphorylate other proteins to coordinate cell cycle progression; must be activated and inactivated at appropriate times for cell cycle to progress.	
Tumor suppressors	p53 and hypophosphorylated Rb normally inhibit G_1-to-S progression; mutations in these genes result in unrestrained cell division (e.g., Li-Fraumeni syndrome).	Rb, p53 modulate G_1 restriction point

CELL TYPES

Permanent	Remain in G_0, regenerate from stem cells.	Neurons, skeletal and cardiac muscle, RBCs.
Stable (quiescent)	Enter G_1 from G_0 when stimulated.	Hepatocytes, lymphocytes.
Labile	Never go to G_0, divide rapidly with a short G_1. Most affected by chemotherapy.	Bone marrow, gut epithelium, skin, hair follicles, germ cells.

Rough endoplasmic reticulum	Site of synthesis of secretory (exported) proteins and of N-linked oligosaccharide addition to many proteins. Nissl bodies (RER in neurons)—synthesize peptide neurotransmitters for secretion. Free ribosomes—unattached to any membrane; site of synthesis of cytosolic and organellar proteins.	Mucus-secreting goblet cells of the small intestine and antibody-secreting plasma cells are rich in RER.
Smooth endoplasmic reticulum	Site of steroid synthesis and detoxification of drugs and poisons. Lacks surface ribosomes.	Liver hepatocytes and steroid hormone–producing cells of the adrenal cortex and gonads are rich in SER.

Cell trafficking
Golgi is the distribution center for proteins and lipids from the ER to the vesicles and plasma membrane. Modifies N-oligosaccharides on asparagine. Adds O-oligosaccharides on serine and threonine. Adds mannose-6-phosphate to proteins for trafficking to lysosomes.

Endosomes are sorting centers for material from outside the cell or from the Golgi, sending it to lysosomes for destruction or back to the membrane/Golgi for further use.

I-cell disease (inclusion cell disease)—inherited lysosomal storage disorder; defect in N-acetylglucosaminyl-1-phosphotransferase → failure of the Golgi to phosphorylate mannose residues (i.e., ↓ mannose-6-phosphate) on glycoproteins → proteins are secreted extracellularly rather than delivered to lysosomes. Results in coarse facial features, clouded corneas, restricted joint movement, and high plasma levels of lysosomal enzymes. Often fatal in childhood.

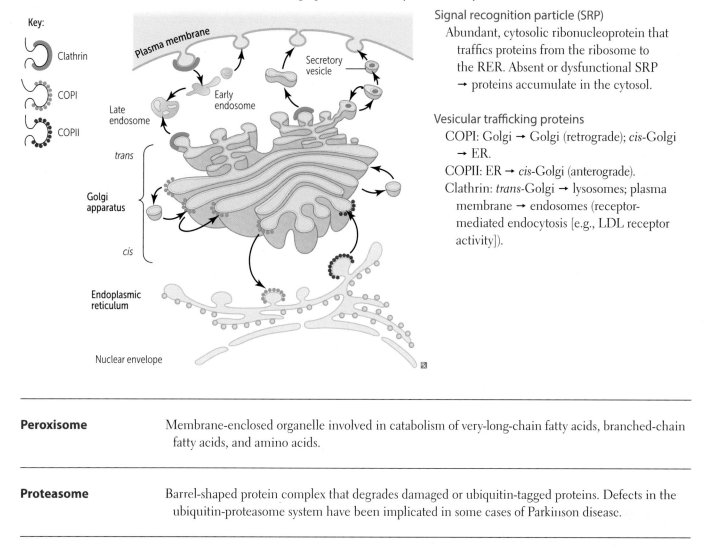

Signal recognition particle (SRP)
Abundant, cytosolic ribonucleoprotein that traffics proteins from the ribosome to the RER. Absent or dysfunctional SRP → proteins accumulate in the cytosol.

Vesicular trafficking proteins
COPI: Golgi → Golgi (retrograde); *cis*-Golgi → ER.
COPII: ER → *cis*-Golgi (anterograde).
Clathrin: *trans*-Golgi → lysosomes; plasma membrane → endosomes (receptor-mediated endocytosis [e.g., LDL receptor activity]).

Peroxisome
Membrane-enclosed organelle involved in catabolism of very-long-chain fatty acids, branched-chain fatty acids, and amino acids.

Proteasome
Barrel-shaped protein complex that degrades damaged or ubiquitin-tagged proteins. Defects in the ubiquitin-proteasome system have been implicated in some cases of Parkinson disease.

Cytoskeletal elements

A network of protein fibers within the cytoplasm that supports cell structure, cell and organelle movement, and cell division.

TYPE OF FILAMENT	PREDOMINANT FUNCTION	EXAMPLES
Microfilaments	Muscle contraction, cytokinesis	Actin.
Intermediate filaments	Maintain cell structure	Vimentin, desmin, cytokeratin, lamins, glial fibrillary acid proteins (GFAP), neurofilaments.
Microtubules	Movement, cell division	Cilia, flagella, mitotic spindle, axonal trafficking, centrioles.

Immunohistochemical stains for intermediate filaments

STAIN	CELL TYPE
Vimentin	Connective tissue
DesMin	Muscle
Cytokeratin	Epithelial cells
GFAP	NeuroGlia
Neurofilaments	Neurons

Microtubule

Positive end (+)

Heterodimer

Protofilament

Negative end (-)

Cylindrical structure composed of a helical array of polymerized heterodimers of α- and β-tubulin. Each dimer has 2 GTP bound. Incorporated into flagella, cilia, mitotic spindles. Grows slowly, collapses quickly. Also involved in slow axoplasmic transport in neurons.

Molecular motor proteins—transport cellular cargo toward opposite ends of microtubule tracks.
- Dynein—retrograde to microtubule (+ → −).
- Kinesin—anterograde to microtubule (− → +).

Drugs that act on microtubules (**M**icrotubules **G**et **C**onstructed **V**ery **P**oorly):
- **M**ebendazole (antihelminthic)
- **G**riseofulvin (antifungal)
- **C**olchicine (antigout)
- **V**incristine/**V**inblastine (anticancer)
- **P**aclitaxel (anticancer)

Cilia structure

9 + 2 arrangement of microtubule doublets (arrows in A).

Axonemal dynein—ATPase that links peripheral 9 doublets and causes bending of cilium by differential sliding of doublets.

Kartagener syndrome (1° ciliary dyskinesia)— immotile cilia due to a dynein arm defect. Results in male and female infertility due to immotile sperm and dysfunctional fallopian tube cilia, respectively; ↑ risk of ectopic pregnancy. Can cause bronchiectasis, recurrent sinusitis, and situs inversus (e.g., dextrocardia on CXR).

| **Plasma membrane composition** | Asymmetric lipid bilayer. Contains cholesterol, phospholipids, sphingolipids, glycolipids, and proteins. Fungal membranes contain ergosterol. | |

| **Sodium-potassium pump** | Na^+-K^+ ATPase is located in the plasma membrane with ATP site on cytosolic side. For each ATP consumed, $3Na^+$ go out of the cell (pump phosphorylated) and $2K^+$ come into the cell (pump dephosphorylated). | Ouabain inhibits by binding to K^+ site. Cardiac glycosides (digoxin and digitoxin) directly inhibit the Na^+-K^+ ATPase, which leads to indirect inhibition of Na^+/Ca^{2+} exchange → ↑ $[Ca^{2+}]_i$ → ↑ cardiac contractility. |

Extracellular space — $3Na^+$ — $2K^+$ — Cytosol — $3Na^+$ — ATP — ADP — P — P — $2K^+$

Collagen	Most abundant protein in the human body. Extensively modified by posttranslational modification. Organizes and strengthens extracellular matrix.	Be (So Totally) Cool, Read Books.
Type I	Most common (90%)—Bone (made by osteoblasts), Skin, Tendon, dentin, fascia, cornea, late wound repair.	Type I: bone. ↓ production in osteogenesis imperfecta type I.
Type II	Cartilage (including hyaline), vitreous body, nucleus pulposus.	Type II: cartwolage.
Type III	Reticulin—skin, blood vessels, uterus, fetal tissue, granulation tissue.	Type III: deficient in the uncommon, vascular type of Ehlers-Danlos syndrome (ThreE D).
Type IV	Basement membrane, basal lamina, lens.	Type IV: under the floor (basement membrane). Defective in Alport syndrome; targeted by autoantibodies in Goodpasture syndrome.

Collagen synthesis and structure

Inside fibroblasts

1. Synthesis (RER)	Translation of collagen α chains (preprocollagen)—usually Gly-X-Y (X and Y are proline or lysine). Glycine content best reflects collagen synthesis (collagen is ⅓ glycine).
2. Hydroxylation (RER)	Hydroxylation of specific proline and lysine residues (requires vitamin C; deficiency → scurvy).
3. Glycosylation (RER)	Glycosylation of pro-α-chain hydroxylysine residues and formation of procollagen via hydrogen and disulfide bonds (triple helix of 3 collagen α chains). Problems forming triple helix → osteogenesis imperfecta.
4. Exocytosis	Exocytosis of procollagen into extracellular space.

Outside fibroblasts

5. Proteolytic processing	Cleavage of disulfide-rich terminal regions of procollagen, transforming it into insoluble tropocollagen.
6. Cross-linking	Reinforcement of many staggered tropocollagen molecules by covalent lysine-hydroxylysine cross-linkage (by copper-containing lysyl oxidase) to make collagen fibrils. Problems with cross-linking → Ehlers-Danlos syndrome, Menkes disease.

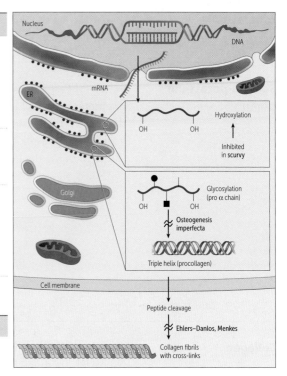

Osteogenesis imperfecta 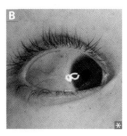	Genetic bone disorder (brittle bone disease **A**) caused by a variety of gene defects. Most common form is autosomal dominant with ↓ production of otherwise normal type I collagen. Manifestations can include:	May be confused with child abuse. 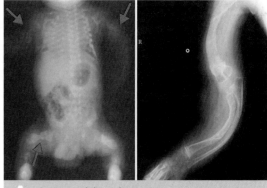

- Multiple fractures with minimal trauma; may occur during the birth process
- Blue sclerae **B** due to the translucency of the connective tissue over the choroidal veins
- Hearing loss (abnormal ossicles)
- Dental imperfections due to lack of dentin

A **Osteogenesis imperfecta.** Severe skeletal deformity and limb shortening due to multiple fractures in a child (left, arrows). On the right, note severe bone deformities of the upper extremity. ✲

Ehlers-Danlos syndrome 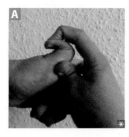	Faulty collagen synthesis causing hyperextensible skin, tendency to bleed (easy bruising), and hypermobile joints A. Multiple types. Inheritance and severity vary. Can be autosomal dominant or recessive. May be associated with joint dislocation, berry and aortic aneurysms, organ rupture.	Hypermobility type (joint instability): most common type. Classical type (joint and skin symptoms): caused by a mutation in type V collagen. Vascular type (vascular and organ rupture): deficient type III collagen.

Menkes disease

X-linked recessive connective tissue disease caused by impaired copper absorption and transport due to defective Menkes protein (ATP7A). Leads to ↓ activity of lysyl oxidase (copper is a necessary cofactor). Results in brittle, "kinky" hair, growth retardation, and hypotonia.

Elastin 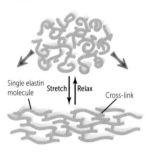 Single elastin molecule — Stretch ↕ Relax — Cross-link	Stretchy protein within skin, lungs, large arteries, elastic ligaments, vocal cords, ligamenta flava (connect vertebrae → relaxed and stretched conformations). Rich in nonhydroxylated proline, glycine, and lysine residues. Tropoelastin with fibrillin scaffolding. Cross-linking takes place extracellularly and gives elastin its elastic properties. Broken down by elastase, which is normally inhibited by α_1-antitrypsin.	Marfan syndrome—caused by a defect in fibrillin, a glycoprotein that forms a sheath around elastin. Emphysema—can be caused by α_1-antitrypsin deficiency, resulting in excess elastase activity. Wrinkles of aging are due to ↓ collagen and elastin production.

▶ BIOCHEMISTRY—LABORATORY TECHNIQUES

Polymerase chain reaction

Molecular biology laboratory procedure used to amplify a desired fragment of DNA. Useful as a diagnostic tool (e.g., neonatal HIV, herpes encephalitis).

Steps:

1. Denaturation—DNA is denatured by heating to generate 2 separate strands.
2. Annealing—during cooling, excess premade DNA primers anneal to a specific sequence on each strand to be amplified.
3. Elongation—heat-stable DNA polymerase replicates the DNA sequence following each primer.

These steps are repeated multiple times for DNA sequence amplification.

Agarose gel electrophoresis—used for size separation of PCR products (smaller molecules travel further); compared against DNA ladder.

Blotting procedures

Southern blot	A **DNA** sample is enzymatically cleaved into smaller pieces, electrophoresed on a gel, and then transferred to a filter. The filter is then soaked in a denaturant and subsequently exposed to a radiolabeled DNA probe that recognizes and anneals to its complementary strand. The resulting double-stranded, labeled piece of DNA is visualized when the filter is exposed to film.	SNoW DRoP: Southern = DNA Northern = RNA Western = Protein
Northern blot	Similar to Southern blot, except that an **RNA** sample is electrophoresed. Useful for studying mRNA levels, which are reflective of gene expression.	
Western blot	Sample protein is separated via gel electrophoresis and transferred to a filter. Labeled antibody is used to bind to relevant **protein**. Confirmatory test for HIV after ⊕ ELISA.	
Southwestern blot	Identifies **DNA-binding proteins** (e.g., transcription factors) using labeled oligonucleotide probes.	

Microarrays	Thousands of nucleic acid sequences are arranged in grids on glass or silicon. DNA or RNA probes are hybridized to the chip, and a scanner detects the relative amounts of complementary binding. Used to profile gene expression levels of thousands of genes simultaneously to study certain diseases and treatments. Able to detect single nucleotide polymorphisms (SNPs) and copy number variations (CNVs) for a variety of applications including genotyping, clinical genetic testing, forensic analysis, cancer mutations, and genetic linkage analysis.

Enzyme-linked immunosorbent assay 	Used to detect the presence of either a specific antigen or a specific antibody in a patient's blood sample. Patient's blood sample is probed with either: ▪ Direct ELISA: uses a test antibody to see if a specific antigen is present. The antibody is directly coupled to a color-generating enzyme to detect the antigen. ▪ Indirect ELISA: uses either a test antigen or antibody to see if a specific antibody or antigen, respectively, is present. A secondary antibody coupled to a color-generating enzyme is added to detect the antibody-antigen complex. Target antigen or antibody present → ⊕ color/fluorescence.	Used in many laboratories to determine whether a particular antibody (e.g., anti-HIV) is present in a patient's blood sample. Both the sensitivity and specificity of ELISA approach 100%, but both false-positive and false-negative results occur.

Karyotyping	A process in which metaphase chromosomes are stained, ordered, and numbered according to morphology, size, arm-length ratio, and banding pattern. Can be performed on a sample of blood, bone marrow, amniotic fluid, or placental tissue. Used to diagnose chromosomal imbalances (e.g., autosomal trisomies, sex chromosome disorders).
Fluorescence in situ hybridization	Fluorescent DNA or RNA probe binds to specific gene site of interest on chromosomes. Used for specific localization of genes and direct visualization of anomalies (e.g., microdeletions) at molecular level (when deletion is too small to be visualized by karyotype). Fluorescence = gene is present; no fluorescence = gene is absent/deleted.
Cloning methods	Cloning is the production of a recombinant DNA molecule that is self-perpetuating. Steps: 1. Isolate eukaryotic mRNA (post-RNA processing steps) of interest. 2. Expose mRNA to reverse transcriptase to produce cDNA (lacks introns). 3. Insert cDNA fragments into bacterial plasmids containing antibiotic resistance genes. 4. Transform recombinant plasmid into bacteria. 5. Surviving bacteria on antibiotic medium produce cloned DNA (copies of cDNA).

Gene expression modifications	Transgenic strategies in mice involve: ▪ Random insertion of gene into mouse genome ▪ Targeted insertion or deletion of gene through homologous recombination with mouse gene	Knock-out = removing a gene, taking it out. Knock-in = inserting a gene.
Cre-lox system	Can inducibly manipulate genes at specific developmental points (e.g., to study a gene whose deletion causes embryonic death).	
RNA interference	dsRNA is synthesized that is complementary to the mRNA sequence of interest. When transfected into human cells, dsRNA separates and promotes degradation of target mRNA, "knocking down" gene expression.	

▶ BIOCHEMISTRY—GENETICS

Genetic terms

TERM	DEFINITION	EXAMPLE
Codominance	Both alleles contribute to the phenotype of the heterozygote.	Blood groups A, B, AB; α_1-antitrypsin deficiency.
Variable expressivity	Phenotype varies among individuals with same genotype.	2 patients with neurofibromatosis type 1 (NF1) may have varying disease severity.
Incomplete penetrance	Not all individuals with a mutant genotype show the mutant phenotype.	BRCA1 gene mutations do not always result in breast or ovarian cancer.
Pleiotropy	One gene contributes to multiple phenotypic effects.	Untreated phenylketonuria (PKU) manifests with light skin, intellectual disability, and musty body odor.
Anticipation	Increased severity or earlier onset of disease in succeeding generations.	Trinucleotide repeat diseases (e.g., Huntington disease).
Loss of heterozygosity	If a patient inherits or develops a mutation in a tumor suppressor gene, the complementary allele must be deleted/mutated before cancer develops. This is not true of oncogenes.	Retinoblastoma and the "two-hit hypothesis."
Dominant negative mutation	Exerts a dominant effect. A heterozygote produces a nonfunctional altered protein that also prevents the normal gene product from functioning.	Mutation of a transcription factor in its allosteric site. Nonfunctioning mutant can still bind DNA, preventing wild-type transcription factor from binding.
Linkage disequilibrium	Tendency for certain alleles at 2 linked loci to occur together more or less often than expected by chance. Measured in a population, not in a family, and often varies in different populations.	
Mosaicism	Presence of genetically distinct cell lines in the same individual. Somatic mosaicism—mutation arises from mitotic errors after fertilization and propagates through multiple tissues or organs. Gonadal mosaicism—mutation only in egg or sperm cells.	**McCune-Albright syndrome**—due to mutation affecting G-protein signaling. Presents with unilateral café-au-lait spots, polyostotic fibrous dysplasia, precocious puberty, multiple endocrine abnormalities. Lethal if mutation occurs before fertilization (affecting all cells), but survivable in patients with mosaicism.
Locus heterogeneity	Mutations at different loci can produce a similar phenotype.	Albinism.
Allelic heterogeneity	Different mutations in the same locus produce the same phenotype.	β-thalassemia.
Heteroplasmy	Presence of both normal and mutated mtDNA, resulting in variable expression in mitochondrially inherited disease.	

Genetic terms (continued)

TERM	DEFINITION	EXAMPLE
Uniparental disomy	Offspring receives 2 copies of a chromosome from 1 parent and no copies from the other parent. Heterodisomy (heterozygous) indicates a meiosis I error. Isodisomy (homozygous) indicates a meiosis II error or postzygotic chromosomal duplication of one of a pair of chromosomes, and loss of the other of the original pair.	Uniparental is eUploid (correct number of chromosomes), not aneuploid. Most occurrences of UPD → normal phenotype. Consider UPD in an individual manifesting a recessive disorder when only one parent is a carrier.
Hardy-Weinberg population genetics	If a population is in Hardy-Weinberg equilibrium and if p and q are the frequencies of separate alleles, then: $p^2 + 2pq + q^2 = 1$ and $p + q = 1$, which implies that: p^2 = frequency of homozygosity for allele p q^2 = frequency of homozygosity for allele q $2pq$ = frequency of heterozygosity (carrier frequency, if an autosomal recessive disease). The frequency of an X-linked recessive disease in males = q and in females = q^2.	Hardy-Weinberg law assumptions include: ▪ No mutation occurring at the locus ▪ Natural selection is not occurring ▪ Completely random mating ▪ No net migration

	pA	qa
pA	AA $p \times p = p^2$	Aa $p \times q$
qa	Aa $p \times q$	aa $q \times q = q^2$

TERM	DEFINITION	EXAMPLE
Imprinting	At some loci, only one allele is active; the other is inactive (imprinted/inactivated by methylation). With one allele inactivated, deletion of the active allele → disease.	Both Prader-Willi and Angelman syndromes are due to mutation or deletion of genes on chromosome 15.
Prader-Willi syndrome	Maternal imprinting: gene from mom is normally silent and **P**aternal gene is deleted/mutated. Results in hyperphagia, obesity, intellectual disability, hypogonadism, and hypotonia.	25% of cases due to maternal uniparental disomy (two maternally imprinted genes are received; no paternal gene received).
AngelMan syndrome	Paternal imprinting: gene from dad is normally silent and **M**aternal gene is deleted/mutated. Results in inappropriate laughter ("happy puppet"), seizures, ataxia, and severe intellectual disability.	5% of cases due to paternal uniparental disomy (two paternally imprinted genes are received; no maternal gene received).

Modes of inheritance

Autosomal dominant	Often due to defects in structural genes. Many generations, both male and female, affected.	Often pleiotropic (multiple apparently unrelated effects) and variably expressive (different between individuals). Family history crucial to diagnosis. With one affected (heterozygous) parent, on average, ½ of children affected.
Autosomal recessive	Often due to enzyme deficiencies. Usually seen in only 1 generation.	Commonly more severe than dominant disorders; patients often present in childhood. ↑ risk in consanguineous families. With 2 carrier (heterozygous) parents, on average: ¼ of children will be affected (homozygous), ½ of children will be carriers, and ¼ of children will be neither affected nor carriers.
X-linked recessive	Sons of heterozygous mothers have a 50% chance of being affected. No male-to-male transmission. Skips generations.	Commonly more severe in males. Females usually must be homozygous to be affected.
X-linked dominant	Transmitted through both parents. Mothers transmit to 50% of daughters and sons; fathers transmit to all daughters but no sons.	**Hypophosphatemic rickets**—formerly known as vitamin D–resistant rickets. Inherited disorder resulting in ↑ phosphate wasting at proximal tubule. Results in rickets-like presentation.
Mitochondrial inheritance	Transmitted only through the mother. All offspring of affected females may show signs of disease.	Variable expression in a population or even within a family due to heteroplasmy. **Mitochondrial myopathies**—rare disorders; often present with myopathy, lactic acidosis and CNS disease. 2° to failure in oxidative phosphorylation. Muscle biopsy often shows "ragged red fibers."

☐ = unaffected male; ■ = affected male; ○ = unaffected female; ● = affected female.

Autosomal dominant diseases

Autosomal dominant polycystic kidney disease (ADPKD)	Bilateral, massive enlargement of kidneys due to multiple large cysts. 85% of cases are due to mutation in *PKD1* (chromosome 16; 16 letters in "polycystic kidney"); remainder due to mutation in *PKD2* (chromosome 4).
Familial adenomatous polyposis	Colon becomes covered with adenomatous polyps after puberty. Progresses to colon cancer unless colon is resected. Mutations on chromosome 5q (*APC* gene); 5 letters in "polyp."
Familial hypercholesterolemia	Elevated LDL due to defective or absent LDL receptor. Leads to severe atherosclerotic disease early in life, corneal arcus, tendon xanthomas (classically in the Achilles tendon).
Hereditary hemorrhagic telangiectasia	Inherited disorder of blood vessels. Findings: branching skin lesions (telangiectasias), recurrent epistaxis, skin discolorations, arteriovenous malformations (AVMs), GI bleeding, hematuria. Also known as Osler-Weber-Rendu syndrome.
Hereditary spherocytosis	Spheroid erythrocytes due to spectrin or ankyrin defect; hemolytic anemia; ↑ MCHC, ↑ RDW. Treatment: splenectomy.
Huntington disease	Findings: depression, progressive dementia, choreiform movements, and caudate atrophy. ↑ dopamine, ↓ GABA, ↓ ACh in the brain. Gene on chromosome 4; trinucleotide repeat disorder: $(CAG)_n$. Demonstrates anticipation: ↑ repeats → ↓ age of onset. "**Hunting 4** food."
Li-Fraumeni syndrome	Abnormalities in *TP53* → multiple malignancies at an early age. Also known as SBLA cancer syndrome (sarcoma, breast, leukemia, adrenal gland).
Marfan syndrome	*FBN1* gene mutation on chromosome 15 → defective fibrin (scaffold for elastin) → connective tissue disorder affecting skeleton, heart, and eyes. Findings: tall with long extremities, pectus excavatum, hypermobile joints, and long, tapering fingers and toes (arachnodactyly); cystic medial necrosis of aorta → aortic incompetence and dissecting aortic aneurysms; floppy mitral valve. Subluxation of lenses, typically upward and temporally.
Multiple endocrine neoplasias (MEN)	Several distinct syndromes (1, 2A, 2B) characterized by familial tumors of endocrine glands, including those of the pancreas, parathyroid, pituitary, thyroid, and adrenal medulla. MEN 1 is associated with *MEN1* gene, MEN 2A and 2B are associated with *RET* gene.
Neurofibromatosis type 1 (von Recklinghausen disease)	Neurocutaneous disorder characterized by café-au-lait spots, cutaneous neurofibromas, optic gliomas, pheochromocytomas, Lisch nodules (pigmented iris hamartomas). Autosomal dominant, 100% penetrance, variable expression. Caused by mutations in the *NF1* gene on chromosome 17; 17 letters in "von Recklinghausen."
Neurofibromatosis type 2	Findings: bilateral acoustic schwannomas, juvenile cataracts, meningiomas, and ependymomas. *NF2* gene on chromosome 22; type 2 = 22.
Tuberous sclerosis	Neurocutaneous disorder with multi-organ system involvement, characterized by numerous benign hamartomas. Incomplete penetrance, variable expression.
von Hippel-Lindau disease	Disorder characterized by development of numerous tumors, both benign and malignant. Associated with deletion of *VHL* gene (tumor suppressor) on chromosome 3 (3p). Von Hippel-Lindau = 3 words for chromosome 3.

Autosomal recessive diseases	Albinism, autosomal recessive polycystic kidney disease (ARPKD), cystic fibrosis, glycogen storage diseases, hemochromatosis, Kartagener syndrome, mucopolysaccharidoses (except Hunter syndrome), phenylketonuria, sickle cell anemia, sphingolipidoses (except Fabry disease), thalassemias, Wilson disease.

Cystic fibrosis

GENETICS	Autosomal recessive; defect in *CFTR* gene on chromosome 7; commonly a deletion of Phe508. Most common lethal genetic disease in Caucasian population.
PATHOPHYSIOLOGY	*CFTR* encodes an ATP-gated Cl^- channel that secretes Cl^- in lungs and GI tract, and reabsorbs Cl^- in sweat glands. Most common mutation → misfolded protein → protein retained in RER and not transported to cell membrane, causing ↓ Cl^- (and H_2O) secretion; ↑ intracellular Cl^- results in compensatory ↑ Na^+ reabsorption via epithelial Na^+ channels → ↑ H_2O reabsorption → abnormally thick mucus secreted into lungs and GI tract. ↑ Na^+ reabsorption also causes more negative transepithelial potential difference.
DIAGNOSIS	↑ Cl^- concentration (> 60 mEq/L) in sweat is diagnostic. Can present with contraction alkalosis and hypokalemia (ECF effects analogous to a patient taking a loop diuretic) because of ECF H_2O/Na^+ losses and concomitant renal K^+/H^+ wasting. ↑ immunoreactive trypsinogen (newborn screening).
COMPLICATIONS	Recurrent pulmonary infections (e.g., *Pseudomonas*), chronic bronchitis and bronchiectasis → reticulonodular pattern on CXR, pancreatic insufficiency, malabsorption with steatorrhea, and nasal polyps. Meconium ileus in newborns. Infertility in males (absence of vas deferens), and subfertility in females (amenorrhea, abnormally thick cervical mucus). Fat-soluble vitamin deficiencies (A, D, E, K).
TREATMENT	N-acetylcysteine to loosen mucus plugs (cleaves disulfide bonds within mucus glycoproteins), dornase alfa (DNAse) to clear leukocytic debris.

X-linked recessive disorders	Bruton agammaglobulinemia, Wiskott-Aldrich syndrome, Fabry disease, G6PD deficiency, Ocular albinism, Lesch-Nyhan syndrome, Duchenne (and Becker) muscular dystrophy, Hunter Syndrome, Hemophilia A and B, Ornithine transcarbamylase deficiency. Female carriers can be variably affected depending on the percentage inactivation of the X chromosome carrying the mutant vs. normal gene.	Be Wise, Fool's **GOLD** Heeds Silly **HO**pe.

Muscular dystrophies

Duchenne	X-linked disorder typically due to **frameshift** (deletions, duplications, or nonsense) mutations → truncated dystrophin protein → inhibited muscle regeneration. Weakness begins in pelvic girdle muscles and progresses superiorly. Pseudohypertrophy of calf muscles due to fibrofatty replacement of muscle A. Gower maneuver—patients use upper extremities to help them stand up. Waddling gait. Onset before 5 years of age. Dilated cardiomyopathy is common cause of death.	Duchenne = deleted dystrophin. Dystrophin gene (*DMD*) is the largest protein-coding human gene → ↑ chance of spontaneous mutation. Dystrophin helps anchor muscle fibers, primarily in skeletal and cardiac muscle. It connects the intracellular cytoskeleton (actin) to the transmembrane proteins α- and β-dystroglycan, which are connected to the extracellular matrix (ECM). Loss of dystrophin results in myonecrosis. ↑ CPK and aldolase are seen; Western blot and muscle biopsy confirm diagnosis.
Becker	X-linked disorder typically due to **non-frameshift** insertions in dystrophin gene (partially functional instead of truncated). Less severe than Duchenne. Onset in adolescence or early adulthood.	Deletions can cause both Duchenne and Becker.
Myotonic type 1	Autosomal dominant. CTG trinucleotide repeat expansion in the *DMPK* gene → abnormal expression of myotonin protein kinase → myotonia, muscle wasting, cataracts, testicular atrophy, frontal balding, arrhythmia.	**My** Tonia, **My** Testicles (testicular atrophy), **My** Toupee (frontal balding), **My** Ticker (arrhythmia).

Fragile X syndrome	X-linked defect affecting the methylation and expression of the *FMR1* gene. The 2nd most common cause of genetic intellectual disability (after Down syndrome). Findings: post-pubertal macroorchidism (enlarged testes), long face with a large jaw, large everted ears, autism, mitral valve prolapse.	Trinucleotide repeat disorder $(CGG)_n$. Fragile **X** = e**X**tra large testes, jaw, ears.

Trinucleotide repeat expansion diseases	Huntington disease, myotonic dystrophy, Friedreich ataxia, fragile **X** syndrome. Fragile X syndrome = $(CGG)_n$. Friedreich ataxia = $(GAA)_n$. Huntington disease = $(CAG)_n$. Myotonic dystrophy = $(CTG)_n$.	**Try** (trinucleotide) **hunting** for **my fried eggs** (X). **X**-Girlfriend's **F**irst **A**id **H**elped **A**ce **M**y **T**est. May show genetic anticipation (disease severity ↑ and age of onset ↓ in successive generations).

Autosomal trisomies

Down syndrome (trisomy 21), 1:700	Findings: intellectual disability, flat facies, prominent epicanthal folds, single palmar crease, gap between 1st 2 toes, duodenal atresia, Hirschsprung disease, congenital heart disease (atrial septal defect [ASD]), Brushfield spots. Associated with early-onset Alzheimer disease (chromosome 21 codes for amyloid precursor protein) and ↑ risk of ALL and AML. 95% of cases due to meiotic nondisjunction (associated with advanced maternal age; from 1:1500 in women < 20 to 1:25 in women > 45 years old). 4% of cases due to Robertsonian translocation. 1% of cases due to mosaicism (no maternal association; post-fertilization mitotic error).	Drinking age (21). Most common viable chromosomal disorder and most common cause of genetic intellectual disability. First-trimester ultrasound commonly shows ↑ nuchal translucency and hypoplastic nasal bone; serum PAPP-A is ↓, free β-hCG is ↑. Second-trimester quad screen shows ↓ α-fetoprotein, ↑ β-hCG, ↓ estriol, ↑ inhibin A.
Edwards syndrome (trisomy 18), 1:8000	Findings: severe intellectual disability, rocker-bottom feet, micrognathia (small jaw), low-set Ears, clenched hands with overlapping fingers, prominent occiput, congenital heart disease. Death usually occurs within 1 year of birth.	Election age (18). 2nd most common trisomy resulting in live birth (most common is Down syndrome). PAPP-A and free β-hCG are ↓ in first trimester. Quad screen shows ↓ α-fetoprotein, ↓ β-hCG, ↓ estriol, ↓ or normal inhibin A.
Patau syndrome (trisomy 13), 1:15,000	Findings: severe intellectual disability, rocker-bottom feet, microphthalmia, microcephaly, cleft liP/Palate, holoProsencephaly, Polydactyly, congenital heart disease, cutis aplasia. Death usually occurs within 1 year of birth.	Puberty (13). First-trimester pregnancy screen shows ↓ free β-hCG, ↓ PAPP-A, and ↑ nuchal translucency.

Meiotic nondisjunction

Chromosomal disorders	CHROMOSOME	SELECTED EXAMPLES
	3	von Hippel-Lindau disease, renal cell carcinoma
	4	ADPKD with PKD2 defect, Huntington disease
	5	Cri-du-chat syndrome, familial adenomatous polyposis
	7	Williams syndrome, cystic fibrosis
	9	Friedreich ataxia
	11	Wilms tumor
	13	Patau syndrome, Wilson disease
	15	Prader-Willi syndrome, Angelman syndrome
	16	ADPKD with PKD1 defect
	17	Neurofibromatosis type 1
	18	Edwards syndrome
	21	Down syndrome
	22	Neurofibromatosis type 2, DiGeorge syndrome (22q11)
	X	Fragile X syndrome, X-linked agammaglobulinemia, Klinefelter syndrome (XXY)

Robertsonian translocation	Chromosomal translocation that commonly involves chromosome pairs 13, 14, 15, 21, and 22. One of the most common types of translocation. Occurs when the long arms of 2 acrocentric chromosomes (chromosomes with centromeres near their ends) fuse at the centromere and the 2 short arms are lost. Balanced translocations normally do not cause any abnormal phenotype. Unbalanced translocations can result in miscarriage, stillbirth, and chromosomal imbalance (e.g., Down syndrome, Patau syndrome).	
Cri-du-chat syndrome	Congenital microdeletion of short arm of chromosome 5 (46,XX or XY, 5p−). Findings: microcephaly, moderate to severe intellectual disability, high-pitched crying/**mewing**, epicanthal folds, cardiac abnormalities (VSD).	*Cri du chat* = cry of the **cat**.
Williams syndrome	Congenital microdeletion of long arm of chromosome 7 (deleted region includes elastin gene). Findings: distinctive "elfin" facies, intellectual disability, hypercalcemia (↑ sensitivity to vitamin D), well-developed verbal skills, extreme friendliness with strangers, cardiovascular problems.	

22q11 deletion syndromes	Microdeletion at chromosome 22q11 → variable presentations including Cleft palate, Abnormal facies, Thymic aplasia → T-cell deficiency, Cardiac defects, and Hypocalcemia 2° to parathyroid aplasia. DiGeorge syndrome—thymic, parathyroid, and cardiac defects. Velocardiofacial syndrome—palate, facial, and cardiac defects.	CATCH-22. Due to aberrant development of 3rd and 4th branchial pouches.

▶ BIOCHEMISTRY—NUTRITION

Vitamins: fat soluble	A, D, E, K. Absorption dependent on gut and pancreas. Toxicity more common than for water-soluble vitamins because fat-soluble vitamins accumulate in fat.	Malabsorption syndromes with steatorrhea, such as cystic fibrosis and sprue, or mineral oil intake can cause fat-soluble vitamin deficiencies.
Vitamins: water soluble	B_1 (thiamine: TPP) B_2 (riboflavin: FAD, FMN) B_3 (niacin: NAD^+) B_5 (pantothenic acid: CoA) B_6 (pyridoxine: PLP) B_7 (biotin) B_9 (folate) B_{12} (cobalamin) C (ascorbic acid)	All wash out easily from body except B_{12} and folate (stored in liver). B-complex deficiencies often result in dermatitis, glossitis, and diarrhea.

Vitamin A (retinol)

FUNCTION	Antioxidant; constituent of visual pigments (**retinal**); essential for normal differentiation of epithelial cells into specialized tissue (pancreatic cells, mucus-secreting cells); prevents squamous metaplasia. Used to treat measles and AML subtype M3.	Retinol is vitamin A, so think **retin-A** (used topically for wrinkles and acne). Found in liver and leafy vegetables.
DEFICIENCY	Night blindness (nyctalopia); dry, scaly skin (xerosis cutis); corneal degeneration (keratomalacia); Bitot spots on conjunctiva; immunosuppression.	
EXCESS	Acute toxicity—nausea, vomiting, vertigo, and blurred vision. Chronic toxicity—alopecia, dry skin (e.g., scaliness), hepatic toxicity and enlargement, arthralgias, and pseudotumor cerebri. Teratogenic (cleft palate, cardiac abnormalities), therefore a ⊖ pregnancy test and reliable contraception are required before isotretinoin (vitamin A derivative) is prescribed for severe acne.	

Vitamin B_1 (thiamine)

FUNCTION	In thiamine pyrophosphate (TPP), a cofactor for several dehydrogenase enzyme reactions: ▪ Pyruvate dehydrogenase (links glycolysis to TCA cycle) ▪ α-ketoglutarate dehydrogenase (TCA cycle) ▪ Transketolase (HMP shunt) ▪ Branched-chain ketoacid dehydrogenase	Think **ATP**: α-ketoglutarate dehydrogenase, Transketolase, and Pyruvate dehydrogenase. Spell beriberi as Ber1Ber1 to remember vitamin B_1. Wernicke-Korsakoff syndrome—confusion, ophthalmoplegia, ataxia (classic triad) + confabulation, personality change, memory loss (permanent). Damage to medial dorsal nucleus of thalamus, mammillary bodies.
DEFICIENCY	Impaired glucose breakdown → ATP depletion worsened by glucose infusion; highly aerobic tissues (e.g., brain, heart) are affected first. Wernicke-Korsakoff syndrome and beriberi. Seen in malnutrition and alcoholism (2° to malnutrition and malabsorption). Diagnosis made by ↑ in RBC transketolase activity following vitamin B_1 administration.	Dry beriberi—polyneuritis, symmetrical muscle wasting. Wet beriberi—high-output cardiac failure (dilated cardiomyopathy), edema.

Vitamin B_2 (riboflavin)

FUNCTION	Component of flavins FAD and FMN, used as cofactors in redox reactions, e.g., the succinate dehydrogenase reaction in the TCA cycle.	FAD and FMN are derived from riboFlavin ($B_2 \approx 2$ ATP).
DEFICIENCY	Cheilosis (inflammation of lips, scaling and fissures at the corners of the mouth), Corneal vascularization.	The 2 C's of B_2.

Vitamin B$_3$ (niacin)

FUNCTION	Constituent of NAD$^+$, NADP$^+$ (used in redox reactions). Derived from tryptophan. Synthesis requires vitamins B$_2$ and B$_6$. Used to treat dyslipidemia; lowers levels of VLDL and raises levels of HDL.	NAD derived from Niacin (B$_3$ ≈ 3 ATP).
DEFICIENCY	Glossitis. Severe deficiency leads to pellagra, which can be caused by Hartnup disease (↓ tryptophan absorption), malignant carcinoid syndrome (↑ tryptophan metabolism), and isoniazid (↓ vitamin B$_6$). Symptoms of pellagra: **D**iarrhea, **D**ementia (also hallucinations), **D**ermatitis (C3/C4 dermatome circumferential "broad collar" rash [Casal necklace], hyperpigmentation of sun-exposed limbs **A**).	The **3 D's** of B$_3$
EXCESS	Facial flushing (induced by prostaglandin, not histamine; can avoid by taking aspirin with niacin), hyperglycemia, hyperuricemia.	

Vitamin B$_5$ (pantothenic acid)

FUNCTION	Essential component of coenzyme A (CoA, a cofactor for acyl transfers) and fatty acid synthase.	B$_5$ is "**pento**"thenic acid.
DEFICIENCY	Dermatitis, enteritis, alopecia, adrenal insufficiency.	

Vitamin B$_6$ (pyridoxine)

FUNCTION	Converted to pyridoxal phosphate (PLP), a cofactor used in transamination (e.g., ALT and AST), decarboxylation reactions, glycogen phosphorylase. Synthesis of cystathionine, heme, niacin, histamine, and neurotransmitters including serotonin, epinephrine, norepinephrine (NE), dopamine, and GABA.
DEFICIENCY	Convulsions, hyperirritability, peripheral neuropathy (deficiency inducible by isoniazid and oral contraceptives), sideroblastic anemias due to impaired hemoglobin synthesis and iron excess.

Vitamin B$_7$ (biotin)

FUNCTION	Cofactor for carboxylation enzymes (which add a 1-carbon group): ■ Pyruvate carboxylase: pyruvate (3C) → oxaloacetate (4C) ■ Acetyl-CoA carboxylase: acetyl-CoA (2C) → malonyl-CoA (3C) ■ Propionyl-CoA carboxylase: propionyl-CoA (3C) → methylmalonyl-CoA (4C)	"**Avid**in in egg whites **avid**ly binds biotin."
DEFICIENCY	Relatively rare. Dermatitis, alopecia, enteritis. Caused by antibiotic use or excessive ingestion of raw egg whites.	

Vitamin B$_9$ (folate)

FUNCTION	Converted to tetrahydrofolic acid (THF), a coenzyme for 1-carbon transfer/methylation reactions. Important for the synthesis of nitrogenous bases in DNA and RNA.	Found in leafy green vegetables. Absorbed in jejunum. Folate from **fol**iage. Small reserve pool stored primarily in the liver.
DEFICIENCY	Macrocytic, megaloblastic anemia; hypersegmented polymorphonuclear cells (PMNs); glossitis; no neurologic symptoms (as opposed to vitamin B$_{12}$ deficiency). Labs: ↑ homocysteine, normal methylmalonic acid levels. Most common vitamin deficiency in the United States. Seen in alcoholism and pregnancy.	Deficiency can be caused by several drugs (e.g., phenytoin, sulfonamides, methotrexate). Supplemental maternal folic acid in early pregnancy decreases risk of neural tube defects.

Vitamin B₁₂ (cobalamin)

FUNCTION	Cofactor for homocysteine methyltransferase (transfers CH_3 groups as methylcobalamin) and methylmalonyl-CoA mutase.	Found in animal products. Synthesized only by microorganisms. Very large reserve pool (several years) stored primarily in the liver. Deficiency is usually caused by insufficient intake (e.g., veganism), malabsorption (e.g., sprue, enteritis, *Diphyllobothrium latum*), lack of intrinsic factor (pernicious anemia, gastric bypass surgery), or absence of terminal ileum (Crohn disease).
DEFICIENCY	Macrocytic, megaloblastic anemia; hypersegmented PMNs; paresthesias and subacute combined degeneration (degeneration of dorsal columns, lateral corticospinal tracts, and spinocerebellar tracts) due to abnormal myelin. Associated with ↑ serum homocysteine and methylmalonic acid levels. Prolonged deficiency → irreversible nerve damage.	Anti-intrinsic factor antibodies diagnostic for pernicious anemia.

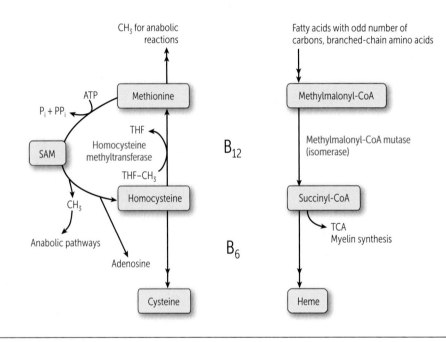

Vitamin C (ascorbic acid)

FUNCTION	Antioxidant; also facilitates iron absorption by reducing it to Fe^{2+} state. Necessary for hydroxylation of proline and lysine in collagen synthesis. Necessary for dopamine β-hydroxylase, which converts dopamine to NE.	Found in fruits and vegetables. Pronounce "**absorbic**" acid. Ancillary treatment for methemoglobinemia by reducing Fe^{3+} to Fe^{2+}.
DEFICIENCY	Scurvy—swollen gums, bruising, petechiae, hemarthrosis, anemia, poor wound healing, perifollicular and subperiosteal hemorrhages, "corkscrew" hair. Weakened immune response.	Vitamin C deficiency causes sCurvy due to a Collagen synthesis defect.
EXCESS	Nausea, vomiting, diarrhea, fatigue, calcium oxalate nephrolithiasis. Can ↑ risk of iron toxicity in predisposed individuals (e.g., those with transfusions, hereditary hemochromatosis).	

Vitamin D

	D_2 = ergocalciferol—ingested from plants. D_3 = cholecalciferol—consumed in milk, formed in sun-exposed skin (stratum basale). 25-OH D_3 = storage form. 1,25-$(OH)_2$ D_3 (calcitriol) = active form.	Drinking milk (fortified with vitamin D) is good for bones.
FUNCTION	↑ intestinal absorption of calcium and phosphate, ↑ bone mineralization.	
DEFICIENCY	Rickets **A** in children (bone pain and deformity), osteomalacia in adults (bone pain and muscle weakness), hypocalcemic tetany. Breastfed infants should receive oral vitamin D. Deficiency is exacerbated by low sun exposure, pigmented skin, prematurity.	
EXCESS	Hypercalcemia, hypercalciuria, loss of appetite, stupor. Seen in granulomatous disease (↑ activation of vitamin D by epithelioid macrophages).	**A** **Rickets.** X-ray of legs in toddler shows medial angulation and outward bowing of femurs and tibia (genu varum).✱

Vitamin E (tocopherol/tocotrienol)

FUNCTION	Antioxidant (protects RBCs and membranes from free radical damage).	Can enhance anticoagulant effects of warfarin.
DEFICIENCY	Hemolytic anemia, acanthocytosis, muscle weakness, posterior column and spinocerebellar tract demyelination.	Neurologic presentation may appear similar to vitamin B_{12} deficiency, but without megaloblastic anemia, hypersegmented neutrophils, or ↑ serum methylmalonic acid levels.

Vitamin K (phytomenadione, phylloquinone, phytonadione)

FUNCTION	Cofactor for the γ-carboxylation of glutamic acid residues on various proteins required for blood clotting. Synthesized by intestinal flora.	K is for Koagulation. Necessary for the maturation of clotting factors II, VII, IX, X, and proteins C and S. Warfarin—vitamin K antagonist.
DEFICIENCY	Neonatal hemorrhage with ↑ PT and ↑ aPTT but normal bleeding time (neonates have sterile intestines and are unable to synthesize vitamin K). Can also occur after prolonged use of broad-spectrum antibiotics.	Not in breast milk; neonates are given vitamin K injection at birth to prevent hemorrhagic disease of the newborn.

Zinc

FUNCTION	Mineral essential for the activity of 100+ enzymes. Important in the formation of zinc fingers (transcription factor motif).	
DEFICIENCY	Delayed wound healing, hypogonadism, ↓ adult hair (axillary, facial, pubic), dysgeusia, anosmia, acrodermatitis enteropathica A. May predispose to alcoholic cirrhosis.	

Zinc deficiency. Well-demarcated, scaly plaques in intertriginous area. RU

Malnutrition

Kwashiorkor	Protein malnutrition resulting in skin lesions, edema due to ↓ plasma oncotic pressure, liver malfunction (fatty change due to ↓ apolipoprotein synthesis). Clinical picture is small child with swollen abdomen A.	Kwashiorkor results from a protein-deficient **MEAL**: Malnutrition Edema Anemia Liver (fatty)
Marasmus	Total calorie malnutrition resulting in tissue and muscle wasting, loss of subcutaneous fat, and variable edema.	Marasmus results in Muscle wasting.

Ethanol metabolism

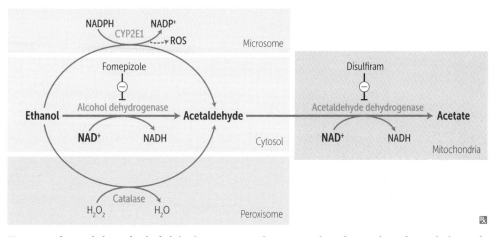

Fomepizole—inhibits alcohol dehydrogenase and is an antidote for methanol or ethylene glycol poisoning.

Disulfiram—inhibits acetaldehyde dehydrogenase (acetaldehyde accumulates, contributing to hangover symptoms).

NAD^+ is the limiting reagent.

Alcohol dehydrogenase operates via zero-order kinetics.

Ethanol metabolism ↑ $NADH/NAD^+$ ratio in liver, causing:

- Pyruvate → lactate (lactic acidosis).
- Oxaloacetate → malate (prevents gluconeogenesis → fasting hypoglycemia)
- Dihydroxyacetone phosphate → glycerol-3-phosphate (combines with fatty acids to make triglycerides → hepatosteatosis)

End result is clinical picture seen in chronic alcoholism.

Additionally, ↑ $NADH/NAD^+$ ratio disfavors TCA production of NADH → ↑ utilization of acetyl-CoA for ketogenesis (→ ketoacidosis) and lipogenesis (→ hepatosteatosis).

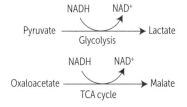

▶ BIOCHEMISTRY—METABOLISM

Metabolism sites

Mitochondria	Fatty acid oxidation (β-oxidation), acetyl-CoA production, TCA cycle, oxidative phosphorylation, ketogenesis.
Cytoplasm	Glycolysis, fatty acid synthesis, HMP shunt, protein synthesis (RER), steroid synthesis (SER), cholesterol synthesis.
Both	Heme synthesis, Urea cycle, Gluconeogenesis. **HUG**s take **two** (i.e., both).

Enzyme terminology	An enzyme's name often describes its function. For example, glucokinase is an enzyme that catalyzes the phosphorylation of glucose using a molecule of ATP. The following are commonly used enzyme descriptors.
Kinase	Uses ATP to add high-energy phosphate group onto substrate (e.g., phosphofructokinase).
Phosphorylase	Adds inorganic phosphate onto substrate without using ATP (e.g., glycogen phosphorylase).
Phosphatase	Removes phosphate group from substrate (e.g., fructose-1,6-bisphosphatase).
Dehydrogenase	Catalyzes oxidation-reduction reactions (e.g., pyruvate dehydrogenase).
Hydroxylase	Adds hydroxyl group (−OH) onto substrate (e.g., tyrosine hydroxylase).
Carboxylase	Transfers CO_2 groups with the help of biotin (e.g., pyruvate carboxylase).
Mutase	Relocates a functional group within a molecule (e.g., vitamin B_{12}–dependent methylmalonyl-CoA mutase).

Rate-determining enzymes of metabolic processes

PROCESS	ENZYME	REGULATORS
Glycolysis	Phosphofructokinase-1 (PFK-1)	AMP ⊕, fructose-2,6-bisphosphate ⊕ ATP ⊖, citrate ⊖
Gluconeogenesis	Fructose-1,6-bisphosphatase	ATP ⊕, acetyl-CoA ⊕ AMP ⊖, fructose-2,6-bisphosphate ⊖
TCA cycle	Isocitrate dehydrogenase	ADP ⊕ ATP ⊖, NADH ⊖
Glycogenesis	Glycogen synthase	Glucose-6-phosphate ⊕, insulin ⊕, cortisol ⊕ Epinephrine ⊖, glucagon ⊖
Glycogenolysis	Glycogen phosphorylase	Epinephrine ⊕, glucagon ⊕, AMP ⊕ Glucose-6-phosphate ⊖, insulin ⊖, ATP ⊖
HMP shunt	Glucose-6-phosphate dehydrogenase (G6PD)	$NADP^+$ ⊕ NADPH ⊖
De novo pyrimidine synthesis	Carbamoyl phosphate synthetase II	ATP ⊕ UTP ⊖
De novo purine synthesis	Glutamine-phosphoribosylpyrophosphate (PRPP) amidotransferase	AMP ⊖, inosine monophosphate (IMP) ⊖, GMP ⊖
Urea cycle	Carbamoyl phosphate synthetase I	N-acetylglutamate ⊕
Fatty acid synthesis	Acetyl-CoA carboxylase (ACC)	Insulin ⊕, citrate ⊕ Glucagon ⊖, palmitoyl-CoA ⊖
Fatty acid oxidation	Carnitine acyltransferase I	Malonyl-CoA ⊖
Ketogenesis	HMG-CoA synthase	
Cholesterol synthesis	HMG-CoA reductase	Insulin ⊕, thyroxine ⊕ Glucagon ⊖, cholesterol ⊖

Summary of pathways

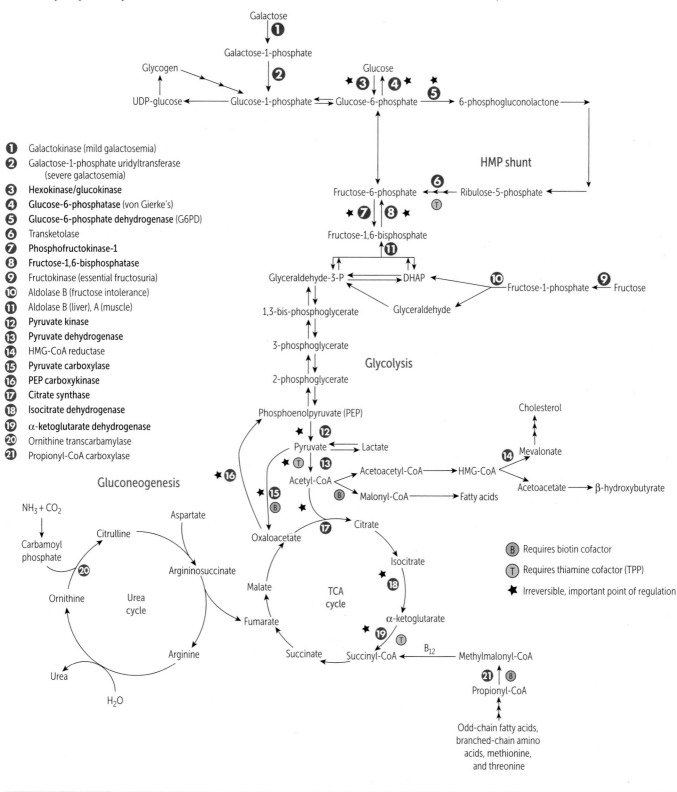

1. Galactokinase (mild galactosemia)
2. Galactose-1-phosphate uridyltransferase (severe galactosemia)
3. **Hexokinase/glucokinase**
4. **Glucose-6-phosphatase** (von Gierke's)
5. **Glucose-6-phosphate dehydrogenase** (G6PD)
6. Transketolase
7. **Phosphofructokinase-1**
8. **Fructose-1,6-bisphosphatase**
9. Fructokinase (essential fructosuria)
10. Aldolase B (fructose intolerance)
11. Aldolase B (liver), A (muscle)
12. **Pyruvate kinase**
13. **Pyruvate dehydrogenase**
14. **HMG-CoA reductase**
15. **Pyruvate carboxylase**
16. **PEP carboxykinase**
17. **Citrate synthase**
18. **Isocitrate dehydrogenase**
19. **α-ketoglutarate dehydrogenase**
20. Ornithine transcarbamylase
21. Propionyl-CoA carboxylase

Ⓑ Requires biotin cofactor

Ⓣ Requires thiamine cofactor (TPP)

★ Irreversible, important point of regulation

ATP production

Aerobic metabolism of glucose produces 32 net ATP via malate-aspartate shuttle (heart and liver), 30 net ATP via glycerol-3-phosphate shuttle (muscle).

Anaerobic glycolysis produces only 2 net ATP per glucose molecule.

ATP hydrolysis can be coupled to energetically unfavorable reactions.

Arsenic causes glycolysis to produce zero net ATP.

Activated carriers

CARRIER MOLECULE	CARRIED IN ACTIVATED FORM
ATP	Phosphoryl groups
NADH, NADPH, $FADH_2$	Electrons
CoA, lipoamide	Acyl groups
Biotin	CO_2
Tetrahydrofolates	1-carbon units
S-adenosylmethionine (SAM)	CH_3 groups
TPP	Aldehydes

Universal electron acceptors

Nicotinamides (NAD^+ from vitamin B_3, $NADP^+$) and flavin nucleotides (FAD^+ from vitamin B_2).

NAD^+ is generally used in **catabolic** processes to carry reducing equivalents away as NADH.

NADPH is used in **anabolic** processes (steroid and fatty acid synthesis) as a supply of reducing equivalents.

NADPH is a product of the HMP shunt.

NADPH is used in:
- Anabolic processes
- Respiratory burst
- Cytochrome P-450 system
- Glutathione reductase

Hexokinase vs. glucokinase

Phosphorylation of glucose to yield glucose-6-phosphate serves as the 1st step of glycolysis (also serves as the 1st step of glycogen synthesis in the liver). Reaction is catalyzed by either hexokinase or glucokinase, depending on the tissue. At low glucose concentrations, hexokinase sequesters glucose in the tissue. At high glucose concentrations, excess glucose is stored in the liver.

	Hexokinase	**Glucokinase**
Location	Most tissues, except liver and pancreatic β cells	Liver, β cells of pancreas
K_m	Lower (↑ affinity)	Higher (↓ affinity)
V_{max}	Lower (↓ capacity)	Higher (↑ capacity)
Induced by insulin	No	Yes
Feedback-inhibited by glucose-6-phosphate	Yes	No
Gene mutation associated with maturity-onset diabetes of the young (MODY)	No	Yes

Glycolysis regulation, key enzymes	Net glycolysis (cytoplasm): Glucose + 2 P_i + 2 ADP + 2 NAD^+ → 2 pyruvate + 2 ATP + 2 NADH + 2 H^+ + 2 H_2O. Equation not balanced chemically, and exact balanced equation depends on ionization state of reactants and products.	

REQUIRE ATP	Glucose ——————→ Glucose-6-P Hexokinase/glucokinase[a]	Glucose-6-P ⊖ hexokinase. Fructose-6-P ⊖ glucokinase.
	Fructose-6-P ——————→ Fructose-1,6-BP Phosphofructokinase-1 (rate-limiting step)	AMP ⊕, fructose-2,6-bisphosphate ⊕. ATP ⊖, citrate ⊖.
	[a]Glucokinase in liver and β cells of pancreas; hexokinase in all other tissues.	

PRODUCE ATP	1,3-BPG ⇌ 3-PG Phosphoglycerate kinase	
	Phosphoenolpyruvate ——————→ Pyruvate Pyruvate kinase	Fructose-1,6-bisphosphate ⊕. ATP ⊖, alanine ⊖.

Regulation by fructose-2,6-bisphosphate		

FBPase-2 (fructose bisphosphatase-2) and PFK-2 (phosphofructokinase-2) are the same bifunctional enzyme whose function is reversed by phosphorylation by protein kinase A.

Fasting state: ↑ glucagon → ↑ cAMP → ↑ protein kinase A → ↑ FBPase-2, ↓ PFK-2, less glycolysis, more gluconeogenesis.

Fed state: ↑ insulin → ↓ cAMP → ↓ protein kinase A → ↓ FBPase-2, ↑ PFK-2, more glycolysis, less gluconeogenesis.

Pyruvate dehydrogenase complex	Mitochondrial enzyme complex linking glycolysis and TCA cycle. Differentially regulated in fed/fasting states (active in fed state).
	Reaction: pyruvate + NAD^+ + CoA → acetyl-CoA + CO_2 + NADH.
	The complex contains 3 enzymes that require 5 cofactors:
	  1. Pyrophosphate (B_1, thiamine; TPP)
	  2. FAD (B_2, riboflavin)
	  3. NAD (B_3, niacin)
	  4. CoA (B_5, pantothenic acid)
	  5. Lipoic acid
	Activated by exercise, which:
	  ↑ NAD^+/NADH ratio
	  ↑ ADP
	  ↑ Ca^{2+}
		The complex is similar to the α-ketoglutarate dehydrogenase complex (same cofactors, similar substrate and action), which converts α-ketoglutarate → succinyl-CoA (TCA cycle).
		
		Arsenic inhibits lipoic acid. Findings: vomiting, rice-water stools, garlic breath.

Pyruvate dehydrogenase complex deficiency	Causes a buildup of pyruvate that gets shunted to lactate (via LDH) and alanine (via ALT). X-linked.	
FINDINGS	Neurologic defects, lactic acidosis, ↑ serum alanine starting in infancy.	
TREATMENT	↑ intake of ketogenic nutrients (e.g., high fat content or ↑ lysine and leucine).	Lysine and Leucine—the onLy pureLy ketogenic amino acids.

Pyruvate metabolism

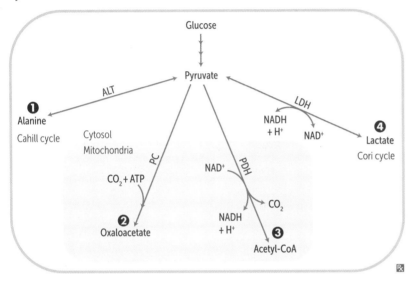

Functions of different pyruvate metabolic pathways (and their associated cofactors):

❶ Alanine aminotransferase (B_6): alanine carries amino groups to the liver from muscle

❷ Pyruvate carboxylase (biotin): oxaloacetate can replenish TCA cycle or be used in gluconeogenesis

❸ Pyruvate dehydrogenase (B_1, B_2, B_3, B_5, lipoic acid): transition from glycolysis to the TCA cycle

❹ Lactic acid dehydrogenase (B_3): end of anaerobic glycolysis (major pathway in RBCs, WBCs, kidney medulla, lens, testes, and cornea)

TCA cycle (Krebs cycle)

Pyruvate → acetyl-CoA produces 1 NADH, 1 CO_2.

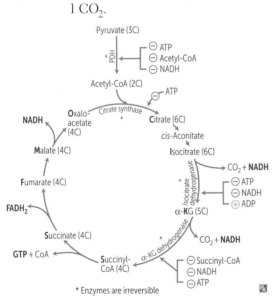

* Enzymes are irreversible

The TCA cycle produces 3 NADH, 1 $FADH_2$, 2 CO_2, 1 GTP per acetyl-CoA = 10 ATP/ acetyl-CoA (2× everything per glucose). TCA cycle reactions occur in the mitochondria.

α-ketoglutarate dehydrogenase complex requires the same cofactors as the pyruvate dehydrogenase complex (B_1, B_2, B_3, B_5, lipoic acid).

Citrate Is Krebs' Starting Substrate For Making Oxaloacetate.

Electron transport chain and oxidative phosphorylation

NADH electrons from glycolysis enter mitochondria via the malate-aspartate or glycerol-3-phosphate shuttle. $FADH_2$ electrons are transferred to complex II (at a lower energy level than NADH). The passage of electrons results in the formation of a proton gradient that, coupled to oxidative phosphorylation, drives the production of ATP.

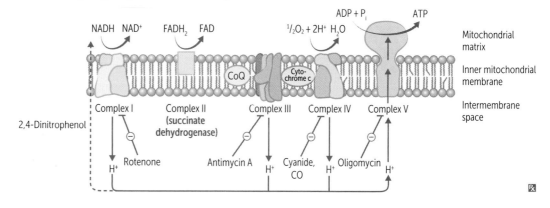

ATP PRODUCED VIA ATP SYNTHASE		
	1 NADH → 2.5 ATP; 1 $FADH_2$ → 1.5 ATP.	
OXIDATIVE PHOSPHORYLATION POISONS		
Electron transport inhibitors	Directly inhibit electron transport, causing a ↓ proton gradient and block of ATP synthesis.	Rotenone, cyanide, antimycin A, CO.
ATP synthase inhibitors	Directly inhibit mitochondrial ATP synthase, causing an ↑ proton gradient. No ATP is produced because electron transport stops.	Oligomycin.
Uncoupling agents	↑ permeability of membrane, causing a ↓ proton gradient and ↑ O_2 consumption. ATP synthesis stops, but electron transport continues. Produces heat.	2,4-Dinitrophenol (used illicitly for weight loss), aspirin (fevers often occur after aspirin overdose), thermogenin in brown fat.

Gluconeogenesis, irreversible enzymes		Pathway Produces Fresh Glucose.
Pyruvate carboxylase	In mitochondria. Pyruvate → oxaloacetate.	Requires biotin, ATP. Activated by acetyl-CoA.
Phosphoenolpyruvate carboxykinase	In cytosol. Oxaloacetate → phosphoenolpyruvate.	Requires GTP.
Fructose-1,6-bisphosphatase	In cytosol. Fructose-1,6-bisphosphate → fructose-6-phosphate.	Citrate ⊕, fructose 2,6-bisphosphate ⊖.
Glucose-6-phosphatase	In ER. Glucose-6-phosphate → glucose.	

Occurs primarily in liver; serves to maintain euglycemia during fasting. Enzymes also found in kidney, intestinal epithelium. Deficiency of the key gluconeogenic enzymes causes hypoglycemia. (Muscle cannot participate in gluconeogenesis because it lacks glucose-6-phosphatase).

Odd-chain fatty acids yield 1 propionyl-CoA during metabolism, which can enter the TCA cycle (as succinyl-CoA), undergo gluconeogenesis, and serve as a glucose source. Even-chain fatty acids cannot produce new glucose, since they yield only acetyl-CoA equivalents.

HMP shunt (pentose phosphate pathway)	Provides a source of NADPH from abundantly available glucose-6-P (NADPH is required for reductive reactions, e.g., glutathione reduction inside RBCs, fatty acid and cholesterol biosynthesis). Additionally, this pathway yields ribose for nucleotide synthesis and glycolytic intermediates. 2 distinct phases (oxidative and nonoxidative), both of which occur in the cytoplasm. No ATP is used or produced. Sites: lactating mammary glands, liver, adrenal cortex (sites of fatty acid or steroid synthesis), RBCs.

REACTIONS	KEY ENZYMES	PRODUCTS
Oxidative (irreversible)	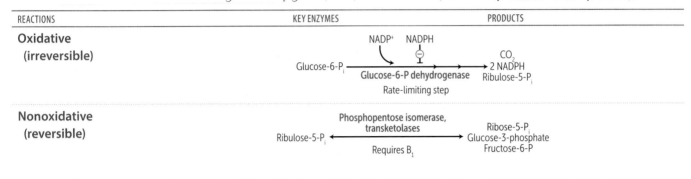	
Nonoxidative (reversible)	Phosphopentose isomerase, transketolases Requires B_1	Ribose-5-P_i Glucose-3-phosphate Fructose-6-P

Oxidative: Glucose-6-P_i → (Glucose-6-P dehydrogenase, Rate-limiting step; NADP$^+$ → NADPH ⊖) → CO_2, 2 NADPH, Ribulose-5-P_i

Nonoxidative: Ribulose-5-P_i ⇌ Ribose-5-P_i, Glucose-3-phosphate, Fructose-6-P

Glucose-6-phosphate dehydrogenase deficiency	NADPH is necessary to keep glutathione reduced, which in turn detoxifies free radicals and peroxides. ↓ NADPH in RBCs leads to hemolytic anemia due to poor RBC defense against oxidizing agents (e.g., fava beans, sulfonamides, primaquine, antituberculosis drugs). Infection can also precipitate hemolysis (free radicals generated via inflammatory response can diffuse into RBCs and cause oxidative damage).	X-linked recessive disorder; most common human enzyme deficiency; more prevalent among blacks. ↑ malarial resistance. **Heinz bodies**—denatured **H**emoglobin precipitates within RBCs due to oxidative stress. **Bite cells**—result from the phagocytic removal of **Heinz** bodies by splenic macrophages. Think, "**Bite** into some **Heinz** ketchup."

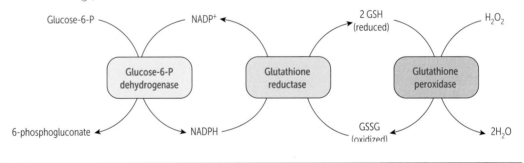

Disorders of fructose metabolism

Essential fructosuria	Involves a defect in **fructokinase**. Autosomal recessive. A benign, asymptomatic condition, since fructose is not trapped in cells. Symptoms: fructose appears in blood and urine. Disorders of fructose metabolism cause milder symptoms than analogous disorders of galactose metabolism.
Fructose intolerance	Hereditary deficiency of **aldolase B**. Autosomal recessive. Fructose-1-phosphate accumulates, causing a ↓ in available phosphate, which results in inhibition of glycogenolysis and gluconeogenesis. Symptoms present following consumption of fruit, juice, or honey. Urine dipstick will be ⊖ (tests for glucose only); reducing sugar can be detected in the urine (nonspecific test for inborn errors of carbohydrate metabolism). Symptoms: hypoglycemia, jaundice, cirrhosis, vomiting. Treatment: ↓ intake of both fructose and sucrose (glucose + fructose).

Fructose metabolism (liver)

❶ Deficiency = essential fructosuria
❷ Deficiency = fructose intolerance
❸ Fructose bypasses rate-limiting step of glycolysis (PFK) via this pathway

Disorders of galactose metabolism

Galactokinase deficiency	Hereditary deficiency of **galactokinase**. Galactitol accumulates if galactose is present in diet. Relatively mild condition. Autosomal recessive. Symptoms: galactose appears in blood and urine, infantile cataracts. May present as failure to track objects or to develop a social smile.
Classic galactosemia	Absence of **galactose-1-phosphate uridyltransferase**. Autosomal recessive. Damage is caused by accumulation of toxic substances (including galactitol, which accumulates in the lens of the eye). Symptoms: failure to thrive, jaundice, hepatomegaly, infantile cataracts, intellectual disability. Can lead to *E. coli* sepsis in neonates. Treatment: exclude galactose and lactose (galactose + glucose) from diet.

Galactose metabolism

Fructose is to Aldolase B as Galactose is to UridylTransferase (**FAB GUT**).
The more serious defects lead to PO_4^{3-} depletion.

Sorbitol	An alternative method of trapping glucose in the cell is to convert it to its alcohol counterpart, called sorbitol, via aldose reductase. Some tissues then convert sorbitol to fructose using sorbitol dehydrogenase; tissues with an insufficient amount of this enzyme are at risk for intracellular sorbitol accumulation, causing osmotic damage (e.g., cataracts, retinopathy, and peripheral neuropathy seen with chronic hyperglycemia in diabetes). High blood levels of galactose also result in conversion to the osmotically active galactitol via aldose reductase.

Liver, ovaries, and seminal vesicles have both enzymes.

$$\text{Glucose} \xrightarrow[\text{NADPH}]{\text{Aldose reductase}} \text{Sorbitol} \xrightarrow[\text{NAD}^+]{\text{Sorbitol dehydrogenase}} \text{Fructose}$$

Schwann cells, retina, and kidneys have only aldose reductase. Lens has primarily aldose reductase.

$$\text{Glucose} \xrightarrow[\text{NADPH}]{\text{Aldose reductase}} \text{Sorbitol}$$

Lactase deficiency	Insufficient lactase enzyme → dietary lactose intolerance. Lactase functions on the brush border to digest lactose (in human and cow milk) into glucose and galactose. Primary: age-dependent decline after childhood (absence of lactase-persistent allele), common in people of Asian, African, or Native American descent. Secondary: loss of brush border due to gastroenteritis (e.g., rotavirus), autoimmune disease, etc. Congenital lactase deficiency: rare, due to defective gene. Stool demonstrates ↓ pH and breath shows ↑ hydrogen content with lactose tolerance test. Intestinal biopsy reveals normal mucosa in patients with hereditary lactose intolerance.
FINDINGS	Bloating, cramps, flatulence, osmotic diarrhea.
TREATMENT	Avoid dairy products or add lactase pills to diet; lactose-free milk.

Amino acids	Only L-amino acids are found in proteins.	
Essential	Glucogenic: methionine (Met), valine (Val), histidine (His). Glucogenic/ketogenic: isoleucine (Ile), phenylalanine (Phe), threonine (Thr), tryptophan (Trp). Ketogenic: leucine (Leu), lysine (Lys).	All essential amino acids need to be supplied in the diet.
Acidic	Aspartic acid (Asp) and glutamic acid (Glu). Negatively charged at body pH.	
Basic	Arginine (Arg), lysine (Lys), histidine (His). Arg is most basic. His has no charge at body pH.	Arg and His are required during periods of growth. Arg and Lys are ↑ in histones, which bind negatively charged DNA.

Urea cycle

Amino acid catabolism results in the formation of common metabolites (e.g., pyruvate, acetyl-CoA), which serve as metabolic fuels. Excess nitrogen (NH_3) generated by this process is converted to urea and excreted by the kidneys.

Ordinarily, Careless Crappers Are Also Frivolous About Urination.

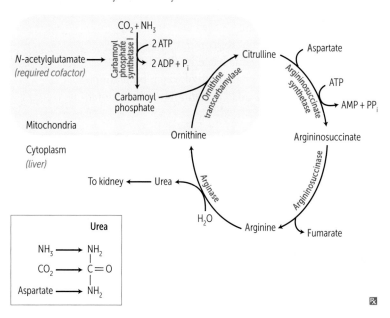

Transport of ammonia by alanine and glutamate

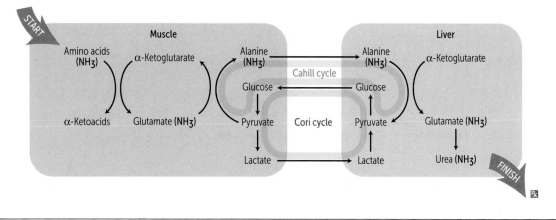

Hyperammonemia	Can be acquired (e.g., liver disease) or hereditary (e.g., urea cycle enzyme deficiencies). Results in excess NH_4^+, which depletes α-ketoglutarate, leading to inhibition of TCA cycle. Treatment: limit protein in diet. Lactulose to acidify the GI tract and trap NH_4^+ for excretion. Rifaximin to ↓ colonic ammoniagenic bacteria. Benzoate or phenylbutyrate (both of which bind amino acid and lead to excretion) may be given to ↓ ammonia levels.	Ammonia intoxication—tremor (asterixis), slurring of speech, somnolence, vomiting, cerebral edema, blurring of vision.
N-acetylglutamate synthase deficiency	Required cofactor for carbamoyl phosphate synthetase I. Absence of N-acetylglutamate → hyperammonemia. Presents in neonates as poorly regulated respiration and body temperature, poor feeding, developmental delay, intellectual disability (identical to presentation of carbamoyl phosphate synthetase I deficiency).	
Ornithine transcarbamylase deficiency	Most common urea cycle disorder. X-linked recessive (vs. other urea cycle enzyme deficiencies, which are autosomal recessive). Interferes with the body's ability to eliminate ammonia. Often evident in the first few days of life, but may present later. Excess carbamoyl phosphate is converted to orotic acid (part of the pyrimidine synthesis pathway). Findings: ↑ orotic acid in blood and urine, ↓ BUN, symptoms of hyperammonemia. No megaloblastic anemia (vs. orotic aciduria).	

Amino acid derivatives

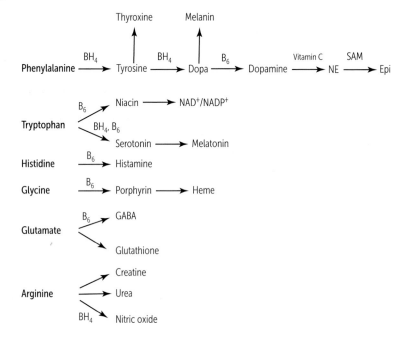

Catecholamine synthesis/tyrosine catabolism

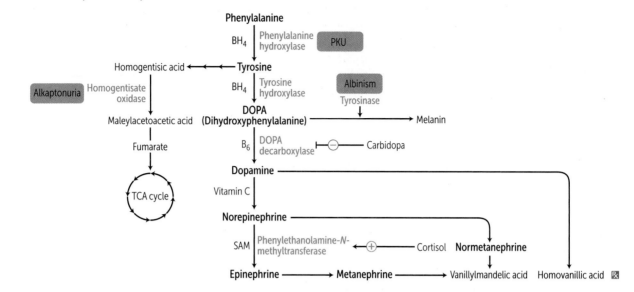

Phenylketonuria	Due to ↓ phenylalanine hydroxylase or ↓ tetrahydrobiopterin cofactor (malignant PKU). Tyrosine becomes essential. ↑ phenylalanine → excess phenylketones in urine. Findings: intellectual disability, growth retardation, seizures, fair skin, eczema, musty body odor. Treatment: ↓ phenylalanine and ↑ tyrosine in diet, tetrahydrobiopterin supplementation. **Maternal PKU**—lack of proper dietary therapy during pregnancy. Findings in infant: microcephaly, intellectual disability, growth retardation, congenital heart defects.	Autosomal recessive. Incidence ≈ 1:10,000. Screening occurs 2–3 days after birth (normal at birth because of maternal enzyme during fetal life). Phenylketones—phenylacetate, phenyllactate, and phenylpyruvate. Disorder of **aromatic** amino acid metabolism → musty body **odor.** PKU patients must avoid the artificial sweetener aspartame, which contains phenylalanine.
Maple syrup urine disease	Blocked degradation of **branched** amino acids (Isoleucine, Leucine, Valine) due to ↓ α-ketoacid dehydrogenase (B$_1$). Causes ↑ α-ketoacids in the blood, especially those of leucine. Causes severe CNS defects, intellectual disability, and death. Treatment: restriction of isoleucine, leucine, valine in diet, and thiamine supplementation.	Autosomal recessive. Urine smells like maple syrup/burnt sugar. **I L**ove **V**ermont **maple syrup** from maple trees (with **branches**).

Alkaptonuria (ochronosis)

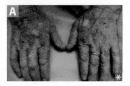

Congenital deficiency of homogentisate oxidase in the degradative pathway of tyrosine to fumarate → pigment-forming homogentisic acid accumulates in tissue 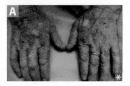. Autosomal recessive. Usually benign.

Findings: dark connective tissue, brown pigmented sclerae, urine turns black on prolonged exposure to air. May have debilitating arthralgias (homogentisic acid toxic to cartilage).

Homocystinuria

Types (all autosomal recessive):
- Cystathionine synthase deficiency (treatment: ↓ methionine, ↑ cysteine, ↑ B_{12} and folate in diet)
- ↓ affinity of cystathionine synthase for pyridoxal phosphate (treatment: ↑↑ B_6 and ↑ cysteine in diet)
- Homocysteine methyltransferase (methionine synthase) deficiency (treatment: ↑ methionine in diet)

All forms result in excess homocysteine.

Findings: ↑↑ homocysteine in urine, intellectual disability, osteoporosis, marfanoid habitus, kyphosis, lens subluxation (downward and inward), thrombosis, and atherosclerosis (stroke and MI).

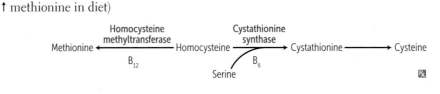

Cystinuria

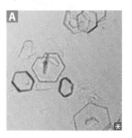

Hereditary defect of renal PCT and intestinal amino acid transporter that prevents reabsorption of **C**ysteine, **O**rnithine, **L**ysine, and **A**rginine (**COLA**).

Excess cystine in the urine can lead to recurrent precipitation of hexagonal cystine stones .

Treatment: urinary alkalinization (e.g., potassium citrate, acetazolamide) and chelating agents (e.g., penicillamine) ↑ solubility of cystine stones; good hydration.

Autosomal recessive. Common (1:7000). Urinary cyanide-nitroprusside test is diagnostic.

Cystine is made of 2 cysteines connected by a disulfide bond.

Glycogen regulation by insulin and glucagon/epinephrine

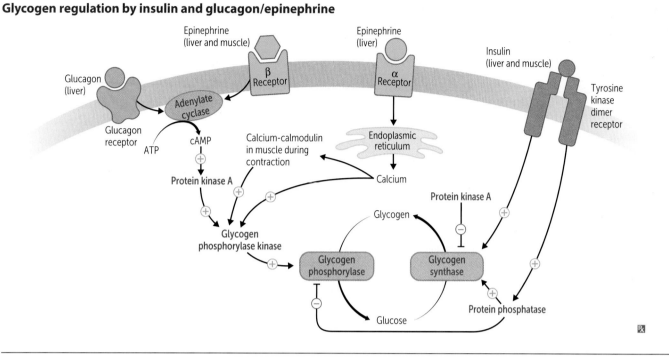

Glycogen	Branches have α-(1,6) bonds; linkages have α-(1,4) bonds.
Skeletal muscle	Glycogen undergoes glycogenolysis → glucose-1-phosphate → glucose-6-phosphate, which is rapidly metabolized during exercise.
Hepatocytes	Glycogen is stored and undergoes glycogenolysis to maintain blood sugar at appropriate levels. Glycogen phosphorylase liberates glucose-1-phosphate residues off branched glycogen until 4 glucose units remain on a branch. Then 4-α-D-glucanotransferase (debranching enzyme ❺) moves 3 molecules of glucose-1-phosphate from the branch to the linkage. Then α-1,6-glucosidase (debranching enzyme ❻) cleaves off the last residue, liberating glucose. "Limit dextrin" refers to the one to four residues remaining on a branch after glycogen phosphorylase has already shortened it.

❶ UDP-glucose pyrophosphorylase
❷ Glycogen synthase
❸ Branching enzyme
❹ Glycogen phosphorylase
❺ Debranching enzyme (4-α-D-glucanotransferase)
❻ Debranching enzyme (α-1,6-glucosidase)

Glucose-6-P
Glucose-1-P
❶
UDP-glucose
❷
Glycogen
❸
❹
❺
❻
Limit dextrin

Note: A small amount of glycogen is degraded in lysosomes by α-1,4-glucosidase (acid maltase).

Glycogen storage diseases

12 types, all resulting in abnormal glycogen metabolism and an accumulation of glycogen within cells.

Very Poor Carbohydrate Metabolism.

DISEASE	FINDINGS	DEFICIENT ENZYME	COMMENTS
Von Gierke disease (type I)	Severe fasting hypoglycemia, ↑↑ glycogen in liver, ↑ blood lactate, ↑ triglycerides, ↑ uric acid, and hepatomegaly	Glucose-6-phosphatase	Autosomal recessive Treatment: frequent oral glucose/cornstarch; avoidance of fructose and galactose
Pompe disease (type II)	Cardiomegaly, hypertrophic cardiomyopathy, exercise intolerance, and systemic findings leading to early death	Lysosomal α-1,4-glucosidase (acid maltase)	Autosomal recessive Pompe trashes the Pump (heart, liver, and muscle)
Cori disease (type III)	Milder form of type I with normal blood lactate levels	Debranching enzyme (α-1,6-glucosidase)	Autosomal recessive Gluconeogenesis is intact
McArdle disease (type V)	↑ glycogen in muscle, but muscle cannot break it down → painful muscle cramps, myoglobinuria (red urine) with strenuous exercise, and arrhythmia from electrolyte abnormalities	Skeletal muscle glycogen phosphorylase (myophosphorylase)	Autosomal recessive Blood glucose levels typically unaffected McArdle = Muscle Treat with vitamin B_6 (cofactor)

Lysosomal storage diseases

Each is caused by a deficiency in one of the many lysosomal enzymes. Results in an accumulation of abnormal metabolic products.

DISEASE	FINDINGS	DEFICIENT ENZYME	ACCUMULATED SUBSTRATE	INHERITANCE
Sphingolipidoses				
Fabry disease	Peripheral neuropathy of hands/feet, angiokeratomas, cardiovascular/renal disease. *, telangiectasia, hypohydrosis*	α-galactosidase A	Ceramide trihexoside *(Gb3) (globotriaosylceramide)*	XR
Gaucher disease	Most common. Hepatosplenomegaly, pancytopenia, osteoporosis, aseptic necrosis of femur, bone crises, Gaucher cells A (lipid-laden macrophages resembling crumpled tissue paper); treatment is recombinant glucocerebrosidase.	Glucocerebrosidase (β-glucosidase)	Glucocerebroside	AR
Niemann-Pick disease	Progressive neurodegeneration, hepatosplenomegaly, foam cells (lipid-laden macrophages) B, "cherry-red" spot on macula C.	Sphingomyelinase	Sphingomyelin	AR
Tay-Sachs disease	Progressive neurodegeneration, developmental delay, "cherry-red" spot on macula C, lysosomes with onion skin, no hepatosplenomegaly (vs. Niemann-Pick).	Hexosaminidase A	GM_2 ganglioside	AR
Krabbe disease	Peripheral neuropathy, developmental delay, optic atrophy, globoid cells.	Galactocerebrosidase	Galactocerebroside, psychosine	AR
Metachromatic leukodystrophy	Central and peripheral demyelination with ataxia, dementia.	Arylsulfatase A	Cerebroside sulfate	AR
Mucopolysaccharidoses				
Hurler syndrome	Developmental delay, gargoylism, airway obstruction, corneal clouding, hepatosplenomegaly.	α-L-iduronidase	Heparan sulfate, dermatan sulfate	AR
Hunter syndrome	Mild Hurler + aggressive behavior, no corneal clouding.	Iduronate sulfatase	Heparan sulfate, dermatan sulfate	XR

No man picks (Niemann-Pick) his nose with his **sphinger** (**sphingomyelinase**).

Tay-Sa**X** lacks he**X**osaminidase.

Hunters see clearly (no corneal clouding) and aggressively aim for the **X** (**X**-linked recessive).

↑ incidence of Tay-Sachs, Niemann-Pick, and some forms of Gaucher disease in Ashkenazi Jews.

Fatty acid metabolism

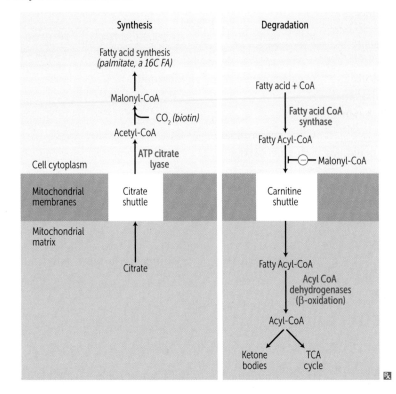

Fatty acid synthesis requires transport of citrate from mitochondria to cytosol. Predominantly occurs in liver, lactating mammary glands, and adipose tissue.

Long-chain fatty acid (LCFA) degradation requires carnitine-dependent transport into the mitochondrial matrix.

"SYtrate" = SYnthesis.
CARnitine = CARnage of fatty acids.

Systemic 1° carnitine deficiency—inherited defect in transport of LCFAs into the mitochondria → toxic accumulation. Causes weakness, hypotonia, and hypoketotic hypoglycemia.

Medium-chain acyl-CoA dehydrogenase deficiency	Autosomal recessive disorder of fatty acid oxidation. ↓ ability to break down fatty acids into acetyl-CoA → accumulation of 8- to 10-carbon fatty acyl carnitines in the blood and hypoketotic hypoglycemia. May present in infancy or early childhood with vomiting, lethargy, seizures, coma, and liver dysfunction.	Minor illness can lead to sudden death. Treat by avoiding fasting.
Ketone bodies	In the liver, fatty acids and amino acids are metabolized to acetoacetate and β-hydroxybutyrate (to be used in muscle and brain). In prolonged starvation and diabetic ketoacidosis, oxaloacetate is depleted for gluconeogenesis. In alcoholism, excess NADH shunts oxaloacetate to malate. Both processes cause a buildup of acetyl-CoA, which shunts glucose and FFA toward the production of ketone bodies.	Breath smells like acetone (fruity odor). Urine test for ketones does not detect β-hydroxybutyrate.

Metabolic fuel use

Exercise

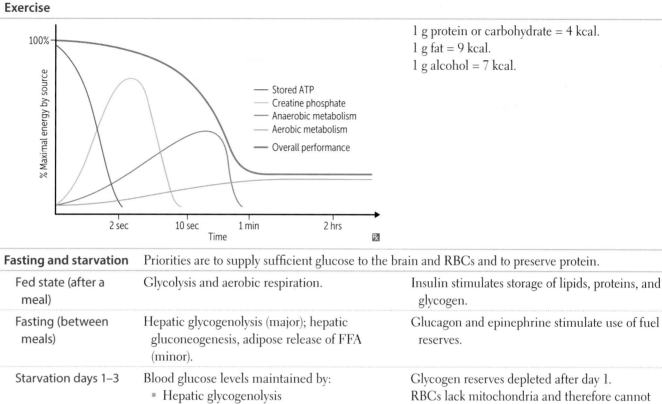

1 g protein or carbohydrate = 4 kcal.
1 g fat = 9 kcal.
1 g alcohol = 7 kcal.

Fasting and starvation	Priorities are to supply sufficient glucose to the brain and RBCs and to preserve protein.	
Fed state (after a meal)	Glycolysis and aerobic respiration.	Insulin stimulates storage of lipids, proteins, and glycogen.
Fasting (between meals)	Hepatic glycogenolysis (major); hepatic gluconeogenesis, adipose release of FFA (minor).	Glucagon and epinephrine stimulate use of fuel reserves.
Starvation days 1–3	Blood glucose levels maintained by: ▪ Hepatic glycogenolysis ▪ Adipose release of FFA ▪ Muscle and liver, which shift fuel use from glucose to FFA ▪ Hepatic gluconeogenesis from peripheral tissue lactate and alanine, and from adipose tissue glycerol and propionyl-CoA (from odd-chain FFA—the only triacylglycerol components that contribute to gluconeogenesis)	Glycogen reserves depleted after day 1. RBCs lack mitochondria and therefore cannot use ketones. 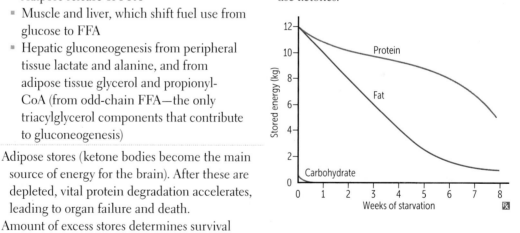
Starvation after day 3	Adipose stores (ketone bodies become the main source of energy for the brain). After these are depleted, vital protein degradation accelerates, leading to organ failure and death. Amount of excess stores determines survival time.	

Cholesterol synthesis

Cholesterol needed to maintain cell membrane integrity and to synthesize bile acid, steroids, and vitamin D.

Rate-limiting step catalyzed by HMG-CoA reductase (induced by insulin), which converts HMG-CoA to mevalonate. ⅔ of plasma cholesterol esterified by lecithin-cholesterol acyltransferase (LCAT).

Statins (e.g., atorvastatin) competitively and reversibly inhibit HMG-CoA reductase.

Lipid transport, key enzymes

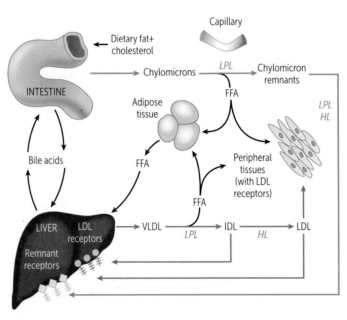

Pancreatic lipase—degradation of dietary triglycerides (TGs) in small intestine.
Lipoprotein lipase (LPL)—degradation of TGs circulating in chylomicrons and VLDLs. Found on vascular endothelial surface.
Hepatic TG lipase (HL)—degradation of TGs remaining in IDL.
Hormone-sensitive lipase—degradation of TGs stored in adipocytes.

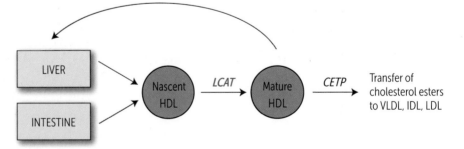

LCAT—catalyzes esterification of cholesterol.
Cholesterol ester transfer protein (CETP)—mediates transfer of cholesterol esters to other lipoprotein particles.

Major apolipoproteins

Apolipoprotein	Function	Chylomicron	Chylomicron remnant	VLDL	IDL	LDL	HDL
E	Mediates remnant uptake	✓	✓	✓	✓		✓
A-I	Activates LCAT	✓					✓
C-II	Lipoprotein lipase cofactor	✓		✓			✓
B-48	Mediates chylomicron secretion	✓	✓				
B-100	Binds LDL receptor			✓	✓	✓	

Lipoprotein functions

Lipoprotein functions — Lipoproteins are composed of varying proportions of cholesterol, TGs, and phospholipids. LDL and HDL carry the most cholesterol.

LDL transports cholesterol from liver to tissues.   LDL is Lousy.
HDL transports cholesterol from periphery to liver.   HDL is Healthy.

Chylomicron — Delivers dietary TGs to peripheral tissue. Delivers cholesterol to liver in the form of chylomicron remnants, which are mostly depleted of their TGs. Secreted by intestinal epithelial cells.

VLDL — Delivers hepatic TGs to peripheral tissue. Secreted by liver.

IDL — Formed in the degradation of VLDL. Delivers TGs and cholesterol to liver.

LDL — Delivers hepatic cholesterol to peripheral tissues. Formed by hepatic lipase modification of IDL in the peripheral tissue. Taken up by target cells via receptor-mediated endocytosis.

HDL — Mediates reverse cholesterol transport from periphery to liver. Acts as a repository for apolipoproteins C and E (which are needed for chylomicron and VLDL metabolism). Secreted from both liver and intestine. Alcohol ↑ synthesis.

Familial dyslipidemias

TYPE	INCREASED BLOOD LEVEL	PATHOPHYSIOLOGY
I—hyper-chylomicronemia	Chylomicrons, TG, cholesterol	Autosomal recessive. Lipoprotein lipase deficiency or altered apolipoprotein C-II. Causes pancreatitis, hepatosplenomegaly, and eruptive/pruritic xanthomas (no ↑ risk for atherosclerosis). Creamy layer in supernatant.
IIa—familial hyper-cholesterolemia	LDL, cholesterol	Autosomal dominant. Absent or defective LDL receptors. Heterozygotes (1:500) have cholesterol ≈ 300 mg/dL; homozygotes (very rare) have cholesterol ≈ 700+ mg/dL. Causes accelerated atherosclerosis (may have MI before age 20), tendon (Achilles) xanthomas, and corneal arcus.
IV—hyper-triglyceridemia	VLDL, TG	Autosomal dominant. Hepatic overproduction of VLDL. Hypertriglyceridemia (> 1000 mg/dL) can cause acute pancreatitis.

▶ NOTES

Microbiology

"*Support bacteria. They're the only culture some people have.*"
—Steven Wright

"*What lies behind us and what lies ahead of us are tiny matters compared to what lies within us.*"
—Henry S. Haskins

This high-yield material covers the basic concepts of microbiology. The emphasis in previous examinations has been approximately 40% bacteriology (20% basic, 20% quasi-clinical), 25% immunology, 25% virology (10% basic, 15% quasi-clinical), 5% parasitology, and 5% mycology.

Microbiology questions on the Step 1 exam often require two (or more) steps: Given a certain clinical presentation, you will first need to identify the most likely causative organism, and you will then need to provide an answer regarding some feature of that organism. For example, a description of a child with fever and a petechial rash will be followed by a question that reads, "From what site does the responsible organism usually enter the blood?"

This section therefore presents organisms in two major ways: in individual microbial "profiles" and in the context of the systems they infect and the clinical presentations they produce. You should become familiar with both formats. When reviewing the systems approach, remind yourself of the features of each microbe by returning to the individual profiles. Also be sure to memorize the laboratory characteristics that allow you to identify microbes.

▶ MICROBIOLOGY—BASIC BACTERIOLOGY

Bacterial structures

STRUCTURE	FUNCTION	CHEMICAL COMPOSITION
Peptidoglycan	Gives rigid support, protects against osmotic pressure.	Sugar backbone with peptide side chains cross-linked by transpeptidase.
Cell wall	Major surface antigen.	Peptidoglycan for support. Lipoteichoic acid induces TNF and IL-1.
Outer membrane (gram negatives)	Site of endotoxin (lipopolysaccharide [LPS]); major surface antigen.	Lipid A induces TNF and IL-1; O polysaccharide is the antigen.
Plasma membrane	Site of oxidative and transport enzymes.	Phospholipid bilayer.
Ribosome	Protein synthesis.	50S and 30S subunits.
Periplasm	Space between the cytoplasmic membrane and outer membrane in gram-negative bacteria.	Contains many hydrolytic enzymes, including β-lactamases.
Pilus/fimbria	Mediate adherence of bacteria to cell surface; sex pilus forms attachment between 2 bacteria during conjugation.	Glycoprotein.
Flagellum	Motility.	Protein.
Spore	Resistant to dehydration, heat, and chemicals.	Keratin-like coat; dipicolinic acid; peptidoglycan.
Plasmid	Contains a variety of genes for antibiotic resistance, enzymes, and toxins.	DNA.
Capsule	Protects against phagocytosis.	Organized, discrete polysaccharide layer (except *Bacillus anthracis*, which contains D-glutamate).
Glycocalyx	Mediates adherence to surfaces, especially foreign surfaces (e.g., indwelling catheters).	Loose network of polysaccharides.

Cell walls

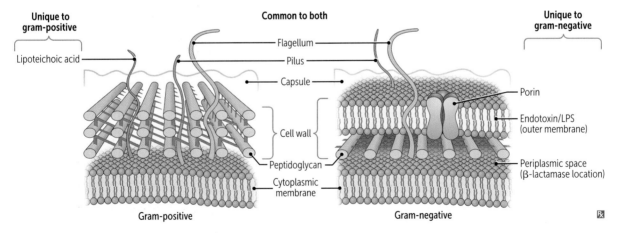

Bacterial taxonomy

MORPHOLOGY	Gram-positive examples	Gram-negative examples
Spherical (coccus)	*Staphylococcus* *Streptococcus*	*Moraxella catarrhalis* *Neisseria*
Rod (bacillus)	*Bacillus* *Clostridium* *Corynebacterium* *Gardnerella* (gram variable) *Lactobacillus* *Listeria* *Mycobacterium* (acid fast) *Propionibacterium*	Enterics: ▪ *Bacteroides* ▪ *Campylobacter* ▪ *E. coli* ▪ *Enterobacter* ▪ *Helicobacter* ▪ *Klebsiella* ▪ *Proteus* ▪ *Pseudomonas* ▪ *Salmonella* ▪ *Serratia* ▪ *Shigella* ▪ *Vibrio* ▪ *Yersinia* Respiratory: ▪ *Bordetella* ▪ *Haemophilus* (pleomorphic) ▪ *Legionella* (silver stain) Zoonotic: ▪ *Bartonella* ▪ *Brucella* ▪ *Francisella* ▪ *Pasteurella*
Branching filamentous	*Actinomyces* *Nocardia* (weakly acid fast)	
Pleomorphic		Chlamydiae (Giemsa) Rickettsiae (Giemsa)
Spiral		Spirochetes: ▪ *Borrelia* (Giemsa) ▪ *Leptospira* ▪ *Treponema*
No cell wall	*Mycoplasma*, *Ureaplasma* (contain sterols, which do not Gram stain)	

Gram stain limitations	These bugs do not Gram stain well:	These Microbes May Lack Real Color.
	Treponema (too thin to be visualized).	Treponemes—dark-field microscopy and fluorescent antibody staining.
	Mycobacteria (high lipid content; mycolic acids in cell wall detected by carbolfuchsin in acid-fast stain).	
	Mycoplasma (no cell wall).	
	Legionella pneumophila (primarily intracellular).	*Legionella*—silver stain.
	Rickettsia (intracellular parasite).	
	Chlamydia (intracellular parasite; lacks classic peptidoglycan because of low muramic acid).	

Stains

Giemsa	*Chlamydia, Borrelia, Rickettsia,* Trypanosomes, *Plasmodium.*	Certain Bugs Really Try my Patience.
PAS (periodic acid–Schiff)	Stains glycogen, mucopolysaccharides; used to diagnose Whipple disease (*Tropheryma whipplei*).	PASs the sugar.
Ziehl-Neelsen (carbol fuchsin)	Acid-fast bacteria (*Nocardia*, Mycobacteria), protozoa (*Cryptosporidium* oocysts).	Alternative is auramine-rhodamine stain for screening (inexpensive, more sensitive but less specific).
India ink	*Cryptococcus neoformans* (mucicarmine can also be used to stain thick polysaccharide capsule red).	
Silver stain	Fungi (e.g., *Pneumocystis*), *Legionella, Helicobacter pylori.*	

Special culture requirements

BUG	MEDIA USED FOR ISOLATION	MEDIA CONTENTS/OTHER
H. influenzae	Chocolate agar	Factors V (NAD^+) and X (hematin)
N. gonorrhoeae, N. meningitidis	Thayer-Martin agar	Vancomycin (inhibits gram-positive organisms), Trimethoprim, Colistin (inhibits gram-negative organisms except *Neisseria*), and Nystatin (inhibits fungi) Very Typically Cultures *Neisseria*
B. pertussis	Bordet-Gengou agar (**Bordet** for *Bordetella*) Regan-Lowe medium	Potato Charcoal, blood, and antibiotic
C. diphtheriae	Tellurite agar, Löffler medium	
M. tuberculosis	Löwenstein-Jensen agar	
M. pneumoniae	Eaton agar	Requires cholesterol
Lactose-fermenting enterics	MacConkey agar	Fermentation produces acid, causing colonies to turn pink
E. coli	Eosin–methylene blue (EMB) agar	Colonies with green metallic sheen
Legionella	Charcoal yeast extract agar buffered with cysteine and iron	
Fungi	Sabouraud agar	"Sab's a **fun guy**!"

Aerobes	Use an O_2-dependent system to generate ATP. Examples include *Nocardia*, *Pseudomonas aeruginosa*, and **Myco***Bacterium tuberculosis*. Reactivation of *M. tuberculosis* (e.g., after immunocompromise or TNF-α inhibitor use) has a predilection for the apices of the lung, which have the highest Po_2.	Nagging Pests Must Breathe.
Anaerobes	Examples include *Fusobacterium*, *Clostridium*, *Bacteroides*, and *Actinomyces*. They lack catalase and/or superoxide dismutase and are thus susceptible to oxidative damage. Generally foul smelling (short-chain fatty acids), are difficult to culture, and produce gas in tissue (CO_2 and H_2).	Anaerobes Frankly Can't Breathe Air. Anaerobes are normal flora in GI tract, typically pathogenic elsewhere. AminO_2glycosides are ineffective against anaerobes because these antibiotics require O_2 to enter into bacterial cell.

Intracellular bugs

Obligate intracellular	*Rickettsia, CHlamydia, COxiella.* Rely on host ATP.	Stay inside (cells) when it is Really CHilly and COld.
Facultative intracellular	*Salmonella, Neisseria, Brucella, Mycobacterium, Listeria, Francisella, Legionella, Yersinia pestis.*	Some Nasty Bugs May Live FacultativeLY.

Encapsulated bacteria	Examples are *Streptococcus pneumoniae, Haemophilus influenzae* type B, *Neisseria meningitidis, Escherichia coli, Salmonella, Klebsiella pneumoniae,* and group B Strep. Their capsules serve as an antiphagocytic virulence factor. Capsule + protein conjugate serves as an antigen in vaccines.	SHiNE SKiS. Are opsonized, and then cleared by spleen. Asplenics have ↓ opsonizing ability and thus ↑ risk for severe infections. Give *S. pneumoniae, H. influenzae, N. meningitidis* vaccines.
Encapsulated bacteria vaccines	Some vaccines containing polysaccharide capsule antigens are conjugated to a carrier protein, enhancing immunogenicity by promoting T-cell activation and subsequent class switching. A polysaccharide antigen alone cannot be presented to T cells.	Pneumococcal vaccine: PCV (pneumococcal conjugate vaccine, i.e., Prevnar); PPSV (pneumococcal polysaccharide vaccine with no conjugated protein, i.e., Pneumovax) *H. influenzae* type B (conjugate vaccine) Meningococcal vaccine (conjugate vaccine)
Urease-positive organisms	*Cryptococcus, H. pylori, Proteus, Ureaplasma, Nocardia, Klebsiella, S. epidermidis, S. saprophyticus.*	CHuck Norris hates PUNKSS.
Catalase-positive organisms	Catalase degrades H_2O_2 into H_2O and bubbles of O_2 **A** before it can be converted to microbicidal products by the enzyme myeloperoxidase. People with chronic granulomatous disease (NADPH oxidase deficiency) have recurrent infections with certain catalase ⊕ organisms. Examples: *Nocardia, Pseudomonas, Listeria, Aspergillus, Candida, E. coli,* Staphylococci, *Serratia.*	Cats Need PLACESS to hide.

Pigment-producing bacteria	*Actinomyces israelii*—yellow "sulfur" granules, which are composed of filaments of bacteria.	Israel has yellow sand.
	S. aureus—yellow pigment.	*Aureus* (Latin) = gold.
	Pseudomonas aeruginosa—blue-green pigment.	Aerugula is green.
	Serratia marcescens—red pigment.	*Serratia marcescens*—think red maraschino cherries.

Bacterial virulence factors	These promote evasion of host immune response.
Protein A	Binds Fc region of IgG. Prevents opsonization and phagocytosis. Expressed by *S. aureus*.
IgA protease	Enzyme that cleaves IgA. Secreted by *S. pneumoniae*, *H. influenzae* type B, and *Neisseria* (SHiN) in order to colonize respiratory mucosa.
M protein	Helps prevent phagocytosis. Expressed by group A streptococci. Shares similar epitopes to human cellular proteins (molecular mimicry); possibly underlies the autoimmune response seen in acute rheumatic fever.

Type III secretion system	Also known as "injectisome." Needle-like protein appendage facilitating direct delivery of toxins from certain gram-negative bacteria (e.g., *Pseudomonas*, *Salmonella*, *Shigella*, *E. coli*) to eukaryotic host cell.

Main features of exotoxins and endotoxins

PROPERTY	Exotoxin	Endotoxin
SOURCE	Certain species of gram-positive and gram-negative bacteria	Outer cell membrane of most gram-negative bacteria
SECRETED FROM CELL	Yes	No
CHEMISTRY	Polypeptide	Lipopolysaccharide (structural part of bacteria; released when lysed)
LOCATION OF GENES	Plasmid or bacteriophage	Bacterial chromosome
TOXICITY	High (fatal dose on the order of 1 μg)	Low (fatal dose on the order of hundreds of micrograms)
CLINICAL EFFECTS	Various effects (see following pages)	Fever, shock (hypotension), DIC
MODE OF ACTION	Various modes (see following pages)	Induces TNF, IL-1, and IL-6
ANTIGENICITY	Induces high-titer antibodies called antitoxins	Poorly antigenic
VACCINES	Toxoids used as vaccines	No toxoids formed and no vaccine available
HEAT STABILITY	Destroyed rapidly at 60°C (except staphylococcal enterotoxin)	Stable at 100°C for 1 hr
TYPICAL DISEASES	Tetanus, botulism, diphtheria	Meningococcemia; sepsis by gram-negative rods

Bugs with exotoxins

BACTERIA	TOXIN	MECHANISM	MANIFESTATION
Inhibit protein synthesis			
Corynebacterium diphtheriae	Diphtheria toxin[a]	Inactivate elongation factor (EF-2)	Pharyngitis with pseudomembranes in throat and severe lymphadenopathy (bull neck)
Pseudomonas aeruginosa	Exotoxin A[a]		Host cell death
Shigella spp.	Shiga toxin (ST)[a]	Inactivate 60S ribosome by removing adenine from rRNA	GI mucosal damage → dysentery; ST also enhances cytokine release, causing hemolytic-uremic syndrome (HUS)
Enterohemorrhagic *E. coli* (EHEC)	Shiga-like toxin (SLT)[a]		SLT enhances cytokine release, causing HUS (prototypically in EHEC serotype O157:H7). Unlike *Shigella*, EHEC does not invade host cells
Increase fluid secretion			
Enterotoxigenic *E. coli* (ETEC)	Heat-**labile** toxin (LT)[a]	Overactivates adenylate cyclase ($\uparrow$ cAMP) → $\uparrow$ Cl⁻ secretion in gut and H_2O efflux	Watery diarrhea: "**labile** in the Air (Adenylate cyclase), **stable** on the Ground (Guanylate cyclase)"
	Heat-**stable** toxin (ST)	Overactivates guanylate cyclase ($\uparrow$ cGMP) → $\downarrow$ resorption of NaCl and H_2O in gut	
Bacillus anthracis	Edema toxin[a]	Mimics the adenylate cyclase enzyme ($\uparrow$ cAMP)	Likely responsible for characteristic edematous borders of black eschar in cutaneous anthrax
Vibrio cholerae	Cholera toxin[a]	Overactivates adenylate cyclase ($\uparrow$ cAMP) by permanently activating G_s → $\uparrow$ Cl⁻ secretion in gut and H_2O efflux	Voluminous "rice-water" diarrhea
Inhibit phagocytic ability			
Bordetella pertussis	Pertussis toxin[a]	Overactivates adenylate cyclase ($\uparrow$ cAMP) by disabling G_i, impairing phagocytosis to permit survival of microbe	Whooping cough—child coughs on expiration and "whoops" on inspiration (toxin may not actually be a cause of cough; can cause "100-day cough" in adults)
Inhibit release of neurotransmitter			
Clostridium tetani	Tetanospasmin[a]	Both are proteases that cleave SNARE (soluble NSF attachment protein receptor), a set of proteins required for neurotransmitter release via vesicular fusion	Spasticity, risus sardonicus, and "lockjaw"; toxin prevents release of **inhibitory** (GABA and glycine) neurotransmitters from Renshaw cells in spinal cord
Clostridium botulinum	Botulinum toxin[a]		Flaccid paralysis, floppy baby; toxin prevents release of **stimulatory** (ACh) signals at neuromuscular junctions → flaccid paralysis

[a]Toxin is an ADP ribosylating A-B toxin: B (binding) component binds to host cell surface receptor, enabling endocytosis; A (active) component attaches ADP-ribosyl to disrupt host cell proteins.

Bugs with exotoxins *(continued)*

BACTERIA	TOXIN	MECHANISM	MANIFESTATION
Lyse cell membranes			
Clostridium perfringens	Alpha toxin	Phospholipase (lecithinase) that degrades tissue and cell membranes	Degradation of phospholipids → myonecrosis ("gas gangrene") and hemolysis ("double zone" of hemolysis on blood agar)
Streptococcus pyogenes	Streptolysin O	Protein that degrades cell membrane	Lyses RBCs; contributes to β-hemolysis; host antibodies against toxin (ASO) used to diagnose rheumatic fever (do not confuse with immune complexes of poststreptococcal glomerulonephritis)
Superantigens causing shock			
Staphylococcus aureus	Toxic shock syndrome toxin (TSST-1)	Binds to MHC II and TCR outside of antigen binding site to cause overwhelming release of IL-1, IL-2, IFN-γ, and TNF-α → shock	Toxic shock syndrome: fever, rash, shock; other toxins cause scalded skin syndrome (exfoliative toxin) and food poisoning (enterotoxin)
Streptococcus pyogenes	Exotoxin A		Toxic shock syndrome: fever, rash, shock

Endotoxin

LPS found in outer membrane of gram-negative bacteria (both cocci and rods).

ENDOTOXIN:
Edema
Nitric oxide
DIC/Death
Outer membrane
TNF-α
O-antigen
eXtremely heat stable
IL-1
Neutrophil chemotaxis

Bacterial genetics

Transformation	Ability to take up naked DNA (i.e., from cell lysis) from environment (also known as "competence"). A feature of many bacteria, especially *S. pneumoniae*, *H. influenzae* type B, and *Neisseria* (SHiN). Any DNA can be used. Adding deoxyribonuclease to environment will degrade naked DNA in medium → no transformation seen.

Conjugation

F⁺ × F⁻	F⁺ plasmid contains genes required for sex pilus and conjugation. Bacteria without this plasmid are termed F⁻. Sex pilus on F⁺ bacterium contacts F⁻ bacterium. A single strand of plasmid DNA is transferred across the conjugal bridge (also known as the "mating bridge"). No transfer of chromosomal DNA.
Hfr × F⁻	F⁺ plasmid can become incorporated into bacterial chromosomal DNA, termed high-frequency recombination (Hfr) cell. Replication of incorporated plasmid DNA may include some flanking chromosomal DNA. Transfer of plasmid and chromosomal genes.
Transposition	Segment of DNA (e.g., transposon) that can "jump" (excision and reintegration) from one location to another, can transfer genes from plasmid to chromosome and vice versa. When excision occurs, may include some flanking chromosomal DNA, which can be incorporated into a plasmid and transferred to another bacterium (e.g., *vanA* gene from vancomycin-resistant *Enterococcus* to *S. aureus*).

Transduction

Generalized	A "packaging" event. Lytic phage infects bacterium, leading to cleavage of bacterial DNA. Parts of bacterial chromosomal DNA may become packaged in viral capsid. Phage infects another bacterium, transferring these genes.
Specialized	An "excision" event. Lysogenic phage infects bacterium; viral DNA incorporates into bacterial chromosome. When phage DNA is excised, flanking bacterial genes may be excised with it. DNA is packaged into phage viral capsid and can infect another bacterium. Genes for the following 5 bacterial toxins are encoded in a lysogenic phage (**ABCDE**): ▪ Shig**A**-like toxin ▪ **B**otulinum toxin (certain strains) ▪ **C**holera toxin ▪ **D**iphtheria toxin ▪ **E**rythrogenic toxin of *Streptococcus pyogenes*

▶ MICROBIOLOGY—CLINICAL BACTERIOLOGY

Gram-positive lab algorithm

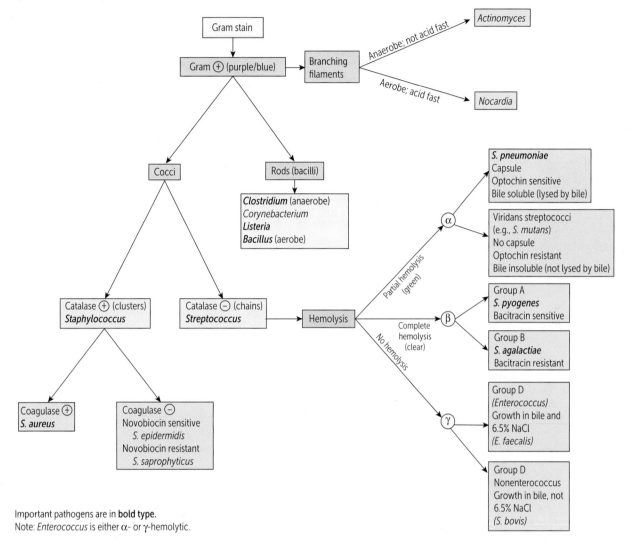

Important pathogens are in **bold type.**
Note: *Enterococcus* is either α- or γ-hemolytic.

Identification of gram-positive cocci

Staphylococci	NOvobiocin—*Saprophyticus* is Resistant; *Epidermidis* is Sensitive.	On the office's "**staph**" retreat, there was NO StRESs.
Streptococci	Optochin—*Viridans* is Resistant; *Pneumoniae* is Sensitive.	OVRPS (overpass).
	Bacitracin—group **B** strep are Resistant; group **A** strep are Sensitive.	B-BRAS.

α-hemolytic bacteria

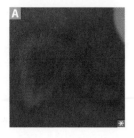

Form green ring around colonies on blood agar 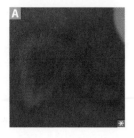. Include the following organisms:
- *Streptococcus pneumoniae* (catalase ⊖ and optochin sensitive)
- Viridans streptococci (catalase ⊖ and optochin resistant)

β-hemolytic bacteria

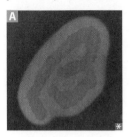

Form clear area of hemolysis on blood agar . Include the following organisms:
- *Staphylococcus aureus* (catalase and coagulase ⊕)
- *Streptococcus pyogenes*—group A strep (catalase ⊖ and bacitracin sensitive)
- *Streptococcus agalactiae*—group B strep (catalase ⊖ and bacitracin resistant)
- *Listeria monocytogenes* (tumbling motility, meningitis in newborns, unpasteurized milk)

Staphylococcus aureus

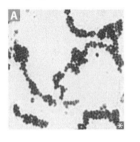

Gram-positive cocci in clusters . Protein A (virulence factor) binds Fc-IgG, inhibiting complement activation and phagocytosis. Commonly colonizes the nares.
Causes:
- Inflammatory disease—skin infections, organ abscesses, pneumonia (often after influenza virus infection), endocarditis, septic arthritis, and osteomyelitis.
- Toxin-mediated disease—toxic shock syndrome (TSST-1), scalded skin syndrome (exfoliative toxin), rapid-onset food poisoning (enterotoxins).
- MRSA (methicillin-resistant *S. aureus*) infection—important cause of serious nosocomial and community-acquired infections; resistant to methicillin and nafcillin because of altered penicillin-binding protein.

TSST is a superantigen that binds to MHC II and T-cell receptor, resulting in polyclonal T-cell activation. Staphylococcal toxic shock syndrome (TSS) presents as fever, vomiting, rash, desquamation, shock, end-organ failure. Associated with prolonged use of vaginal tampons or nasal packing. Compare with *Streptococcus pyogenes* TSS (a toxic shock–like syndrome associated with painful skin infection).

S. aureus food poisoning due to ingestion of preformed toxin → short incubation period (2–6 hr) followed by nonbloody diarrhea and emesis. Enterotoxin is heat stable → not destroyed by cooking.

Staph make catalase because they have more "**staff**." Bad staph (*aureus*) make coagulase and toxins. Forms fibrin clot around self → abscess.

Staphylococcus epidermidis

Infects prosthetic devices (e.g., hip implant, heart valve) and intravenous catheters by producing adherent biofilms. Component of normal skin flora; contaminates blood cultures. Novobiocin sensitive.

Staphylococcus saprophyticus

Second most common cause of uncomplicated UTI in young women (first is *E. coli*). Novobiocin resistant.

Streptococcus pneumoniae	Most common cause of: ■ Meningitis ■ Otitis media (in children) ■ Pneumonia ■ Sinusitis Lancet-shaped, gram-positive diplococci Ⓐ. Encapsulated. IgA protease.	*S. pneumoniae* **MOPS** are **M**ost **OP**tochin **S**ensitive. Pneumococcus is associated with "rusty" sputum, sepsis in sickle cell disease and splenectomy. No virulence without capsule.
Viridans group streptococci	α-hemolytic. They are normal flora of the oropharynx that cause dental caries (*Streptococcus mutans*) and subacute bacterial endocarditis at damaged **heart** valves (*S. sanguinis*). Resistant to optochin, differentiating them from S. *pneumoniae*, which is α-hemolytic but is optochin sensitive.	*Sanguinis* = **blood**. Think, "there is lots of **blood** in the **heart**" (endocarditis). S. *sanguinis* makes dextrans, which bind to fibrin-platelet aggregates on damaged heart valves. Viridans group strep live in the mouth because they are not afraid **of-the-chin** (**op-to-chin** resistant).
***Streptococcus pyogenes* (group A streptococci)**	Group A strep Ⓐ cause: ■ Pyogenic—pharyngitis, cellulitis, impetigo, erysipelas ■ Toxigenic—scarlet fever, toxic shock–like syndrome, necrotizing fasciitis ■ Immunologic—rheumatic fever, acute glomerulonephritis Bacitracin sensitive, β-hemolytic, pyrrolidonyl arylamidase (PYR) ⊕. Antibodies to M protein enhance host defenses against S. *pyogenes* but can give rise to rheumatic fever. ASO titer detects recent S. *pyogenes* infection.	J♥NES (major criteria for acute rheumatic fever): Joints—polyarthritis ♥—carditis Nodules (subcutaneous) Erythema marginatum Sydenham chorea **Pharyngitis** can result in rheumatic "**phever**" and glomerulone**phritis**. Impetigo more commonly precedes glomerulonephritis than pharyngitis. Scarlet fever—scarlet rash with sandpaper-like texture, strawberry tongue, circumoral pallor, subsequent desquamation.
***Streptococcus agalactiae* (group B streptococci)**	Bacitracin resistant, β-hemolytic, colonizes vagina; causes pneumonia, meningitis, and sepsis, mainly in **babies**. Produces CAMP factor, which enlarges the area of hemolysis formed by S. *aureus*. (Note: CAMP stands for the authors of the test, not cyclic AMP.) Hippurate test ⊕. Screen pregnant women at 35–37 weeks of gestation. Patients with ⊕ culture receive intrapartum penicillin prophylaxis.	Group **B** for **B**abies!

Enterococci (group D streptococci)	Enterococci (*E. faecalis* and *E. faecium*) are normal colonic flora that are penicillin G resistant and cause UTI, biliary tract infections, and subacute endocarditis (following GI/GU procedures). Lancefield group D includes the enterococci and the nonenterococcal group D streptococci. Lancefield grouping is based on differences in the C carbohydrate on the bacterial cell wall. Variable hemolysis. VRE (vancomycin-resistant enterococci) are an important cause of nosocomial infection.	Enterococci, hardier than nonenterococcal group D, can grow in 6.5% NaCl and bile (lab test). *Entero* = intestine, *faecalis* = feces, *strepto* = twisted (chains), *coccus* = berry.
***Streptococcus bovis* (group D streptococci)**	Colonizes the gut. *S. gallolyticus* (*S. bovis* biotype 1) can cause bacteremia and subacute endocarditis and is associated with colon cancer.	Bovis in the blood = cancer in the colon.

Corynebacterium diphtheriae
 	
	Causes diphtheria via exotoxin encoded by β-prophage. Potent exotoxin inhibits protein synthesis via ADP-ribosylation of EF-2. Symptoms include pseudomembranous pharyngitis (grayish-white membrane **A**) with lymphadenopathy, myocarditis, and arrhythmias.
	
	Lab diagnosis based on gram-positive rods with metachromatic (blue and red) granules and ⊕ Elek test for toxin.
	
	Toxoid vaccine prevents diphtheria.
		Coryne = club shaped.
		Black colonies on cystine-tellurite agar.
		ABCDEFG:
		  ADP-ribosylation
		  β-prophage
		  Corynebacterium
		  Diphtheriae
		  Elongation Factor 2
		  Granules

Spores: bacterial	Some bacteria can form spores at the end of the stationary phase when nutrients are limited. Spores are highly resistant to heat and chemicals. Have dipicolinic acid in their core. Have no metabolic activity. Must autoclave to potentially kill spores (as is done to surgical equipment) by steaming at 121°C for 15 minutes.	**Species** *Bacillus anthracis* *Bacillus cereus* *Clostridium botulinum* *Clostridium difficile* *Clostridium perfringens* *Clostridium tetani* *Coxiella burnetii* **Disease** Anthrax Food poisoning Botulism Antibiotic-associated colitis Gas gangrene Tetanus Q fever

Clostridia (with exotoxins)	Gram-positive, spore-forming, obligate anaerobic bacilli.	
C. tetani	Produces tetanospasmin, an exotoxin causing tetanus. Tetanus toxin (and botulinum toxin) are proteases that cleave SNARE proteins for neurotransmitters. Blocks release of inhibitory neurotransmitters, GABA and glycine, from Renshaw cells in spinal cord. Causes **spastic** paralysis, trismus (lockjaw), risus sardonicus (raised eyebrows and open grin). Prevent with tetanus vaccine. Treat with antitoxin +/– vaccine booster, diazepam (for muscle spasms).	Tetanus is **tetanic** paralysis.
C. botulinum	Produces a preformed, heat-labile toxin that inhibits ACh release at the neuromuscular junction, causing botulism. In adults, disease is caused by ingestion of preformed toxin. In babies, ingestion of spores in honey causes disease (**floppy** baby syndrome). Treat with antitoxin.	*Botulinum* is from bad **bott**les of food and honey (causes a **flaccid** paralysis).
C. perfringens	Produces α toxin (lecithinase, a phospholipase) that can cause myonecrosis (gas gangrene 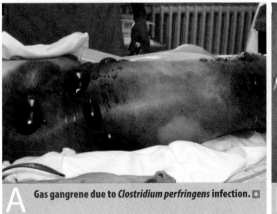) and hemolysis.	*Perfringens* **perf**orates a gangrenous leg.
C. difficile	Produces 2 toxins. Toxin A, enterotoxin, binds to the brush border of the gut. Toxin B, cytotoxin, causes cytoskeletal disruption via actin depolymerization → pseudomembranous colitis 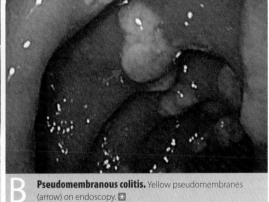 → diarrhea. Often 2° to antibiotic use, especially clindamycin or ampicillin. Diagnosed by detection one or both toxins in stool by PCR.	*Difficile* causes **di**arrhea. Treatment: metronidazole or oral vancomycin. For recurrent cases, consider repeating prior regimen, fidaxomicin, or fecal microbiota transplant.

A **Gas gangrene due to *Clostridium perfringens* infection.** ✴

B **Pseudomembranous colitis.** Yellow pseudomembranes (arrow) on endoscopy. ✴

Anthrax	Caused by *Bacillus anthracis*, a gram-positive, spore-forming rod (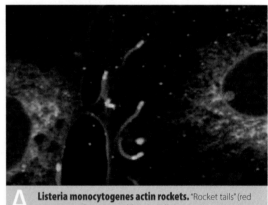, left) that produces anthrax toxin. The only bacterium with a polypeptide capsule (contains D-glutamate).	
Cutaneous anthrax	Painless papule surrounded by vesicles → ulcer with black eschar (A, right) (painless, necrotic) → uncommonly progresses to bacteremia and death.	
Pulmonary anthrax	Inhalation of spores → flu-like symptoms that rapidly progress to fever, pulmonary hemorrhage, mediastinitis, and shock.	

A **Anthrax.** Gram-positive rods (left). ❇ Ulcer with black eschar/crust (right). ❇

Bacillus cereus	Causes food poisoning. Spores survive cooking rice. Keeping rice warm results in germination of spores and enterotoxin formation. Emetic type usually seen with rice and pasta. Nausea and vomiting within 1–5 hr. Caused by cereulide, a preformed toxin. Diarrheal type causes watery, nonbloody diarrhea and GI pain within 8–18 hr.	Reheated rice syndrome.

Listeria monocytogenes	Facultative intracellular microbe; acquired by ingestion of unpasteurized dairy products and cold deli meats, via transplacental transmission, or by vaginal transmission during birth. Forms "rocket tails" A (via actin polymerization) that allow intracellular movement and cell-to-cell spread across cell membranes, thereby avoiding antibody. Characteristic tumbling motility; is only gram-positive organism to produce endotoxin. Can cause amnionitis, septicemia, and spontaneous abortion in pregnant women; granulomatosis infantiseptica; neonatal meningitis; meningitis in immunocompromised patients; mild gastroenteritis in healthy individuals. Treatment: gastroenteritis is usually self limited; ampicillin in infants, immunocompromised, and the elderly as empirical treatment of meningitis.	

A **Listeria monocytogenes actin rockets.** "Rocket tails" (red structures) of *Listeria* enable intracellular movement and spread between two cells (green structures). ❇

Actinomyces vs. *Nocardia*

Both form long, branching filaments resembling fungi.

Actinomyces	*Nocardia*
Gram-positive anaerobe 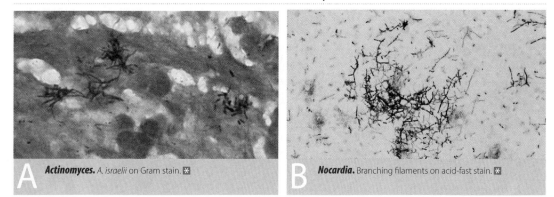	Gram-positive aerobe
Not acid fast	Acid fast (weak)
Normal oral flora	Found in soil
Causes oral/facial abscesses that drain through sinus tracts, forms yellow "sulfur granules"	Causes pulmonary infections in immunocompromised and cutaneous infections after trauma in immunocompetent
Treat with penicillin	Treat with sulfonamides

Treatment is a **SNAP**: Sulfonamides—Nocardia; Actinomyces—Penicillin

A **Actinomyces.** *A. israelii* on Gram stain. ✳

B **Nocardia.** Branching filaments on acid-fast stain. ✳

1° and 2° tuberculosis

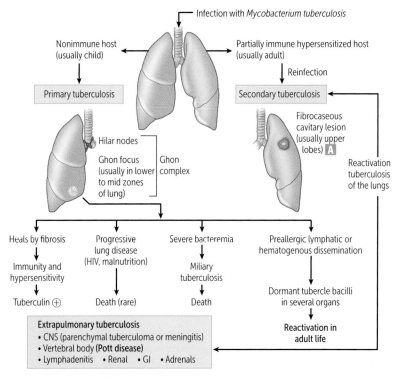

Infection with *Mycobacterium tuberculosis*

Nonimmune host (usually child)

Partially immune hypersensitized host (usually adult)

Primary tuberculosis

Reinfection

Secondary tuberculosis

Hilar nodes

Ghon focus (usually in lower to mid zones of lung)

Ghon complex

Fibrocaseous cavitary lesion (usually upper lobes) **A**

Reactivation tuberculosis of the lungs

Heals by fibrosis

Progressive lung disease (HIV, malnutrition)

Severe bacteremia

Preallergic lymphatic or hematogenous dissemination

Immunity and hypersensitivity

Miliary tuberculosis

Dormant tubercle bacilli in several organs

Tuberculin ⊕

Death (rare)

Death

Reactivation in adult life

Extrapulmonary tuberculosis
- CNS (parenchymal tuberculoma or meningitis)
- Vertebral body (**Pott disease**)
- Lymphadenitis • Renal • GI • Adrenals

PPD ⊕ if current infection or past exposure. False positives with BCG vaccination (further workup required).

PPD ⊖ if no infection or anergic (steroids, malnutrition, immunocompromise) and in sarcoidosis.

Interferon-γ release assay (IGRA) has fewer false positives from BCG vaccination.

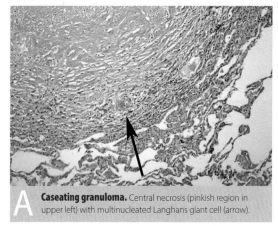

A **Caseating granuloma.** Central necrosis (pinkish region in upper left) with multinucleated Langhans giant cell (arrow).

Mycobacteria

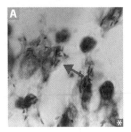

Mycobacterium tuberculosis (TB, often resistant to multiple drugs).

M. avium–intracellulare (causes disseminated, non-TB disease in AIDS; often resistant to multiple drugs). Prophylaxis with azithromycin when CD4+ count < 50 cells/mm^3.

M. scrofulaceum (cervical lymphadenitis in children).

M. marinum (hand infection in aquarium handlers).

All mycobacteria are acid-fast organisms (pink rods; arrow in A).

TB symptoms include fever, night sweats, weight loss, cough (nonproductive or productive), hemoptysis.

Cord factor in virulent strains inhibits macrophage maturation and induces release of TNF-α. Sulfatides (surface glycolipids) inhibit phagolysosomal fusion.

Leprosy (Hansen disease)

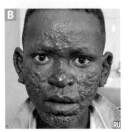

Caused by *Mycobacterium leprae*, an acid-fast bacillus that likes cool temperatures (infects skin and superficial nerves—"glove and stocking" loss of sensation A) and cannot be grown in vitro. Reservoir in United States: armadillos.

Hansen disease has 2 forms:

- Lepromatous—presents diffusely over the skin, with leonine (lion-like) facies B, and is communicable; characterized by low cell-mediated immunity with a humoral Th2 response.

- Tuberculoid—limited to a few hypoesthetic, hairless skin plaques; characterized by high cell-mediated immunity with a largely Th1-type immune response.

Treatment: dapsone and rifampin for tuberculoid form; clofazimine is added for lepromatous form.

Lepromatous can be lethal.

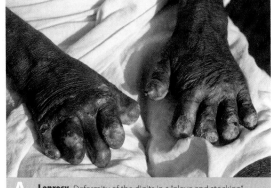

Leprosy. Deformity of the digits in a "glove and stocking" distribution due to sensory loss and repeated trauma.

Gram-negative lab algorithm

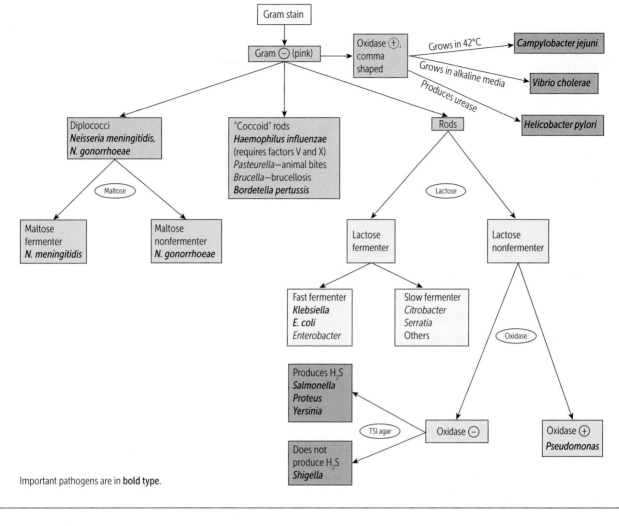

Important pathogens are in **bold type**.

| **Lactose-fermenting enteric bacteria** | Fermentation of **lactose** → pink colonies on MacConkey agar. Examples include *Citrobacter, Klebsiella, E. coli, Enterobacter,* and *Serratia* (weak fermenter). *E. coli* produces β-galactosidase, which breaks down lactose into glucose and galactose. | **Lactose** is key. Test with MacCon**KEE'S** agar. EMB agar—lactose fermenters grow as purple/black colonies. *E. coli* grows colonies with a green sheen. |

Neisseria

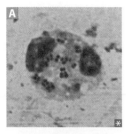

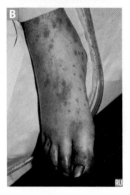

Gram-negative diplococci. Both ferment glucose and produce IgA proteases. *N. gonorrhoeae* is often intracellular (within neutrophils) .

MeninGococci ferment Maltose and Glucose. Gonococci ferment Glucose.

Gonococci	Meningococci
No polysaccharide capsule	Polysaccharide capsule
No maltose fermentation	Maltose fermentation
No vaccine due to antigenic variation of pilus proteins	Vaccine (type B vaccine not widely available)
Sexually or perinatally transmitted	Transmitted via respiratory and oral secretions
Causes gonorrhea, septic arthritis, neonatal conjunctivitis, pelvic inflammatory disease (PID), and Fitz-Hugh–Curtis syndrome	Causes meningococcemia 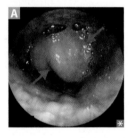 and meningitis, Waterhouse-Friderichsen syndrome
Condoms ↓ sexual transmission. Erythromycin ointment prevents neonatal transmission	Rifampin, ciprofloxacin, or ceftriaxone prophylaxis in close contacts
Treatment: ceftriaxone + (azithromycin or doxycycline) for possible chlamydial coinfection	Treatment: ceftriaxone or penicillin G

Haemophilus influenzae

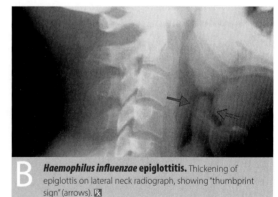

Small gram-negative (coccobacillary) rod. Aerosol transmission. Nontypeable strains are the most common cause of mucosal infections (otitis media, conjunctivitis, bronchitis) as well as invasive infections since the vaccine for capsular type b was introduced. Produces IgA protease. Culture on chocolate agar, which contains factors V (NAD$^+$) and X (hematin) for growth; can also be grown with *S. aureus*, which provides factor V through the hemolysis of RBCs. *HaEMOPhilus* causes **E**piglottitis (["cherry red" in children), **M**eningitis, **O**titis media, and **P**neumonia.

Treat mucosal infections with amoxicillin +/– clavulanate.

Treat meningitis with ceftriaxone. Rifampin prophylaxis for close contacts.

Vaccine contains type b capsular polysaccharide (polyribosylribitol phosphate) conjugated to diphtheria toxoid or other protein. Given between 2 and 18 months of age.

Does not cause the flu (influenza virus does).

B ***Haemophilus influenzae* epiglottitis.** Thickening of epiglottis on lateral neck radiograph, showing "thumbprint sign" (arrows). ℞

Legionella pneumophila

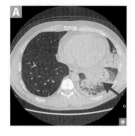

Gram-negative rod. Gram stains poorly—use **silver** stain. Grow on **charcoal** yeast extract culture with **iron** and **cysteine**. Detected by presence of antigen in urine. Labs may show hyponatremia. Aerosol transmission from environmental water source habitat (e.g., air conditioning systems, hot water tanks). No person-to-person transmission. Treatment: macrolide or quinolone.

Legionnaires' disease—severe pneumonia (often unilateral and lobar **A**), fever, GI and CNS symptoms.

Pontiac fever—mild flu-like syndrome.

Think of a French **legionnaire** (soldier) with his **silver** helmet, sitting around a campfire (**charcoal**) with his **iron** dagger—he is no **sissy** (cysteine).

Pseudomonas aeruginosa

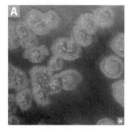

Aerobic, motile, gram-negative rod. Non-lactose fermenting, oxidase ⊕. Produces pyocyanin (blue-green pigment **A**); has a grape-like odor. Produces endotoxin (fever, shock) and exotoxin A (inactivates EF-2).

PSEUDDOmonas is associated with:
- Pneumonia
- Sepsis
- Otitis **E**xterna (swimmer's ear)
- UTIs
- **D**rug use
- **D**iabetes
- **O**steomyelitis (e.g., puncture wounds)

Depending on source and severity, treatment may include:
- Extended-spectrum β-lactams (e.g., piperacillin, ticarcillin, cefepime)
- Carbapenems (e.g., imipenem, meropenem)
- Monobactams (e.g., aztreonam)
- Fluoroquinolones (e.g., ciprofloxacin)
- Aminoglycosides (e.g., gentamicin, tobramycin)
- For multidrug-resistant strains: colistin, polymyxin B

Ecthyma gangrenosum—rapidly progressive, necrotic cutaneous lesion **B** caused by *Pseudomonas* bacteremia. Typically seen in immunocompromised patients.

Aeruginosa—aerobic.

Think *Pseudomonas* in burn victims.

Mucoid polysaccharide capsule may contribute to chronic pneumonia in cystic fibrosis patients due to biofilm formation.

Can cause wound infection in burn victims.

Frequently found in water → hot tub folliculitis.

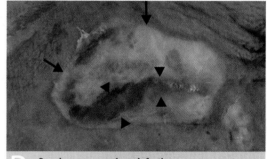

B ***Pseudomonas aeruginosa* infection.** Ecthyma gangrenosum of the chest. Large ulcer (arrows) with necrotic region (arrowheads). ✱

E. coli

E. coli virulence factors: fimbriae—cystitis and pyelonephritis; K capsule—pneumonia, neonatal meningitis; LPS endotoxin—septic shock.

STRAIN	TOXIN AND MECHANISM	PRESENTATION
EIEC	Microbe invades intestinal mucosa and causes necrosis and inflammation. Clinical manifestations similar to *Shigella*.	Invasive; dysentery.
ETEC	Produces heat-labile and heat-stable enteroToxins. No inflammation or invasion.	Travelers' diarrhea (watery).
EPEC	No toxin produced. Adheres to apical surface, flattens villi, prevents absorption.	Diarrhea, usually in children (Pediatrics).
EHEC	Also called STEC (Shiga toxin–producing *E. coli*). O157:H7 is most common serotype in U.S. Shiga-like toxin causes **hemolytic-uremic syndrome**: triad of anemia, thrombocytopenia, and acute renal failure due to microthrombi forming on damaged endothelium → mechanical hemolysis (with schistocytes on peripheral blood smear), platelet consumption, and ↓ renal blood flow.	Dysentery (toxin alone causes necrosis and inflammation). Does not ferment sorbitol (distinguishes EHEC from other *E. coli*).

Klebsiella

An intestinal flora that causes lobar pneumonia in alcoholics and diabetics when aspirated. Very mucoid colonies caused by abundant polysaccharide capsules. Dark red "currant jelly" sputum (blood/mucus). Also cause of nosocomial UTIs.

4 A's of *KlebsiellA*:
Aspiration pneumonia
Abscess in lungs and liver
Alcoholics
di-A-betics

Campylobacter jejuni

Major cause of bloody diarrhea, especially in children. Fecal-oral transmission through person-to-person contact or via ingestion of poultry, meat, unpasteurized milk. Contact with infected animals (dogs, cats, pigs) is also a risk factor. Comma- or S-shaped, oxidase ⊕, grows at 42°C ("*Campylobacter* likes the hot **camp**fire"). Common antecedent to Guillain-Barré syndrome and reactive arthritis.

Salmonella* vs. *Shigella Both *Salmonella* and *Shigella* are gram-negative bacilli that are non-lactose fermenters and oxidase ⊖.

	Salmonella typhi	*Salmonella* spp. (except *S. typhi*)	*Shigella*
RESERVOIRS	Humans only	Humans and animals	Humans only
SPREAD	Can disseminate hematogenously	Can disseminate hematogenously	Cell to cell; no hematogenous spread
H$_2$S PRODUCTION	Yes	Yes	No
FLAGELLA	Yes (**salmon swim**)	Yes (**salmon swim**)	No
VIRULENCE FACTORS	Endotoxin; Vi capsule	Endotoxin	Endotoxin; Shiga toxin (enterotoxin)
INFECTIOUS DOSE (ID$_{50}$)	High—large inoculum required because organism inactivated by gastric acids	High	Low—very small inoculum required; resistant to gastric acids
EFFECT OF ANTIBIOTICS ON FECAL EXCRETION	Prolongs duration	Prolongs duration	Shortens duration
IMMUNE RESPONSE	Primarily monocytes	PMNs in disseminated disease	Primarily PMN infiltration
GI MANIFESTATIONS	Constipation, followed by diarrhea	Bloody diarrhea	Bloody diarrhea (bacillary dysentery)
VACCINE	Oral vaccine contains live attenuated *S. typhi* IM vaccine contains Vi capsular polysaccharide	No vaccine	No vaccine
UNIQUE PROPERTIES	▪ Causes typhoid fever (rose spots on abdomen, constipation, abdominal pain, fever); treat with ceftriaxone or fluoroquinolone ▪ Carrier state with gallbladder colonization	▪ Poultry, eggs, pets, and turtles are common sources ▪ Gastroenteritis is usually caused by non-typhoidal *Salmonella*	▪ **Four F's:** **F**ingers, **F**lies, **F**ood, **F**eces ▪ In order of decreasing severity (less toxin produced): *S. dysenteriae*, *S. flexneri*, *S. boydii*, *S. sonnei* ▪ Invasion is the key to pathogenicity; organisms that produce little toxin can cause disease due to invasion

Vibrio cholerae Produces profuse rice-water diarrhea via enterotoxin that permanently activates G$_s$, ↑ cAMP. Comma shaped 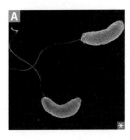, oxidase ⊕, grows in alkaline media. Endemic to developing countries. Prompt oral rehydration is necessary.

Yersinia enterocolitica Usually transmitted from pet feces (e.g., puppies), contaminated milk, or pork. Causes acute diarrhea or pseudoappendicitis (right lower abdominal pain due to mesenteric adenitis and/or terminal ileitis).

Helicobacter pylori

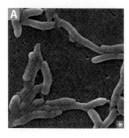

Causes gastritis and peptic ulcers (especially duodenal). Risk factor for peptic ulcer, gastric adenocarcinoma, and MALT lymphoma. Curved gram-negative rod A that is catalase, oxidase, and urease ⊕ (can use urea breath test or fecal antigen test for diagnosis). Creates alkaline environment.

Most common initial treatment is triple therapy: proton pump inhibitor + clarithromycin + amoxicillin (or metronidazole if penicillin allergy).

Spirochetes

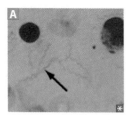

Spiral-shaped bacteria with axial filaments. Includes *Borrelia* (big size), *Leptospira*, and *Treponema*. Only *Borrelia* can be visualized using aniline dyes (Wright or Giemsa stain) in light microscopy A due to size. *Treponema* is visualized by dark-field microscopy.

BLT.
Borrelia is Big.

Leptospira interrogans

Found in water contaminated with animal urine, causes **leptospirosis**—flu-like symptoms, myalgias (classically of calves), jaundice, photophobia with conjunctival suffusion (erythema without exudate). Prevalent among surfers and in tropics (i.e., Hawaii).

Weil disease (icterohemorrhagic leptospirosis)—severe form with jaundice and azotemia from liver and kidney dysfunction, fever, hemorrhage, and anemia.

Lyme disease

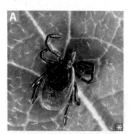

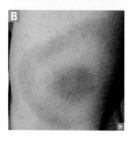

Caused by *Borrelia burgdorferi*, which is transmitted by the *Ixodes* deer tick A (also vector for *Anaplasma* spp. and protozoa *Babesia*). Natural reservoir is the mouse. Mice are important to tick life cycle. Common in northeastern United States.

- Initial symptoms—erythema chronicum migrans B, flu-like symptoms, +/– facial nerve palsy.
- Later symptoms—monoarthritis (large joints) and migratory polyarthritis, cardiac (AV nodal block), neurologic (meningitis, facial nerve palsy, polyneuropathy).

Treatment: doxycycline, ceftriaxone.

A Key **Lyme** pie to the **FACE**:
Facial nerve palsy (typically bilateral)
Arthritis
Cardiac block
Erythema chronicum migrans

Syphilis	Caused by spirochete *Treponema pallidum*.
1° syphilis	Localized disease presenting with **painless** chancre **A**. If available, use dark-field microscopy to visualize treponemes in fluid from chancre **B**. VDRL ⊕ in ~ 80%.
2° syphilis	Disseminated disease with constitutional symptoms, maculopapular rash **C** (including palms and soles **D**), condylomata lata **E** (smooth, moist, painless, wart-like white lesions on genitals); also confirmable with dark-field microscopy. Serologic testing: VDRL/RPR (nonspecific), confirm diagnosis with specific test (e.g., FTA-ABS). Secondary syphilis = Systemic. Latent syphilis (⊕ serology without symptoms) follows.
3° syphilis	Gummas **F** (chronic granulomas), aortitis (vasa vasorum destruction), neurosyphilis (tabes dorsalis, "general paresis"), Argyll Robertson pupil (constricts with accommodation but is not reactive to light; also called "prostitute's pupil" since it accommodates but does not react). Signs: broad-based ataxia, ⊕ Romberg, Charcot joint, stroke without hypertension. For neurosyphilis: test spinal fluid with VDRL and PCR.
Congenital syphilis	Presents with facial abnormalities such as rhagades (linear scars at angle of mouth, black arrow in **G**), snuffles (nasal discharge, red arrow in **G**), saddle nose, notched (Hutchinson) teeth **H**, mulberry molars, and short maxilla; saber shins; CN VIII deafness. To prevent, treat mother early in pregnancy, as placental transmission typically occurs after first trimester.

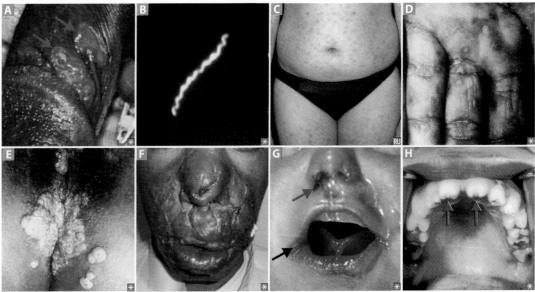

VDRL false positives	VDRL detects nonspecific antibody that reacts with beef cardiolipin. Inexpensive, widely available test for syphilis, quantitative, sensitive but not specific. False-positive results on **VDRL** with: **V**iral infection (mono, hepatitis) **D**rugs **R**heumatic fever **L**upus and leprosy
Jarisch-Herxheimer reaction	Flu-like syndrome (fever, chills, headache, myalgia) after antibiotics are started; due to killed bacteria (usually spirochetes) releasing endotoxins.

Zoonotic bacteria Zoonosis: infectious disease transmitted between animals and humans.

SPECIES	DISEASE	TRANSMISSION AND SOURCE
Anaplasma spp.	Anaplasmosis	*Ixodes* ticks (live on deer and mice)
Bartonella spp.	Cat scratch disease, bacillary angiomatosis	Cat scratch
Borrelia burgdorferi	Lyme disease	*Ixodes* ticks (live on deer and mice)
Borrelia recurrentis	**Relapsing** fever	Louse (recurrent due to variable surface antigens)
Brucella spp.	Brucellosis/undulant fever	Unpasteurized dairy
Campylobacter	Bloody diarrhea	Puppies, livestock (fecal-oral, ingestion of undercooked meat)
Chlamydophila psittaci	Psittacosis	Parrots, other birds
Coxiella burnetii	Q fever	Aerosols of cattle/sheep amniotic fluid
Ehrlichia chaffeensis	Ehrlichiosis	*Ambylomma* (Lone Star tick)
Francisella tularensis	Tularemia	Ticks, rabbits, deer fly
Leptospira spp.	Leptospirosis	Animal urine
Mycobacterium leprae	Leprosy	Humans with lepromatous leprosy; armadillo (rare)
Pasteurella multocida	Cellulitis, osteomyelitis	Animal bite, cats, dogs
Rickettsia prowazekii	Epidemic typhus	Louse
Rickettsia rickettsii	Rocky Mountain spotted fever	*Dermacentor* (dog tick)
Rickettsia typhi	Endemic typhus	Fleas
Salmonella	Diarrhea (which may be bloody), vomiting, fever, abdominal cramps	Reptiles and poultry
Yersinia pestis	Plague	Fleas (rats and prairie dogs are reservoirs)

Gardnerella vaginalis

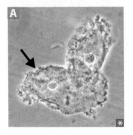

A pleomorphic, gram-variable rod involved in bacterial vaginosis. Presents as a gray vaginal discharge with a **fishy** smell; nonpainful (vs. vaginitis). Associated with sexual activity, but not sexually transmitted. Bacterial vaginosis is also characterized by overgrowth of certain anaerobic bacteria in vagina. **Clue** cells, or vaginal epithelial cells covered with *Gardnerella* bacteria ("stippled" appearance along outer margins), are visible under the microscope (arrow in A).

Treatment: metronidazole or clindamycin.

I don't have a **clue** why I smell **fish** in the **vagina** garden!

Amine whiff test—mixing discharge with 10% KOH enhances fishy odor.

Rickettsial diseases and vector-borne illness	Treatment for all: doxycycline.	
RASH COMMON		
Rocky Mountain spotted fever	*Rickettsia rickettsii*, vector is tick. Despite its name, disease occurs primarily in the South Atlantic states, especially North Carolina. Rash typically starts at wrists **A** and ankles and then spreads to trunk, palms, and soles.	Classic triad—headache, fever, rash (vasculitis). **Palms** and **soles** rash is seen in Coxsackievirus **A** infection (hand, foot, and mouth disease), Rocky Mountain spotted fever, and 2° Syphilis (you drive **CARS** using your **palms** and **soles**).
Typhus	Endemic (fleas)—*R. typhi*. Epidemic (human body louse)—*R. prowazekii*. Rash starts centrally and spreads out, sparing palms and soles.	*Rickettsii* on the w**R**ists, **T**yphus on the **T**runk.
RASH RARE		
Ehrlichiosis	*Ehrlichia*, vector is tick. Monocytes with morulae **B** (berry-like inclusions) in cytoplasm.	
Anaplasmosis	*Anaplasma*, vector is tick. Granulocytes with morulae in cytoplasm.	
Q fever	*Coxiella burnetii*, no arthropod vector. Spores inhaled as aerosols from cattle/sheep amniotic fluid. Presents as pneumonia. Most common cause of culture ⊖ endocarditis.	**Q** fever is **Q**ueer because it has no rash or vector and its causative organism can survive outside in its endospore form. Not in the *Rickettsia* genus, but closely related.

A **Rickettsial diseases.** Rocky Mountain spotted fever. ✳

B **Rickettsial diseases.** *Ehrlichia* morulae (arrows) in cytoplasm of monocyte. ✳

Chlamydiae

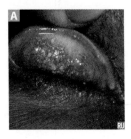

Chlamydiae cannot make their own ATP. They are obligate intracellular organisms that cause mucosal infections. 2 forms:
- Elementary body (small, dense) is "Enfectious" and Enters cell via Endocytosis; transforms into reticulate body.
- Reticulate body Replicates in cell by fission; Reorganizes into elementary bodies.

Chlamydia trachomatis causes reactive arthritis (Reiter syndrome), follicular conjunctivitis 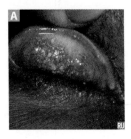, nongonococcal urethritis, and PID.

C. pneumoniae and *C. psittaci* cause atypical pneumonia; transmitted by aerosol.

Treatment: azithromycin (favored because one-time treatment) or doxycycline.

Chlamys = cloak (intracellular).
Chlamydophila psittaci—notable for an avian reservoir.

Lab diagnosis: cytoplasmic inclusions seen on Giemsa or fluorescent antibody–stained smear.

The chlamydial cell wall lacks classic peptidoglycan (due to reduced muramic acid), rendering β-lactam antibiotics less effective.

Chlamydia trachomatis serotypes

Types A, B, and C	Chronic infection, cause blindness due to follicular conjunctivitis in Africa.	**ABC** = **A**frica, **B**lindness, **C**hronic infection.
Types D–K	Urethritis/PID, ectopic pregnancy, neonatal pneumonia (staccato cough) with eosinophilia, neonatal conjunctivitis.	D–K = everything else. Neonatal disease can be acquired during passage through infected birth canal.
Types L1, L2, and L3	Lymphogranuloma venereum—small, painless ulcers on genitals → swollen, painful inguinal lymph nodes that ulcerate (buboes). Treat with doxycycline.	

Mycoplasma pneumoniae

Classic cause of atypical "walking" pneumonia (insidious onset, headache, nonproductive cough, patchy or diffuse interstitial infiltrate). X-ray looks worse than patient. High titer of cold agglutinins (IgM), which can agglutinate or lyse RBCs. Grown on Eaton agar.

Treatment: macrolides, doxycycline, or fluoroquinolone (penicillin ineffective since *Mycoplasma* have no cell wall).

No cell wall. Not seen on Gram stain. Pleomorphic .

Bacterial membrane contains sterols for stability.

Mycoplasmal pneumonia is more common in patients < 30 years old.

Frequent outbreaks in military recruits and prisons.

▶ MICROBIOLOGY—MYCOLOGY

Systemic mycoses
All of the following can cause pneumonia and can disseminate. All are caused by dimorphic fungi: cold (20°C) = mold; heat (37°C) = yeast. The only exception is coccidioidomycosis, which is a spherule (not yeast) in tissue. Treatment: fluconazole or itraconazole for **local** infection; amphotericin B for **systemic** infection. Systemic mycoses can mimic TB (granuloma formation), except, unlike TB, have no person-person transmission.

DISEASE	ENDEMIC LOCATION AND PATHOLOGIC FEATURES	NOTES
Histoplasmosis 	Mississippi and Ohio River valleys. Causes pneumonia. Macrophage filled with *Histoplasma* (smaller than RBC) **A**.	Histo hides (within macrophages). Bird or bat droppings.
Blastomycosis 	States east of Mississippi River and Central America. Causes inflammatory lung disease and can disseminate to skin and bone. Forms granulomatous nodules. Broad-base budding (same size as RBC) **B**.	Blasto buds broadly.
Coccidioidomycosis 	Southwestern United States, California. Causes pneumonia and meningitis; can disseminate to bone and skin. Case rate ↑ after earthquakes (spores in dust thrown into air → inhaled → spherules in lung). Spherule (much larger than RBC) filled with endospores **C**.	Coccidio crowds. "(San Joaquin) Valley fever". "Desert bumps" = erythema nodosum "Desert rheumatism" = arthralgias
Paracoccidioidomycosis 	Latin America. Budding yeast with "**captain's wheel**" formation (much larger than RBC) **D**.	Paracoccidio **parasails** with the **captain's wheel** all the way to **Latin America**.

Cutaneous mycoses

Tinea (dermatophytes)	Tinea is the clinical name given to dermatophyte (cutaneous fungal) infections. Dermatophytes include *Microsporum*, *Trichophyton*, and *Epidermophyton*. Branching septate hyphae visible on KOH preparation with blue fungal stain **A**.
Tinea capitis	Occurs on head, scalp. Associated with lymphadenopathy, alopecia, scaling **B**.
Tinea corporis	Occurs on body. Characterized by erythematous scaling rings ("ringworm") and central clearing **C**. Can be acquired from contact with an infected cat or dog.
Tinea cruris	Occurs in inguinal area **D**. Often does not show the central clearing seen in tinea corporis.

Tinea pedis	Three varieties:
	  ▪ Interdigital **E**; most common
	  ▪ Moccasin distribution **F**
	  ▪ Vesicular type

Tinea unguium	Onychomycosis; occurs on nails.
Tinea versicolor	Caused by *Malassezia* spp. (*Pityrosporum* spp.), a yeast-like fungus (not a dermatophyte despite being called tinea). Degradation of lipids produces acids that damage melanocytes and cause hypopigmented **G** and/or pink patches. Can occur any time of year but common in summer (hot, humid weather). "Spaghetti and meatballs" appearance on microscopy **H**. Treatment: topical and/or oral antifungal medications, selenium sulfide.

Opportunistic fungal infections

Candida albicans A

alba = white.
Systemic or superficial fungal infection.
Oral B and esophageal thrush in immunocompromised (neonates, steroids, diabetes, AIDS), vulvovaginitis (diabetes, use of antibiotics), diaper rash, endocarditis in IV drug users, disseminated candidiasis (to any organ), chronic mucocutaneous candidiasis.
Treatment: topical azole for vaginal; nystatin, fluconazole, or caspofungin for oral/esophageal; fluconazole, caspofungin, or amphotericin B for systemic.

Candida albicans. Pseudohyphae and budding yeasts at 20°C (left). ✖ Germ tubes at 37°C (right). ✖

Aspergillus fumigatus C

Invasive aspergillosis, especially in immunocompromised and those with chronic granulomatous disease.
Allergic bronchopulmonary aspergillosis (ABPA): associated with asthma and cystic fibrosis; may cause bronchiectasis and eosinophilia.
Aspergillomas in lung cavities, especially after TB infection.
Some species of *Aspergillus* produce aflatoxins, which are associated with hepatocellular carcinoma.
Think "**A**" for Acute Angles in *Aspergillus*. Not dimorphic.

Aspergillus fumigatus. Septate hyphae that branch at 45° angle (left). ✖ Conidiophore with radiating chains of spores (right). ✖

Cryptococcus neoformans D

Cryptococcal meningitis, cryptococcosis.
Heavily encapsulated yeast. Not dimorphic.
Found in soil, pigeon droppings. Acquired through inhalation with hematogenous dissemination to meninges. Culture on Sabouraud agar. Stains with India ink and mucicarmine. Latex agglutination test detects polysaccharide capsular antigen and is more specific. "Soap bubble" lesions in brain.

Cryptococcus neoformans. 5-10 μm yeasts with wide capsular halos and unequal budding in India ink stain. ✖

Mucor E and *Rhizopus* spp.

Mucormycosis. Disease mostly in ketoacidotic diabetic and/or neutropenic patients (e.g., leukemia). Fungi proliferate in blood vessel walls, penetrate cribriform plate, and enter brain. Rhinocerebral, frontal lobe abscess; cavernous sinus thrombosis. Headache, facial pain, black necrotic eschar on face; may have cranial nerve involvement.
Treatment: surgical debridement, amphotericin B.

Mucor. Irregular, broad, nonseptate hyphae branching at wide angles. ✖

Pneumocystis jirovecii

Causes *Pneumocystis* pneumonia (PCP), a diffuse interstitial pneumonia. Yeast-like fungus (originally classified as protozoan). Inhaled. Most infections are asymptomatic. Immunosuppression (e.g., AIDS) predisposes to disease. Diffuse, bilateral ground-glass opacities on CXR/CT A. Diagnosed by lung biopsy or lavage. Disc-shaped yeast forms on methenamine silver stain of lung tissue B.

Treatment/prophylaxis: TMP-SMX, pentamidine, dapsone (prophylaxis only), atovaquone (prophylaxis only). Start prophylaxis when CD4+ count drops to < 200 cells/mm^3 in HIV patients.

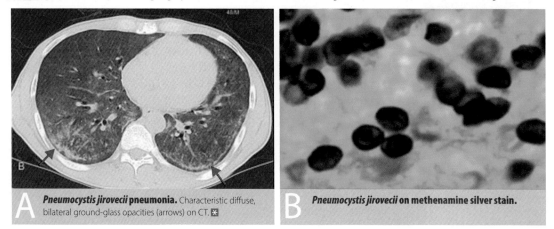

A **Pneumocystis jirovecii pneumonia.** Characteristic diffuse, bilateral ground-glass opacities (arrows) on CT. ✱

B **Pneumocystis jirovecii on methenamine silver stain.**

Sporothrix schenckii

Sporotrichosis. Dimorphic, cigar-shaped budding yeast that lives on vegetation. When spores are traumatically introduced into the skin, typically by a thorn ("**rose** gardener's" disease), causes local pustule or ulcer A with nodules along draining lymphatics (ascending lymphangitis). Disseminated disease possible in immunocompromised host.

Treatment: itraconazole or **pot**assium iodide. "Plant a **rose** in the **pot**."

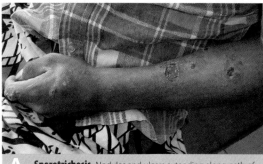

A **Sporotrichosis.** Nodules and ulcers extending along path of lymphatic drainage. RU

Protozoa—GI infections

ORGANISM	DISEASE	TRANSMISSION	DIAGNOSIS	TREATMENT
Giardia lamblia 	**Giardiasis**—bloating, flatulence, foul-smelling, fatty diarrhea (often seen in campers/hikers)—think fat-rich **Ghirardelli** chocolates for **fatty** stools of *Giardia*	Cysts in water	Trophozoites A or cysts B in stool 	Metronidazole
Entamoeba histolytica 	**Amebiasis**—bloody diarrhea (dysentery), liver abscess ("anchovy paste" exudate), RUQ pain; histology shows flask-shaped ulcer	Cysts in water	Serology and/or trophozoites (with RBCs in the cytoplasm) C or cysts (with up to 4 nuclei) D in stool 	Metronidazole; iodoquinol for asymptomatic cyst passers
Cryptosporidium 	Severe diarrhea in AIDS Mild disease (watery diarrhea) in immunocompetent hosts	Oocysts in water	Oocysts on acid-fast stain E	Prevention (by filtering city water supplies); nitazoxanide in immunocompetent hosts

Protozoa—CNS infections

ORGANISM	DISEASE	TRANSMISSION	DIAGNOSIS	TREATMENT
Toxoplasma gondii	Congenital toxoplasmosis = classic triad of chorioretinitis, hydrocephalus, and intracranial calcifications; reactivation in AIDS → brain abscess seen as ring-enhancing lesions on CT/MRI **A**	Cysts in meat (most common); oocysts in cat feces; crosses placenta (pregnant women should avoid cats)	Serology, biopsy (tachyzoite) **B**	Sulfadiazine + pyrimethamine
Naegleria fowleri	Rapidly fatal meningoencephalitis	Swimming in **freshwater** lakes (think **Nalgene** bottle filled with **fresh water** containing *Naegleria*); enters via cribriform plate	Amoebas in spinal fluid **C**	Amphotericin B has been effective for a few survivors
Trypanosoma brucei	**African sleeping sickness**— enlarged lymph nodes, recurring fever (due to antigenic variation), somnolence, coma Two subspecies: *Trypanosoma brucei rhodesiense, Trypanosoma brucei gambiense*	Tsetse fly, a painful bite	Blood smear **D**	**Suramin** for blood-borne disease or **mela**rsoprol for CNS penetration ("it **sure** is nice to go to sleep"; **mela**tonin helps with sleep)

Protozoa—Hematologic infections

ORGANISM	DISEASE	TRANSMISSION	DIAGNOSIS	TREATMENT

Plasmodium
  P. vivax/ovale
  P. falciparum
  P. malariae
 	
	Malaria—fever, headache, anemia, splenomegaly
	P. vivax/ovale—48-hr cycle (tertian; includes fever on first day and third day, thus fevers are actually 48 hr apart); dormant form (hypnozoite) in liver
	P. falciparum—severe; irregular fever patterns; parasitized RBCs occlude capillaries in brain (cerebral malaria), kidneys, lungs
	P. malariae—72-hr cycle (quartan)
		Anopheles mosquito	Blood smear: trophozoite ring form within RBC **A**, schizont containing merozoites **B**; red granules (Schüffner stippling) throughout RBC cytoplasm seen with *P. vivax/ovale*
			
				Chloroquine (for sensitive species), which blocks *Plasmodium* heme polymerase; if resistant, use mefloquine or atovaquone/proguanil
				If life-threatening, use intravenous quinidine or artesunate (test for G6PD deficiency)
				For *P. vivax/ovale*, add primaquine for hypnozoite (test for G6PD deficiency)

Babesia 	**Babesiosis**—fever and hemolytic anemia; predominantly in northeastern United States; asplenia ↑ risk of severe disease	*Ixodes* tick (same as *Borrelia burgdorferi* of Lyme disease; may often coinfect humans)	Blood smear: ring form **C1**, "Maltese cross" **C2**; PCR	Atovaquone + azithromycin

Protozoa—Others

ORGANISM	DISEASE	TRANSMISSION	DIAGNOSIS	TREATMENT
Visceral infections				
Trypanosoma cruzi	**Chagas disease**—dilated cardiomyopathy with apical atrophy, megacolon, megaesophagus; predominantly in South America. Unilateral periorbital swelling (Romaña sign) characteristic of acute stage	Reduviid bug ("**kissing** bug") feces, deposited in a painless bite (much like a **kiss**)	Blood smear A	Benznidazole or nifurtimox
Leishmania donovani	**Visceral leishmaniasis (kala-azar)**—spiking fevers, hepatosplenomegaly, pancytopenia	Sandfly	Macrophages containing amastigotes B	Amphotericin B, sodium stibogluconate
Sexually transmitted infections				
Trichomonas vaginalis	**Vaginitis**—foul-smelling, greenish discharge; itching and burning; do not confuse with *Gardnerella vaginalis*, a gram-variable bacterium associated with bacterial vaginosis	Sexual (cannot exist outside human because it cannot form cysts)	Trophozoites (motile) C on wet mount; "strawberry cervix"	Metronidazole for patient and partner (prophylaxis)

Nematodes (roundworms)

ORGANISM	TRANSMISSION	DISEASE	TREATMENT
Intestinal			
Enterobius vermicularis (pinworm)	Fecal-oral	Intestinal infection causing anal pruritus (diagnosed by seeing egg **A** via the tape test)	**Bend**azoles (because worms are **bend**y)
Ascaris lumbricoides (giant roundworm)	Fecal-oral; eggs visible in feces under microscope **B**	Intestinal infection with possible obstruction at ileocecal valve	Bendazoles
Strongyloides stercoralis	Larvae in soil penetrate the skin	Intestinal infection causing vomiting, diarrhea, epigastric pain (may feel like peptic ulcer)	Ivermectin or bendazoles
Ancylostoma duodenale, Necator americanus (hookworms)	Larvae penetrate skin	Intestinal infection causing anemia by sucking blood from intestinal walls	Bendazoles or pyrantel pamoate
Trichinella spiralis	Fecal-oral; undercooked meat (esp. pork)	Intestinal infection; larvae enter bloodstream and encyst in striated muscle cells → inflammation of muscle. **Trichinosis**—fever, vomiting, nausea, periorbital edema, myalgia	Bendazoles
Tissue			
Onchocerca volvulus	Female blackfly bite	Hyperpigmented skin and river blindness (**black** flies, **black** skin nodules, "**black** sight"); allergic reaction to microfilaria possible	Ivermectin (**iver**mectin for **river** blindness)
Loa loa	Deer fly, horse fly, mango fly	Swelling in skin, worm in conjunctiva	Diethylcarbamazine
Wuchereria bancrofti	Female mosquito	**Elephantiasis**—worms block lymphatic vessels **C**, takes 9 mo–1 yr after bite to become symptomatic	Diethylcarbamazine
Toxocara canis	Fecal-oral	Visceral larva migrans	Bendazoles

Nematode routes of infection	Ingested—*Enterobius, Ascaris, Toxocara, Trichinella*	You'll get sick if you **EATT** these!
	Cutaneous—*Strongyloides, Ancylostoma, Necator*	These get into your feet from the **SAN**d.
	Bites—*Loa loa, Onchocerca volvulus, Wuchereria bancrofti*	Lay **LOW** to avoid getting bitten.

Cestodes (tapeworms)

ORGANISM	TRANSMISSION	DISEASE	TREATMENT
Taenia solium A	Ingestion of larvae encysted in undercooked pork	Intestinal infection	Praziquantel
	Ingestion of eggs	Cysticercosis, neurocysticercosis B	Praziquantel; albendazole for neurocysticercosis
Diphyllobothrium latum	Ingestion of larvae from raw freshwater fish	Vitamin B_{12} deficiency (tapeworm competes for B_{12} in intestine) → megaloblastic anemia	Praziquantel
Echinococcus granulosus C	Ingestion of eggs from dog feces Sheep are an intermediate host	Hydatid cysts D in liver E, causing anaphylaxis if antigens released (hydatid cyst injected with ethanol or hypertonic saline to kill daughter cysts before removal)	Albendazole

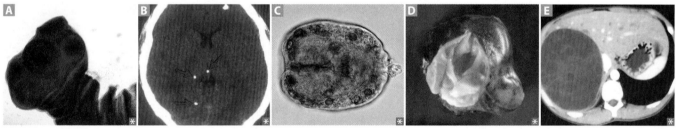

Trematodes (flukes)

ORGANISM	TRANSMISSION	DISEASE	TREATMENT
Schistosoma	Snails are host; cercariae penetrate skin of humans	Liver and spleen enlargement (*S. mansoni*, egg with lateral spine A), fibrosis, and inflammation Chronic infection with *S. haematobium* (egg with terminal spine B) can lead to squamous cell carcinoma of the bladder (painless hematuria) and pulmonary hypertension	Praziquantel
Clonorchis sinensis	Undercooked fish	Biliary tract inflammation → pigmented gallstones Associated with cholangiocarcinoma	Praziquantel

Parasite hints

ASSOCIATIONS	ORGANISM
Biliary tract disease, cholangiocarcinoma	*Clonorchis sinensis*
Brain cysts, seizures	*Taenia solium* (cysticercosis)
Hematuria, squamous cell bladder cancer	*Schistosoma haematobium*
Liver (hydatid) cysts	*Echinococcus granulosus*
Microcytic anemia	*Ancylostoma, Necator*
Myalgias, periorbital edema	*Trichinella spiralis*
Perianal pruritus	*Enterobius*
Portal hypertension	*Schistosoma mansoni, Schistosoma japonicum*
Vitamin B_{12} deficiency	*Diphyllobothrium latum*

▸ MICROBIOLOGY—VIROLOGY

Viral structure—general features

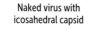

Naked virus with icosahedral capsid

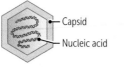

Enveloped virus with icosahedral capsid

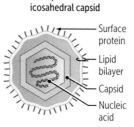

Enveloped virus with helical capsid

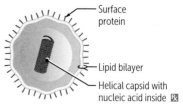

Viral genetics

Recombination	Exchange of genes between 2 chromosomes by crossing over within regions of significant base sequence homology.
Reassortment	When viruses with segmented genomes (e.g., influenza virus) exchange genetic material. For example, the 2009 novel H1N1 influenza A pandemic emerged via complex viral reassortment of genes from human, swine, and avian viruses.
Complementation	When 1 of 2 viruses that infect the cell has a mutation that results in a nonfunctional protein. The nonmutated virus "complements" the mutated one by making a functional protein that serves both viruses. For example, hepatitis D virus requires the presence of replicating hepatitis B virus to supply HBsAg, the envelope protein for HDV.
Phenotypic mixing	Occurs with simultaneous infection of a cell with 2 viruses. Genome of virus A can be partially or completely coated (forming pseudovirion) with the surface proteins of virus B. Type B protein coat determines the tropism (infectivity) of the hybrid virus. However, the progeny from this infection have a type A coat that is encoded by its type A genetic material.

Viral vaccines

Live attenuated vaccines	Induce humoral and cell-mediated immunity but have reverted to virulence on rare occasions. Killed/inactivated vaccines induce only humoral immunity but are stable. **Live** attenuated: **small**pox, **yellow** fever, **rota**virus, **chicken**pox (VZV), **Sabin** polio virus, **MMR**, Influenza (intranasal).	No booster needed for live attenuated vaccines. Dangerous to give live vaccines to immunocompromised patients or their close contacts. "**Live!** One night only! See **small yellow rota**ting **chicken**s get vaccinated with **Sabin** and **MMR!** It's incredible!" MMR = measles, mumps, rubella; live attenuated vaccine that can be given to HIV-positive patients who do not show signs of immunodeficiency.
Killed	Rabies, Influenza (injected), Salk Polio, and HAV vaccines.	Sal**K** = **K**illed. **RIP** Always.
Subunit	HBV (antigen = HBsAg), HPV (types 6, 11, 16, and 18).	

DNA viral genomes	All DNA viruses except the Parvoviridae are dsDNA. All are linear except papilloma-, polyoma-, and hepadnaviruses (circular).	All are dsDNA (like our cells), except "**part-of-a-virus**" (**parvo**virus) is ssDNA. *Parvus* = small.
RNA viral genomes	All RNA viruses except Reoviridae are ssRNA. Positive-stranded RNA viruses: I went to a **retro** (**retro**virus) **toga** (**toga**virus) party, where I drank flavored (**flavi**virus) **Corona** (**corona**virus) and ate **hippy** (**hepe**virus) California (**calici**virus) pickles (**picorna**virus).	All are ssRNA (like our mRNA), except "**repeato-virus**" (**reo**virus) is dsRNA.
Naked viral genome infectivity	Purified nucleic acids of most dsDNA (except poxviruses and HBV) and ⊕ strand ssRNA (≈ mRNA) viruses are infectious. Naked nucleic acids of ⊖ strand ssRNA and dsRNA viruses are not infectious. They require polymerases contained in the complete virion.	

Viral replication

DNA viruses	All replicate in the nucleus (except poxvirus).
RNA viruses	All replicate in the cytoplasm (except influenza virus and retroviruses).

Viral envelopes	**Naked** (nonenveloped) viruses include **P**apillomavirus, **A**denovirus, **P**arvovirus, **P**olyomavirus, **C**alicivirus, **P**icornavirus, **R**eovirus, and **Hep**evirus. Generally, enveloped viruses acquire their envelopes from plasma membrane when they exit from cell. Exceptions include herpesviruses, which acquire envelopes from nuclear membrane.	Give **PAPP** smears and **CPR** to a **naked Heppy** (hippy). DNA = **PAPP**; RNA = **CPR** and **hepe**virus.

DNA virus characteristics

Some general rules—all DNA viruses:

GENERAL RULE	COMMENTS
Are **HHAPPPP**y viruses	Hepadna, Herpes, Adeno, Pox, Parvo, Papilloma, Polyoma.
Are double stranded	Except parvo (single stranded).
Are linear	Except papilloma and polyoma (circular, supercoiled) and hepadna (circular, incomplete).
Are icosahedral	Except pox (complex).
Replicate in the nucleus	Except pox (carries own DNA-dependent RNA polymerase).

DNA viruses

VIRAL FAMILY	ENVELOPE	DNA STRUCTURE	MEDICAL IMPORTANCE
Herpesviruses	Yes	DS and linear	HSV-1—oral (and some genital) lesions, spontaneous temporal lobe encephalitis, keratoconjunctivitis HSV-2—genital (and some oral) lesions VZV (HHV-3)—chickenpox, zoster (shingles) EBV (HHV-4)—mononucleosis, Burkitt lymphoma, Hodgkin lymphoma, nasopharyngeal carcinoma CMV (HHV-5)—infection in immunosuppressed patients (AIDS **retinitis** ["**sight**omegalovirus"]), especially transplant recipients; congenital defects HHV-6—roseola (exanthem subitum) HHV-7—less common cause of roseola HHV-8—Kaposi sarcoma
Hepadnavirus	Yes	Partially DS and circular	HBV: ▪ Acute or chronic hepatitis ▪ Not a retrovirus but has reverse transcriptase
Adenovirus	No	DS and linear	Febrile pharyngitis 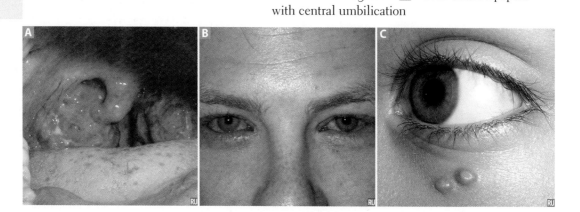—sore throat Acute hemorrhagic cystitis Pneumonia Conjunctivitis **B**—"pink eye"
Parvovirus	No	SS and linear (smallest DNA virus)	B19 virus—aplastic crises in sickle cell disease, "slapped cheeks" rash in children (erythema infectiosum, or fifth disease) RBC destruction in fetus leads to hydrops fetalis and death, in adults leads to pure RBC aplasia and rheumatoid arthritis–like symptoms
Papillomavirus	No	DS and circular	HPV–warts (serotypes 1, 2, 6, 11), CIN, cervical cancer (most commonly 16, 18)
Polyomavirus	No	DS and circular	JC virus—progressive multifocal leukoencephalopathy (PML) in HIV BK virus—transplant patients, commonly targets kidney **JC: J**unky **C**erebrum; **BK: B**ad **K**idney
Poxvirus	Yes	DS and linear (largest DNA virus)	Smallpox eradicated by use of live attenuated vaccine. Eradication was achieved by world-wide use of the live attenuated vaccine Cowpox ("milkmaid blisters") Molluscum contagiosum **C**—flesh-colored papule with central umbilication

Herpesviruses

HSV-1	Gingivostomatitis, keratoconjunctivitis A, herpes labialis B, temporal lobe encephalitis (most common cause of sporadic encephalitis, can present with altered mental status, seizures, and/or aphasia). Transmitted by respiratory secretions, saliva.
HSV-2	Herpes genitalis C, neonatal herpes. Latent in sacral ganglia. Transmitted by sexual contact, perinatally.
VZV	Varicella-zoster (chickenpox D, shingles E), encephalitis, pneumonia. Latent in dorsal root or trigeminal ganglia. Most common complication of shingles is post-herpetic neuralgia. Transmitted by respiratory secretions.
EBV	Mononucleosis. Characterized by fever, hepatosplenomegaly, pharyngitis, and lymphadenopathy (especially posterior cervical nodes F). Transmitted by respiratory secretions and saliva; also called "kissing disease" since commonly seen in teens, young adults. Infects B cells through CD21. Atypical lymphocytes seen on peripheral blood smear G are not infected B cells but rather reactive cytotoxic T cells. Detect by ⊕ Monospot test—heterophile antibodies detected by agglutination of sheep or horse RBCs. Associated with lymphomas (e.g., endemic Burkitt lymphoma), nasopharyngeal carcinoma.
CMV	Congenital infection, mononucleosis (⊖ Monospot), pneumonia, retinitis. Infected cells have characteristic "owl eye" inclusions H. Latent in mononuclear cells. Transmitted congenitally and by transfusion, sexual contact, saliva, urine, transplant.
HHV-6/HHV-7	Roseola: high fevers for several days that can cause seizures, followed by a diffuse macular rash I. Transmitted by saliva.
HHV-8	Kaposi sarcoma, a neoplasm of endothelial cells. Seen in HIV/AIDS and transplant patients. Dark/violaceous plaques or nodules J representing vascular proliferations. Can also affect GI tract and lungs. Transmitted by sexual contact.

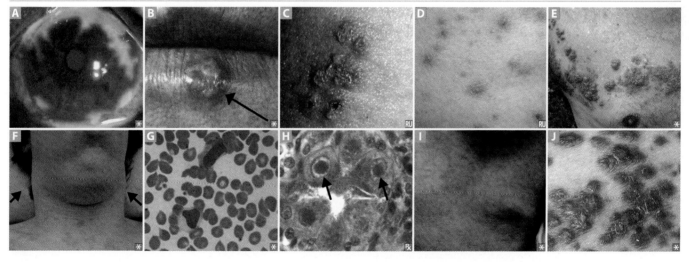

HSV identification

Viral culture for skin/genitalia.
CSF PCR for herpes encephalitis.
Tzanck test—a smear of an opened skin vesicle
to detect multinucleated giant cells commonly
seen in HSV-1, HSV-2, and VZV infection 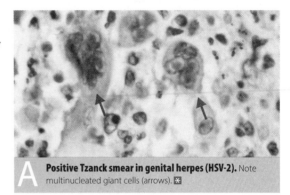.
Intranuclear inclusions also seen with HSV-1,
HSV-2, VZV.

Tzanck heavens I do not have herpes.

A **Positive Tzanck smear in genital herpes (HSV-2).** Note multinucleated giant cells (arrows). ✶

RNA viruses

VIRAL FAMILY	ENVELOPE	RNA STRUCTURE	CAPSID SYMMETRY	MEDICAL IMPORTANCE
Reoviruses	No	DS linear 10–12 segments	Icosahedral (double)	Coltivirus[a]—Colorado tick fever Rotavirus—#1 cause of fatal diarrhea in children
Picornaviruses	No	SS ⊕ linear	Icosahedral	**P**oliovirus—polio-Salk/Sabin vaccines—IPV/OPV **E**chovirus—aseptic meningitis **R**hinovirus—"common cold" **C**oxsackievirus—aseptic meningitis; herpangina (mouth blisters, fever); hand, foot, and mouth disease; myocarditis; pericarditis **H**AV—acute viral hepatitis **PERCH**
Hepevirus	No	SS ⊕ linear	Icosahedral	HEV
Caliciviruses	No	SS ⊕ linear	Icosahedral	Norovirus—viral gastroenteritis
Flaviviruses	Yes	SS ⊕ linear	Icosahedral	HCV Yellow fever[a] Dengue[a] St. Louis encephalitis[a] West Nile virus[a]
Togaviruses	Yes	SS ⊕ linear	Icosahedral	Rubella Eastern equine encephalitis[a] Western equine encephalitis[a]
Retroviruses	Yes	SS ⊕ linear 2 copies	Icosahedral (HTLV), complex and conical (HIV)	Have reverse transcriptase HTLV—T-cell leukemia HIV—AIDS
Coronaviruses	Yes	SS ⊕ linear	Helical	Coronavirus—"common cold" and SARS
Orthomyxoviruses	Yes	SS ⊖ linear 8 segments	Helical	Influenza virus

Paramyxoviruses	Yes	SS ⊖ linear Nonsegmented	Helical	**PaRaM**yxovirus:
				  Parainfluenza—croup
				  RSV—bronchiolitis in babies; **R**x—ribavirin
				  Measles, **M**umps

Rhabdoviruses	Yes	SS ⊖ linear	Helical	Rabies
Filoviruses	Yes	SS ⊖ linear	Helical	Ebola/Marburg hemorrhagic fever—often fatal!
Arenaviruses	Yes	SS ⊖ circular 2 segments	Helical	LCMV—lymphocytic choriomeningitis virus Lassa fever encephalitis—spread by rodents
Bunyaviruses	Yes	SS ⊖ circular 3 segments	Helical	California encephalitis[a] Sandfly/Rift Valley fevers[a] Crimean-Congo hemorrhagic fever[a] Hantavirus—hemorrhagic fever, pneumonia
Delta virus	Yes	SS ⊖ circular	Uncertain	HDV is a "defective" virus that requires the presence of HBV to replicate

SS, single-stranded; DS, double-stranded; ⊕, positive sense; ⊖, negative sense; [a]= **arbo**virus, **arth**ropod **bo**rne (mosquitoes, ticks).

Negative-stranded viruses	Must transcribe ⊖ strand to ⊕. Virion brings its own RNA-dependent RNA polymerase. They include **A**renaviruses, **B**unyaviruses, **P**aramyxoviruses, **O**rthomyxoviruses, **F**iloviruses, and **R**habdoviruses.	Always Bring Polymerase Or Fail Replication.
Segmented viruses	All are RNA viruses. They include **B**unyaviruses, **O**rthomyxoviruses (influenza viruses), **A**renaviruses, and **R**eoviruses.	BOAR.
Picornavirus	Includes **P**oliovirus, **E**chovirus, **R**hinovirus, **C**oxsackievirus, and **H**AV. RNA is translated into 1 large polypeptide that is cleaved by proteases into functional viral proteins. Can cause aseptic (viral) meningitis (except rhinovirus and HAV). All are enteroviruses (fecal-oral spread) except rhinovirus.	Pico**RNA**virus = small **RNA** virus. **PERCH** on a "peak" (pico).
Rhinovirus	A picornavirus. Nonenveloped RNA virus. Cause of common cold; > 100 serologic types. Acid labile—destroyed by stomach acid; therefore, does not infect the GI tract (unlike the other picornaviruses).	**Rhino** has a runny **nose**.
Yellow fever virus	A flavivirus (also an arbovirus) transmitted by *Aedes* mosquitoes **A**. Virus has a monkey or human reservoir. Symptoms: high fever, black vomitus, and jaundice. May see Councilman bodies (eosinophilic apoptotic globules) on liver biopsy.	*Flavi* = yellow, jaundice.
Rotavirus	Rotavirus **A**, the most important global cause of infantile gastroenteritis, is a segmented dsRNA virus (a reovirus). Major cause of acute diarrhea in the United States during winter, especially in day care centers, kindergartens. Villous destruction with atrophy leads to ↓ absorption of Na⁺ and loss of K⁺.	**ROTA**virus = Right Out The Anus. CDC recommends routine vaccination of all infants.

Influenza viruses	Orthomyxoviruses. Enveloped, ⊖ ssRNA viruses with 8-segment genome. Contain hemagglutinin (promotes viral entry) and neuraminidase (promotes progeny virion release) antigens. Patients at risk for fatal bacterial superinfection, most commonly *S. aureus*, *S. pneumoniae*, and *H. influenzae*. Rapid genetic changes.	Reformulated vaccine ("the flu shot") contains viral strains most likely to appear during the flu season. Killed viral vaccine is most frequently used. Live attenuated vaccine contains temperature-sensitive mutant that replicates in the nose but not in the lung; administered intranasally.
Genetic shift/ antigenic shift	Causes pandemics. Reassortment of viral genome segments, such as when segments of human flu A virus reassort with swine flu A virus.	Sudden shift is more deadly than gradual drift.
Genetic drift/ antigenic drift	Causes epidemics. Minor (antigenic drift) changes based on random mutation in hemagglutinin or neuraminidase genes.	

Rubella virus   A togavirus. Causes rubella, once known as German (3-day) measles. Fever, postauricular and other lymphadenopathy, arthralgias, and fine rash **A**. Causes mild disease in children but serious congenital disease (a ToRCHeS infection). Congenital rubella findings include "blueberry muffin" appearance, indicative of extramedullary hematopoiesis **B**.

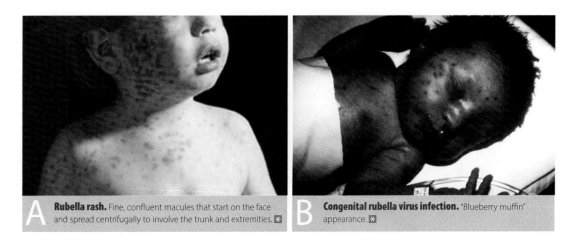

A **Rubella rash.** Fine, confluent macules that start on the face and spread centrifugally to involve the trunk and extremities. ✳

B **Congenital rubella virus infection.** "Blueberry muffin" appearance. ✳

Paramyxoviruses   Paramyxoviruses cause disease in children. They include those that cause parainfluenza (croup: seal-like barking cough), mumps, and measles as well as RSV, which causes respiratory tract infection (bronchiolitis, pneumonia) in infants. All contain surface F (fusion) protein, which causes respiratory epithelial cells to fuse and form multinucleated cells. Palivizumab (monoclonal antibody against F protein) prevents pneumonia caused by RSV infection in premature infants.

Croup (acute laryngo-tracheobronchitis)

Caused by parainfluenza viruses (paramyxovirus). Results in a "seal-like" barking cough and inspiratory stridor. Narrowing of upper trachea and subglottis leads to characteristic steeple sign on X-ray 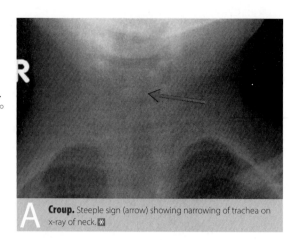. Severe croup can result in pulsus paradoxus 2° to upper airway obstruction.

A **Croup.** Steeple sign (arrow) showing narrowing of trachea on x-ray of neck. ✱

Measles (rubeola) virus

A paramyxovirus that causes measles. Usual presentation involves prodromal fever with cough, coryza, and conjunctivitis, then eventually Koplik spots **A**, followed by a maculopapular rash **B** that starts at the head/neck and spreads downward. Lymphadenitis with Warthin-Finkeldey giant cells (fused lymphocytes) in a background of paracortical hyperplasia. SSPE (subacute sclerosing panencephalitis, occurring years later), encephalitis (1:2000), and giant cell pneumonia (rarely, in immunosuppressed) are possible sequelae.

3 C's of measles:
Cough
Coryza
Conjunctivitis
Vitamin A supplementation can reduce measles mortality in malnourished or vitamin-deficient children.

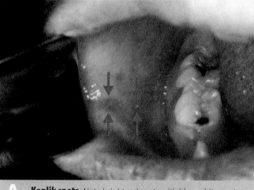

A **Koplik spots.** Note bright red spots with blue-white center on buccal mucosa (arrows) that precede the measles rash by 1–2 days. ✱

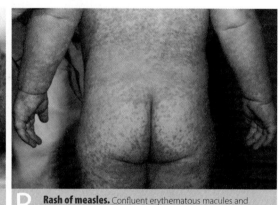

B **Rash of measles.** Confluent erythematous macules and papules, presents late, and includes limbs as it spreads downward. ✱

Mumps virus

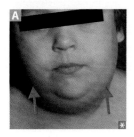

A paramyxovirus that causes mumps, uncommon due to effectiveness of MMR vaccine.

Symptoms: **P**arotitis 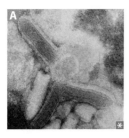, **O**rchitis (inflammation of testes), and aseptic **M**eningitis. Can cause sterility (especially after puberty).

Mumps makes your parotid glands and testes as big as **POM**-poms.

Rabies virus

Bullet-shaped virus A. Negri bodies B commonly found in Purkinje cells of cerebellum and in hippocampal neurons. Rabies has long incubation period (weeks to months) before symptom onset. Postexposure prophylaxis is wound cleaning plus immunization with killed vaccine and rabies immunoglobulin. Example of passive-active immunity.

Travels to the CNS by migrating in a retrograde fashion up nerve axons after binding to ACh receptors.

Progression of disease: fever, malaise → agitation, photophobia, hydrophobia, hypersalivation → paralysis, coma → death.

More commonly from bat, raccoon, and skunk bites than from dog bites in the United States.

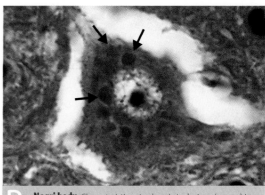

B **Negri body.** Characteristic cytoplasmic inclusions (arrows) in neurons infected by rabies virus. ✶

Ebola virus

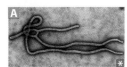

A filovirus A that targets endothelial cells, phagocytes, hepatocytes. Presents with abrupt onset of flu-like symptoms, diarrhea/vomiting, high fever, myalgia. Can progress to DIC, diffuse hemorrhage, shock. High mortality rate, no definitive treatment. Supportive care. Strict isolation of infected individuals and barrier practices for health care workers are key to preventing transmission.

Transmission requires direct contact with bodily fluids or fomites (including dead bodies); high incidence of nosocomial infection.

Hepatitis viruses

	VIRUS	TRANSMISSION	CARRIER	INCUBATION	HCC RISK	NOTES
HAV[a]	RNA picornavirus	Fecal-oral	No	Short (weeks)	No	Asymptomatic (usually), Acute, Alone (no carriers)
HBV[b]	DNA hepadnavirus	Parenteral, sexual, perinatal	Yes	Long (months)	Yes	Blood, Baby-making, Birthing
HCV	RNA flavivirus	Primarily blood (IVDU, post-transfusion)	Yes	Long	Yes	Chronic, Cirrhosis, Carcinoma, Carrier
HDV	RNA delta virus	Parenteral, sexual, perinatal	Yes	Superinfection (HDV after HBV)—short Coinfection (HDV with HBV)—long	Yes	Defective virus Dependent on HBV; superinfection → ↓ prognosis
HEV[a]	RNA hepevirus	Fecal-oral, especially waterborne	No	Short	No	High mortality in pregnant women; Enteric, Expectant mothers, Epidemic

Signs and symptoms of all hepatitis viruses: episodes of fever, jaundice, ↑ ALT and AST. May see Councilman bodies (eosinophilic apoptotic globules) on liver biopsy.

[a]HAV and HEV are fecal-oral: The **vowels** hit your **bowels**. Naked viruses do not rely on an envelope, so they are not destroyed by the gut.

[b]In HBV, the DNA polymerase has both DNA- and RNA-dependent activities. Upon entry into the nucleus, the polymerase functions to complete the partial dsDNA. The host RNA polymerase transcribes mRNA from viral DNA to make viral proteins. The DNA polymerase then reverse transcribes viral RNA to DNA, which is the genome of the progeny virus.

Hepatitis serologic markers

Anti-HAV (IgM)	IgM antibody to HAV; best test to detect acute hepatitis A.
Anti-HAV (IgG)	IgG antibody indicates prior HAV infection and/or prior vaccination; protects against reinfection.
HBsAg	Antigen found on surface of HBV; indicates hepatitis B infection.
Anti-HBs	Antibody to HBsAg; indicates immunity to hepatitis B.
HBcAg	Antigen associated with core of HBV.
Anti-HBc	Antibody to HBcAg; IgM = acute/recent infection; IgG = prior exposure or chronic infection. IgM anti-HBc may be the sole positive marker of infection during window period.
HBeAg	A second, different antigenic determinant in the HBV core. HBeAg indicates active viral replication and therefore high transmissibility.
Anti-HBe	Antibody to HBeAg; indicates low transmissibility.

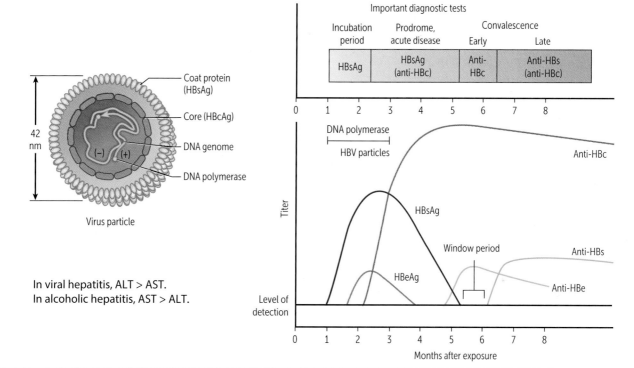

In viral hepatitis, ALT > AST.
In alcoholic hepatitis, AST > ALT.

	HBsAg	Anti-HBs	HBeAg	Anti-HBe	Anti-HBc
Acute HBV	✓		✓		IgM
Window				✓	IgM
Chronic HBV (high infectivity)	✓		✓		IgG
Chronic HBV (low infectivity)	✓			✓	IgG
Recovery		✓		✓	IgG
Immunized		✓			

HIV

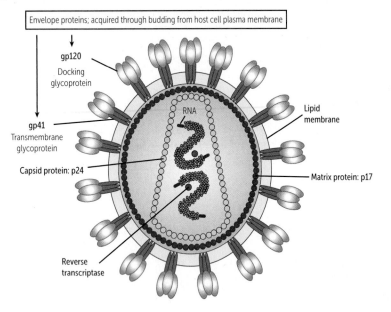

Envelope proteins; acquired through budding from host cell plasma membrane

gp120
Docking glycoprotein

gp41
Transmembrane glycoprotein

Capsid protein: p24

RNA

Lipid membrane

Matrix protein: p17

Reverse transcriptase

Diploid genome (2 molecules of RNA).
The 3 structural genes (protein coded for):
- *env* (gp120 and gp41):
  - Formed from cleavage of gp160 to form envelope glycoproteins.
  - gp120—attachment to host CD4+ T cell.
  - gp41—fusion and entry.
- *gag* (p24)—capsid protein.
- *pol*—reverse transcriptase, aspartate protease, integrase.

Reverse transcriptase synthesizes dsDNA from genomic RNA; dsDNA integrates into host genome.

Virus binds CD4 as well as a coreceptor, either CCR5 on macrophages (early infection) or CXCR4 on T cells (late infection).

Homozygous CCR5 mutation = immunity.
Heterozygous CCR5 mutation = slower course.

HIV diagnosis

Presumptive diagnosis made with ELISA (sensitive, high false-positive rate and low threshold, **rule out** test); ⊕ results are then confirmed with Western blot assay (specific, low false-positive rate and high threshold, rule in test).

Viral load tests determine the amount of viral RNA in the plasma. High viral load associated with poor prognosis. Also use viral load to monitor effect of drug therapy.

AIDS diagnosis ≤ 200 CD4+ cells/mm³ (normal: 500–1500 cells/mm³). HIV-positive with AIDS-defining condition (e.g., *Pneumocystis* pneumonia) or CD4+ percentage < 14%.

ELISA/Western blot tests look for antibodies to viral proteins; these tests often are falsely negative in the first 1–2 months of HIV infection and falsely positive initially in babies born to infected mothers (anti-gp120 crosses placenta).

Time course of untreated HIV infection

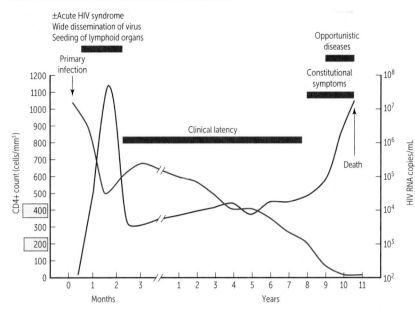

Four stages of untreated infection:
1. Flu-like (acute)
2. Feeling fine (latent)
3. Falling count
4. Final crisis

During latent phase, virus replicates in lymph nodes.

Red line = CD4+ T cell count (cells/mm³); blue line = HIV RNA copies/mL plasma.

Blue boxes on vertical CD4+ count axis indicate moderate immunocompromise (< 400 CD4+ cells/mm³) and when AIDS-defining illnesses emerge (< 200 CD4+ cells/mm³).

Common diseases of HIV-positive adults

As CD4+ count ↓, risks of reactivation of past infections (e.g., TB, HSV, shingles), dissemination of bacterial infections and fungal infections (e.g., coccidioidomycosis), and non-Hodgkin lymphomas ↑.

PATHOGEN	PRESENTATION	FINDINGS
< 500 cells/mm³		
Candida albicans	Oral thrush	Scrapable white plaque, pseudohyphae on microscopy
EBV	Oral hairy leukoplakia	Unscrapable white plaque on lateral tongue
Bartonella henselae	Bacillary angiomatosis	Biopsy with neutrophilic inflammation
HHV-8	Kaposi sarcoma	Biopsy with lymphocytic inflammation
Cryptosporidium spp.	Chronic, watery diarrhea	Acid-fast oocysts in stool
HPV	Squamous cell carcinoma, commonly of anus (men who have sex with men) or cervix (women)	
< 200 cells/mm³		
Toxoplasma gondii	Brain abscesses	Multiple ring-enhancing lesions on MRI
HIV	Dementia	
JC virus (reactivation)	Progressive multifocal leukoencephalopathy	Nonenhancing areas of demyelination on MRI
Pneumocystis jirovecii	*Pneumocystis* pneumonia	"Ground-glass" opacities on CXR
< 100 cells/mm³		
Aspergillus fumigatus	Hemoptysis, pleuritic pain	Cavitation or infiltrates on chest imaging
Cryptococcus neoformans	Meningitis	Thickly encapsulated yeast on India ink stain
Candida albicans	Esophagitis	White plaques on endoscopy; yeast and pseudohyphae on biopsy
CMV	Retinitis, esophagitis, colitis, pneumonitis, encephalitis	Linear ulcers on endoscopy, cotton-wool spots on fundoscopy. Biopsy reveals cells with intranuclear (owl eye) inclusion bodies
EBV	B-cell lymphoma (e.g., non-Hodgkin lymphoma, CNS lymphoma)	CNS lymphoma—ring enhancing, may be solitary (vs. *Toxoplasma*)
Histoplasma capsulatum	Fever, weight loss, fatigue, cough, dyspnea, nausea, vomiting, diarrhea	Oval yeast cells within macrophages
Mycobacterium avium–intracellulare, Mycobacterium avium complex	Nonspecific systemic symptoms (fever, night sweats, weight loss) or focal lymphadenitis	

Prions

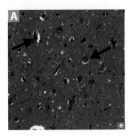

Prion diseases are caused by the conversion of a normal (predominantly α-helical) protein termed prion protein (PrP^c) to a β-pleated form (PrP^{sc}), which is transmissible via CNS-related tissue (iatrogenic CJD) or food contaminated by BSE-infected animal products (variant CJD). PrP^{sc} resists protease degradation and facilitates the conversion of still more PrP^c to PrP^{sc}. Resistant to standard sterilizing procedures, including standard autoclaving. Accumulation of PrP^{sc} results in spongiform encephalopathy and dementia, ataxia, and death.

Creutzfeldt-Jakob disease—rapidly progressive dementia, typically sporadic (some familial forms).
Bovine spongiform encephalopathy (BSE)—also known as "mad cow disease."
Kuru—acquired prion disease noted in tribal populations practicing human cannibalism.

▸ MICROBIOLOGY—SYSTEMS

Normal flora: dominant

LOCATION	MICROORGANISM
Skin	*S. epidermidis*
Nose	*S. epidermidis*; colonized by *S. aureus*
Oropharynx	Viridans group streptococci
Dental plaque	*S. mutans*
Colon	*B. fragilis* > *E. coli*
Vagina	*Lactobacillus*, colonized by *E. coli* and group B strep

Neonates delivered by C-section have no flora but are rapidly colonized after birth.

Bugs causing food poisoning

S. aureus and *B. cereus* food poisoning starts quickly and ends quickly.

MICROORGANISM	SOURCE OF INFECTION
B. cereus	Reheated rice. "Food poisoning from reheated rice? **Be serious!**" (***B. cereus***)
C. botulinum	Improperly canned foods, raw honey
C. perfringens	Reheated meat
E. coli O157:H7	Undercooked meat
Salmonella	Poultry, meat, and eggs
S. aureus	Meats, mayonnaise, custard; preformed toxin
V. parahaemolyticus and *V. vulnificus*[a]	Contaminated seafood

[a]*V. vulnificus* can also cause wound infections from contact with contaminated water or shellfish.

Bugs causing diarrhea

Bloody diarrhea

Campylobacter	Comma- or S-shaped organisms; growth at 42°C
E. histolytica	Protozoan; amebic dysentery; liver abscess
Enterohemorrhagic *E. coli*	O157:H7; can cause HUS; makes Shiga-like toxin
Enteroinvasive *E. coli*	Invades colonic mucosa
Salmonella	Lactose ⊖; flagellar motility; has animal reservoir, especially poultry and eggs
Shigella	Lactose ⊖; very low ID_{50}; produces Shiga toxin (human reservoir only); bacillary dysentery
Y. enterocolitica	Day care outbreaks, pseudoappendicitis

Watery diarrhea

C. difficile	Pseudomembranous colitis; caused by antibiotics; occasionally bloody diarrhea
C. perfringens	Also causes gas gangrene
Enterotoxigenic *E. coli*	Travelers' diarrhea; produces heat-labile (LT) and heat-stable (ST) toxins
Protozoa	*Giardia, Cryptosporidium*
V. cholerae	Comma-shaped organisms; rice-water diarrhea; often from infected seafood
Viruses	Rotavirus, norovirus, adenovirus

Common causes of pneumonia

NEONATES (< 4 WK)	CHILDREN (4 WK–18 YR)	ADULTS (18–40 YR)	ADULTS (40–65 YR)	ELDERLY
Group B streptococci *E. coli*	Viruses (**RSV**) *Mycoplasma* *C. trachomatis* (infants–3 yr) *C. pneumoniae* (school-aged children) *S. pneumoniae* Runts May Cough Chunky Sputum	*Mycoplasma* *C. pneumoniae* *S. pneumoniae*	*S. pneumoniae* *H. influenzae* Anaerobes Viruses *Mycoplasma*	*S. pneumoniae* Influenza virus Anaerobes *H. influenzae* Gram-negative rods

Special groups

Alcoholic/IV drug user	*S. pneumoniae, Klebsiella, S. aureus*
Aspiration	Anaerobes (e.g., *Peptostreptococcus, Fusobacterium, Prevotella, Bacteroides*)
Atypical	*Mycoplasma, Legionella, Chlamydia*
Cystic fibrosis	*Pseudomonas, S. aureus, S. pneumoniae*
Immunocompromised	*S. aureus*, enteric gram-negative rods, fungi, viruses, *P. jirovecii* (with HIV)
Nosocomial (hospital acquired)	*S. aureus, Pseudomonas*, other enteric gram-negative rods
Postviral	*S. aureus, H. influenzae, S. pneumoniae*

Common causes of meningitis

NEWBORN (0–6 MO)	CHILDREN (6 MO–6 YR)	6–60 YR	60 YR +
Group B streptococci	*S. pneumoniae*	*S. pneumoniae*	*S. pneumoniae*
E. coli	*N. meningitidis*	*N. meningitidis* (#1 in teens)	Gram-negative rods
Listeria	*H. influenzae* type B	Enteroviruses	*Listeria*
	Enteroviruses	HSV	

Give ceftriaxone and vancomycin empirically (add ampicillin if *Listeria* is suspected).

Viral causes of meningitis: enteroviruses (especially coxsackievirus), HSV-2 (HSV-1 = encephalitis), HIV, West Nile virus (also causes encephalitis), VZV.

In HIV: *Cryptococcus* spp.

Note: Incidence of *H. influenzae* meningitis has ↓ greatly with introduction of the conjugate *H. influenzae* vaccine in last 10–15 years. Today, cases are usually seen in unimmunized children.

CSF findings in meningitis

	OPENING PRESSURE	CELL TYPE	PROTEIN	SUGAR
Bacterial	↑	↑ PMNs	↑	↓
Fungal/TB	↑	↑ lymphocytes	↑	↓
Viral	Normal/↑	↑ lymphocytes	Normal/↑	Normal

Infections causing brain abscess

Most commonly viridans streptococci and *Staphylococcus aureus*. If dental infection or extraction precedes abscess, oral anaerobes commonly involved.

Multiple abscesses are usually from bacteremia; single lesions from contiguous sites: otitis media and mastoiditis → temporal lobe and cerebellum; sinusitis or dental infection → frontal lobe. *Toxoplasma* reactivation in AIDS.

Osteomyelitis

RISK FACTOR	ASSOCIATED INFECTION
Assume if no other information is available	*S. aureus* (most common overall)
Sexually active	*Neisseria gonorrhoeae* (rare), septic arthritis more common
Sickle cell disease	*Salmonella* and *S. aureus*
Prosthetic joint replacement	*S. aureus* and *S. epidermidis*
Vertebral involvement	*S. aureus, Mycobacterium tuberculosis* (Pott disease)
Cat and dog bites	*Pasteurella multocida*
IV drug abuse	*Pseudomonas, Candida, S. aureus* are most common

Elevated C-reactive protein (CRP) and erythrocyte sedimentation rate common but nonspecific. MRI is best for detecting acute infection and detailing anatomic involvement **A**. Radiographs are insensitive early but can be useful in chronic osteomyelitis **B**.

Urinary tract infections

Cystitis presents with dysuria, frequency, urgency, suprapubic pain, and WBCs (but not WBC casts) in urine. Primarily caused by ascension of microbes from urethra to bladder. Males—infants with congenital defects, vesicoureteral reflux. Elderly—enlarged prostate. Ascension to kidney results in pyelonephritis, which presents with fever, chills, flank pain, costovertebral angle tenderness, hematuria, and WBC casts.

Ten times more common in women (shorter urethras colonized by fecal flora). Other predisposing factors: obstruction, kidney surgery, catheterization, GU malformation, diabetes, pregnancy.

UTI bugs

SPECIES	FEATURES	COMMENTS
Escherichia coli	Leading cause of UTI. Colonies show green metallic sheen on EMB agar.	Diagnostic markers:
Staphylococcus saprophyticus	2nd leading cause of UTI in sexually active women.	⊕ Leukocyte esterase = evidence of WBC activity.
Klebsiella pneumoniae	3rd leading cause of UTI. Large mucoid capsule and viscous colonies.	⊕ Nitrite test = reduction of urinary nitrates by bacterial species (e.g., *E. coli*).
Serratia marcescens	Some strains produce a red pigment; often nosocomial and drug resistant.	⊕ Urease test = urease-producing bugs (e.g., *Proteus, Klebsiella*).
Enterococcus	Often nosocomial and drug resistant.	
Proteus mirabilis	Motility causes "swarming" on agar; produces urease; associated with struvite stones.	
Pseudomonas aeruginosa	Blue-green pigment and fruity odor; usually nosocomial and drug resistant.	

Common vaginal infections

	Bacterial vaginosis	**Trichomoniasis**	***Candida* vulvovaginitis**
SIGNS AND SYMPTOMS	No inflammation Thin, white discharge 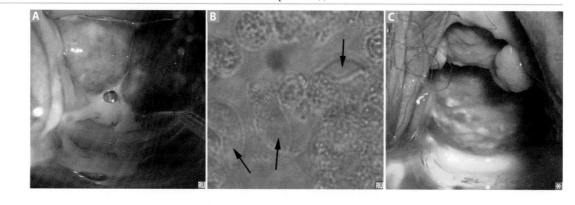 **A** with fishy odor	Inflammation ("strawberry cervix") Frothy, grey-green, foul-smelling discharge	Inflammation Thick, white, "cottage cheese" discharge **C**
LAB FINDINGS	Clue cells pH > 4.5	Motile trichomonads **B** pH > 4.5	Pseudohyphae pH normal (4.0–4.5)
TREATMENT	Metronidazole	Metronidazole Treat sexual partner(s)	-azoles

ToRCHeS infections   Microbes that may pass from mother to fetus. Transmission is transplacental in most cases, or via delivery (especially HSV-2). Nonspecific signs common to many **ToRCHeS** infections include hepatosplenomegaly, jaundice, thrombocytopenia, and growth retardation.

Other important infectious agents include *Streptococcus agalactiae* (group B streptococci), *E. coli*, and *Listeria monocytogenes*—all causes of meningitis in neonates. Parvovirus B19 causes hydrops fetalis.

AGENT	MODE OF TRANSMISSION	MATERNAL MANIFESTATIONS	NEONATAL MANIFESTIONS
Toxoplasma gondii	Cat feces or ingestion of undercooked meat	Usually asymptomatic; lymphadenopathy (rarely)	Classic triad: chorioretinitis, hydrocephalus, and intracranial calcifications, +/– "blueberry muffin" rash
Rubella	Respiratory droplets	Rash, lymphadenopathy, arthritis	Classic triad: PDA (or pulmonary artery hypoplasia), cataracts, and deafness, +/– "blueberry muffin" rash
CMV	Sexual contact, organ transplants	Usually asymptomatic; mononucleosis-like illness	Hearing loss, seizures, petechial rash, "blueberry muffin" rash, periventricular calcifications
HIV	Sexual contact, needlestick	Variable presentation depending on CD4+ count	Recurrent infections, chronic diarrhea
Herpes simplex virus-2	Skin or mucous membrane contact	Usually asymptomatic; herpetic (vesicular) lesions	Encephalitis, herpetic (vesicular) lesions
Syphilis	Sexual contact	Chancre (1°) and disseminated rash (2°) are the two stages likely to result in fetal infection	Often results in stillbirth, hydrops fetalis; if child survives, presents with facial abnormalities (e.g., notched teeth, saddle nose, short maxilla), saber shins, CN VIII deafness

Red rashes of childhood

AGENT	ASSOCIATED SYNDROME/DISEASE	CLINICAL PRESENTATION
Coxsackievirus type A	Hand-foot-mouth disease	Oval-shaped vesicles on palms and soles **A**; vesicles and ulcers in oral mucosa
HHV-6	Roseola (exanthem subitum)	Asymptomatic rose-colored macules appear on body after several days of high fever; can present with febrile seizures; usually affects infants
Measles virus	Measles (rubeola)	Beginning at head and moving down; rash is preceded by cough, coryza, conjunctivitis, and blue-white (Koplik) spots on buccal mucosa
Parvovirus B19	Erythema infectiosum (fifth disease)	"Slapped cheek" rash on face **B** (can cause hydrops fetalis in pregnant women)
Rubella virus	Rubella (German measles)	Pink coalescing macules begin at head and move down → fine desquamating truncal rash; postauricular lymphadenopathy
Streptococcus pyogenes	Scarlet fever	Erythematous, sandpaper-like rash with fever and sore throat
VZV	Chickenpox	Vesicular rash begins on trunk; spreads to face and extremities with lesions of different ages

A Hand-foot-mouth disease. RU

B Erythema infectiosum. RU

Sexually transmitted infections

DISEASE	CLINICAL FEATURES	ORGANISM
AIDS	Opportunistic infections, Kaposi sarcoma, lymphoma	HIV
Chancroid	Painful genital ulcer with exudate, inguinal adenopathy	*Haemophilus **ducreyi*** (it's so painful, you "**do cry**")
Chlamydia	Urethritis, cervicitis, conjunctivitis, reactive arthritis, PID	*Chlamydia trachomatis* (D–K)
Condylomata acuminata	Genital warts, koilocytes	HPV-6 and -11
Genital herpes	Painful penile, vulvar, or cervical vesicles and ulcers; can cause systemic symptoms such as fever, headache, myalgia	HSV-2, less commonly HSV-1
Gonorrhea	Urethritis, cervicitis, PID, prostatitis, epididymitis, arthritis, creamy purulent discharge	*Neisseria gonorrhoeae*
Hepatitis B	Jaundice	HBV
Lymphogranuloma venereum	Infection of lymphatics; painless genital ulcers, painful lymphadenopathy (i.e., buboes)	*C. trachomatis* (L1–L3)
1° syphilis	Painless chancre	*Treponema pallidum*
2° syphilis	Fever, lymphadenopathy, skin rashes, condylomata lata	
3° syphilis	Gummas, tabes dorsalis, general paresis, aortitis, Argyll Robertson pupil	
Trichomoniasis	Vaginitis, strawberry cervix, motile in wet prep	*Trichomonas vaginalis*

Pelvic inflammatory disease

Top bugs—*Chlamydia trachomatis* (subacute, often undiagnosed), *Neisseria gonorrhoeae* (acute). *C. trachomatis*—most common bacterial STI in the United States. Cervical motion tenderness (chandelier sign), purulent cervical discharge A. PID may include salpingitis, endometritis, hydrosalpinx, and tubo-ovarian abscess.

Salpingitis is a risk factor for ectopic pregnancy, infertility, chronic pelvic pain, and adhesions. Can lead to Fitz-Hugh–Curtis syndrome—infection of the liver capsule and "violin string" adhesions of peritoneum to liver B.

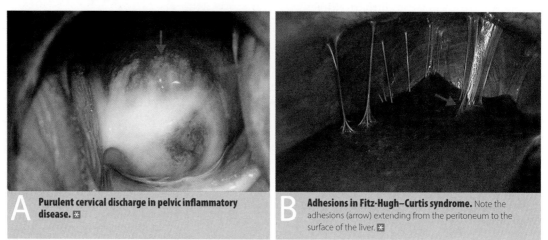

A **Purulent cervical discharge in pelvic inflammatory disease.** ✳

B **Adhesions in Fitz-Hugh–Curtis syndrome.** Note the adhesions (arrow) extending from the peritoneum to the surface of the liver. ✳

Nosocomial infections   *E. coli* (UTI) and *S. aureus* (wound infection) are the two most common causes.

RISK FACTOR	PATHOGEN	UNIQUE SIGNS/SYMPTOMS
Altered mental status, old age, aspiration	Polymicrobial, gram-negative bacteria, often anaerobes	Right lower lobe infiltrate or right upper/middle lobe (patient recumbent); purulent malodorous sputum
Antibiotic use	*Clostridium difficile*	Watery diarrhea, leukocytosis
Decubitus ulcers, surgical wounds, drains	*S. aureus* (including MRSA), gram-negative anaerobes	Erythema, tenderness, induration, drainage from surgical wound sites
Intravascular catheters	*S. aureus* (including MRSA), *S. epidermidis* (long term), *Enterobacter*	Erythema, induration, tenderness, drainage from access sites
Mechanical ventilation, endotracheal intubation	Late onset: *P. aeruginosa*, *Klebsiella*, *Acinetobacter*, *S. aureus*	New infiltrate on CXR, ↑ sputum production; sweet odor (*Pseudomonas*)
Renal dialysis unit, needlestick	HBV	
Urinary catheterization	*E. coli*, *Klebsiella*, *Proteus* spp.	Dysuria, leukocytosis, flank pain or costovertebral angle tenderness
Water aerosols	*Legionella*	Signs of pneumonia, GI symptoms (nausea, vomiting)

Bugs affecting unimmunized children

CLINICAL PRESENTATION	FINDINGS/LABS	PATHOGEN
Dermatologic		
Rash	Beginning at head and moving down with postauricular lymphadenopathy	Rubella virus
	Beginning at head and moving down; rash preceded by cough, coryza, conjunctivitis, and blue-white (Koplik) spots on buccal mucosa	Measles virus
Neurologic		
Meningitis	Microbe colonizes nasopharynx	*H. influenzae* type B
	Can also lead to myalgia and paralysis	Poliovirus
Respiratory		
Epiglottitis	Fever with dysphagia, drooling, and difficulty breathing due to edematous "cherry red" epiglottis; "thumbprint sign" on X-ray	*H. influenzae* type B (also capable of causing epiglottitis in fully immunized children)
Pharyngitis	Grayish oropharyngeal exudate ("pseudomembranes" may obstruct airway); painful throat	*Corynebacterium diphtheriae* (elaborates toxin that causes necrosis in pharynx, cardiac, and CNS tissue)

	CHARACTERISTIC	ORGANISM
Bug hints (if all else fails)	Asplenic patient (due to surgical splenectomy or autosplenectomy, e.g., chronic sickle cell disease)	Encapsulated microbes, especially **SHiN** (**S.** *pneumoniae* >> *H. influenzae* type B > *N. meningitidis*)
	Branching rods in oral infection, sulfur granules	*Actinomyces israelii*
	Chronic granulomatous disease	Catalase ⊕ microbes, especially S. *aureus*
	"Currant jelly" sputum	*Klebsiella*
	Dog or cat bite	*Pasteurella multocida*
	Facial nerve palsy	*Borrelia burgdorferi* (Lyme disease)
	Fungal infection in diabetic or immunocompromised patient	*Mucor* or *Rhizopus* spp.
	Health care provider	HBV (from needlestick)
	Neutropenic patients	*Candida albicans* (systemic), *Aspergillus*
	Organ transplant recipient	CMV
	PAS ⊕	*Tropheryma whipplei* (Whipple disease)
	Pediatric infection	*Haemophilus influenzae* (including epiglottitis)
	Pneumonia in cystic fibrosis, burn infection	*Pseudomonas aeruginosa*
	Pus, empyema, abscess	S. *aureus*
	Rash on hands and feet	Coxsackie A virus, *Treponema pallidum*, *Rickettsia rickettsii*
	Sepsis/meningitis in newborn	Group B strep
	Surgical wound	S. *aureus*
	Traumatic open wound	*Clostridium perfringens*

▸ MICROBIOLOGY—ANTIMICROBIALS

Antimicrobial therapy

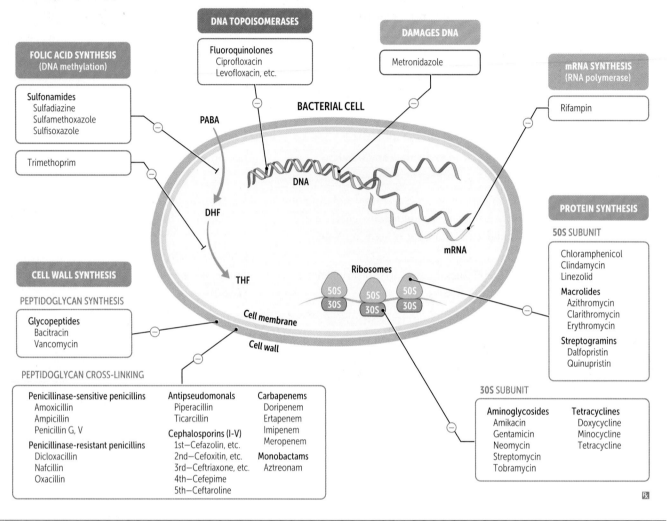

Penicillin G, V	Penicillin G (IV and IM form), penicillin V (oral). Prototype β-lactam antibiotics.
MECHANISM	Bind penicillin-binding proteins (transpeptidases). Block transpeptidase cross-linking of peptidoglycan in cell wall. Activate autolytic enzymes.
CLINICAL USE	Mostly used for gram-positive organisms (*S. pneumoniae, S. pyogenes, Actinomyces*). Also used for gram-negative cocci (mainly *N. meningitidis*) and spirochetes (namely *T. pallidum*). Bactericidal for gram-positive cocci, gram-positive rods, gram-negative cocci, and spirochetes. Penicillinase sensitive.
TOXICITY	Hypersensitivity reactions, hemolytic anemia.
RESISTANCE	Penicillinase in bacteria (a type of β-lactamase) cleaves β-lactam ring.

Amoxicillin, ampicillin (aminopenicillins, penicillinase-sensitive penicillins)

MECHANISM	Same as penicillin. Wider spectrum; penicillinase sensitive. Also combine with clavulanic acid to protect against destruction by β-lactamase.	AMinoPenicillins are AMPed-up penicillin. AmOxicillin has greater Oral bioavailability than ampicillin.
CLINICAL USE	Extended-spectrum penicillin—*H. influenzae*, *H. pylori*, *E. coli*, *Listeria monocytogenes*, *Proteus mirabilis*, *Salmonella*, *Shigella*, enterococci.	Coverage: ampicillin/amoxicillin **HHELPSS** kill enterococci.
TOXICITY	Hypersensitivity reactions; rash; pseudomembranous colitis.	
MECHANISM OF RESISTANCE	Penicillinase in bacteria (a type of β-lactamase) cleaves β-lactam ring.	

Dicloxacillin, nafcillin, oxacillin (penicillinase-resistant penicillins)

MECHANISM	Same as penicillin. Narrow spectrum; penicillinase resistant because bulky R group blocks access of β-lactamase to β-lactam ring.	
CLINICAL USE	*S. aureus* (except MRSA; resistant because of altered penicillin-binding protein target site).	"Use **naf** (nafcillin) for **staph**."
TOXICITY	Hypersensitivity reactions, interstitial nephritis.	

Piperacillin, ticarcillin (antipseudomonals)

MECHANISM	Same as penicillin. Extended spectrum.
CLINICAL USE	*Pseudomonas* spp. and gram-negative rods; susceptible to penicillinase; use with β-lactamase inhibitors.
TOXICITY	Hypersensitivity reactions.

β-lactamase inhibitors	Include Clavulanic Acid, Sulbactam, Tazobactam. Often added to penicillin antibiotics to protect the antibiotic from destruction by β-lactamase (penicillinase).	CAST.

Cephalosporins (generations I–V)

MECHANISM	β-lactam drugs that inhibit cell wall synthesis but are less susceptible to penicillinases. Bactericidal.	Organisms typically not covered by cephalosporins are **LAME**: *Listeria*, Atypicals (*Chlamydia*, *Mycoplasma*), MRSA, and Enterococci. Exception: ceftaroline covers MRSA.
CLINICAL USE	1st generation (cefazolin, cephalexin)—gram-positive cocci, *Proteus mirabilis*, *E. coli*, *Klebsiella pneumoniae*. Cefazolin used prior to surgery to prevent *S. aureus* wound infections.	1st generation—**PEcK**.
	2nd generation (cefoxitin, cefaclor, cefuroxime)—gram-positive cocci, *Haemophilus influenzae*, *Enterobacter aerogenes*, *Neisseria* spp., *Proteus mirabilis*, *E. coli*, *Klebsiella pneumoniae*, *Serratia marcescens*.	2nd generation—**HEN PEcKS**.
	3rd generation (ceftriaxone, cefotaxime, ceftazidime)—serious gram-negative infections resistant to other β-lactams.	Ceftriaxone—meningitis, gonorrhea, disseminated Lyme disease. Ceftazidime—*Pseudomonas*.
	4th generation (cefepime)—gram-negative organisms, with ↑ activity against *Pseudomonas* and gram-positive organisms.	
	5th generation (ceftaroline)—broad gram-positive and gram-negative organism coverage, including MRSA; does not cover *Pseudomonas*.	
TOXICITY	Hypersensitivity reactions, autoimmune hemolytic anemia, disulfiram-like reaction, vitamin K deficiency. Exhibit cross-reactivity with penicillins. ↑ nephrotoxicity of aminoglycosides.	
MECHANISM OF RESISTANCE	Structural change in penicillin-binding proteins (transpeptidases).	

Carbapenems

Imipenem, meropenem, ertapenem, doripenem.

MECHANISM	Imipenem is a broad-spectrum, β-lactamase–resistant carbapenem. Always administered with cilastatin (inhibitor of renal dehydropeptidase I) to ↓ inactivation of drug in renal tubules.	With imipenem, "the kill is **lastin'** with ci**lastatin**." Newer carbapenems include ertapenem (limited *Pseudomonas* coverage) and doripenem.
CLINICAL USE	Gram-positive cocci, gram-negative rods, and anaerobes. Wide spectrum, but significant side effects limit use to life-threatening infections or after other drugs have failed. Meropenem has a ↓ risk of seizures and is stable to dehydropeptidase I.	
TOXICITY	GI distress, skin rash, and CNS toxicity (seizures) at high plasma levels.	

Monobactams

Aztreonam

MECHANISM	Less susceptible to β-lactamases. Prevents peptidoglycan cross-linking by binding to penicillin-binding protein 3. Synergistic with aminoglycosides. No cross-allergenicity with penicillins.
CLINICAL USE	Gram-negative rods only—no activity against gram-positives or anaerobes. For penicillin-allergic patients and those with renal insufficiency who cannot tolerate aminoglycosides.
TOXICITY	Usually nontoxic; occasional GI upset.

Vancomycin

MECHANISM	Inhibits cell wall peptidoglycan formation by binding D-ala D-ala portion of cell wall precursors. Bactericidal. Not susceptible to β-lactamases.
CLINICAL USE	Gram-positive bugs only—serious, multidrug-resistant organisms, including MRSA, *S. epidermidis*, sensitive *Enteroccocus* species, and *Clostridium difficile* (oral dose for pseudomembranous colitis).
TOXICITY	Well tolerated in general—but **NOT** trouble free. Nephrotoxicity, Ototoxicity, Thrombophlebitis, diffuse flushing—red man syndrome (can largely prevent by pretreatment with antihistamines and slow infusion rate).
MECHANISM OF RESISTANCE	Occurs in bacteria via amino acid modification of **D-ala D-ala** to D-ala D-lac. "Pay back **2 D-alas** (dollars) for **van**dalizing (**van**comycin)."

Protein synthesis inhibitors

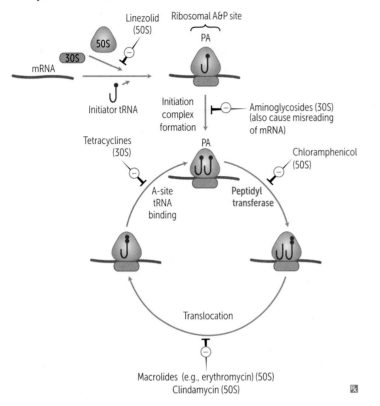

Specifically target smaller bacterial ribosome (70S, made of 30S and 50S subunits), leaving human ribosome (80S) unaffected.

30S inhibitors

A = Aminoglycosides [bactericidal]
T = Tetracyclines [bacteriostatic]

50S inhibitors

C = Chloramphenicol, Clindamycin [bacteriostatic]
E = Erythromycin (macrolides) [bacteriostatic]
L = Linezolid [variable]
"Buy **AT 30**, **CCEL** (sell) at **50**."

Aminoglycosides	Gentamicin, Neomycin, Amikacin, Tobramycin, Streptomycin.	"Mean" (aminoglycoside) GNATS caNNOT kill anaerobes.
MECHANISM	Bactericidal; irreversible inhibition of initiation complex through binding of the 30S subunit. Can cause misreading of mRNA. Also block translocation. Require O_2 for uptake; therefore ineffective against anaerobes.	
CLINICAL USE	Severe gram-negative rod infections. Synergistic with β-lactam antibiotics. Neomycin for bowel surgery.	
TOXICITY	Nephrotoxicity, Neuromuscular blockade, Ototoxicity (especially when used with loop diuretics). Teratogen.	
MECHANISM OF RESISTANCE	Bacterial transferase enzymes inactivate the drug by acetylation, phosphorylation, or adenylation.	

Tetracyclines	Tetracycline, doxycycline, minocycline.
MECHANISM	Bacteriostatic; bind to 30S and prevent attachment of aminoacyl-tRNA; limited CNS penetration. Doxycycline is fecally eliminated and can be used in patients with renal failure. Do not take tetracyclines with milk (Ca^{2+}), antacids (Ca^{2+} or Mg^{2+}), or iron-containing preparations because divalent cations inhibit drugs' absorption in the gut.
CLINICAL USE	*Borrelia burgdorferi, M. pneumoniae.* Drugs' ability to accumulate intracellularly makes them very effective against *Rickettsia* and *Chlamydia.* Also used to treat acne.
TOXICITY	GI distress, discoloration of teeth and inhibition of bone growth in children, photosensitivity. Contraindicated in pregnancy.
MECHANISM OF RESISTANCE	↓ uptake or ↑ efflux out of bacterial cells by plasmid-encoded transport pumps.

Chloramphenicol	
MECHANISM	Blocks peptidyltransferase at 50S ribosomal subunit. Bacteriostatic.
CLINICAL USE	Meningitis (*Haemophilus influenzae, Neisseria meningitidis, Streptococcus pneumoniae*) and Rocky Mountain spotted fever (*Rickettsia rickettsii*). Limited use owing to toxicities but often still used in developing countries because of low cost.
TOXICITY	Anemia (dose dependent), aplastic anemia (dose independent), gray baby syndrome (in premature infants because they lack liver UDP-glucuronyl transferase).
MECHANISM OF RESISTANCE	Plasmid-encoded acetyltransferase inactivates the drug.

Clindamycin		
MECHANISM	Blocks peptide transfer (translocation) at 50S ribosomal subunit. Bacteriostatic.	
CLINICAL USE	Anaerobic infections (e.g., *Bacteroides* spp., *Clostridium perfringens*) in aspiration pneumonia, lung abscesses, and oral infections. Also effective against invasive group A streptococcal infection.	Treats anaerobic infections **above** the diaphragm vs. metronidazole (anaerobic infections **below** diaphragm).
TOXICITY	Pseudomembranous colitis (*C. difficile* overgrowth), fever, diarrhea.	

Oxazolidinones	Linezolid
MECHANISM	Inhibit protein synthesis by binding to 50S subunit and preventing formation of the initiation complex.
CLINICAL USE	Gram-positive species including MRSA and VRE.
TOXICITY	Bone marrow suppression (especially thrombocytopenia), peripheral neuropathy, serotonin syndrome.
MECHANISM OF RESISTANCE	Point mutation of ribosomal RNA.

Macrolides	Azithromycin, clarithromycin, erythromycin.
MECHANISM	Inhibit protein synthesis by blocking translocation ("macro**slides**"); bind to the 23S rRNA of the 50S ribosomal subunit. Bacteriostatic.
CLINICAL USE	Atypical pneumonias (*Mycoplasma*, *Chlamydia*, *Legionella*), STIs (*Chlamydia*), gram-positive cocci (streptococcal infections in patients allergic to penicillin), and *B. pertussis*.
TOXICITY	**MACRO**: Gastrointestinal **M**otility issues, **A**rrhythmia caused by prolonged QT interval, acute **C**holestatic hepatitis, **R**ash, e**O**sinophilia. Increases serum concentration of theophyllines, oral anticoagulants. Clarithromycin and erythromycin inhibit cytochrome P-450.
MECHANISM OF RESISTANCE	Methylation of 23S rRNA-binding site prevents binding of drug.

Trimethoprim	
MECHANISM	Inhibits bacterial dihydrofolate reductase. Bacteriostatic.
CLINICAL USE	Used in combination with sulfonamides (trimethoprim-sulfamethoxazole [TMP-SMX]), causing sequential block of folate synthesis. Combination used for UTIs, *Shigella*, *Salmonella*, *Pneumocystis jirovecii* pneumonia treatment and prophylaxis, toxoplasmosis prophylaxis.
TOXICITY	Megaloblastic anemia, leukopenia, granulocytopenia. (May alleviate with supplemental folinic acid). **TMP T**reats **M**arrow **P**oorly.

Sulfonamides	Sulfamethoxazole (SMX), sulfisoxazole, sulfadiazine.
MECHANISM	Inhibit folate synthesis. *Para*-aminobenzoic acid (PABA) antimetabolites inhibit dihydropteroate synthase. Bacteriostatic (bactericidal when combined with trimethoprim). (Dapsone, used to treat lepromatous leprosy, is a closely related drug that also inhibits folate synthesis.)
CLINICAL USE	Gram-positives, gram-negatives, *Nocardia*, *Chlamydia*. Triple sulfas or SMX for simple UTI.
TOXICITY	Hypersensitivity reactions, hemolysis if G6PD deficient, nephrotoxicity (tubulointerstitial nephritis), photosensitivity, kernicterus in infants, displace other drugs from albumin (e.g., warfarin).
MECHANISM OF RESISTANCE	Altered enzyme (bacterial dihydropteroate synthase), ↓ uptake, or ↑ PABA synthesis.

PABA + Pteridine

Dihydropteroate synthase — **Sulfonamides**

Dihydropteroic acid

Dihydrofolic acid

Dihydrofolate reductase — **Trimethoprim, pyrimethamine**

Tetrahydrofolic acid (THF)

Purines → DNA, RNA

Thymidine → DNA

Methionine → Protein

Fluoroquinolones	Ciprofloxacin, norfloxacin, levofloxacin, ofloxacin, moxifloxacin, gemifloxacin, enoxacin.	
MECHANISM	Inhibit prokaryotic enzymes topoisomerase II (DNA gyrase) and topoisomerase IV. Bactericidal. Must not be taken with antacids.	
CLINICAL USE	Gram-negative rods of urinary and GI tracts (including *Pseudomonas*), *Neisseria*, some gram-positive organisms.	
TOXICITY	GI upset, superinfections, skin rashes, headache, dizziness. Less commonly, can cause leg cramps and myalgias. Contraindicated in pregnant women, nursing mothers, and children < 18 years old due to possible damage to cartilage. Some may prolong QT interval. May cause tendonitis or tendon rupture in people > 60 years old and in patients taking prednisone.	**Fluoroquinolones** hurt attachments to your **bones**.
MECHANISM OF RESISTANCE	Chromosome-encoded mutation in DNA gyrase, plasmid-mediated resistance, efflux pumps.	

Daptomycin		
MECHANISM	Lipopeptide that disrupts cell membrane of gram-positive cocci.	
CLINICAL USE	*S. aureus* skin infections (especially MRSA), bacteremia, endocarditis, VRE.	Not used for pneumonia (avidly binds to and is inactivated by surfactant).
TOXICITY	Myopathy, rhabdomyolysis.	

Metronidazole		
MECHANISM	Forms toxic free radical metabolites in the bacterial cell that damage DNA. Bactericidal, antiprotozoal.	
CLINICAL USE	Treats *Giardia*, *Entamoeba*, *Trichomonas*, *Gardnerella vaginalis*, Anaerobes (*Bacteroides*, *C. difficile*). Used with a proton pump inhibitor and clarithromycin for "triple therapy" against *H. Pylori*.	**GET GAP** on the **Metro** with **metro**nidazole! Treats anaerobic infection **below** the diaphragm vs. clindamycin (anaerobic infections **above** diaphragm).
TOXICITY	Disulfiram-like reaction (severe flushing, tachycardia, hypotension) with alcohol; headache, metallic taste.	

Antimycobacterial drugs

BACTERIUM	PROPHYLAXIS	TREATMENT
M. tuberculosis	Isoniazid	Rifampin, Isoniazid, Pyrazinamide, Ethambutol (**RIPE** for treatment)
M. avium–intracellulare	Azithromycin, rifabutin	More drug resistant than *M. tuberculosis*. Azithromycin or clarithromycin + ethambutol. Can add rifabutin or ciprofloxacin.
M. leprae	N/A	Long-term treatment with dapsone and rifampin for tuberculoid form. Add clofazimine for lepromatous form.

MYCOBACTERIAL CELL

Rifamycins — Rifampin, rifabutin.

MECHANISM	Inhibit DNA-dependent RNA polymerase.	Rifampin's 4 R's:
CLINICAL USE	*Mycobacterium tuberculosis*; delay resistance to dapsone when used for leprosy. Used for meningococcal prophylaxis and chemoprophylaxis in contacts of children with *Haemophilus influenzae* type B.	RNA polymerase inhibitor Ramps up microsomal cytochrome P-450 Red/orange body fluids Rapid resistance if used alone Rifampin **ramps** up cytochrome P-450, but rifabutin does not.
TOXICITY	Minor hepatotoxicity and drug interactions (↑ cytochrome P-450); orange body fluids (nonhazardous side effect). Rifabutin favored over rifampin in patients with HIV infection due to less cytochrome P-450 stimulation.	
MECHANISM OF RESISTANCE	Mutations reduce drug binding to RNA polymerase. Monotherapy rapidly leads to resistance.	

Isoniazid

MECHANISM	↓ synthesis of mycolic acids. Bacterial catalase-peroxidase (encoded by KatG) needed to convert INH to active metabolite.
CLINICAL USE	*Mycobacterium tuberculosis*. The only agent used as solo prophylaxis against TB.	Different INH half-lives in fast vs. slow acetylators.
TOXICITY	Neurotoxicity, hepatotoxicity. Pyridoxine (vitamin B_6) can prevent neurotoxicity.	**INH** Injures Neurons and Hepatocytes.
MECHANISM OF RESISTANCE	Mutations leading to underexpression of KatG.

Pyrazinamide

MECHANISM	Mechanism uncertain. Pyrazinamide is a prodrug that is converted to the active compound pyrazinoic acid.
CLINICAL USE	*Mycobacterium tuberculosis*.
TOXICITY	Hyperuricemia, hepatotoxicity.

Ethambutol

MECHANISM	↓ carbohydrate polymerization of mycobacterium cell wall by blocking arabinosyltransferase.
CLINICAL USE	*Mycobacterium tuberculosis*.
TOXICITY	**Optic** neuropathy (red-green color blindness). Pronounce "eyethambutol."

Antimicrobial prophylaxis

CLINICAL SCENARIO	MEDICATION
High risk for endocarditis and undergoing surgical or dental procedures	Amoxicillin
Exposure to gonorrhea	Ceftriaxone
History of recurrent UTIs	TMP-SMX
Exposure to meningococcal infection	Ceftriaxone, ciprofloxacin, or rifampin
Pregnant woman carrying group B strep	Penicillin G
Prevention of gonococcal conjunctivitis in newborn	Erythromycin ointment
Prevention of postsurgical infection due to *S. aureus*	Cefazolin
Prophylaxis of strep pharyngitis in child with prior rheumatic fever	Benzathine penicillin G or oral penicillin V
Exposure to syphilis	Benzathine penicillin G

Prophylaxis in HIV patients

CELL COUNT	PROPHYLAXIS	INFECTION
CD4 < 200 cells/mm³	TMP-SMX	*Pneumocystis* pneumonia
CD4 < 100 cells/mm³	TMP-SMX	*Pneumocystis* pneumonia and toxoplasmosis
CD4 < 50 cells/mm³	Azithromycin or clarithromycin	*Mycobacterium avium* complex

Treatment of highly resistant bacteria

MRSA: vancomycin, daptomycin, linezolid, tigecycline, ceftaroline.

VRE: linezolid and streptogramins (quinupristin, dalfopristin).

Multidrug-resistant *P. aeruginosa*, multidrug-resistant *Acinetobacter baumannii*: polymyxins B and E (colistin).

Antifungal therapy

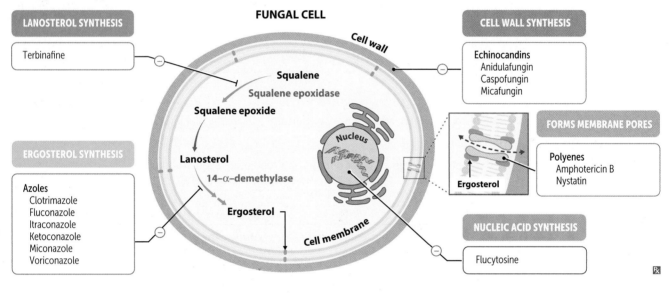

Amphotericin B

MECHANISM	Binds ergosterol (unique to fungi); forms membrane pores that allow leakage of electrolytes.	Amphotericin "tears" holes in the fungal membrane by forming pores.
CLINICAL USE	Serious, systemic mycoses. *Cryptococcus* (amphotericin B with/without flucytosine for cryptococcal meningitis), *Blastomyces*, *Coccidioides*, *Histoplasma*, *Candida*, *Mucor*. Intrathecally for fungal meningitis. Supplement K⁺ and Mg²⁺ because of altered renal tubule permeability.	
TOXICITY	Fever/chills ("shake and bake"), hypotension, nephrotoxicity, arrhythmias, anemia, IV phlebitis ("**amphoterrible**"). Hydration ↓ nephrotoxicity. Liposomal amphotericin ↓ toxicity.	

Nystatin

MECHANISM	Same as amphotericin B. Topical use only as too toxic for systemic use.
CLINICAL USE	"Swish and swallow" for oral candidiasis (thrush); topical for diaper rash or vaginal candidiasis.

Flucytosine

MECHANISM	Inhibits DNA and RNA biosynthesis by conversion to 5-fluorouracil by cytosine deaminase.
CLINICAL USE	Systemic fungal infections (especially meningitis caused by *Cryptococcus*) in combination with amphotericin B.
TOXICITY	Bone marrow suppression.

Azoles

	Clotrimazole, fluconazole, itraconazole, ketoconazole, miconazole, voriconazole.
MECHANISM	Inhibit fungal sterol (ergosterol) synthesis by inhibiting the cytochrome P-450 enzyme that converts lanosterol to ergosterol.
CLINICAL USE	Local and less serious systemic mycoses. Fluconazole for chronic suppression of cryptococcal meningitis in AIDS patients and candidal infections of all types. Itraconazole for *Blastomyces*, *Coccidioides*, *Histoplasma*. Clotrimazole and miconazole for topical fungal infections.
TOXICITY	Testosterone synthesis inhibition (gynecomastia, especially with ketoconazole), liver dysfunction (inhibits cytochrome P-450).

Terbinafine

MECHANISM	Inhibits the fungal enzyme squalene epoxidase.
CLINICAL USE	Dermatophytoses (especially onychomycosis—fungal infection of finger or toe nails).
TOXICITY	GI upset, headaches, hepatotoxicity, taste disturbance.

Echinocandins

	Anidulafungin, caspofungin, micafungin.
MECHANISM	Inhibit cell wall synthesis by inhibiting synthesis of β-glucan.
CLINICAL USE	Invasive aspergillosis, *Candida*.
TOXICITY	GI upset, flushing (by histamine release).

Griseofulvin

MECHANISM	Interferes with microtubule function; disrupts mitosis. Deposits in keratin-containing tissues (e.g., nails).
CLINICAL USE	Oral treatment of superficial infections; inhibits growth of dermatophytes (tinea, ringworm).
TOXICITY	Teratogenic, carcinogenic, confusion, headaches, ↑ cytochrome P-450 and warfarin metabolism.

Antiprotozoan therapy	Pyrimethamine (toxoplasmosis), suramin and melarsoprol (*Trypanosoma brucei*), nifurtimox (*T. cruzi*), sodium stibogluconate (leishmaniasis).

Anti-mite/louse therapy	Permethrin (blocks Na$^+$ channels → neurotoxicity), malathion (acetylcholinesterase inhibitor), lindane (blocks GABA channels → neurotoxicity). Used to treat scabies (*Sarcoptes scabiei*) and lice (*Pediculus* and *Pthirus*).

Chloroquine

MECHANISM	Blocks detoxification of heme into hemozoin. Heme accumulates and is toxic to plasmodia.
CLINICAL USE	Treatment of plasmodial species other than *P. falciparum* (frequency of resistance in *P. falciparum* is too high). Resistance due to membrane pump that ↓ intracellular concentration of drug. Treat *P. falciparum* with artemether/lumefantrine or atovaquone/proguanil. For life-threatening malaria, use quinidine in U.S. (quinine elsewhere) or artesunate.
TOXICITY	Retinopathy; pruritus (especially in dark-skinned individuals).

Antihelminthic therapy	Mebendazole, pyrantel pamoate, ivermectin, diethylcarbamazine, praziquantel.

Antiviral therapy

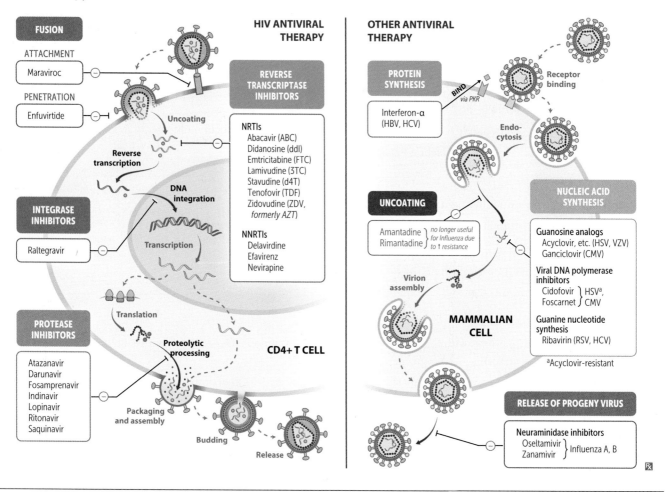

Oseltamivir, zanamivir

MECHANISM	Inhibit influenza neuraminidase → ↓ release of progeny virus.
CLINICAL USE	Treatment and prevention of both influenza A and B.

Acyclovir, famciclovir, valacyclovir

MECHANISM	Guanosine analogs. Monophosphorylated by HSV/VZV thymidine kinase and not phosphorylated in uninfected cells → few adverse effects. Triphosphate formed by cellular enzymes. Preferentially inhibit viral DNA polymerase by chain termination.
CLINICAL USE	HSV and VZV. Weak activity against EBV. No activity against CMV. Used for HSV-induced mucocutaneous and genital lesions as well as for encephalitis. Prophylaxis in immunocompromised patients. No effect on latent forms of HSV and VZV. Valacyclovir, a prodrug of acyclovir, has better oral bioavailability. For herpes zoster, use famciclovir.
TOXICITY	Obstructive crystalline nephropathy and acute renal failure if not adequately hydrated.
MECHANISM OF RESISTANCE	Mutated viral thymidine kinase.

Ganciclovir

MECHANISM	5′-monophosphate formed by a CMV viral kinase. Guanosine analog. Triphosphate formed by cellular kinases. Preferentially inhibits viral DNA polymerase. Preferentially inhibit viral DNA polymerase by chain termination.
CLINICAL USE	CMV, especially in immunocompromised patients. Valganciclovir, a prodrug of ganciclovir, has better oral bioavailability.
TOXICITY	Leukopenia, neutropenia, thrombocytopenia, renal toxicity. More toxic to host enzymes than acyclovir.
MECHANISM OF RESISTANCE	Mutated viral kinase.

Foscarnet

MECHANISM	Viral DNA/RNA polymerase inhibitor and HIV reverse transcriptase inhibitor. Binds to pyrophosphate-binding site of enzyme. Does not require activation by viral kinase.	Foscarnet = pyrofosphate analog.
CLINICAL USE	CMV retinitis in immunocompromised patients when ganciclovir fails; acyclovir-resistant HSV.	
TOXICITY	Nephrotoxicity, electrolyte abnormalities (hypo- or hypercalcemia, hypo- or hyperphosphatemia, hypokalemia, hypomagnesemia) can lead to seizures.	
MECHANISM OF RESISTANCE	Mutated DNA polymerase.	

Cidofovir

MECHANISM	Preferentially inhibits viral DNA polymerase. Does not require phosphorylation by viral kinase.
CLINICAL USE	CMV retinitis in immunocompromised patients; acyclovir-resistant HSV. Long half-life.
TOXICITY	Nephrotoxicity (coadminister with probenecid and IV saline to ↓ toxicity).

HIV therapy

Highly active antiretroviral therapy (HAART): often initiated at the time of HIV diagnosis. Strongest indication for patients presenting with AIDS-defining illness, low CD4+ cell counts (< 500 cells/mm^3), or high viral load. Regimen consists of 3 drugs to prevent resistance: 2 NRTIs *and* 1 of the following: NNRTI *or* protease inhibitor *or* integrase inhibitor.

DRUG	MECHANISM	TOXICITY
Protease inhibitors		
Atazanavir Darunavir Fosamprenavir Indinavir Lopinavir Ritonavir Saquinavir	Assembly of virions depends on HIV-1 protease (*pol* gene), which cleaves the polypeptide products of HIV mRNA into their functional parts. Thus, protease inhibitors prevent maturation of new viruses. Ritonavir can "boost" other drug concentrations by inhibiting cytochrome P-450. All protease inhibitors end in -*navir*. **Navir** (never) **tease** a **protease**.	Hyperglycemia, GI intolerance (nausea, diarrhea), lipodystrophy. Nephropathy, hematuria (indinavir). Rifampin (a potent CYP/UGT inducer) contraindicated with protease inhibitors because it can decrease protease inhibitor concentration.
NRTIs		
Abacavir (ABC) Didanosine (ddI) Emtricitabine (FTC) Lamivudine (3TC) Stavudine (d4T) Tenofovir (TDF) Zidovudine (ZDV, formerly AZT)	Competitively inhibit nucleotide binding to reverse transcriptase and terminate the DNA chain (lack a 3′ OH group). Tenofovir is a nucleoTide; the others are nucleosides and need to be phosphorylated to be active. ZDV is used for general prophylaxis and during pregnancy to ↓ risk of fetal transmission. Have **you dined** (vudine) with my **nuclear** (nucleosides) family?	Bone marrow suppression (can be reversed with granulocyte colony-stimulating factor [G-CSF] and erythropoietin), peripheral neuropathy, lactic acidosis (nucleosides), anemia (ZDV), pancreatitis (didanosine).
NNRTIs		
Delavirdine Efavirenz Nevirapine	Bind to reverse transcriptase at site different from NRTIs. Do not require phosphorylation to be active or compete with nucleotides.	Rash and hepatotoxicity are common to all NNRTIs. Vivid dreams and CNS symptoms are common with efavirenz. Delavirdine and efavirenz are contraindicated in pregnancy.
Integrase inhibitors		
Raltegravir	Inhibits HIV genome integration into host cell chromosome by reversibly inhibiting HIV integrase.	↑ creatine kinase.
Fusion inhibitors		
Enfuvirtide	Binds gp41, inhibiting viral entry.	Skin reaction at injection sites.
Maraviroc	Binds CCR-5 on surface of T cells/monocytes, inhibiting interaction with gp120.	

Interferons

MECHANISM	Glycoproteins normally synthesized by virus-infected cells, exhibiting a wide range of antiviral and antitumoral properties.
CLINICAL USE	IFN-α: chronic hepatitis B and C, Kaposi sarcoma, hairy cell leukemia, condyloma acuminatum, renal cell carcinoma, malignant melanoma. IFN-β: multiple sclerosis. IFN-γ: chronic granulomatous disease.
TOXICITY	Neutropenia, myopathy.

Hepatitis C therapy

DRUG	MECHANISM	CLINICAL USE
Ribavirin	Inhibits synthesis of guanine nucleotides by competitively inhibiting inosine monophosphate dehydrogenase.	Chronic HCV, also used in RSV (palivizumab preferred in children) Toxicity: hemolytic anemia; severe teratogen.
Simeprevir	HCV protease inhibitor; prevents viral replication.	Chronic HCV in combination with ribavirin and peginterferon alfa. Do not use as monotherapy. Toxicity: photosensitivity reactions, rash.
Sofosbuvir	Inhibits HCV RNA-dependent RNA polymerase acting as a chain terminator.	Chronic HCV in combination with ribavirin, +/– peginterferon alfa. Do not use as monotherapy. Toxicity: fatigue, headache, nausea.

Infection control techniques

	Goals include the reduction of pathogenic organism counts to safe levels (disinfection) and the inactivation of self-propagating biological entities (sterilization).
Autoclave	Pressurized steam at > 120°C. May be sporicidal.
Alcohols	Denature proteins and disrupt cell membranes. Not sporicidal.
Chlorhexidine	Denatures proteins and disrupts cell membranes. Not sporicidal.
Hydrogen peroxide	Free radical oxidation. Sporicidal.
Iodine and iodophors	Halogenation of DNA, RNA, and proteins. May be sporicidal.

Antibiotics to avoid in pregnancy

ANTIBIOTIC	ADVERSE EFFECT
Sulfonamides	Kernicterus
Aminoglycosides	Ototoxicity
Fluoroquinolones	Cartilage damage
Clarithromycin	Embryotoxic
Tetracyclines	Discolored teeth, inhibition of bone growth
Ribavirin (antiviral)	Teratogenic
Griseofulvin (antifungal)	Teratogenic
Chloramphenicol	Gray baby syndrome

SAFe Children Take Really Good Care.

Immunology

"I hate to disappoint you, but my rubber lips are immune to your charms."
—Batman & Robin

"No State shall make or enforce any law which shall abridge the privileges or immunities of citizens of the United States . . ."
—The United States Constitution

Mastery of the basic principles and facts in the immunology section will be useful for the Step 1 exam. Cell surface markers are important to know because they are clinically useful (e.g., in identifying specific types of immunodeficiency or cancer) and are functionally critical to the jobs immune cells carry out. By spending a little extra effort here, it is possible to turn a traditionally difficult subject into one that is high yield.

▶ IMMUNOLOGY—LYMPHOID STRUCTURES

Lymph node	A 2° lymphoid organ that has many afferents, 1 or more efferents. Encapsulated, with trabeculae. Functions are nonspecific filtration by macrophages, storage of B and T cells, and immune response activation.
Follicle	Site of B-cell localization and proliferation. In outer cortex. 1° follicles are dense and dormant. 2° follicles have pale central germinal centers and are active.
Medulla	Consists of medullary cords (closely packed lymphocytes and plasma cells) and medullary sinuses. Medullary sinuses communicate with efferent lymphatics and contain reticular cells and macrophages.
Paracortex	Houses T cells. Region of cortex between follicles and medulla. Contains high endothelial venules through which T and B cells enter from blood. Not well developed in patients with DiGeorge syndrome.

Paracortex enlarges in an extreme cellular immune response (e.g., viral infection).

Lymph drainage

LYMPH NODE CLUSTER	AREA OF BODY DRAINED
Cervical	Head and neck
Hilar	Lungs
Mediastinal	Trachea and esophagus
Axillary	Upper limb, breast, skin above umbilicus
Celiac	Liver, stomach, spleen, pancreas, upper duodenum
Superior mesenteric	Lower duodenum, jejunum, ileum, colon to splenic flexure
Inferior mesenteric	Colon from splenic flexure to upper rectum
Internal iliac	Lower rectum to anal canal (above pectinate line), bladder, vagina (middle third), prostate
Para-aortic	Testes, ovaries, kidneys, uterus
Superficial inguinal	Anal canal (below pectinate line), skin below umbilicus (except popliteal territory), scrotum
Popliteal	Dorsolateral foot, posterior calf

Right lymphatic duct drains right side of body above diaphragm.
Thoracic duct drains everything else into junction of left subclavian and internal jugular veins.

Sinusoids of spleen	Long, vascular channels in red pulp with fenestrated "barrel hoop" basement membrane 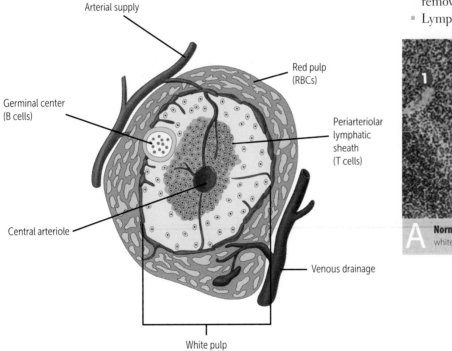.	Splenic dysfunction (e.g., postsplenectomy, sickle cell disease): ↓ IgM → ↓ complement activation → ↓ C3b opsonization → ↑ susceptibility to encapsulated organisms (SHiNE SKiS):

- T cells are found in the periarteriolar lymphatic sheath (PALS) within the white pulp of the spleen.
- B cells are found in follicles within the white pulp of the spleen.
- The marginal zone, in between the red pulp and white pulp, contains APCs and specialized B cells, and is where APCs capture blood-borne antigens for recognition by lymphocytes.

Macrophages found nearby in spleen remove encapsulated bacteria.

- *Streptococcus pneumoniae*
- *Haemophilus influenzae* type b
- *Neisseria meningitidis*
- *Escherichia coli*
- *Salmonella* spp.
- *Klebsiella pneumoniae*
- Group B Streptococci

Postsplenectomy:
- Howell-Jolly bodies (nuclear remnants)
- Target cells
- Thrombocytosis (loss of sequestration and removal)
- Lymphocytosis (loss of sequestration)

Arterial supply

Red pulp (RBCs)

Germinal center (B cells)

Periarteriolar lymphatic sheath (T cells)

Central arteriole

Venous drainage

White pulp

Normal spleen. The red pulp is seen peripherally (1) and the white pulp is seen centrally (2).

Thymus	Site of T-cell differentiation and maturation. Encapsulated. **Th**ymus is derived from the **Th**ird pharyngeal pouch. Lymphocytes of mesenchymal origin. Cortex is dense with immature T cells; medulla is pale with mature T cells and Hassall corpuscles containing epithelial reticular cells.	T cells = **T**hymus B cells = **B**one marrow

▶ IMMUNOLOGY—LYMPHOCYTES

Innate vs. adaptive immunity

	Innate immunity	Adaptive immunity
COMPONENTS	Neutrophils, macrophages, monocytes, dendritic cells, natural killer (NK) cells (lymphoid origin), complement	T cells, B cells, circulating antibodies
MECHANISM	Germline encoded	Variation through V(D)J recombination during lymphocyte development
RESISTANCE	Resistance persists through generations; does not change within an organism's lifetime	Microbial resistance not heritable
RESPONSE TO PATHOGENS	Nonspecific Occurs rapidly (minutes to hours)	Highly specific, refined over time Develops over long periods; memory response is faster and more robust
PHYSICAL BARRIERS	Epithelial tight junctions, mucus	—
SECRETED PROTEINS	Lysozyme, complement, C-reactive protein (CRP), defensins	Immunoglobulins
KEY FEATURES IN PATHOGEN RECOGNITION	Toll-like receptors (TLRs): pattern recognition receptors that recognize pathogen-associated molecular patterns (PAMPs). Examples of PAMPs include LPS (gram-negative bacteria), flagellin (bacteria), ssRNA (viruses)	Memory cells: activated B and T cells; subsequent exposure to a previously encountered antigen → stronger, quicker immune response

MHC I and II

MHC encoded by HLA genes. Present antigen fragments to T cells and bind T-cell receptors (TCRs).

	MHC I	MHC II
LOCI	HLA-A, HLA-B, HLA-C	HLA-DR, HLA-DP, HLA-DQ
BINDING	TCR and CD8	TCR and CD4
EXPRESSION	Expressed on all nucleated cells Not expressed on RBCs	Expressed on APCs
FUNCTION	Present **endogenously** synthesized **antigens** (e.g., viral or cytosolic proteins) to **CD8+ cytotoxic T cells**	Present **exogenously** synthesized **antigens** (e.g., bacterial proteins) to **CD4+ helper T cells**
ANTIGEN LOADING	Antigen peptides loaded onto MHC I in RER after delivery via TAP (transporter associated with antigen processing)	Antigen loaded following release of invariant chain in an acidified endosome
ASSOCIATED PROTEINS	β_2-microglobulin	Invariant chain

HLA subtypes associated with diseases

A3	Hemochromatosis.	
B27	**P**soriatic arthritis, **A**nkylosing spondylitis, arthritis of **I**nflammatory bowel disease, **R**eactive arthritis (formerly Reiter syndrome).	**PAIR.** Also known as seronegative arthropathies.
DQ2/DQ8	Celiac disease.	
DR2	Multiple sclerosis, hay fever, SLE, Goodpasture syndrome.	
DR3	Diabetes mellitus type 1, SLE, Graves disease, Hashimoto thyroiditis.	
DR4	**Rheum**atoid arthritis, diabetes mellitus type 1.	There are **4** walls in a "**rheum**" (room).
DR5	Pernicious anemia → vitamin B_{12} deficiency, Hashimoto thyroiditis.	

Natural killer cells	Use perforin and granzymes to induce apoptosis of virally infected cells and tumor cells. Lymphocyte member of innate immune system. Activity enhanced by IL-2, IL-12, IFN-α, and IFN-β. Induced to kill when exposed to a nonspecific activation signal on target cell and/or to an absence of class I MHC on target cell surface. Also kills via antibody-dependent cell-mediated cytotoxicity (CD16 binds Fc region of bound Ig, activating the NK cell).

Major functions of B and T cells

B-cell functions	Recognize antigen—undergo somatic hypermutation to optimize antigen specificity. Produce antibody—differentiate into plasma cells to secrete specific immunoglobulins. Maintain immunologic memory—memory B cells persist and accelerate future response to antigen.
T-cell functions	CD4+ T cells help B cells make antibodies and produce cytokines to recruit phagocytes and activate other leukocytes. CD8+ T cells directly kill virus-infected cells. Delayed cell-mediated hypersensitivity (type IV). Acute and chronic cellular organ rejection. **Rule of 8:** MHC **II** × CD4 = 8; MHC **I** × CD8 = 8.

Differentiation of T cells

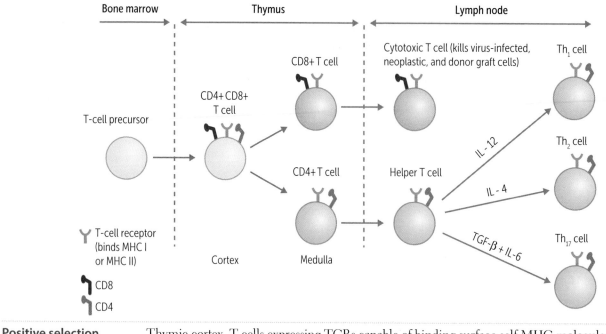

Positive selection	Thymic cortex. T cells expressing TCRs capable of binding surface self-MHC molecules survive.
Negative selection	Medulla. T cells expressing TCRs with high affinity for self antigens undergo apoptosis.

Helper T cells

Th1 cell	Th2 cell
Secretes IFN-γ	Secretes IL-4, IL-5, IL-10, IL-13
Activates macrophages and cytotoxic T cells	Recruits eosinophils for parasite defense and promotes IgE production by B cells
Activated by INF-γ and IL-12	Activated by IL-4
Inhibited by IL-4 and IL-10 (from Th2 cell)	Inhibited by IFN-γ (from Th1 cell)

Macrophage-lymphocyte interaction—macrophages release IL-12, which stimulates T cells to differentiate into Th1 cells. Th1 cells release IFN-γ to stimulate macrophages.
Helper T cells have CD4, which binds to MHC II on APCs.

Cytotoxic T cells

Kill virus-infected, neoplastic, and donor graft cells by inducing apoptosis.
Release cytotoxic granules containing preformed proteins (e.g., perforin, granzyme B).
Cytotoxic T cells have CD8, which binds to MHC I on virus-infected cells.

Regulatory T cells

Help maintain specific immune tolerance by suppressing CD4 and CD8 T-cell effector functions.
Identified by expression of CD3, CD4, CD25, and FOXP3.
Activated regulatory T cells produce anti-inflammatory cytokines (e.g., IL-10, TGF-β).

T- and B-cell activation	Antigen-presenting cells (APCs): B cells, macrophages, dendritic cells. Two signals are required for T-cell activation, B-cell activation, and class switching.
Naive T-cell activation	1. Dendritic cell (specialized APC) samples and processes antigen. 2. Dendritic cell migrates to the draining lymph node. 3. Foreign antigen is presented on MHC II and recognized by TCR on Th (CD4+) cell. Antigen is presented on MHC I to Tc (CD8+) cell. 4. "Costimulatory signal" is given by interaction of B7 and CD28 (signal 2). 5. Th cell activates and produces cytokines. Tc cell activates and is able to recognize and kill virus-infected cell.
B-cell activation and class switching	1. Th-cell activation as above. 2. B-cell receptor–mediated endocytosis; foreign antigen is presented on MHC II and recognized by TCR on Th cell (signal 1). 3. CD40 receptor on B cell binds CD40 ligand (CD40L) on Th cell (signal 2). 4. Th cell secretes cytokines that determine Ig class switching of B cell. B cell activates and undergoes class switching, affinity maturation, and antibody production.

Antibody structure and function

Fab (variable) region consisting of light (L) and heavy (H) chains recognizes antigens. Fc region of IgM and IgG fixes complement. Heavy chain contributes to Fc and Fab regions. Light chain contributes only to Fab region.

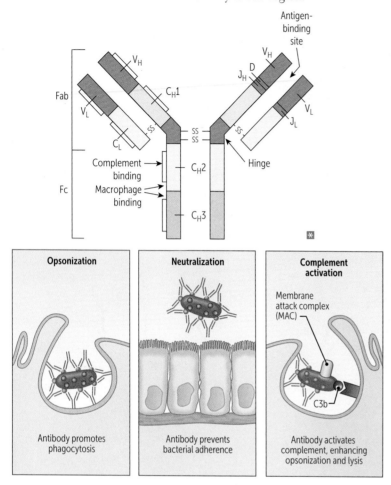

Fab:
- Fragment, antigen binding
- Determines idiotype: unique antigen-binding pocket; only 1 antigenic specificity expressed per B cell

Fc:
- Constant
- Carboxy terminal
- Complement binding
- Carbohydrate side chains
- Determines isotype (IgM, IgD, etc.)

Antibody diversity is generated by:
- Random recombination of VJ (light-chain) or V(D)J (heavy-chain) genes
- Random combination of heavy chains with light chains
- Somatic hypermutation (following antigen stimulation)
- Addition of nucleotides to DNA during recombination by terminal deoxynucleotidyl transferase

Opsonization	Neutralization	Complement activation
Antibody promotes phagocytosis	Antibody prevents bacterial adherence	Antibody activates complement, enhancing opsonization and lysis

Immunoglobulin isotypes	Mature B cells express IgM and IgD on their surfaces. They may differentiate in germinal centers of lymph nodes by isotype switching (gene rearrangement; mediated by cytokines and CD40L) into plasma cells that secrete IgA, IgE, or IgG.
IgG	Main antibody in 2° (**delayed**) response to an antigen. Most abundant isotype in serum. Fixes complement, crosses the placenta (provides infants with passive immunity), opsonizes bacteria, neutralizes bacterial toxins and viruses.
IgA	Prevents attachment of bacteria and viruses to mucous membranes; does not fix complement. Monomer (in circulation) or dimer (when secreted). Crosses epithelial cells by transcytosis. Produced in GI tract (e.g., by Peyer patches) and protects against gut infections (e.g., *Giardia*). Most produced antibody overall, but has lower serum concentrations. Released into secretions (tears, saliva, mucus) and breast milk. Picks up secretory component from epithelial cells before secretion.
IgM	Produced in the 1° (**immediate**) response to an antigen. Fixes complement but does not cross the placenta. Antigen receptor on the surface of B cells. Monomer on B cell, pentamer when secreted. Pentamer enables avid binding to antigen while humoral response evolves.
IgD	Unclear function. Found on surface of many B cells and in serum.
IgE	Binds mast cells and basophils; cross-links when exposed to allergen, mediating immediate (type I) hypersensitivity through release of inflammatory mediators such as histamine. Mediates immunity to worms by activating eosinophils. Lowest concentration in serum.

Antigen type and memory

Thymus-independent antigens	Antigens lacking a peptide component (e.g., lipopolysaccharides from gram-negative bacteria); cannot be presented by MHC to T cells. Weakly or nonimmunogenic; vaccines often require boosters and adjuvants (e.g., pneumococcal polysaccharide vaccine).
Thymus-dependent antigens	Antigens containing a protein component (e.g., diphtheria vaccine). Class switching and immunologic memory occur as a result of direct contact of B cells with Th cells (CD40–CD40L interaction).

▶ IMMUNOLOGY—IMMUNE RESPONSES

Acute-phase reactants	Factors whose serum concentrations change significantly in response to inflammation; produced by the liver in both acute and chronic inflammatory states. Notably induced by IL-6.
POSITIVE (UPREGULATED)	
C-reactive protein	Opsonin; fixes complement and facilitates phagocytosis. Measured clinically as a sign of ongoing inflammation.
Ferritin	Binds and sequesters iron to inhibit microbial iron scavenging.
Fibrinogen	Coagulation factor; promotes endothelial repair; correlates with ESR.
Hepcidin	Prevents release of iron bound by ferritin → anemia of chronic disease.
Serum amyloid A	Prolonged elevation can lead to amyloidosis.
NEGATIVE (DOWNREGULATED)	
Albumin	Reduction conserves amino acids for positive reactants.
Transferrin	Internalized by macrophages to sequester iron.

Complement	System of hepatically synthesized plasma proteins that play a role in innate immunity and inflammation. Membrane attack complex (MAC) defends against gram-negative bacteria.	
ACTIVATION	**Classic** pathway—IgG or IgM mediated. Alternative pathway—microbe surface molecules. Lectin pathway—mannose or other sugars on microbe surface.	**GM** makes **classic** cars.
FUNCTIONS	C3b—opsonization. C3a, C4a, C5a—anaphylaxis. C5a—neutrophil chemotaxis. C5b-9—cytolysis by MAC.	C3b binds bacteria.
	Opsonins—C3b and IgG are the two 1° opsonins in bacterial defense; enhance phagocytosis. C3b also helps clear immune complexes.	*Opsonin* (Greek) = to prepare for eating.
	Inhibitors—decay-accelerating factor (DAF, aka CD55) and C1 esterase inhibitor help prevent complement activation on self cells (e.g., RBCs).	

*Historically, the larger fragment of C2 was called C2a but is now referred to as C2b.

Complement disorders

C1 esterase inhibitor deficiency	Causes hereditary angioedema. ACE inhibitors are contraindicated.
C3 deficiency	Increases risk of severe, recurrent pyogenic sinus and respiratory tract infections; ↑ susceptibility to type III hypersensitivity reactions.
C5–C9 deficiencies	Terminal complement deficiency increases susceptibility to recurrent *Neisseria* bacteremia.
DAF (GPI-anchored enzyme) deficiency	Causes complement-mediated lysis of RBCs and paroxysmal nocturnal hemoglobinuria.

Important cytokines

SECRETED BY MACROPHAGES		
IL-1	Also called osteoclast-activating factor. Causes fever, acute inflammation. Activates endothelium to express adhesion molecules. Induces chemokine secretion to recruit WBCs.	"Hot T-bone stEAK": IL-1: fever (**hot**). IL-2: stimulates **T** cells. IL-3: stimulates **bone** marrow. IL-4: stimulates Ig**E** production. IL-5: stimulates Ig**A** production. IL-6: stimulates a**K**ute-phase protein production.
IL-6	Causes fever and stimulates production of acute-phase proteins.	
IL-8	Major chemotactic factor for neutrophils.	"**Clean up** on **aisle 8**." Neutrophils are recruited by **IL-8** to **clear** infections.
IL-12	Induces differentiation of T cells into Th1 cells. Activates NK cells.	
TNF-α	Mediates septic shock. Activates endothelium. Causes WBC recruitment, vascular leak.	Causes cachexia in malignancy.
SECRETED BY ALL T CELLS		
IL-2	Stimulates growth of helper, cytotoxic, and regulatory T cells, and NK cells.	
IL-3	Supports growth and differentiation of bone marrow stem cells. Functions like GM-CSF.	
FROM Th1 CELLS		
Interferon-γ	Secreted by NK cells in response to IL-12 from macrophages; stimulates macrophages to kill phagocytosed pathogens.	Also activates NK cells to kill virus-infected cells. Increases MHC expression and antigen presentation by all cells.
FROM Th2 CELLS		
IL-4	Induces differentiation into Th2 cells. Promotes growth of B cells. Enhances class switching to IgE and IgG.	
IL-5	Promotes differentiation of B cells. Enhances class switching to IgA. Stimulates growth and differentiation of eosinophils.	
IL-10	Modulates inflammatory response. Decreases expression of MHC class II and Th1 cytokines. Inhibits activated macrophages and dendritic cells. Also secreted by regulatory T cells.	TGF-β and IL-10 both attenuate the immune response.

Respiratory burst (oxidative burst)

Involves the activation of the phagocyte NADPH oxidase complex (e.g., in neutrophils, monocytes), which utilizes O_2 as a substrate. Plays an important role in the immune response → rapid release of reactive oxygen species (ROS). NADPH plays a role in both the creation and neutralization of ROS. Myeloperoxidase is a blue-green heme-containing pigment that gives sputum its color.

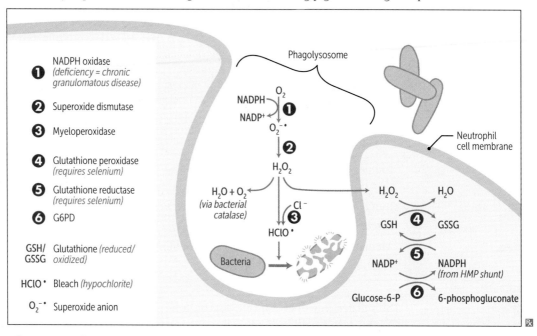

Phagocytes of patients with CGD can utilize H_2O_2 generated by invading organisms and convert it to ROS. Patients are at ↑ risk for infection by catalase ⊕ species (e.g., *S. aureus*, *Aspergillus*) capable of neutralizing their own H_2O_2, leaving phagocytes without ROS for fighting infections. Pyocyanin of *P. aeruginosa* functions to generate ROS to kill competing microbes. Lactoferrin is a protein found in secretory fluids and neutrophils that inhibits microbial growth via iron chelation.

Interferon α and β

A part of innate host defense against both RNA and DNA viruses. **Interfer**ons are glycoproteins synthesized by virus-infected cells that act locally on uninfected cells, "priming them" for viral defense by helping to selectively degrade viral nucleic acid and protein.

Essentially results in apoptosis, thereby disrupting viral amplification.

Interfere with viruses.

Cell surface proteins	MHC I present on all nucleated cells (i.e., not mature RBCs).	
T cells	TCR (binds antigen-MHC complex) CD3 (associated with TCR for signal transduction) CD28 (binds B7 on APC)	
Helper T cells	CD4, CD40L	
Cytotoxic T cells	CD8	
Regulatory T cells	CD4, CD25	
B cells	Ig (binds antigen) CD19, CD20, CD21 (receptor for EBV), CD40 MHC II, B7	You can drink **B**eer at the **B**ar when you're **21**: **B** cells, Epstein-**B**arr virus, CD**21**.
Macrophages	CD14, CD40 MHC II, B7 Fc and C3b receptors (enhanced phagocytosis)	
NK cells	CD16 (binds Fc of IgG), CD56 (unique marker for NK)	
Hematopoietic stem cells	CD34	

Anergy	State during which a cell cannot become activated by exposure to its antigen. T and B cells become anergic when exposed to their antigen without costimulatory signal (signal 2). Another mechanism of self-tolerance.

Effects of bacterial toxins	Superantigens (*S. pyogenes* and *S. aureus*)—cross-link the β region of the T-cell receptor to the MHC class II on APCs. Can activate any CD4+ T cell → massive release of cytokines. Endotoxins/lipopolysaccharide (gram-negative bacteria)—directly stimulate macrophages by binding to endotoxin receptor TLR4/CD14; Th cells are not involved.

Antigenic variation	Classic examples: ■ Bacteria—*Salmonella* (2 flagellar variants), *Borrelia recurrentis* (relapsing fever), *N. gonorrhoeae* (pilus protein) ■ Viruses—influenza, HIV, HCV ■ Parasites—trypanosomes	Some mechanisms for variation include DNA rearrangement and RNA segment reassortment (e.g., influenza major shift).

Passive vs. active immunity

	Passive	Active
MEANS OF ACQUISITION	Receiving preformed antibodies	Exposure to foreign antigens
ONSET	Rapid	Slow
DURATION	Short span of antibodies (half-life = 3 weeks)	Long-lasting protection (memory)
EXAMPLES	IgA in breast milk, maternal IgG crossing placenta, antitoxin, humanized monoclonal antibody	Natural infection, vaccines, toxoid
NOTES	After exposure to Tetanus toxin, Botulinum toxin, HBV, Varicella, or Rabies virus, unvaccinated patients are given preformed antibodies (passive)—"To Be Healed Very Rapidly"	Combined passive and active immunizations can be given for hepatitis B or rabies exposure

Vaccination

Induces an active immune response (humoral and/or cellular) to specific pathogens.

VACCINE TYPE	DESCRIPTION	PROS/CONS	EXAMPLES
Live attenuated vaccine	Microorganism loses its pathogenicity but retains capacity for transient growth within inoculated host. Induces **cellular and humoral responses**. MMR is the only live attenuated vaccine given to persons with HIV.	Pro: induces strong, often lifelong immunity. Con: may revert to virulent form. Often contraindicated in pregnancy and immunodeficiency.	Measles, mumps, rubella, polio (Sabin), influenza (intranasal), varicella, yellow fever.
Inactivated or killed vaccine	Pathogen is inactivated by heat or chemicals. Maintaining epitope structure on surface antigens is important for immune response. Mainly induces a **humoral response**.	Pro: safer than live vaccines. Con: weaker immune response; booster shots usually required.	Rabies, Influenza (injection), Polio (Salk), hepatitis A ("**R.I.P.** Always").

Hypersensitivity types

Type I Mast cell or basophil · Fc receptor · IgE · Ag	Anaphylactic and atopic—free antigen cross-links IgE on presensitized mast cells and basophils, triggering immediate release of vasoactive amines that act at postcapillary venules (i.e., histamine). Reaction develops rapidly after antigen exposure because of preformed antibody. Delayed response follows due to production of arachidonic acid metabolites (e.g., leukotrienes).	First (type) and Fast (anaphylaxis). Types I, II, and III are all antibody mediated. Test: skin test for specific IgE.

Type II
 	
IgG · Cell · IgG · C
 	
C = complement
	Cytotoxic (antibody mediated)—IgM, IgG bind to fixed antigen on "enemy" cell → cellular destruction.
	3 mechanisms:
	▪ Opsonization and phagocytosis
	▪ Complement- and Fc receptor–mediated inflammation
	▪ Antibody-mediated cellular dysfunction
		Type **II** is cy-2-toxic.
		Antibody and complement lead to MAC.
		Direct and indirect Coombs' tests:
		  Direct—detects antibodies that have adhered to patient's RBCs (e.g., test an Rh ⊕ infant of an Rh ⊖ mother).
		  Indirect—detects serum antibodies that can adhere to other RBCs (e.g., test an Rh ⊖ woman for Rh ⊕ antibodies).

Type III Ag · C · Ag	Immune complex—antigen-antibody (IgG) complexes activate complement, which attracts neutrophils; neutrophils release lysosomal enzymes. **Serum sickness**—an immune complex disease in which antibodies to foreign proteins are produced (takes 5 days). Immune complexes form and are deposited in membranes, where they fix complement (leads to tissue damage). More common than Arthus reaction. **Arthus reaction**—a local subacute antibody-mediated hypersensitivity reaction. Intradermal injection of antigen induces antibodies, which form antigen-antibody complexes in the skin. Characterized by edema, necrosis, and activation of complement.	In type **III** reaction, imagine an immune complex as **3** things stuck together: antigen-antibody-complement. Most serum sickness is now caused by drugs (not serum) acting as haptens. Fever, urticaria, arthralgia, proteinuria, lymphadenopathy occur 5–10 days after antigen exposure. Antigen-antibody complexes cause the Arthus reaction. Test: immunofluorescent staining.

Type IV
 	
APC · Th cells
	Delayed (T-cell–mediated) type—sensitized T cells encounter antigen and then release cytokines (leads to macrophage activation; no antibody involved).	**4th** and **last**—delayed. Cell mediated; therefore, it is not transferable by serum.
		4 T's = T cells, Transplant rejections, TB skin tests, Touching (contact dermatitis).
		Test: patch test, PPD.
		
		ACID:
		  Anaphylactic and Atopic (type I)
		  Cytotoxic (antibody mediated) (type II)
		  Immune complex (type III)
		  Delayed (cell mediated) (type IV)

Hypersensitivity disorders

REACTION	EXAMPLES	PRESENTATION
Type I	Allergic and atopic disorders (e.g., rhinitis, hay fever, eczema, hives, asthma) Anaphylaxis (e.g., bee sting, some food/drug allergies)	Immediate, anaphylactic, atopic
Type II	Acute hemolytic transfusion reactions Autoimmune hemolytic anemia Bullous pemphigoid Erythroblastosis fetalis Goodpasture syndrome Graves disease Guillain-Barré syndrome Idiopathic thrombocytopenic purpura Myasthenia gravis Pemphigus vulgaris Pernicious anemia Rheumatic fever	Disease tends to be specific to tissue or site where antigen is found
Type III	Arthus reaction (e.g., swelling and inflammation following tetanus vaccine) SLE Polyarteritis nodosa Poststreptococcal glomerulonephritis Serum sickness	Can be associated with vasculitis and systemic manifestations
Type IV	Contact dermatitis (e.g., poison ivy, nickel allergy) Graft-versus-host disease Multiple sclerosis PPD (test for *M. tuberculosis*)	Response is delayed and does **not** involve antibodies (vs. types I, II, and III)

Blood transfusion reactions

TYPE	PATHOGENESIS	CLINICAL PRESENTATION
Allergic reaction	Type I hypersensitivity reaction against plasma proteins in transfused blood.	Urticaria, pruritus, wheezing, fever. Treat with antihistamines.
Anaphylactic reaction	Severe allergic reaction. IgA-deficient individuals must receive blood products without IgA.	Dyspnea, bronchospasm, hypotension, respiratory arrest, shock. Treat with epinephrine.
Febrile nonhemolytic transfusion reaction	Type II hypersensitivity reaction. Host antibodies against donor HLA antigens and WBCs.	Fever, headaches, chills, flushing.
Acute hemolytic transfusion reaction	Type II hypersensitivity reaction. Intravascular hemolysis (ABO blood group incompatibility) or extravascular hemolysis (host antibody reaction against foreign antigen on donor RBCs).	Fever, hypotension, tachypnea, tachycardia, flank pain, hemoglobinuria (intravascular hemolysis), jaundice (extravascular).

Autoantibodies

AUTOANTIBODY	ASSOCIATED DISORDER
Anti-ACh receptor	Myasthenia gravis
Anti-basement membrane	Goodpasture syndrome
Anticardiolipin, lupus anticoagulant	SLE, antiphospholipid syndrome
Anticentromere	Limited scleroderma (CREST syndrome)
Anti-desmosome (anti-desmoglein)	Pemphigus vulgaris
Anti-dsDNA, anti-Smith	SLE
Anti-glutamic acid decarboxylase (GAD-65)	Type 1 diabetes mellitus
Antihemidesmosome	Bullous pemphigoid
Anti-histone	Drug-induced lupus
Anti-Jo-1, anti-SRP, anti-Mi-2	Polymyositis, dermatomyositis
Antimicrosomal, antithyroglobulin	Hashimoto thyroiditis
Antimitochondrial	1° biliary cirrhosis
Antinuclear antibodies	SLE, nonspecific
Antiparietal cell	Pernicious anemia
Anti-Scl-70 (anti-DNA topoisomerase I)	Scleroderma (diffuse)
Anti-smooth muscle	Autoimmune hepatitis
Anti-SSA, anti-SSB (anti-Ro, anti-La)	Sjögren syndrome
Anti-TSH receptor	Graves disease
Anti-U1 RNP (ribonucleoprotein)	Mixed connective tissue disease
IgA anti-endomysial, IgA anti-tissue transglutaminase	Celiac disease
MPO-ANCA/p-ANCA	Microscopic polyangiitis, eosinophilic granulomatosis with polyangiitis (Churg-Strauss syndrome)
PR3-ANCA/c-ANCA	Granulomatosis with polyangiitis (Wegener)
Rheumatoid factor (IgM antibody that targets IgG Fc region), anti-CCP (more specific)	Rheumatoid arthritis

Immunodeficiencies

DISEASE	DEFECT	PRESENTATION	FINDINGS
B-cell disorders			
X-linked (Bruton) agammaglobulinemia	Defect in *BTK*, a tyrosine kinase gene → no B-cell maturation. X-linked recessive (↑ in Boys).	Recurrent bacterial and enteroviral infections after 6 months (↓ maternal IgG).	Absent B cells in peripheral blood, ↓ Ig of all classes. Absent/scanty lymph nodes and tonsils.
Selective IgA deficiency	Unknown. Most common 1° immunodeficiency.	Majority Asymptomatic. Can see Airway and GI infections, Autoimmune disease, Atopy, Anaphylaxis to IgA-containing products.	↓ IgA with normal IgG, IgM levels.
Common variable immunodeficiency	Defect in B-cell differentiation. Many causes.	Can be acquired in 20s–30s; ↑ risk of autoimmune disease, bronchiectasis, lymphoma, sinopulmonary infections.	↓ plasma cells, ↓ immunoglobulins.
T-cell disorders			
Thymic aplasia (DiGeorge syndrome)	22q11 deletion; failure to develop 3rd and 4th pharyngeal pouches → absent thymus and parathyroids.	Tetany (hypocalcemia), recurrent viral/fungal infections (T-cell deficiency), conotruncal abnormalities (e.g., tetralogy of Fallot, truncus arteriosus).	↓ T cells, ↓ PTH, ↓ Ca^{2+}. Absent thymic shadow on CXR. 22q11 deletion detected by FISH.
IL-12 receptor deficiency	↓ Th1 response. Autosomal recessive.	Disseminated mycobacterial and fungal infections; may present after administration of BCG vaccine.	↓ IFN-γ.
Autosomal dominant hyper-IgE syndrome (Job syndrome)	Deficiency of Th17 cells due to *STAT3* mutation → impaired recruitment of neutrophils to sites of infection.	FATED: coarse Facies, cold (noninflamed) staphylococcal Abscesses, retained primary Teeth, ↑ IgE, Dermatologic problems (eczema).	↑ IgE, ↓ IFN-γ.
Chronic mucocutaneous candidiasis	T-cell dysfunction. Many causes.	Noninvasive *Candida albicans* infections of skin and mucous membranes.	Absent in vitro T-cell proliferation in response to *Candida* antigens. Absent cutaneous reaction to *Candida* antigens.

Immunodeficiencies (continued)

DISEASE	DEFECT	PRESENTATION	FINDINGS
B- and T-cell disorders			
Severe combined immunodeficiency (SCID)	Several types including defective IL-2R gamma chain (most common, X-linked), adenosine deaminase deficiency (autosomal recessive).	Failure to thrive, chronic diarrhea, thrush. Recurrent viral, bacterial, fungal, and protozoal infections. Treatment: bone marrow transplant (no concern for rejection).	↓ T-cell receptor excision circles (TRECs). Absence of thymic shadow (CXR), germinal centers (lymph node biopsy), and T cells (flow cytometry).
Ataxia-telangiectasia	Defects in *ATM* gene → failure to repair DNA double strand breaks → cell cycle arrest.	Triad: cerebellar defects (Ataxia), spider Angiomas (telangiectasia), IgA deficiency.	↑ AFP. ↓ IgA, IgG, and IgE. Lymphopenia, cerebellar atrophy.
Hyper-IgM syndrome	Most commonly due to defective CD40L on Th cells → class switching defect; X-linked recessive.	Severe pyogenic infections early in life; opportunistic infection with *Pneumocystis*, *Cryptosporidium*, CMV.	↑ IgM. ↓↓ IgG, IgA, IgE.
Wiskott-Aldrich syndrome	Mutation in *WAS* gene (X-linked recessive); T cells unable to reorganize actin cytoskeleton.	**WATER**: **W**iskott-Aldrich: **T**hrombocytopenic purpura, **E**czema, **R**ecurrent infections. ↑ risk of autoimmune disease and malignancy.	↓ to normal IgG, IgM. ↑ IgE, IgA. Fewer and smaller platelets.
Phagocyte dysfunction			
Leukocyte adhesion deficiency (type 1)	Defect in LFA-1 integrin (CD18) protein on phagocytes; impaired migration and chemotaxis; autosomal recessive.	Recurrent bacterial skin and mucosal infections, absent pus formation, impaired wound healing, delayed separation of umbilical cord (> 30 days).	↑ neutrophils. Absence of neutrophils at infection sites.
Chédiak-Higashi syndrome	Defect in lysosomal trafficking regulator gene (*LYST*). Microtubule dysfunction in phagosome-lysosome fusion; autosomal recessive.	Recurrent pyogenic infections by staphylococci and streptococci, partial albinism, peripheral neuropathy, progressive neurodegeneration, infiltrative lymphohistiocytosis.	Giant granules in granulocytes Ａ and platelets. Pancytopenia. Mild coagulation defects.
Chronic granulomatous disease	Defect of NADPH oxidase → ↓ reactive oxygen species (e.g., superoxide) and ↓ respiratory burst in neutrophils; X-linked recessive most common.	↑ susceptibility to catalase ⊕ organisms (Need **PLACESS**): *Nocardia*, *Pseudomonas*, *Listeria*, *Aspergillus*, *Candida*, *E. coli*, *S. aureus*, *Serratia*.	Abnormal dihydrorhodamine (flow cytometry) test. Nitroblue tetrazolium dye reduction test is ⊖.

Infections in immunodeficiency

PATHOGEN	↓ T CELLS	↓ B CELLS	↓ GRANULOCYTES	↓ COMPLEMENT
Bacteria	Sepsis	Encapsulated: *Streptococcus pneumoniae, Haemophilus influenzae* type B, *Neisseria meningitidis, Escherichia coli, Salmonella, Klebsiella pneumoniae*, group B Strep (**SHiNE SKiS**)	*Staphylococcus, Burkholderia cepacia, Pseudomonas aeruginosa, Serratia, Nocardia*	Encapsulated species with early component deficiencies *Neisseria* with late component (MAC) deficiencies
Viruses	CMV, EBV, JCV, VZV, chronic infection with respiratory/GI viruses	Enteroviral encephalitis, poliovirus (live vaccine contraindicated)	N/A	N/A
Fungi/parasites	*Candida* (local), PCP	GI giardiasis (no IgA)	*Candida* (systemic), *Aspergillus*	N/A

Note: B-cell deficiencies tend to produce recurrent bacterial infections, whereas T-cell deficiencies produce more fungal and viral infections.

Grafts

Autograft	From self.
Syngeneic graft (isograft)	From identical twin or clone.
Allograft	From nonidentical individual of same species.
Xenograft	From different species.

Transplant rejection

TYPE OF REJECTION	ONSET	PATHOGENESIS	FEATURES
Hyperacute	Within minutes	Pre-existing recipient antibodies react to donor antigen (type II hypersensitivity reaction), activate complement.	Widespread thrombosis of graft vessels → ischemia/necrosis. Graft must be removed.
Acute	Weeks to months	Cellular: CD8+ T cells activated against donor MHCs. Humoral: similar to hyperacute, except antibodies develop after transplant.	Vasculitis of graft vessels with dense interstitial lymphocytic infiltrate. Prevent/reverse with immunosuppressants.
Chronic	Months to years	CD4+ T cells respond to recipient APCs presenting donor peptides, including allogeneic MHC. Both cellular and humoral components.	Recipient T cells react and secrete cytokines → proliferation of vascular smooth muscle and parenchymal fibrosis. Dominated by arteriosclerosis.
Graft-versus-host disease	Varies	Grafted immunocompetent T cells proliferate in the immunocompromised host and reject host cells with "foreign" proteins → severe organ dysfunction.	Maculopapular rash, jaundice, diarrhea, hepatosplenomegaly. Usually in bone marrow and liver transplants (rich in lymphocytes). Potentially beneficial in bone marrow transplant for leukemia (graft-versus-tumor effect).

▶ IMMUNOLOGY—IMMUNOSUPPRESSANTS

Immunosuppressants   Agents that block lymphocyte activation and proliferation. Reduce acute transplant rejection by suppressing cellular immunity. Frequently combined to achieve greater efficacy with ↓ toxicity. Chronic suppression ↑ risk of infection and malignancy.

DRUG	MECHANISM	USE	TOXICITY	NOTES
Cyclosporine	Calcineurin inhibitor; binds **cyclophilin**. Blocks T-cell activation by **preventing IL-2 transcription**.	Transplant rejection prophylaxis, psoriasis, rheumatoid arthritis.	**Nephrotoxicity**, hypertension, hyperlipidemia, neurotoxicity, gingival hyperplasia, hirsutism.	Both calcineurin inhibitors are highly nephrotoxic.
Tacrolimus (FK506)	Calcineurin inhibitor; binds FK506 binding protein (FKBP). Blocks T-cell activation by **preventing IL-2 transcription**.	Transplant rejection prophylaxis.	Similar to cyclosporine, ↑ risk of diabetes and neurotoxicity; no gingival hyperplasia or hirsutism.	
Sirolimus (Rapamycin)	mTOR inhibitor; binds FKBP. Blocks T-cell activation and B-cell differentiation by **preventing response to IL-2**.	Kidney transplant rejection prophylaxis.	Anemia, thrombocytopenia, leukopenia, insulin resistance, hyperlipidemia; **not nephrotoxic**.	Kidney "sir-vives." Synergistic with cyclosporine. Also used in drug-eluting stents.
Daclizumab, basiliximab	Monoclonal antibodies; block IL-2R.	Kidney transplant rejection prophylaxis.	Edema, hypertension, tremor.	
Azathioprine	Antimetabolite precursor of 6-mercaptopurine. Inhibits lymphocyte proliferation by blocking nucleotide synthesis.	Transplant rejection prophylaxis, rheumatoid arthritis, Crohn disease, glomerulonephritis, other autoimmune conditions.	Leukopenia, anemia, thrombocytopenia.	6-MP degraded by xanthine oxidase; toxicity ↑ by allopurinol. Pronounce "azathio-**purine**."
Glucocorticoids	Inhibit NF-κB. Suppress both B- and T-cell function by ↓ transcription of many cytokines.	Transplant rejection prophylaxis (immuno-suppression), many autoimmune disorders, inflammation.	Hyperglycemia, osteoporosis, central obesity, muscle breakdown, psychosis, acne, hypertension, cataracts, avascular necrosis.	Can cause iatrogenic Cushing syndrome.

Immunosuppression targets

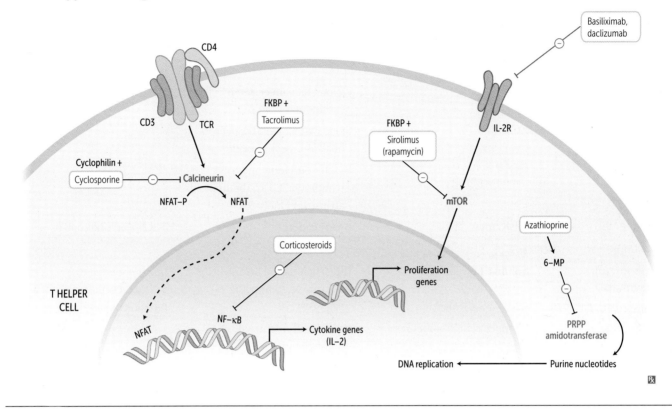

Recombinant cytokines and clinical uses	AGENT	CLINICAL USES
	Aldesleukin (IL-2)	Renal cell carcinoma, metastatic melanoma
	Epoetin alfa (erythropoietin)	Anemias (especially in renal failure)
	Filgrastim (G-CSF)	Recovery of bone marrow
	Sargramostim (GM-CSF)	Recovery of bone marrow
	IFN-α	Chronic hepatitis B and C, Kaposi sarcoma, malignant melanoma
	IFN-β	Multiple sclerosis
	IFN-γ	Chronic granulomatous disease
	Romiplostim, eltrombopag	Thrombocytopenia
	Oprelvekin (IL-11)	Thrombocytopenia

Therapeutic antibodies

AGENT	TARGET	CLINICAL USE	NOTES
Cancer therapy			
Alemtuzumab	CD52	CLL	"Alymtuzumab"—chronic lymphocytic leukemia
Bevacizumab	VEGF	Colorectal cancer, renal cell carcinoma	
Cetuximab	EGFR	Stage IV colorectal cancer, head and neck cancer	
Rituximab	CD20	B-cell non-Hodgkin lymphoma, CLL, rheumatoid arthritis, ITP	
Trastuzumab	HER2/neu	Breast cancer	HER2—"tras2zumab"
Autoimmune disease therapy			
Adalimumab, infliximab	Soluble TNF-α	IBD, rheumatoid arthritis, ankylosing spondylitis, psoriasis	Etanercept is a decoy TNF-α receptor and not a monoclonal antibody
Eculizumab	Complement protein C5	Paroxysmal nocturnal hemoglobinuria	
Natalizumab	α4-integrin	Multiple sclerosis, Crohn disease	α4-integrin: WBC adhesion Risk of PML in patients with JC virus
Other			
Abciximab	Platelet glycoproteins IIb/IIIa	Antiplatelet agent for prevention of ischemic complications in patients undergoing percutaneous coronary intervention	IIb times IIIa equals "absiximab"
Denosumab	RANKL	Osteoporosis; inhibits osteoclast maturation (mimics osteoprotegerin)	Denosumab affects osteoclasts
Digoxin immune Fab	Digoxin	Antidote for digoxin toxicity	
Omalizumab	IgE	Allergic asthma; prevents IgE binding to FcεRI	
Palivizumab	RSV F protein	RSV prophylaxis for high-risk infants	PaliVIzumab—VIrus
Ranibizumab, bevacizumab	VEGF	Neovascular age-related macular degeneration	

Pathology

"Digressions, objections, delight in mockery, carefree mistrust are signs of health; everything unconditional belongs in pathology."
—Friedrich Nietzsche

The fundamental principles of pathology are key to understanding diseases in all organ systems. Major topics such as inflammation and neoplasia appear frequently in questions across different organ systems, and such topics are definitely high yield. For example, the concepts of cell injury and inflammation are key to understanding the inflammatory response that follows myocardial infarction, a very common subject of board questions. Similarly, a familiarity with the early cellular changes that culminate in the development of neoplasias—for example, esophageal or colon cancer—is critical. Finally, make sure you recognize the major tumor-associated genes and are comfortable with key cancer concepts such as tumor staging and metastasis.

▶ PATHOLOGY—INFLAMMATION

Apoptosis

Programmed cell death; ATP required. Intrinsic or extrinsic pathway; both pathways → activation of cytosolic caspases that mediate cellular breakdown.

No significant inflammation (unlike necrosis).

Characterized by deeply eosinophilic cytoplasm, cell shrinkage, nuclear shrinkage (pyknosis) and basophilia, membrane blebbing, nuclear fragmentation (karyorrhexis), and formation of apoptotic bodies, which are then phagocytosed.

DNA laddering is a sensitive indicator of apoptosis; during karyorrhexis, endonucleases cleave at internucleosomal regions, yielding fragments in multiples of 180 bp. Radiation therapy causes apoptosis of tumors and surrounding tissue via free radical formation and dsDNA breakage. Rapidly dividing cells (e.g., skin, GI mucosa) are very susceptible to radiation therapy–induced apoptosis.

Intrinsic pathway

Involved in tissue remodeling in embryogenesis. Occurs when a regulating factor is withdrawn from a proliferating cell population (e.g., ↓ IL-2 after a completed immunologic reaction → apoptosis of proliferating effector cells). Also occurs after exposure to injurious stimuli (e.g., radiation, toxins, hypoxia).

Changes in proportions of anti- and pro-apoptotic factors → ↑ mitochondrial permeability and cytochrome c release. BAX and BAK are proapoptotic proteins; Bcl-2 is antiapoptotic.

Bcl-2 prevents cytochrome c release by binding to and inhibiting Apaf-1. Apaf-1 normally induces the activation of caspases. If Bcl-2 is overexpressed (e.g., follicular lymphoma), then Apaf-1 is overly inhibited, → ↓ caspase activation and tumorigenesis.

Extrinsic pathway

2 pathways:
- Ligand receptor interactions (FasL binding to Fas [CD95])
- Immune cell (cytotoxic T-cell release of perforin and granzyme B)

Fas-FasL interaction is necessary in thymic medullary negative selection. Mutations in Fas ↑ numbers of circulating self-reacting lymphocytes due to failure of clonal deletion.

After Fas crosslinks with FasL, multiple Fas molecules coalesce, forming a binding site for a death domain–containing adapter protein, FADD. FADD binds inactive caspases, activating them.

Defective Fas-FasL interactions contribute to autoimmune disorders.

Necrosis

Enzymatic degradation and protein denaturation of cell due to exogenous injury → intracellular components leak. Inflammatory process (unlike apoptosis).

TYPE	SEEN IN	DUE TO	HISTOLOGY
Coagulative	Ischemia/infarcts in most tissues (except brain)	Ischemia or infarction; proteins denature, then enzymatic degradation	Cell outlines preserved; ↑ cytoplasmic binding of acidophilic dyes **A**
Liquefactive	Bacterial abscesses, brain infarcts (due to ↑ fat content)	Neutrophils releasing lysosomal enzymes that digest the tissue **B**; enzymatic degradation first, then proteins denature	Early: cellular debris and macrophages Late: cystic spaces and cavitation (brain) Neutrophils and cell debris seen with bacterial infection
Caseous	TB, systemic fungi (e.g., *Histoplasma capsulatum*), *Nocardia*	Macrophages wall off the infecting microorganism → granular debris **C**	Fragmented cells and debris surrounded by lymphocytes and macrophages
Fat	Enzymatic: acute pancreatitis (saponification) Nonenzymatic: breast trauma	Damaged cells release lipase, which breaks down fatty acids in cell membranes	Outlines of dead fat cells without peripheral nuclei; saponification of fat (combined with Ca^{2+}) appears dark blue on H&E stain **D**
Fibrinoid	Immune reactions in vessels	Immune complexes combine with fibrin → vessel wall damage	Vessel walls are thick and pink **E**
Gangrenous	Distal extremity, after chronic ischemia	Dry: ischemia **F**	Coagulative
		Wet: superinfection	Liquefactive

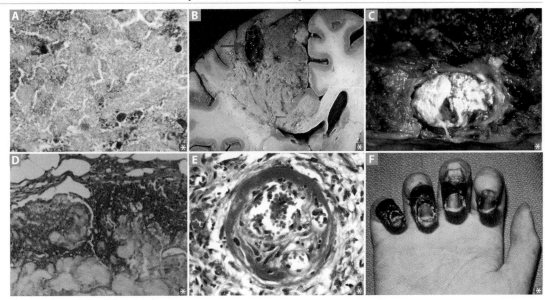

Cell injury

REVERSIBLE WITH O$_2$	IRREVERSIBLE
ATP depletion	Nuclear pyknosis, karyorrhexis, karyolysis
Cellular/mitochondrial swelling (↓ ATP → ↓ activity of Na$^+$/K$^+$ pumps)	Plasma membrane damage (degradation of membrane phospholipid)
Nuclear chromatin clumping	Lysosomal rupture
↓ glycogen	Mitochondrial permeability/vacuolization; phospholipid-containing amorphous densities within mitochondria (swelling alone is reversible)
Fatty change	
Ribosomal/polysomal detachment (↓ protein synthesis)	
Membrane blebbing	

Ischemia: susceptible areas

Areas susceptible to hypoxia/ischemia and infarction:

ORGAN	LOCATION
Brain	ACA/MCA/PCA boundary areas[a,b]
Heart	Subendocardium (LV)
Kidney	Straight segment of proximal tubule (medulla) Thick ascending limb (medulla)
Liver	Area around central vein (zone III)
Colon	Splenic flexure,[a] rectum[a]

[a]Watershed areas (border zones) receive dual blood supply from most distal branches of 2 arteries, which protects these areas from single-vessel focal blockage. However, these areas are susceptible to ischemia from systemic hypoperfusion.

[b]Hypoxic ischemic encephalopathy (HIE) affects pyramidal cells of hippocampus and Purkinje cells of cerebellum.

Infarcts: red vs. pale

Red

Red (hemorrhagic) infarcts (left in **A**) occur in venous occlusion and tissues with multiple blood supplies, such as liver, lung, and intestine; reperfusion (e.g., after angioplasty). Reperfusion injury is due to damage by free radicals.

Red = **r**eperfusion.

Pale

Pale (anemic) infarcts (right in **A**) occur in solid organs with a single (end-arterial) blood supply, such as heart, kidney, and spleen.

A **Infarcts.** Image on left shows red infarct (arrows). ℞ Image on right shows pale infarct (arrows). ✖

Atrophy	Reduction in the size and/or number of cells. Causes include:
	▪ ↓ endogenous hormones (e.g., post-menopausal ovaries)
	▪ ↑ exogenous hormones (e.g., factitious thyrotoxicosis, steroid use)
	▪ ↓ innervation (e.g., motor neuron damage)
	▪ ↓ blood flow/nutrients
	▪ ↓ metabolic demand (e.g., prolonged hospitalization, paralysis)
	▪ ↑ pressure (e.g., nephrolithiasis)
	▪ Occlusion of secretory ducts (e.g., cystic fibrosis, calculus/stone)

Inflammation	Characterized by *rubor* (redness), *dolor* (pain), *calor* (heat), *tumor* (swelling), and *functio laesa* (loss of function).
Vascular component	↑ vascular permeability, vasodilation, endothelial injury.
Cellular component	Neutrophils extravasate from circulation to injured tissue to participate in inflammation through phagocytosis, degranulation, and inflammatory mediator release.
Acute	Neutrophil, eosinophil, and antibody mediated. Acute inflammation is rapid onset (seconds to minutes) and of short duration (minutes to days). Outcomes include complete resolution, abscess formation, or progression to chronic inflammation.
Chronic	Mononuclear cell and fibroblast mediated. Characterized by persistent destruction and repair. Associated with blood vessel proliferation, fibrosis. Granuloma: nodular collections of epithelioid macrophages and giant cells. Outcomes include scarring and amyloidosis.

Chromatolysis	Process involving the neuronal cell body following axonal injury. Changes reflect ↑ protein synthesis in effort to repair the damaged axon. Characterized by:
	▪ Round cellular swelling **A**
	▪ Displacement of the nucleus to the periphery
	▪ Dispersion of Nissl substance throughout cytoplasm

Types of calcification

Dystrophic calcification	Ca^{2+} deposition in **abnormal tissues** 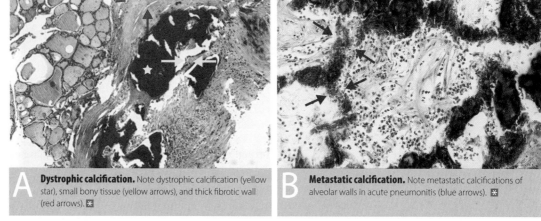A 2° to injury or necrosis. Tends to be localized (e.g., calcific aortic stenosis). Seen in TB (lungs and pericardium), liquefactive necrosis of chronic abscesses, fat necrosis, infarcts, thrombi, schistosomiasis, Mönckeberg arteriolosclerosis, congenital CMV + toxoplasmosis, psammoma bodies. Is not directly associated with serum Ca^{2+} levels (patients are usually **normocalcemic**).
Metastatic calcification	Widespread (i.e., diffuse, metastatic) deposition of Ca^{2+} in **normal tissue** B 2° to hypercalcemia (e.g., 1° hyperparathyroidism, sarcoidosis, hypervitaminosis D) or high calcium-phosphate product levels (e.g., chronic renal failure with 2° hyperparathyroidism, long-term dialysis, calciphylaxis, warfarin). Ca^{2+} deposits predominantly in interstitial tissues of kidney, lung, and gastric mucosa (these tissues lose acid quickly; ↑ pH favors deposition). Patients are usually **not normocalcemic**.

A **Dystrophic calcification.** Note dystrophic calcification (yellow star), small bony tissue (yellow arrows), and thick fibrotic wall (red arrows). ✳

B **Metastatic calcification.** Note metastatic calcifications of alveolar walls in acute pneumonitis (blue arrows). ✳

Leukocyte extravasation

Extravasation predominantly occurs at postcapillary venules.
WBCs exit from blood vessels at sites of tissue injury and inflammation in 4 steps:

STEP	VASCULATURE/STROMA	LEUKOCYTE
❶ Margination and rolling—defective in leukocyte adhesion deficiency type 2 (↓ Sialyl-Lewis^X)	E-selectin P-selectin GlyCAM-1, CD34	Sialyl-Lewis^X Sialyl-Lewis^X L-selectin
❷ Tight-binding—defective in leukocyte adhesion deficiency type 1 (↓ CD18 integrin subunit)	ICAM-1 (CD54) VCAM-1 (CD106)	CD11/18 integrins (LFA-1, Mac-1) VLA-4 integrin
❸ Diapedesis—WBC travels between endothelial cells and exits blood vessel	PECAM-1 (CD31)	PECAM-1 (CD31)
❹ Migration—WBC travels through interstitium to site of injury or infection guided by chemotactic signals	Chemotactic products released in response to bacteria: C5a, IL-8, LTB$_4$, kallikrein, platelet-activating factor	Various

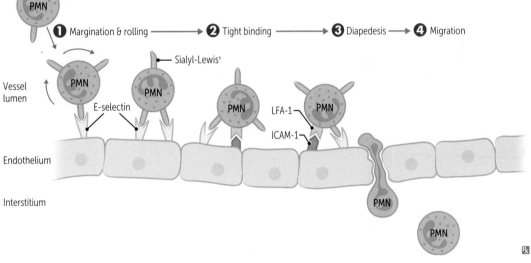

Free radical injury

Free radicals damage cells via membrane lipid peroxidation, protein modification, and DNA breakage.

Initiated via radiation exposure (e.g., cancer therapy), metabolism of drugs (phase I), redox reactions, nitric oxide, transition metals, WBC (e.g., neutrophils, macrophages) oxidative burst.

Free radicals can be eliminated by scavenging enzymes (e.g., catalase, superoxide dismutase, glutathione peroxidase), spontaneous decay, antioxidants (e.g., vitamins A, C, E), and certain metal carrier proteins (e.g., transferrin, ceruloplasmin).

Pathologies include:

- Retinopathy of prematurity (abnormal vascularization)
- Bronchopulmonary dysplasia
- Carbon tetrachloride, leading to liver necrosis (fatty change)
- Acetaminophen overdose (fulminant hepatitis, renal papillary necrosis)
- Iron overload (hemochromatosis)
- Reperfusion injury (e.g., superoxide), especially after thrombolytic therapy

---

Inhalational injury and sequelae

Pulmonary complication associated with smoke and fire. Caused by heat, particulates (< 1 μm diameter), or irritants (e.g., NH_3) → chemical tracheobronchitis, edema 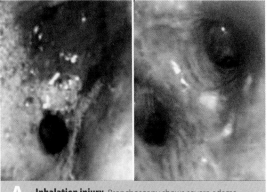, pneumonia, ARDS. Many patients present 2° to burns, CO inhalation, or arsenic poisoning.

A **Inhalation injury.** Bronchoscopy shows severe edema, congestion of bronchus, and carbon soot deposition 18 hours after inhalation injury (left), which have largely resolved by 11 days after injury (right).

Scar formation 70–80% of tensile strength regained at 3 months; little additional tensile strength will be regained afterward.

	Hypertrophic scars A	Keloid scars B
COLLAGEN SYNTHESIS	↑	↑↑↑
COLLAGEN ARRANGEMENT	Parallel	Disorganized
EXTENT	Confined to borders of original wound	Extend beyond borders of original wound
RECURRENCE	Infrequently recur following resection	Frequently recur following resection
NOTES		Higher incidence in African Americans

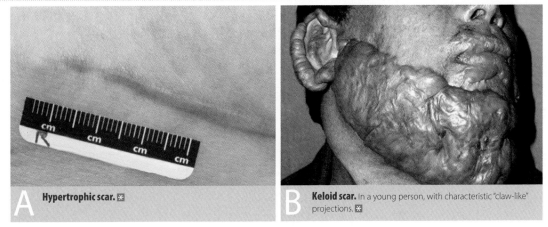

A **Hypertrophic scar.** ✦

B **Keloid scar.** In a young person, with characteristic "claw-like" projections. ✦

Wound healing

Tissue mediators	MEDIATOR	ROLE
	PDGF	Secreted by activated platelets and macrophages Induces vascular remodeling and smooth muscle cell migration Stimulates fibroblast growth for collagen synthesis
	FGF	Stimulates angiogenesis
	EGF	Stimulates cell growth via tyrosine kinases (e.g., EGFR, as expressed by *ERBB2*)
	TGF-β	Angiogenesis, fibrosis, cell cycle arrest
	Metalloproteinases	Tissue remodeling
	VEGF	Stimulates angiogenesis

PHASE OF WOUND HEALING	MEDIATORS	CHARACTERISTICS
Inflammatory (up to 3 days after wound)	Platelets, neutrophils, macrophages	Clot formation, ↑ vessel permeability and neutrophil migration into tissue; macrophages clear debris 2 days later
Proliferative (day 3–weeks after wound)	Fibroblasts, myofibroblasts, endothelial cells, keratinocytes, macrophages	Deposition of granulation tissue and collagen, angiogenesis, epithelial cell proliferation, dissolution of clot, and wound contraction (mediated by myofibroblasts)
Remodeling (1 week–6+ months after wound)	Fibroblasts	Type III collagen replaced by type I collagen, ↑ tensile strength of tissue

Granulomatous diseases

Bartonella henselae (cat scratch disease)

Berylliosis

Eosinophilic granulomatosis with polyangiitis (Churg-Strauss syndrome)

Crohn disease (noncaseating granuloma)

Foreign bodies

Francisella tularensis

Fungal infections (caseous necrosis)

Granulomatosis with polyangiitis (Wegener)

Listeria monocytogenes (granulomatosis infantiseptica)

M. leprae (leprosy; Hansen disease)

M. tuberculosis (caseous necrosis)

Treponema pallidum (3° syphilis)

Sarcoidosis Ⓐ (noncaseating granuloma)

Schistosomiasis

Th1 cells secrete IFN-γ, activating macrophages. TNF-α from macrophages induces and maintains granuloma formation. Anti-TNF drugs can, as a side effect, cause sequestering granulomas to break down, leading to disseminated disease. Always test for latent TB before starting anti-TNF therapy.

Exudate vs. transudate

Exudate ("Thick...")	Transudate ("and thin")
Cellular	Hypocellular
Protein-rich	Protein-poor
Specific gravity > 1.020	Specific gravity < 1.012
Due to:	Due to:
▪ Lymphatic obstruction ▪ Inflammation/infection ▪ Malignancy	▪ ↑ hydrostatic pressure (e.g., HF) ▪ ↓ oncotic pressure (e.g., cirrhosis, nephrotic syndrome) ▪ Na^+ retention

Erythrocyte sedimentation rate

Products of inflammation (e.g., fibrinogen) coat RBCs and cause aggregation. The denser RBC aggregates fall at a faster rate within a pipette tube. Often co-tested with CRP levels.

↑ ESR	↓ ESR
Most anemias	Sickle cell anemia (altered shape)
Infections	Polycythemia (↑ RBCs "dilute" aggregation factors)
Inflammation (e.g., temporal arteritis)	HF
Cancer (e.g., multiple myeloma)	Microcytosis
Pregnancy	Hypofibrinogenemia
Autoimmune disorders (e.g., SLE)	

Amyloidosis	Abnormal aggregation of proteins A B (or their fragments) into β-pleated sheets → damage and apoptosis.
COMMON TYPES	DESCRIPTION
AL (primary)	Due to deposition of proteins from Ig **L**ight chains. Can occur as a plasma cell disorder or associated with multiple myeloma. Often affects multiple organ systems, including renal (nephrotic syndrome), cardiac (restrictive cardiomyopathy, arrhythmia), hematologic (easy bruising, splenomegaly), GI (hepatomegaly), and neurologic (neuropathy).
AA (secondary)	Seen with chronic inflammatory conditions such as rheumatoid arthritis, IBD, spondyloarthropathy, protracted infection. Fibrils composed of serum **A**myloid **A**. Often multisystem like AL amyloidosis.
Dialysis-related	Fibrils composed of β₂-microglobulin in patients with ESRD and/or on long-term dialysis. May present as carpal tunnel syndrome.
Heritable	Heterogeneous group of disorders, including familial amyloid polyneuropathies due to transthyretin gene mutation.
Age-related (senile) systemic	Due to deposition of normal (wild-type) transthyretin in myocardium and other sites. Slower progression of cardiac dysfunction relative to AL amyloidosis.
Organ-specific	Amyloid deposition localized to a single organ. Most important form is amyloidosis in Alzheimer disease due to deposition of β-amyloid protein cleaved from amyloid precursor protein (APP). Islet amyloid polypeptide (IAPP) is commonly seen in diabetes mellitus type 2 and is caused by deposition of amylin in pancreatic islets.

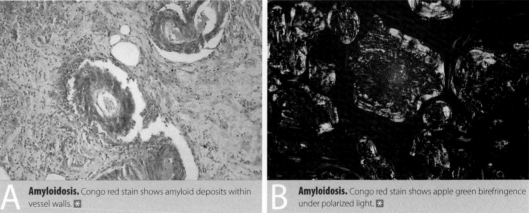

A **Amyloidosis.** Congo red stain shows amyloid deposits within vessel walls. ✲

B **Amyloidosis.** Congo red stain shows apple green birefringence under polarized light. ✲

Lipofuscin	A yellow-brown "wear and tear" pigment A associated with normal aging. Formed by oxidation and polymerization of autophagocytosed organellar membranes. Autopsy of elderly person will reveal deposits in heart, colon, liver, kidney, eye, and other organs.

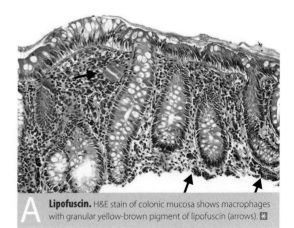

A **Lipofuscin.** H&E stain of colonic mucosa shows macrophages with granular yellow-brown pigment of lipofuscin (arrows). ✲

▶ PATHOLOGY—NEOPLASIA

Neoplastic progression   Hallmarks of cancer: evasion of apoptosis, growth signal self-sufficiency, anti-growth signal insensitivity, sustained angiogenesis, limitless replicative potential, tissue invasion, and metastasis.

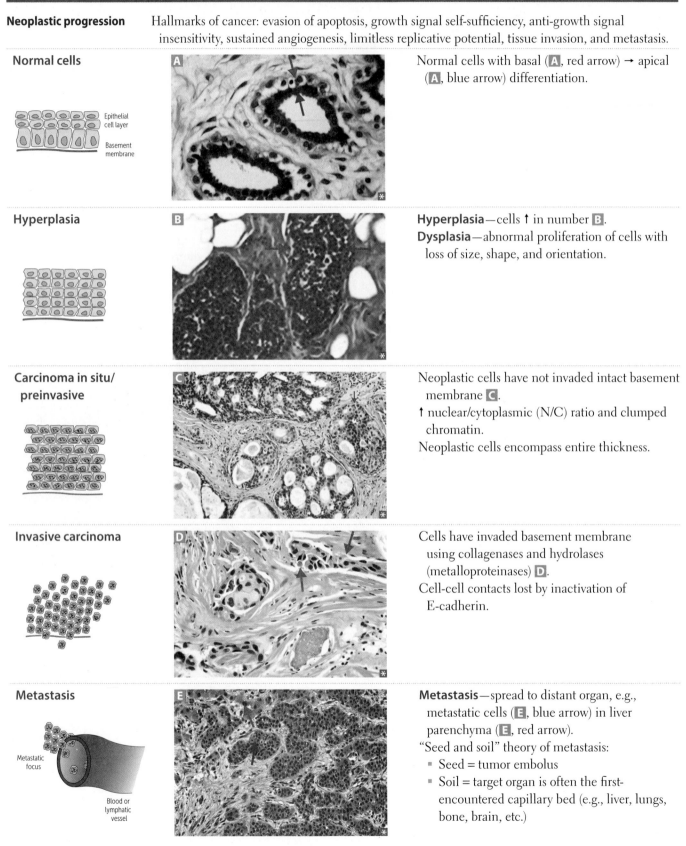

Normal cells

Epithelial cell layer
Basement membrane

Normal cells with basal (**A**, red arrow) → apical (**A**, blue arrow) differentiation.

Hyperplasia

Hyperplasia—cells ↑ in number **B**.
Dysplasia—abnormal proliferation of cells with loss of size, shape, and orientation.

Carcinoma in situ/ preinvasive

Neoplastic cells have not invaded intact basement membrane **C**.
↑ nuclear/cytoplasmic (N/C) ratio and clumped chromatin.
Neoplastic cells encompass entire thickness.

Invasive carcinoma

Cells have invaded basement membrane using collagenases and hydrolases (metalloproteinases) **D**.
Cell-cell contacts lost by inactivation of E-cadherin.

Metastasis

Metastatic focus

Blood or lymphatic vessel

Metastasis—spread to distant organ, e.g., metastatic cells (**E**, blue arrow) in liver parenchyma (**E**, red arrow).
"Seed and soil" theory of metastasis:
- Seed = tumor embolus
- Soil = target organ is often the first-encountered capillary bed (e.g., liver, lungs, bone, brain, etc.)

P-glycoprotein	Also known as multidrug resistance protein 1 (MDR1). Classically seen in adrenal cell carcinoma but also expressed by other cancer cells (e.g., colon, liver). Used to pump out toxins, including chemotherapeutic agents (one mechanism of ↓ responsiveness or resistance to chemotherapy over time).

-plasia definitions

REVERSIBLE	
Hyperplasia	↑ in number of cells. Distinct from hypertrophy (↑ in size of cells).
Metaplasia	One adult cell type is replaced by another. Often 2° to irritation (e.g., Barrett esophagus) and/or environmental exposure (e.g., smoking-induced tracheal/bronchial squamous metaplasia). Also occurs where two different epithelia meet (e.g., squamocolumnar junction of the uterine cervix).
Dysplasia	Abnormal growth with loss of cellular orientation, shape, and size in comparison to normal tissue maturation; commonly preneoplastic.
IRREVERSIBLE	
Anaplasia	Loss of structural differentiation and function of cells, resembling primitive cells of same tissue; often equated with undifferentiated malignant neoplasms. May see "giant cells" with single large nucleus or several nuclei.
Neoplasia	An uncontrolled and excessive clonal proliferation of cells. Neoplasia may be benign or malignant.
Desmoplasia	Fibrous tissue formation in response to neoplasm (e.g., linitis plastica in diffuse stomach cancer).

Tumor grade vs. stage

Grade	Degree of cellular differentiation and mitotic activity on histology. Usually graded 1–4; 1 = low grade, well differentiated; 4 = high grade, poorly differentiated, anaplastic.	Stage almost always has more prognostic value than grade.
Stage	Degree of localization/spread based on site and size of 1° lesion, spread to regional lymph nodes, presence of metastases. Based on clinical (c) or pathology (p) findings. Example: cT3N1M0	TNM staging system (Stage = Spread): **T** = **T**umor size **N** = **N**ode involvement **M** = **M**etastases Each TNM factor has independent prognostic value.

Tumor nomenclature

Carcinoma implies epithelial origin, whereas **sarcoma** denotes mesenchymal origin. Both terms imply malignancy. Most carcinomas spread via lymphatics; most sarcomas spread hematogenously. Terms for non-neoplastic malformations include hamartoma (disorganized overgrowth of tissues in their native location, e.g., Peutz-Jeghers polyps) and choristoma (normal tissue in a foreign location, e.g., gastric tissue located in small bowel in Meckel diverticulum).

CELL TYPE	BENIGN	MALIGNANT
Epithelium	Adenoma, papilloma	Adenocarcinoma, papillary carcinoma
Mesenchyme		
Blood cells		Leukemia, lymphoma
Blood vessels	Hemangioma	Angiosarcoma
Smooth muscle	Leiomyoma	Leiomyosarcoma
Striated muscle	Rhabdomyoma	Rhabdomyosarcoma
Connective tissue	Fibroma	Fibrosarcoma
Bone	Osteoma	Osteosarcoma
Fat	Lipoma	Liposarcoma

Tumor classifications

Benign	Usually well differentiated, well demarcated, low mitotic activity, no metastasis, no necrosis.
Malignant	May show poor differentiation, erratic growth, local invasion, metastasis, and ↓ apoptosis. Upregulation of telomerase prevents chromosome shortening and cell death.

Cachexia

Weight loss, muscle atrophy, and fatigue that occur in chronic disease (e.g., cancer, AIDS, heart failure, TB). Mediated by TNF-α (nicknamed cachectin), IFN-γ, IL-1, and IL-6.

Disease conditions associated with neoplasms

Gastrointestinal	
Acanthosis nigricans	Rare paraneoplastic indicator of visceral malignancy (more commonly associated with insulin resistance)
Barrett esophagus	Precursor to esophageal adenocarcinoma
Chronic atrophic gastritis, postsurgical gastric remnants	Predispose to gastric adenocarcinoma
Cirrhosis	Predisposes to hepatocellular carcinoma
Ulcerative colitis	Predisposes to colon adenocarcinoma

Musculoskeletal and skin	
Actinic keratosis	Precursor to squamous cell carcinoma of the skin
Dermato- and polymyositis	Predispose to visceral malignancies, particularly genitourinary
Dysplastic nevus	Precursor to malignant melanoma
Multiple seborrheic keratoses	GI, breast, lung, and lymphoid malignancies
Paget disease of bone	Predisposes to 2° osteosarcoma and fibrosarcoma
Plummer-Vinson syndrome	Predisposes to squamous cell carcinoma of the esophagus
Tuberous sclerosis	Often manifests with multiple hamartomatous (benign) tumors including giant cell astrocytomas, renal angiomyolipomas, cardiac rhabdomyomas; tumors may become malignant
Xeroderma pigmentosum, albinism	Predispose to squamous cell carcinoma, basal cell carcinoma, melanoma

Hematologic	
AIDS	Predisposes to aggressive lymphoma (non-Hodgkin) and Kaposi sarcoma
Autoimmune diseases (e.g., Hashimoto thyroiditis, SLE)	Predispose to lymphoma
Down syndrome	Predisposes to acute lymphocytic leukemia
Immunodeficiency	Predisposes to lymphoma, melanoma, renal cell carcinoma
Li-Fraumeni syndrome	$p53$ mutation predisposes to various cancer types at a young age (e.g., sarcoma, breast, leukemia, adrenal gland)
Radiation exposure	High risk of developing leukemia, sarcoma, papillary thyroid cancer, breast cancer

Oncogenes

Gain of function → ↑ cancer risk. Need damage to only 1 allele.

GENE	GENE PRODUCT	ASSOCIATED TUMOR
BCR-ABL	Tyrosine kinase	CML, ALL
BCL-2	Antiapoptotic molecule (inhibits apoptosis)	Follicular and undifferentiated lymphomas
BRAF	Serine/threonine kinase	Melanoma, non-Hodgkin lymphoma
c-kit	Cytokine receptor	Gastrointestinal stromal tumor (GIST)
c-myc	Transcription factor	Burkitt lymphoma
HER2/neu (c-erbB2)	Tyrosine kinase	Breast, ovarian, and gastric carcinomas
L-myc	Transcription factor	Lung tumor
N-myc	Transcription factor	Neuroblastoma
RAS	GTPase	Colon cancer, lung cancer, pancreatic cancer
RET	Tyrosine kinase	MEN 2A and 2B, medullary thyroid cancer

Tumor suppressor genes

Loss of function → ↑ cancer risk; both alleles must be lost for expression of disease.

GENE	ASSOCIATED TUMOR	GENE PRODUCT
APC	Colorectal cancer (associated with FAP)	
BRCA1/BRCA2	Breast and ovarian cancer	DNA repair protein
DCC	Colon cancer	DCC—Deleted in Colon Cancer
DPC4/SMAD4	Pancreatic cancer	DPC—Deleted in Pancreatic Cancer
MEN1	MEN 1	Menin
NF1	NeuroFibromatosis type 1	Ras GTPase activating protein (neurofibromin)
NF2	NeuroFibromatosis type 2	Merlin (schwannomin) protein
p16	Melanoma	Cyclin-dependent kinase inhibitor 2A
p53	Most human cancers, Li-Fraumeni syndrome	Transcription factor for p21, blocks G_1 → S phase
PTEN	Breast cancer, prostate cancer, endometrial cancer	
Rb	Retinoblastoma, osteosarcoma	Inhibits E2F; blocks G_1 → S phase
TSC1	Tuberous sclerosis	Hamartin protein
TSC2	Tuberous sclerosis	Tuberin protein
VHL	von Hippel-Lindau disease, renal cell carcinoma	Inhibits hypoxia inducible factor 1a
WT1/WT2	Wilms Tumor (nephroblastoma)	

Tumor markers	Tumor markers should not be used as the 1° tool for cancer diagnosis or screening. They may be used to monitor tumor recurrence and response to therapy, but definitive diagnosis is usually made via biopsy.	
Alkaline phosphatase	Metastases to bone or liver, Paget disease of bone, seminoma (placental ALP).	
α-fetoprotein	Hepatocellular carcinoma, hepatoblastoma, yolk sac (endodermal sinus) tumor, mixed germ cell tumor.	Normally made by fetus. Transiently elevated in pregnancy; high levels associated with neural tube and abdominal wall defects, low levels associated with Down syndrome.
β-hCG	Hydatidiform moles and Choriocarcinomas (Gestational trophoblastic disease), testicular cancer, mixed germ cell tumor.	Produced by syncytiotrophoblasts of the placenta.
CA 15-3/CA 27-29	Breast cancer.	
CA 19-9	Pancreatic adenocarcinoma.	
CA 125	Ovarian cancer.	
Calcitonin	Medullary thyroid carcinoma.	
CEA	CarcinoEmbryonic Antigen. Very nonspecific but produced by ~ 70% of colorectal and pancreatic cancers; also produced by gastric, breast, and medullary thyroid carcinomas.	
Chromogranin	Neuroendocrine tumors/carcinoid.	
PSA	Prostate-specific antigen. Prostate cancer.	Can also be elevated in BPH and prostatitis. Questionable risk/benefit for screening.

Oncogenic microbes	Microbe	Associated cancer
	EBV	Burkitt lymphoma, Hodgkin lymphoma, nasopharyngeal carcinoma, 1° CNS lymphoma (in immunocompromised patients)
	HBV, HCV	Hepatocellular carcinoma
	HHV-8	Kaposi sarcoma
	HPV	Cervical and penile/anal carcinoma (types 16, 18), head and neck cancer
	H. pylori	Gastric adenocarcinoma and MALT lymphoma
	HTLV-1	Adult T-cell leukemia/lymphoma
	Liver fluke (*Clonorchis sinensis*)	Cholangiocarcinoma
	Schistosoma haematobium	Bladder cancer (squamous cell)

Carcinogens

TOXIN	ORGAN	IMPACT
Aflatoxins (*Aspergillus*)	Liver	Hepatocellular carcinoma
Alkylating agents	Blood	Leukemia/lymphoma
Aromatic amines (e.g., benzidine, 2-naphthylamine)	Bladder	Transitional cell carcinoma
Arsenic	Liver	Angiosarcoma
	Lung	Lung cancer
	Skin	Squamous cell carcinoma
Asbestos	Lung	Bronchogenic carcinoma > mesothelioma
Carbon tetrachloride	Liver	Centrilobular necrosis, fatty change
Cigarette smoke	Bladder	Transitional cell carcinoma
	Cervix	Cervical carcinoma
	Esophagus	Squamous cell carcinoma/adenocarcinoma
	Kidney	Renal cell carcinoma
	Larynx	Squamous cell carcinoma
	Lung	Squamous cell and small cell carcinoma
	Pancreas	Pancreatic adenocarcinoma
Ethanol	Esophagus	Squamous cell carcinoma
	Liver	Hepatocellular carcinoma
Ionizing radiation	Thyroid	Papillary thyroid carcinoma
Nitrosamines (smoked foods)	Stomach	Gastric cancer
Radon	Lung	Lung cancer (2nd leading cause after cigarette smoke)
Vinyl chloride	Liver	Angiosarcoma

Paraneoplastic syndromes

HORMONE/AGENT	EFFECT	NEOPLASM(S)
1,25-$(OH)_2 D_3$ (calcitriol)	Hypercalcemia	Hodgkin lymphoma, non-Hodgkin lymphoma
ACTH	Cushing syndrome	Small cell lung carcinoma, renal cell carcinoma
ADH	SIADH	Small cell lung carcinoma, intracranial neoplasms
Antibodies against presynaptic Ca^{2+} channels at NMJ	Lambert-Eaton myasthenic syndrome (muscle weakness)	Small cell lung carcinoma
Erythropoietin	Polycythemia	Renal cell carcinoma, hemangioblastoma, hepatocellular carcinoma, leiomyoma, pheochromocytoma
PTHrP	Hypercalcemia	Squamous cell lung carcinoma, renal cell carcinoma, breast cancer

Psammoma bodies

Laminated, concentric spherules with dystrophic calcification 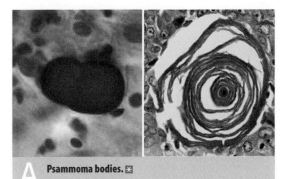, PSaMMoma bodies are seen in:

- Papillary carcinoma of thyroid
- Serous papillary cystadenocarcinoma of ovary
- Meningioma
- Malignant mesothelioma

Psammoma bodies. 🔆

Cancer epidemiology

	MALE	FEMALE	NOTES
Incidence	1. Prostate 2. Lung 3. Colon/rectum	1. Breast 2. Lung 3. Colon/rectum	Lung cancer incidence has dropped in men, but has not changed significantly in women.
Mortality	1. Lung 2. Prostate 3. Colon/rectum	1. Lung 2. Breast 3. Colon/rectum	Cancer is the 2nd leading cause of death in the United States (heart disease is 1st).

Common metastases

SITE OF METASTASIS	1° TUMOR	NOTES
Brain	Lung > breast > prostate > melanoma > GI.	50% of brain tumors are from metastases **A** **B**. Commonly seen as multiple well-circumscribed tumors at gray/white matter junction.
Liver	Colon >> stomach > pancreas.	Liver **C** **D** and lung are the most common sites of metastasis after the regional lymph nodes.
Bone	Prostate, breast > lung, thyroid, kidney.	Bone metastasis **E** **F** >> 1° bone tumors (e.g., multiple myeloma, lytic). Common mets to bone: breast (mixed), lung (mixed), thyroid (lytic), kidney (lytic), prostate (blastic). Predilection for axial skeleton **G**.

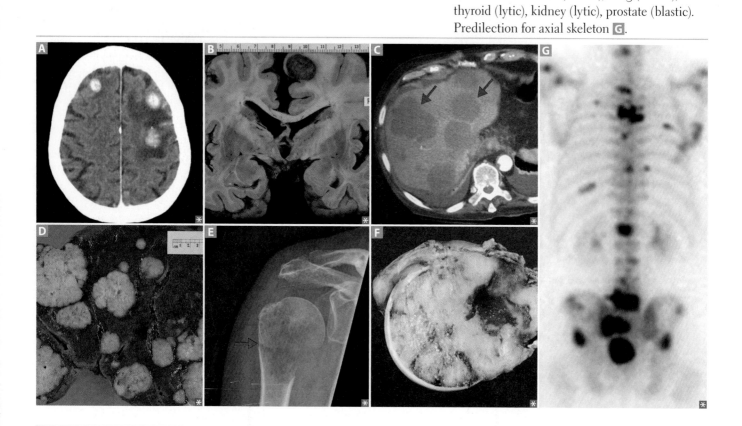

Pharmacology

"Take me, I am the drug; take me, I am hallucinogenic."
—Salvador Dali

"I was under medication when I made the decision not to burn the tapes."
—Richard Nixon

"I wondher why ye can always read a doctor's bill an' ye niver can read his purscription."
—Finley Peter Dunne

"Once you get locked into a serious drug collection, the tendency is to push it as far as you can."
—Hunter S. Thompson

Preparation for questions on pharmacology is straightforward. Memorizing all the key drugs and their characteristics (e.g., mechanisms, clinical use, and important side effects) is high yield. Focus on understanding the prototype drugs in each class. Avoid memorizing obscure derivatives. Learn the "classic" and distinguishing toxicities of the major drugs. Specific drug dosages or trade names are generally not testable. Reviewing associated biochemistry, physiology, and microbiology can be useful while studying pharmacology. There is a strong emphasis on ANS, CNS, antimicrobial, and cardiovascular agents as well as on NSAIDs. Much of the material is clinically relevant. We occasionally mention drugs that are no longer available in the U.S., but help illustrate high-yield pharmacologic or disease mechanisms. They are highlighted as being of historical significance and should not appear on the USMLE. However, recently approved drugs are fair game for the exam.

▶ PHARMACOLOGY—PHARMACOKINETICS & PHARMACODYNAMICS

Enzyme kinetics

Michaelis-Menten kinetics

[S] = concentration of substrate; V = velocity.

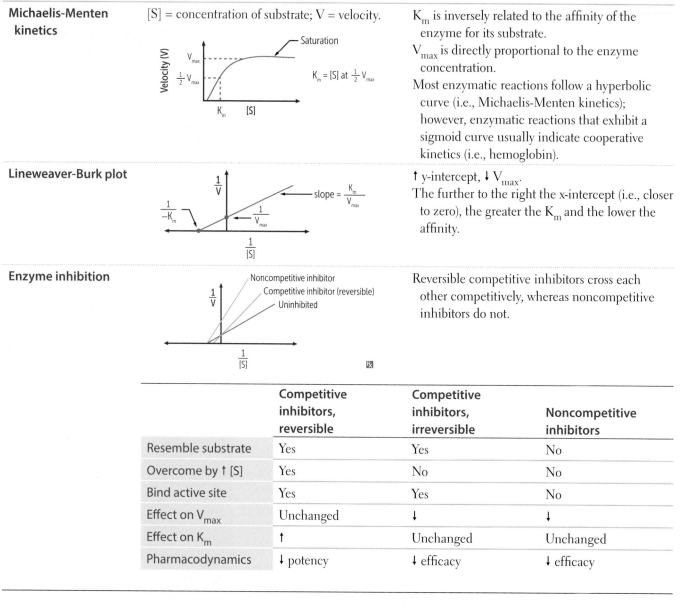

K_m = [S] at $\frac{1}{2}$ V_{max}

K_m is inversely related to the affinity of the enzyme for its substrate.

V_{max} is directly proportional to the enzyme concentration.

Most enzymatic reactions follow a hyperbolic curve (i.e., Michaelis-Menten kinetics); however, enzymatic reactions that exhibit a sigmoid curve usually indicate cooperative kinetics (i.e., hemoglobin).

Lineweaver-Burk plot

slope = $\frac{K_m}{V_{max}}$

↑ y-intercept, ↓ V_{max}.

The further to the right the x-intercept (i.e., closer to zero), the greater the K_m and the lower the affinity.

Enzyme inhibition

Reversible competitive inhibitors cross each other competitively, whereas noncompetitive inhibitors do not.

	Competitive inhibitors, reversible	Competitive inhibitors, irreversible	Noncompetitive inhibitors
Resemble substrate	Yes	Yes	No
Overcome by ↑ [S]	Yes	No	No
Bind active site	Yes	Yes	No
Effect on V_{max}	Unchanged	↓	↓
Effect on K_m	↑	Unchanged	Unchanged
Pharmacodynamics	↓ potency	↓ efficacy	↓ efficacy

Pharmacokinetics

Bioavailability (F)	Fraction of administered drug reaching systemic circulation unchanged. For an IV dose, F = 100%. Orally: F typically < 100% due to incomplete absorption and first-pass metabolism.
Volume of distribution (V_d)	Theoretical volume occupied by the total amount of drug in the body relative to its plasma concentration. Apparent V_d of plasma protein–bound drugs can be altered by liver and kidney disease (↓ protein binding, ↑ V_d). Drugs may distribute in more than one compartment.

$$V_d = \frac{\text{amount of drug in the body}}{\text{plasma drug concentration}}$$

V_d	COMPARTMENT	DRUG TYPES
Low	Blood	Large/charged molecules; plasma protein bound
Medium	ECF	Small hydrophilic molecules
High	All tissues including fat	Small lipophilic molecules, especially if bound to tissue protein

Clearance (CL)	The volume of plasma cleared of drug per unit time. Clearance may be impaired with defects in cardiac, hepatic, or renal function.

$$CL = \frac{\text{rate of elimination of drug}}{\text{plasma drug concentration}} = V_d \times K_e \text{ (elimination constant)}$$

Half-life ($t_{1/2}$)	The time required to change the amount of drug in the body by ½ during elimination (or constant infusion). Property of first-order elimination. A drug infused at a constant rate takes 4–5 half-lives to reach steady state. It takes 3.3 half-lives to reach 90% of the steady-state level.

$$t_{1/2} = \frac{0.693 \times V_d}{CL}$$

# of half-lives	1	2	3	4
% remaining	50%	25%	12.5%	6.25%

Dosage calculations	$$\text{Loading dose} = \frac{C_p \times V_d}{F}$$ $$\text{Maintenance dose} = \frac{C_p \times CL \times \tau}{F}$$ C_p = target plasma concentration at steady state τ = dosage interval (time between doses), if not administered continuously

In renal or liver disease, maintenance dose ↓ and loading dose is usually unchanged.
Time to steady state depends primarily on $t_{1/2}$ and is independent of dose and dosing frequency.

Elimination of drugs

Zero-order elimination	Rate of elimination is constant regardless of C_p (i.e., constant **amount** of drug eliminated per unit time). C_p ↓ linearly with time. Examples of drugs—Phenytoin, Ethanol, and Aspirin (at high or toxic concentrations).	Capacity-limited elimination. **PEA.** (A pea is round, shaped like the "0" in zero-order.)
First-order elimination	Rate of elimination is directly proportional to the drug concentration (i.e., constant **fraction** of drug eliminated per unit time). C_p ↓ exponentially with time.	Flow-dependent elimination.

Urine pH and drug elimination

Urine pH and drug elimination	Ionized species are trapped in urine and cleared quickly. Neutral forms can be reabsorbed.
Weak acids	Examples: phenobarbital, methotrexate, aspirin, TCAs. Trapped in basic environments. Treat overdose with bicarbonate.

$$\underset{\text{(lipid soluble)}}{RCOOH} \rightleftharpoons \underset{\text{(trapped)}}{RCOO^- + H^+}$$

Weak bases	Example: amphetamines. Trapped in acidic environments. Treat overdose with ammonium chloride.

$$\underset{\text{(trapped)}}{RNH_3^+} \rightleftharpoons \underset{\text{(lipid soluble)}}{RNH_2 + H^+}$$

Drug metabolism

Phase I	Reduction, oxidation, hydrolysis with cytochrome P-450 usually yield slightly polar, water-soluble metabolites (often still active).	Geriatric patients lose phase I first.
Phase II	Conjugation (Glucuronidation, Acetylation, Sulfation) usually yields very polar, inactive metabolites (renally excreted).	Geriatric patients have **GAS** (phase II). Patients who are slow acetylators have ↑ side effects from certain drugs because of ↓ rate of metabolism.

Efficacy vs. potency

Efficacy

Maximal effect a drug can produce. Represented by the y-value (V_{max}). ↑ y-value = ↑ V_{max} = ↑ efficacy. Unrelated to potency (i.e., efficacious drugs can have high or low potency). Partial agonists have less efficacy than full agonists.

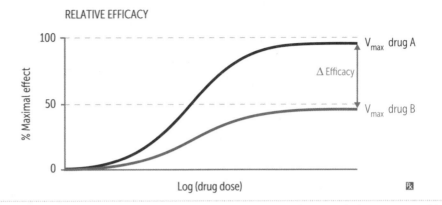

RELATIVE EFFICACY

Potency

Amount of drug needed for a given effect. ↑ potency (EC_{50}) = ↓ drug needed. Represented by the x-value (EC_{50}). Left-shifting = ↓ EC_{50} = ↑ potency. Unrelated to efficacy (i.e., potent drugs can have high or low efficacy).

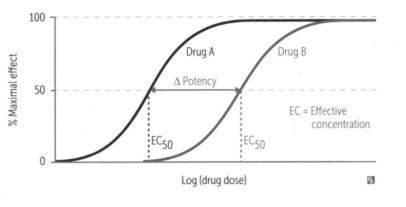

RELATIVE POTENCY

Receptor binding

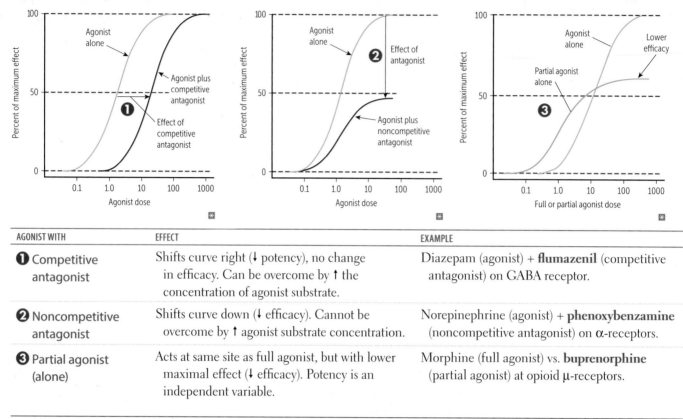

AGONIST WITH	EFFECT	EXAMPLE
❶ Competitive antagonist	Shifts curve right (↓ potency), no change in efficacy. Can be overcome by ↑ the concentration of agonist substrate.	Diazepam (agonist) + **flumazenil** (competitive antagonist) on GABA receptor.
❷ Noncompetitive antagonist	Shifts curve down (↓ efficacy). Cannot be overcome by ↑ agonist substrate concentration.	Norepinephrine (agonist) + **phenoxybenzamine** (noncompetitive antagonist) on α-receptors.
❸ Partial agonist (alone)	Acts at same site as full agonist, but with lower maximal effect (↓ efficacy). Potency is an independent variable.	Morphine (full agonist) vs. **buprenorphine** (partial agonist) at opioid μ-receptors.

Therapeutic index

Measurement of drug safety.

$$\frac{TD_{50}}{ED_{50}} = \frac{\text{median toxic dose}}{\text{median effective dose}}$$

Therapeutic window—measure of clinical drug effectiveness for a patient.

TITE: Therapeutic Index = TD_{50} / ED_{50}.
Safer drugs have higher TI values. Drugs with lower TI values include digoxin, lithium, theophylline, and warfarin.
LD_{50} (lethal median dose) often replaces TD_{50} in animal studies.

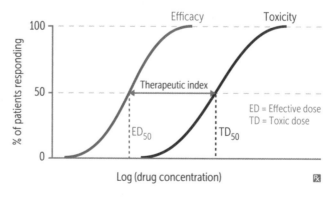

Central and peripheral nervous system

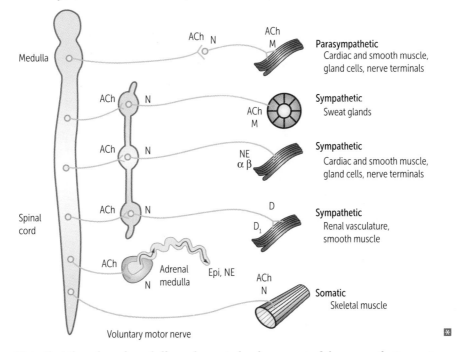

Note that the adrenal medulla and sweat glands are part of the sympathetic nervous system but are
innervated by cholinergic fibers.
Botulinum toxin prevents release of acetylcholine at cholinergic terminals.

ACh receptors	Nicotinic ACh receptors are ligand-gated Na^+/K^+ channels; N_N (found in autonomic ganglia) and N_M (found in neuromuscular junction) subtypes. Muscarinic ACh receptors are G-protein–coupled receptors that usually act through 2nd messengers; 5 subtypes: M_1, M_2, M_3, M_4, and M_5.

G-protein–linked 2nd messengers

RECEPTOR	G-PROTEIN CLASS	MAJOR FUNCTIONS
Sympathetic		
α_1	q	↑ vascular smooth muscle contraction, ↑ pupillary dilator muscle contraction (mydriasis), ↑ intestinal and bladder sphincter muscle contraction
α_2	i	↓ sympathetic outflow, ↓ insulin release, ↓ lipolysis, ↑ platelet aggregation, ↓ aqueous humor production
β_1	s	↑ heart rate, ↑ contractility, ↑ renin release, ↑ lipolysis
β_2	s	Vasodilation, bronchodilation, ↑ lipolysis, ↑ insulin release, ↓ uterine tone (tocolysis), ciliary muscle relaxation, ↑ aqueous humor production
Parasympathetic		
M_1	q	CNS, enteric nervous system
M_2	i	↓ heart rate and contractility of atria
M_3	q	↑ exocrine gland secretions (e.g., lacrimal, salivary, gastric acid), ↑ gut peristalsis, ↑ bladder contraction, bronchoconstriction, ↑ pupillary sphincter muscle contraction (miosis), ciliary muscle contraction (accommodation)
Dopamine		
D_1	s	Relaxes renal vascular smooth muscle
D_2	i	Modulates transmitter release, especially in brain
Histamine		
H_1	q	↑ nasal and bronchial mucus production, ↑ vascular permeability, contraction of bronchioles, pruritus, pain
H_2	s	↑ gastric acid secretion
Vasopressin		
V_1	q	↑ vascular smooth muscle contraction
V_2	s	↑ H_2O permeability and reabsorption in collecting tubules of kidney (V_2 is found in the 2 kidneys)

"**Q**iss (kiss) and **qiq** (kick) till you're **siq** (sick) of **sqs** (super qinky sex)."

H_1, α_1, V_1, M_1, M_3 Receptor $\xrightarrow{G_q}$ Phospholipase **C** ⟶ DAG ⟶ Protein kinase **C**   **HAV**e **1 M&M.**

Lipids ⟶ PIP_2

IP_3 ⟶ ↑ $[Ca^{2+}]_{in}$ ⟶ Smooth muscle contraction

β_1, β_2, D_1, H_2, V_2 Receptor $\overset{G_s}{\diagdown}$

Adenylyl cyclase ⟶ ATP ↓ cAMP ⟶ Protein kinase **A** ⟶ ↑ $[Ca^{2+}]_{in}$ (heart)

M_2, α_2, D_2 Receptor $\overset{G_i}{\diagup}$

Myosin light-chain kinase (smooth muscle)

MAD 2's.

Autonomic drugs

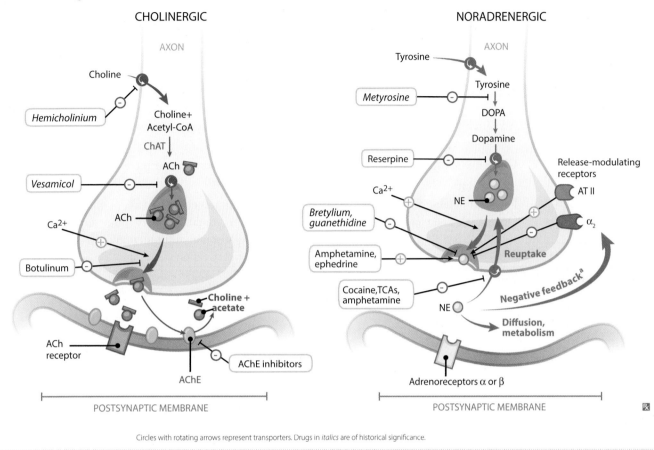

CHOLINERGIC

NORADRENERGIC

Circles with rotating arrows represent transporters. Drugs in *italics* are of historical significance.

[a]Release of norepinephrine from a sympathetic nerve ending is modulated by norepinephrine itself, acting on presynaptic α_2-autoreceptors.

Cholinomimetic agents

DRUG	CLINICAL APPLICATIONS	ACTION
Direct agonists		
Bethanechol	Postoperative ileus, neurogenic ileus, urinary retention	Activates bowel and bladder smooth muscle; resistant to AChE. "**Bethany, call** (**bethanechol**) me to activate your bowels and bladder."
Carbachol	Constricts pupil and relieves intraocular pressure in glaucoma	**Car**bon copy of a**c**etyl**ch**oline.
Methacholine	Challenge test for diagnosis of asthma	Stimulates **m**uscarinic receptors in airway when inhaled.
Pilocarpine	Potent stimulator of sweat, tears, and saliva Open-angle and closed-angle glaucoma	Contracts ciliary muscle of eye (open-angle glaucoma), pupillary sphincter (closed-angle glaucoma); resistant to AChE. "You cry, drool, and sweat on your '**pilow**.'"
Indirect agonists (anticholinesterases)		
Donepezil, galantamine, rivastigmine	Alzheimer disease.	↑ ACh.
Edrophonium	Historically, diagnosis of myasthenia gravis (extremely short acting). Myasthenia now diagnosed by anti-AChR Ab (anti-acetylcholine receptor antibody) test.	↑ ACh.
Neostigmine	Postoperative and neurogenic ileus and urinary retention, myasthenia gravis, reversal of neuromuscular junction blockade (postoperative).	↑ ACh. **Neo** CNS = **No** CNS penetration.
Physostigmine	Anticholinergic toxicity; crosses blood-brain barrier → CNS.	↑ ACh. **Physostigmine** "**phyxes**" atropine overdose.
Pyridostigmine	Myasthenia gravis (long acting); does not penetrate CNS.	↑ ACh; ↑ muscle strength. **Pyridostigmine** gets **rid** of myasthenia gravis.

Note: With all cholinomimetic agents, watch for exacerbation of COPD, asthma, and peptic ulcers when giving to susceptible patients.

Cholinesterase inhibitor poisoning	Often due to organophosphates, such as parathion, that **irreversibly** inhibit AChE. Causes **D**iarrhea, **U**rination, **M**iosis, **B**ronchospasm, **B**radycardia, **E**xcitation of skeletal muscle and CNS, **L**acrimation, **S**weating, and **S**alivation.	**DUMBBELSS.** Organophosphates are often components of insecticides; poisoning usually seen in farmers. Antidote—atropine (competitive inhibitor) + pralidoxime (regenerates AChE if given early).

Muscarinic antagonists

DRUGS	ORGAN SYSTEMS	APPLICATIONS
Atropine, homatropine, tropicamide	Eye	Produce mydriasis and cycloplegia.
Benztropine	CNS	Parkinson disease ("**park** my **Benz**"). Acute dystonia.
Glycopyrrolate	GI, respiratory	Parenteral: preoperative use to reduce airway secretions. Oral: drooling, peptic ulcer.
Hyoscyamine, dicyclomine	GI	Antispasmodics for irritable bowel syndrome.
Ipratropium, tiotropium	Respiratory	COPD, asthma ("**I pray** I can breathe soon!").
Oxybutynin, solifenacin, tolterodine	Genitourinary	Reduce bladder spasms and urge urinary incontinence (overactive bladder).
Scopolamine	CNS	Motion sickness.

Atropine Muscarinic antagonist. Used to treat bradycardia and for ophthalmic applications.

ORGAN SYSTEM	ACTION	NOTES
Eye	↑ pupil dilation, cycloplegia	Blocks **DUMBBeLSS**. Skeletal muscle and CNS excitation mediated by nicotinic receptors. See previous page.
Airway	↓ secretions	
Stomach	↓ acid secretion	
Gut	↓ motility	
Bladder	↓ urgency in cystitis	
TOXICITY	↑ body **temperature** (due to ↓ sweating); rapid pulse; dry mouth; **dry, flushed skin**; **cycloplegia**; constipation; **disorientation** Can cause acute angle-closure glaucoma in elderly (due to mydriasis), urinary retention in men with prostatic hyperplasia, and hyperthermia in infants	Side effects: **Hot** as a hare **Dry** as a bone **Red** as a beet **Blind** as a bat **Mad** as a hatter Jimson weed (*Datura*) → gardener's pupil (mydriasis due to plant alkaloids)

Tetrodotoxin

Highly potent toxin that binds fast voltage-gated Na^+ channels in cardiac and nerve tissue, preventing depolarization (blocks action potential without changing resting potential). Causes nausea, diarrhea, paresthesias, weakness, dizziness, loss of reflexes. Treatment is primarily supportive.

Poisoning can result from ingestion of poorly prepared pufferfish (fugu), a delicacy in Japan.

Ciguatoxin

Causes ciguatera fish poisoning. Opens Na^+ channels causing depolarization. Symptoms easily confused with cholinergic poisoning. Temperature-related dysesthesia (e.g., "cold feels hot; hot feels cold") is regarded as a specific finding of ciguatera. Treatment is primarily supportive.

Caused by consumption of reef fish (e.g., barracuda, snapper, moray eel).

Scombroid poisoning

Acute-onset burning sensation of the mouth, flushing of face, erythema, urticaria, pruritus, headache. May cause anaphylaxis-like presentation (i.e., bronchospasm, angioedema, hypotension). Treat supportively with antihistamines; if needed, antianaphylactics (e.g., bronchodilators, epinephrine).

Caused by consumption of dark-meat fish (e.g., bonito, mackerel, mahi-mahi, tuna) improperly stored at warm temperature. Bacterial histidine decarboxylase converts histidine → histamine. Histamine is not degraded by cooking. Frequently misdiagnosed as allergy to fish.

Sympathomimetics

DRUG	EFFECT	APPLICATIONS
Direct sympathomimetics		
Albuterol, salmeterol	$\beta_2 > \beta_1$	Albuterol for acute asthma; salmeterol for long-term asthma or COPD control.
Dobutamine	$\beta_1 > \beta_2, \alpha$	Heart failure (HF) (inotropic > chronotropic), cardiac stress testing.
Dopamine	$D_1 = D_2 > \beta > \alpha$	Unstable bradycardia, HF, shock; inotropic and chronotropic α effects predominate at high doses.
Epinephrine	$\beta > \alpha$	Anaphylaxis, asthma, open-angle glaucoma; α effects predominate at high doses. Significantly stronger effect at β_2-receptor than norepinephrine.
Isoproterenol	$\beta_1 = \beta_2$	Electrophysiologic evaluation of tachyarrhythmias. Can worsen ischemia.
Norepinephrine	$\alpha_1 > \alpha_2 > \beta_1$	Hypotension (but ↓ renal perfusion). Significantly weaker effect at β_2-receptor than epinephrine.
Phenylephrine	$\alpha_1 > \alpha_2$	Hypotension (vasoconstrictor), ocular procedures (mydriatic), rhinitis (decongestant).
Indirect sympathomimetics		
Amphetamine	Indirect general agonist, reuptake inhibitor, also releases stored catecholamines	Narcolepsy, obesity, ADHD.
Cocaine	Indirect general agonist, reuptake inhibitor	Causes vasoconstriction and local anesthesia. Never give β-blockers if cocaine intoxication is suspected (can lead to unopposed α_1 activation and extreme hypertension).
Ephedrine	Indirect general agonist, releases stored catecholamines	Nasal decongestion, urinary incontinence, hypotension.

Norepinephrine vs. isoproterenol

Norepinephrine ↑ systolic and diastolic pressures as a result of α_1-mediated vasoconstriction → ↑ mean arterial pressure → reflex bradycardia. However, isoproterenol (no longer commonly used) has little α effect but causes β_2-mediated vasodilation, resulting in ↓ mean arterial pressure and ↑ heart rate through β_1 and reflex activity.

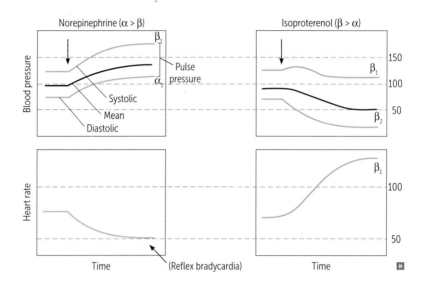

Sympatholytics (α_2-agonists)

DRUG	APPLICATIONS	TOXICITY
Clonidine	Hypertensive urgency (limited situations); does not decrease renal blood flow ADHD, Tourette syndrome	CNS depression, bradycardia, hypotension, respiratory depression, miosis
α-methyldopa	Hypertension in pregnancy	Direct Coombs ⊕ hemolysis, SLE-like syndrome

α-blockers

DRUG	APPLICATIONS	SIDE EFFECTS
Nonselective		
Phenoxybenzamine (irreversible)	Pheochromocytoma (used preoperatively) to prevent catecholamine (hypertensive) crisis	Orthostatic hypotension, reflex tachycardia
Phentolamine (reversible)	Give to patients on MAO inhibitors who eat tyramine-containing foods	
α₁ selective (-osin ending)		
Prazosin, terazosin, doxazosin, tamsulosin	Urinary symptoms of BPH; PTSD (prazosin); hypertension (except tamsulosin)	1st-dose orthostatic hypotension, dizziness, headache
α₂ selective		
Mirtazapine	Depression	Sedation, ↑ serum cholesterol, ↑ appetite

α-blockade of epinephrine vs. phenylephrine

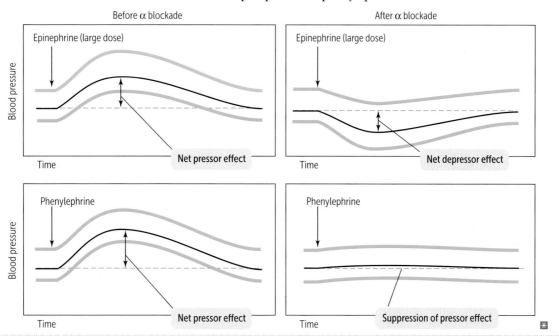

Shown above are the effects of an α-blocker (e.g., phentolamine) on blood pressure responses to epinephrine and phenylephrine. The epinephrine response exhibits reversal of the mean blood pressure change, from a net increase (the α response) to a net decrease (the β₂ response). The response to phenylephrine is suppressed but not reversed because phenylephrine is a "pure" α-agonist without β action.

β-blockers

Acebutolol, atenolol, betaxolol, carvedilol, esmolol, labetalol, metoprolol, nadolol, nebivolol, pindolol, propranolol, timolol.

APPLICATION	EFFECTS	NOTES
Angina pectoris	↓ heart rate and contractility, resulting in ↓ O_2 consumption	
MI	β-blockers (metoprolol, carvedilol, and bisoprolol) ↓ mortality	
SVT (metoprolol, esmolol)	↓ AV conduction velocity (class II antiarrhythmic)	
Hypertension	↓ cardiac output, ↓ renin secretion (due to β_1-receptor blockade on JGA cells)	
HF	↓ mortality in chronic HF	
Glaucoma (timolol)	↓ secretion of aqueous humor	
TOXICITY	Impotence, cardiovascular adverse effects (bradycardia, AV block, HF), CNS adverse effects (seizures, sedation, sleep alterations), dyslipidemia (metoprolol), and asthma/COPD exacerbations	Avoid in cocaine users due to risk of unopposed α-adrenergic receptor agonist activity Despite theoretical concern of masking hypoglycemia in diabetics, benefits likely outweigh risks; not contraindicated
SELECTIVITY	β_1-selective antagonists ($\beta_1 > \beta_2$)—acebutolol (partial agonist), atenolol, betaxolol, esmolol, metoprolol	Selective antagonists mostly go from **A** to **M** (β_1 with 1st half of alphabet)
	Nonselective antagonists ($\beta_1 = \beta_2$)—nadolol, pindolol (partial agonist), propranolol, timolol	Nonselective antagonists mostly go from **N** to **Z** (β_2 with 2nd half of alphabet)
	Nonselective α- and β-antagonists—carvedilol, labetalol	Nonselective α- and β-antagonists have modified suffixes (instead of "-olol")
	Nebivolol combines cardiac-selective β_1-adrenergic blockade with stimulation of β_3-receptors, which activate nitric oxide synthase in the vasculature	

▶ PHARMACOLOGY—TOXICITIES AND SIDE EFFECTS

Specific antidotes

TOXIN	ANTIDOTE/TREATMENT
Acetaminophen	N-acetylcysteine (replenishes glutathione)
AChE inhibitors, organophosphates	Atropine > pralidoxime
Amphetamines (basic)	NH_4Cl (acidify urine)
Antimuscarinic, anticholinergic agents	Physostigmine salicylate, control hyperthermia
Benzodiazepines	Flumazenil
β-blockers	Glucagon
Carbon monoxide	100% O_2, hyperbaric O_2
Copper, arsenic, gold	Penicillamine
Cyanide	Nitrite + thiosulfate, hydroxocobalamin
Digitalis (digoxin)	Anti-dig Fab fragments
Heparin	Protamine sulfate
Iron	Deferoxamine, deferasirox
Lead	EDTA, dimercaprol, succimer, penicillamine
Mercury, arsenic, gold	Dimercaprol (BAL), succimer
Methanol, ethylene glycol (antifreeze)	Fomepizole > ethanol, dialysis
Methemoglobin	**Meth**ylene blue, vitamin C
Opioids	Naloxone, naltrexone
Salicylates	$NaHCO_3$ (alkalinize urine), dialysis
TCAs	$NaHCO_3$ (plasma alkalinization)
tPA, streptokinase, urokinase	Aminocaproic acid
Warfarin	Vitamin K (delayed effect), fresh frozen plasma (immediate)

Drug reactions—cardiovascular

DRUG REACTION	CAUSAL AGENTS
Coronary vasospasm	Cocaine, sumatriptan, ergot alkaloids
Cutaneous flushing	**V**ancomycin, **A**denosine, **N**iacin, **C**a^{2+} channel blockers (**VANC**)
Dilated cardiomyopathy	Anthracyclines (e.g., doxorubicin, daunorubicin); prevent with dexrazoxane
Torsades de pointes	Class III (e.g., sotalol) and class IA (e.g., quinidine) antiarrhythmics, macrolide antibiotics, antipsychotics, TCAs

Drug reactions—endocrine/reproductive

DRUG REACTION	CAUSAL AGENTS	NOTES
Adrenocortical insufficiency	HPA suppression 2° to glucocorticoid withdrawal	
Hot flashes	Tamoxifen, clomiphene	
Hyperglycemia	Tacrolimus, Protease inhibitors, Niacin, HCTZ, Corticosteroids	Taking Pills Necessitates Having blood Checked
Hypothyroidism	Lithium, amiodarone, sulfonamides	

Drug reactions—GI

DRUG REACTION	CAUSAL AGENTS	NOTES
Acute cholestatic hepatitis, jaundice	Erythromycin	
Diarrhea	Metformin, Erythromycin, Colchicine, Orlistat, Acarbose	Might Excite Colon On Accident
Focal to massive hepatic necrosis	Halothane, *Amanita phalloides* (death cap mushroom), Valproic acid, Acetaminophen	Liver "HAVAc"
Hepatitis	Rifampin, isoniazid, pyrazinamide, statins, fibrates	
Pancreatitis	Didanosine, Corticosteroids, Alcohol, Valproic acid, Azathioprine, Diuretics (furosemide, HCTZ)	Drugs Causing A Violent Abdominal Distress
Pseudomembranous colitis	Clindamycin, ampicillin, cephalosporins	Antibiotics predispose to superinfection by resistant C. *difficile*

Drug reactions—hematologic

DRUG REACTION	CAUSAL AGENTS	NOTES
Agranulocytosis	Ganciclovir, Clozapine, Carbamazepine, Colchicine, Methimazole, Propylthiouracil	Gangs CCCrush Myeloblasts and Promyelocytes
Aplastic anemia	Carbamazepine, Methimazole, NSAIDs, Benzene, Chloramphenicol, Propylthiouracil	Can't Make New Blood Cells Properly
Direct Coombs-positive hemolytic anemia	Methyldopa, penicillin	
Gray baby syndrome	Chloramphenicol	
Hemolysis in G6PD deficiency	Isoniazid, Sulfonamides, Dapsone, Primaquine, Aspirin, Ibuprofen, Nitrofurantoin	Hemolysis IS D PAIN
Megaloblastic anemia	Phenytoin, Methotrexate, Sulfa drugs	Having a blast with PMS
Thrombocytopenia	Heparin	
Thrombotic complications	OCPs, hormone replacement therapy	

Drug reactions—musculoskeletal/skin/connective tissue

DRUG REACTION	CAUSAL AGENTS	NOTES
Fat redistribution	Protease inhibitors, Glucocorticoids	Fat PiG
Gingival hyperplasia	Phenytoin, Ca^{2+} channel blockers, cyclosporine	
Hyperuricemia (gout)	Pyrazinamide, Thiazides, Furosemide, Niacin, Cyclosporine	Painful Tophi and Feet Need Care
Myopathy	Fibrates, niacin, colchicine, hydroxychloroquine, interferon-α, penicillamine, statins, glucocorticoids	
Osteoporosis	Corticosteroids, heparin	
Photosensitivity	Sulfonamides, Amiodarone, Tetracyclines, 5-FU	SAT For Photo
Rash (Stevens-Johnson syndrome)	Anti-epileptic drugs (especially lamotrigine), allopurinol, sulfa drugs, penicillin	Steven Johnson has epileptic allergy to sulfa drugs and penicillin
SLE-like syndrome	Sulfa drugs, Hydralazine, Isoniazid, Procainamide, Phenytoin, Etanercept	Having lupus is "SHIPP-E"
Teeth discoloration	Tetracyclines	
Tendonitis, tendon rupture, and cartilage damage	Fluoroquinolones	

Drug reactions—neurologic

DRUG REACTION	CAUSAL AGENTS	NOTES
Cinchonism	Quinidine, quinine	
Parkinson-like syndrome	Antipsychotics, Reserpine, Metoclopramide	Cogwheel rigidity of ARM
Seizures	Isoniazid (vitamin B_6 deficiency), Bupropion, Imipenem/cilastatin, Enflurane	With seizures, I BItE my tongue
Tardive dyskinesia	Antipsychotics, metoclopramide	

Drug reactions—renal/genitourinary

DRUG REACTION	CAUSAL AGENTS	NOTES
Diabetes insipidus	Lithium, demeclocycline	
Fanconi syndrome	Expired tetracycline	
Hemorrhagic cystitis	Cyclophosphamide, ifosfamide	Prevent by coadministering with mesna
Interstitial nephritis	Methicillin, NSAIDs, furosemide	
SIADH	Carbamazepine, Cyclophosphamide, SSRIs	Can't Concentrate Serum Sodium

Drug reactions—respiratory

DRUG REACTION	CAUSAL AGENTS	NOTES
Dry cough	ACE inhibitors	
Pulmonary fibrosis	Bleomycin, Amiodarone, Busulfan, Methotrexate	Breathing Air Badly from Medications

Drug reactions—multiorgan

DRUG REACTION	CAUSAL AGENTS
Antimuscarinic	Atropine, TCAs, H_1-blockers, antipsychotics
Disulfiram-like reaction	Metronidazole, certain cephalosporins, griseofulvin, procarbazine, 1st-generation sulfonylureas
Nephrotoxicity/ ototoxicity	Aminoglycosides, vancomycin, loop diuretics, cisplatin. Cisplatin toxicity may respond to amifostine.

Cytochrome P-450 interactions (selected)	Inducers (+)	Substrates	Inhibitors (−)
	Chronic alcohol use	Anti-epileptics	Acute alcohol abuse
	St. John's wort	Theophylline	Ritonavir
	Phenytoin	Warfarin	Amiodarone
	Phenobarbital	OCPs	Cimetidine
	Nevirapine		Ketoconazole
	Rifampin		Sulfonamides
	Griseofulvin		Isoniazid (INH)
	Carbamazepine		Grapefruit juice
			Quinidine
			Macrolides (except azithromycin)
	Chronic alcoholics Steal Phen-Phen and Never Refuse Greasy Carbs	Always Think When Outdoors	AAA RACKS IN GQ Magazine

Sulfa drugs	Probenecid, Furosemide, Acetazolamide, Celecoxib, Thiazides, Sulfonamide antibiotics, Sulfasalazine, Sulfonylureas. Patients with sulfa allergies may develop fever, urinary tract infection, Stevens-Johnson syndrome, hemolytic anemia, thrombocytopenia, agranulocytosis, and urticaria (hives). Symptoms range from mild to life threatening.	Popular FACTSSS

▸ PHARMACOLOGY—MISCELLANEOUS

Drug names

ENDING	CATEGORY	EXAMPLE
Antimicrobial		
-azole	Ergosterol synthesis inhibitor	Ketoconazole
-bendazole	Antiparasitic/antihelmintic	Mebendazole
-cillin	Peptidoglycan synthesis inhibitor	Ampicillin
-cycline	Protein synthesis inhibitor	Tetracycline
-ivir	Neuraminidase inhibitor	Oseltamivir
-navir	Protease inhibitor	Ritonavir
-ovir	DNA polymerase inhibitor	Acyclovir
-thromycin	Macrolide antibiotic	Azithromycin
CNS		
-ane	Inhalational general anesthetic	Halothane
-azine	Typical antipsychotic	Thioridazine
-barbital	Barbiturate	Phenobarbital
-caine	Local anesthetic	Lidocaine
-etine	SSRI	Fluoxetine
-ipramine, -triptyline	TCA	Imipramine, amitriptyline
-triptan	$5\text{-HT}_{1B/1D}$ agonists	Sumatriptan
-zepam, -zolam	Benzodiazepine	Diazepam, alprazolam
Autonomic		
-chol	Cholinergic agonist	Bethanechol/carbachol
-curium, -curonium	Nondepolarizing paralytic	Atracurium, vecuronium
-olol	β-blocker	Propranolol
-stigmine	AChE inhibitor	Neostigmine
-terol	β_2-agonist	Albuterol
-zosin	α_1-antagonist	Prazosin
Cardiovascular		
-afil	PDE-5 inhibitor	Sildenafil
-dipine	Dihydropyridine CCB	Amlodipine
-pril	ACE inhibitor	Captopril
-sartan	Angiotensin-II receptor blocker	Losartan
-statin	HMG-CoA reductase inhibitor	Atorvastatin
Other		
-dronate	Bisphosphonate	Alendronate
-glitazone	PPAR-γ activator	Rosiglitazone
-prazole	Proton pump inhibitor	Omeprazole
-prost	Prostaglandin analog	Latanoprost
-tidine	H_2-antagonist	Cimetidine
-tropin	Pituitary hormone	Somatotropin
-ximab	Chimeric monoclonal Ab	Basiliximab
-zumab	Humanized monoclonal Ab	Daclizumab

▶ NOTES

SECTION III

High-Yield
Organ Systems

"*Symptoms, then, are in reality nothing but the cry from suffering organs.*"
—Jean-Martin Charcot

"*Man is an intelligence in servitude to his organs.*"
—Aldous Huxley

"*Learn that you are a machine, your heart an engine, your lungs a fanning machine and a sieve, your brain with its two lobes an electric battery.*"
—Andrew T. Still

▶ APPROACHING THE ORGAN SYSTEMS

In this section, we have divided the High-Yield Facts into the major **Organ Systems.** Within each Organ System are several subsections, including **Embryology, Anatomy, Physiology, Pathology,** and **Pharmacology.** As you progress through each Organ System, refer back to information in the previous subsections to organize these basic science subsections into a "vertically integrated" framework for learning. Below is some general advice for studying the organ systems by these subsections.

Embryology

Relevant embryology is included in each organ system subsection. Embryology tends to correspond well with the relevant anatomy, especially with regard to congenital malformations.

Anatomy

Several topics fall under this heading, including gross anatomy, histology, and neuroanatomy. Do not memorize all the small details; however, do not ignore anatomy altogether. Review what you have already learned and what you wish you had learned. Many questions require two or more steps. The first step is to identify a structure on anatomic cross section, electron micrograph, or photomicrograph. The second step may require an understanding of the clinical significance of the structure.

When studying, stress clinically important material. For example, be familiar with gross anatomy and radiologic anatomy related to specific diseases (e.g., Pancoast tumor, Horner syndrome), traumatic injuries (e.g., fractures, sensory and motor nerve deficits), procedures (e.g., lumbar puncture), and common surgeries (e.g., cholecystectomy). There are also many questions on the exam involving X-rays, CT scans, and neuro MRI scans. Many students suggest browsing through a general radiology atlas, pathology atlas, and histology atlas. Focus on learning basic anatomy at key levels in the body (e.g., sagittal brain MRI; axial CT of the midthorax, abdomen, and pelvis). Basic neuroanatomy (especially pathways, blood supply, and functional anatomy), associated neuropathology, and neurophysiology have good yield. Please note that many of the photographic images in this book are for illustrative purposes and are not necessarily reflective of Step 1 emphasis.

Physiology

The portion of the examination dealing with physiology is broad and concept oriented and thus does not lend itself as well to fact-based review. Diagrams are often the best study aids, especially given the increasing number of questions requiring the interpretation of diagrams. Learn to apply basic physiologic relationships in a variety of ways (e.g., the Fick equation, clearance equations). You are seldom asked to perform complex calculations. Hormones are the focus of many questions, so learn their sites of production and action as well as their regulatory mechanisms.

A large portion of the physiology tested on the USMLE Step 1 is clinically relevant and involves understanding physiologic changes associated with pathologic processes (e.g., changes in pulmonary function with COPD). Thus, it is worthwhile to review the physiologic changes that are found with common pathologies of the major organ systems (e.g., heart, lungs, kidneys, GI tract) and endocrine glands.

Pathology

Questions dealing with this discipline are difficult to prepare for because of the sheer volume of material involved. Review the basic principles and hallmark characteristics of the key diseases. Given the clinical orientation of Step 1, it is no longer sufficient to know only the "buzzword" associations of certain diseases (e.g., café-au-lait macules and neurofibromatosis); you must also know the clinical descriptions of these findings.

Given the clinical slant of the USMLE Step 1, it is also important to review the classic presenting signs and symptoms of diseases as well as their associated laboratory findings. Delve into the signs, symptoms, and pathophysiology of major diseases that have a high prevalence in the United States (e.g., alcoholism, diabetes, hypertension, heart failure, ischemic heart disease, infectious disease). Be prepared to think one step beyond the simple diagnosis to treatment or complications.

The examination includes a number of color photomicrographs and photographs of gross specimens that are presented in the setting of a brief clinical history. However, read the question and the choices carefully before looking at the illustration, because the history will help you identify the pathologic process. Flip through an illustrated pathology textbook, color atlases, and appropriate Web sites in order to look at the pictures in the days before the exam. Pay attention to potential clues such as age, sex, ethnicity, occupation, recent activities and exposures, and specialized lab tests.

Pharmacology

Preparation for questions on pharmacology is straightforward. Memorizing all the key drugs and their characteristics (e.g., mechanisms, clinical use, and important side effects) is high yield. Focus on understanding the prototype drugs in each class. Avoid memorizing obscure derivatives. Learn the "classic" and distinguishing toxicities of the major drugs. Do not bother with drug dosages or trade names. Reviewing associated biochemistry, physiology, and microbiology can be useful while studying pharmacology. There is a strong emphasis on ANS, CNS, antimicrobial, and cardiovascular agents as well as NSAIDs. Much of the material is clinically relevant. Newer drugs on the market are also fair game.

▶ NOTES

Cardiovascular

"As for me, except for an occasional heart attack, I feel as young as I ever did."

—Robert Benchley

"Hearts will never be practical until they are made unbreakable."

—The Wizard of Oz

"As the arteries grow hard, the heart grows soft."

—H. L. Mencken

"Nobody has ever measured, not even poets, how much the heart can hold."

—Zelda Fitzgerald

"Only from the heart can you touch the sky."

—Rumi

"It is not the size of the man but the size of his heart that matters."

—Evander Holyfield

▶ CARDIOVASCULAR—EMBRYOLOGY

Heart embryology

EMBRYONIC STRUCTURE	GIVES RISE TO
Truncus arteriosus	Ascending aorta and pulmonary trunk
Bulbus cordis	Smooth parts (outflow tract) of left and right ventricles
Primitive atrium	Trabeculated part of left and right atria
Primitive ventricle	Trabeculated part of left and right ventricles
Primitive pulmonary vein	Smooth part of left atrium
Left horn of sinus venosus	Coronary sinus
Right horn of sinus venosus	Smooth part of right atrium (sinus venarum)
Right common cardinal vein and right anterior cardinal vein	Superior vena cava (SVC)

Heart morphogenesis

First functional organ in vertebrate embryos; beats spontaneously by week 4 of development.

Cardiac looping

Primary heart tube loops to establish left-right polarity; begins in week 4 of gestation.

Defect in left-right dynein (involved in L/R asymmetry) can lead to dextrocardia, as seen in Kartagener syndrome (primary ciliary dyskinesia).

Septation of the chambers

Atria

❶ Septum primum grows toward endocardial cushions, narrowing foramen primum.
❷ Foramen secundum forms in septum primum (foramen primum disappears).
❸ Septum secundum develops as foramen secundum maintains right-to-left shunt.
❹ Septum secundum expands and covers most of the foramen secundum. The residual foramen is the foramen ovale.
❺ Remaining portion of septum primum forms valve of foramen ovale.
6. (Not shown) Septum secundum and septum primum fuse to form the atrial septum.
7. (Not shown) Foramen ovale usually closes soon after birth because of ↑ LA pressure.

Patent foramen ovale—caused by failure of septum primum and septum secundum to fuse after birth; most are left untreated. Can lead to paradoxical emboli (venous thromboemboli that enter systemic arterial circulation), similar to those resulting from an ASD.

Heart morphogenesis (continued)

Ventricles	❶ Muscular ventricular septum forms. Opening is called interventricular foramen. ❷ Aorticopulmonary septum rotates and fuses with muscular ventricular septum to form membranous interventricular septum, closing interventricular foramen. ❸ Growth of endocardial cushions separates atria from ventricles and contributes to both atrial septation and membranous portion of the interventricular septum.	Ventricular septal defect (VSD)—most commonly occurs in the membranous septum.

Outflow tract formation	Truncus arteriosus rotates; neural crest and endocardial cell migrations → truncal and bulbar ridges that spiral and fuse to form aorticopulmonary septum → ascending aorta and pulmonary trunk.	Conotruncal abnormalities: ▪ Transposition of great vessels. ▪ Tetralogy of Fallot. ▪ Persistent truncus arteriosus.
Valve development	Aortic/pulmonary: derived from endocardial cushions of outflow tract. Mitral/tricuspid: derived from fused endocardial cushions of the AV canal.	Valvular anomalies may be stenotic, regurgitant, atretic (e.g., tricuspid atresia), or displaced (e.g., Ebstein anomaly).

Fetal erythropoiesis	Fetal erythropoiesis occurs in: ■ Yolk sac (3–8 weeks) ■ Liver (6 weeks–birth) ■ Spleen (10–28 weeks) ■ Bone marrow (18 weeks to adult)	**Y**oung **L**iver **S**ynthesizes **B**lood.
Hemoglobin development	Embryonic globins: ζ and ϵ. Fetal hemoglobin (HbF) = $\alpha_2\gamma_2$. Adult hemoglobin (HbA$_1$) = $\alpha_2\beta_2$. HbF has higher affinity for O_2 due to less avid binding of 2,3-BPG, allowing HbF to extract O_2 from maternal hemoglobin (HbA$_1$ and HbA$_2$) across the placenta.	From fetal to adult hemoglobin: **A**lpha **A**lways; **G**amma **G**oes, **B**ecomes **B**eta.

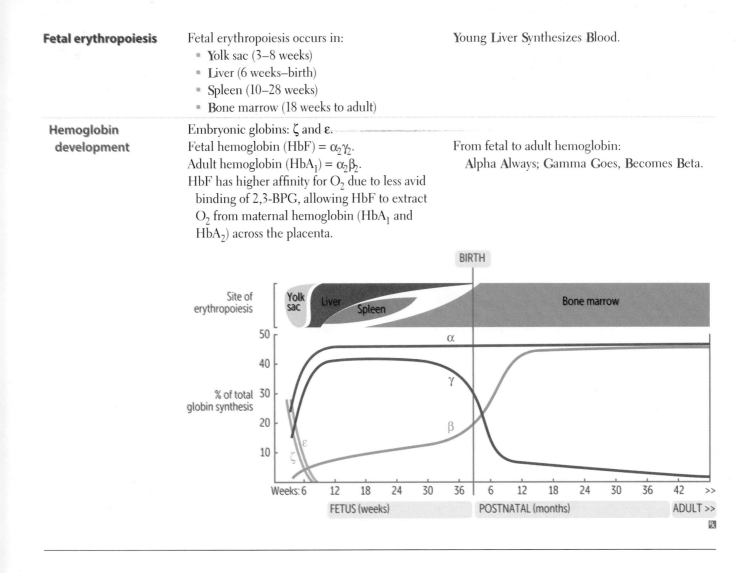

Fetal circulation

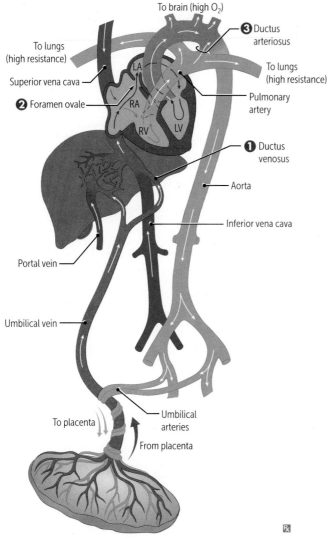

Blood in umbilical vein has a Po_2 of ≈ 30 mmHg and is ≈ 80% saturated with O_2. Umbilical arteries have low O_2 saturation.

3 important shunts:

❶ Blood entering fetus through the umbilical vein is conducted via the **ductus venosus** into the IVC, bypassing hepatic circulation.

❷ Most of the highly oxygenated blood reaching the heart via the IVC is directed through the **foramen ovale** and pumped into the aorta to supply the head and body.

❸ Deoxygenated blood from the SVC passes through the RA → RV → main pulmonary artery → patent ductus arteriosus → descending aorta; shunt is due to high fetal pulmonary artery resistance (due partly to low O_2 tension).

At birth, infant takes a breath; ↓ resistance in pulmonary vasculature → ↑ left atrial pressure vs. right atrial pressure; foramen ovale closes (now called fossa ovalis); ↑ in O_2 (from respiration) and ↓ in prostaglandins (from placental separation) → closure of ductus arteriosus.

Indomethacin helps close PDA → ligamentum arteriosum (remnant of ductus arteriosus).

Prostaglandins E_1 and E_2 kEEp PDA open.

Fetal-postnatal derivatives

AllaNtois → urachus	MediaN umbilical ligament	Urachus is part of allantoic duct between bladder and umbilicus.
Ductus arteriosus	Ligamentum arteriosum	
Ductus venosus	Ligamentum venosum	
Foramen ovale	Fossa ovalis	
Notochord	Nucleus pulposus	
UmbiLical arteries	MediaL umbilical ligaments	
Umbilical vein	Ligamentum teres hepatis	Contained in falciform ligament.

▶ CARDIOVASCULAR—ANATOMY

Coronary artery anatomy

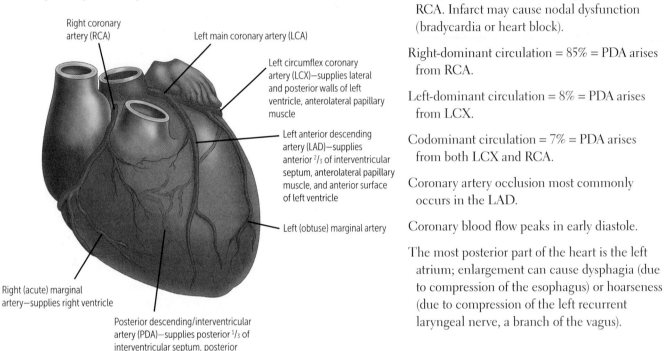

Right coronary artery (RCA)

Left main coronary artery (LCA)

Left circumflex coronary artery (LCX)—supplies lateral and posterior walls of left ventricle, anterolateral papillary muscle

Left anterior descending artery (LAD)—supplies anterior $2/3$ of interventricular septum, anterolateral papillary muscle, and anterior surface of left ventricle

Left (obtuse) marginal artery

Right (acute) marginal artery—supplies right ventricle

Posterior descending/interventricular artery (PDA)—supplies posterior $1/3$ of interventricular septum, posterior walls of ventricles, and posteromedial papillary muscle

SA and AV nodes are usually supplied by RCA. Infarct may cause nodal dysfunction (bradycardia or heart block).

Right-dominant circulation = 85% = PDA arises from RCA.

Left-dominant circulation = 8% = PDA arises from LCX.

Codominant circulation = 7% = PDA arises from both LCX and RCA.

Coronary artery occlusion most commonly occurs in the LAD.

Coronary blood flow peaks in early diastole.

The most posterior part of the heart is the left atrium; enlargement can cause dysphagia (due to compression of the esophagus) or hoarseness (due to compression of the left recurrent laryngeal nerve, a branch of the vagus).

▶ CARDIOVASCULAR—PHYSIOLOGY

Cardiac output

CO = stroke volume (SV) × heart rate (HR).

Fick principle:

$$CO = \frac{\text{rate of } O_2 \text{ consumption}}{\text{arterial } O_2 \text{ content} - \text{venous } O_2 \text{ content}}$$

Mean arterial pressure (MAP) = CO × total peripheral resistance (TPR).

MAP = $2/3$ diastolic pressure + $1/3$ systolic pressure.

Pulse pressure = systolic pressure – diastolic pressure. Pulse pressure is proportional to SV, inversely proportional to arterial compliance.

SV = end-diastolic volume (EDV) – end-systolic volume (ESV).

During the early stages of exercise, CO is maintained by ↑ HR and ↑ SV. During the late stages of exercise, CO is maintained by ↑ HR only (SV plateaus).
Diastole is preferentially shortened with ↑ HR; less filling time → ↓ CO (e.g., ventricular tachycardia).

↑ pulse pressure in hyperthyroidism, aortic regurgitation, aortic stiffening (isolated systolic hypertension in elderly), obstructive sleep apnea (↑ sympathetic tone), exercise (transient).
↓ pulse pressure in aortic stenosis, cardiogenic shock, cardiac tamponade, advanced heart failure (HF).

Cardiac output variables

Stroke volume	Stroke Volume affected by Contractility, Afterload, and Preload. ↑ SV with: • ↑ Contractility (e.g., anxiety, exercise, pregnancy) • ↑ Preload • ↓ Afterload	SV CAP. A failing heart has ↓ SV (systolic and/or diastolic dysfunction)
Contractility	Contractility (and SV) ↑ with: • Catecholamines (↑ activity of Ca^{2+} pump in sarcoplasmic reticulum) • ↑ intracellular Ca^{2+} • ↓ extracellular Na^+ (↓ activity of Na^+/Ca^{2+} exchanger) • Digitalis (blocks Na^+/K^+ pump → ↑ intracellular Na^+ → ↓ Na^+/Ca^{2+} exchanger activity → ↑ intracellular Ca^{2+})	Contractility (and SV) ↓ with: • β_1-blockade (↓ cAMP) • HF with systolic dysfunction • Acidosis • Hypoxia/hypercapnia (↓ Po_2/↑ Pco_2) • Non-dihydropyridine Ca^{2+} channel blockers
Myocardial oxygen demand	↑ MyoCARDial O_2 demand is ↑ by: • ↑ Contractility • ↑ Afterload (proportional to arterial pressure) • ↑ heart Rate • ↑ Diameter of ventricle (↑ wall tension)	Wall tension follows Laplace's law: $$\text{Wall tension} = \frac{\text{pressure} \times \text{radius}}{2 \times \text{wall thickness}}$$
Preload	Preload approximated by ventricular EDV; depends on venous tone and circulating blood volume.	VEnodilators (e.g., nitroglycerin) ↓ prEload.
Afterload	Afterload approximated by MAP. ↑ afterload → ↑ pressure → ↑ wall tension per Laplace's law. LV compensates for ↑ afterload by thickening (hypertrophy) in order to ↓ wall tension.	VAsodilators (e.g., hydrAlAzine) ↓ Afterload (Arterial). ACE inhibitors and ARBs ↓ both preload and afterload. Chronic hypertension (↑ MAP) → LV hypertrophy.
Ejection fraction	$$EF = \frac{SV}{EDV} = \frac{EDV - ESV}{EDV}$$ Left ventricular EF is an index of ventricular contractility; normal EF is ≥ 55%.	EF ↓ in systolic HF. EF normal in diastolic HF.

Starling curve

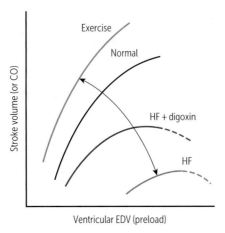

Force of contraction is proportional to end-diastolic length of cardiac muscle fiber (preload).

↑ contractility with catecholamines, positive inotropes (e.g., digoxin).

↓ contractility with loss of myocardium (e.g., MI), β-blockers (acutely), non-dihydropyridine Ca^{2+} channel blockers, dilated cardiomyopathy.

Resistance, pressure, flow

$\Delta P = Q \times R$

Similar to Ohm's law: $\Delta V = IR$

Volumetric flow rate (Q) = flow velocity (v) × cross-sectional area (A)

Resistance

$$= \frac{\text{driving pressure } (\Delta P)}{\text{flow (Q)}} = \frac{8\eta \text{ (viscosity)} \times \text{length}}{\pi r^4}$$

Total resistance of vessels in series:

$TR = R_1 + R_2 + R_3 \ldots$

Total resistance of vessels in parallel:

$$\frac{1}{TR} = \frac{1}{R_1} + \frac{1}{R_2} + \frac{1}{R_3} \ldots$$

Viscosity depends mostly on hematocrit

Viscosity ↑ in hyperproteinemic states (e.g., multiple myeloma), polycythemia

Viscosity ↓ in anemia

Capillaries have highest total cross-sectional area and lowest flow velocity.

Organ removal (e.g., nephrectomy) → ↑ TPR and ↓ CO.

Pressure gradient drives flow from high pressure to low pressure.

Arterioles account for most of TPR. Veins provide most of blood storage capacity.

Cardiac and vascular function curves

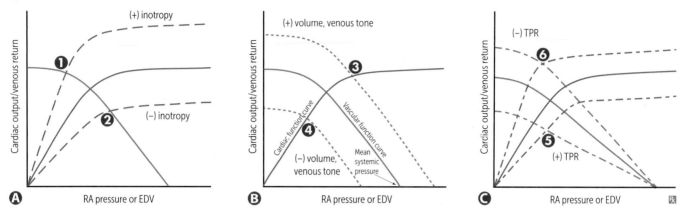

Intersection of curves = operating point of heart (i.e., venous return and CO are equal).

CURVE	EFFECT	EXAMPLES
Ⓐ Inotropy	Changes in contractility → altered CO for a given RA pressure (preload).	❶ Catecholamines, digoxin ⊕ ❷ Uncompensated HF, narcotic overdose ⊖
Ⓑ Venous return	Changes in circulating volume or venous tone → altered RA pressure for a given CO. Mean systemic pressure (x-intercept) changes with volume/venous tone.	❸ Fluid infusion, sympathetic activity ⊕ ❹ Acute hemorrhage, spinal anesthesia ⊖
Ⓒ Total peripheral resistance	Changes in TPR → altered CO at a given RA pressure; however, mean systemic pressure (x-intercept) is unchanged.	❺ Vasopressors ⊕ ❻ Exercise, AV shunt ⊖

Changes often occur in tandem, and may be reinforcing (e.g., exercise ↑ inotropy and ↓ TPR to maximize CO) or compensatory (e.g., HF ↓ inotropy → fluid retention to ↑ preload to maintain CO).

Pressure-volume loops and cardiac cycle

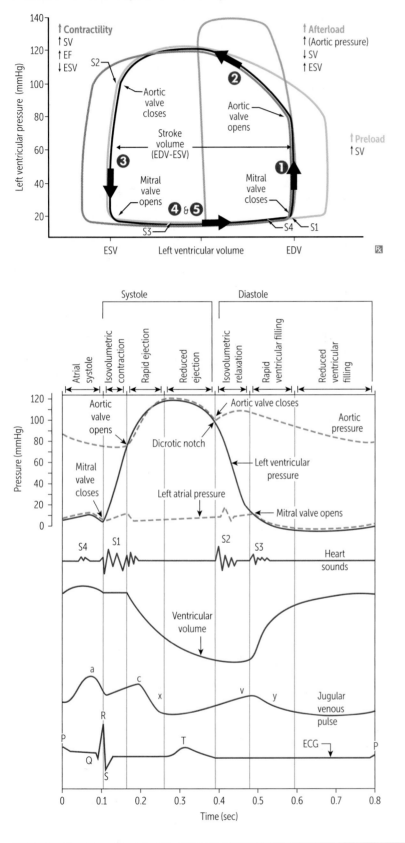

The black loop represents normal cardiac physiology.

Phases—left ventricle:
❶ Isovolumetric contraction—period between mitral valve closing and aortic valve opening; period of highest O_2 consumption
❷ Systolic ejection—period between aortic valve opening and closing
❸ Isovolumetric relaxation—period between aortic valve closing and mitral valve opening
❹ Rapid filling—period just after mitral valve opening
❺ Reduced filling—period just before mitral valve closing

Sounds:
S1—mitral and tricuspid valve closure. Loudest at mitral area.
S2—aortic and pulmonary valve closure. Loudest at left upper sternal border.
S3—in early diastole during rapid ventricular filling phase. Associated with ↑ filling pressures (e.g., mitral regurgitation, HF) and more common in dilated ventricles (but normal in children and pregnant women).
S4—in late diastole ("atrial kick"). Best heard at apex with patient in left lateral decubitus position. High atrial pressure. Associated with ventricular hypertrophy. Left atrium must push against stiff LV wall.

Jugular venous pulse (JVP):
a wave—atrial contraction. Absent in atrial fibrillation.
c wave—RV contraction (closed tricuspid valve bulging into atrium).
x descent—atrial relaxation and downward displacement of closed tricuspid valve during ventricular contraction. Absent in tricuspid regurgitation.
v wave—↑ right atrial pressure due to filling ("villing") against closed tricuspid valve.
y descent—RA emptying into RV.

Splitting

Normal splitting	Inspiration → drop in intrathoracic pressure → ↑ venous return → ↑ RV filling → ↑ RV stroke volume → ↑ RV ejection time → delayed closure of pulmonic valve. ↓ pulmonary impedance (↑ capacity of the pulmonary circulation) also occurs during inspiration, which contributes to delayed closure of pulmonic valve.	Expiration Inspiration	| || S1 A2 P2 | | |
Wide splitting	Seen in conditions that delay RV emptying (e.g., pulmonic stenosis, right bundle branch block). Delay in RV emptying causes delayed pulmonic sound (regardless of breath). An exaggeration of normal splitting.	Expiration Inspiration	| | | S1 A2 P2 | | |
Fixed splitting	Seen in ASD. ASD → left-to-right shunt → ↑ RA and RV volumes → ↑ flow through pulmonic valve such that, regardless of breath, pulmonic closure is greatly delayed.	Expiration Inspiration	| | | S1 A2 P2 | | |
Paradoxical splitting	Seen in conditions that delay aortic valve closure (e.g., aortic stenosis, left bundle branch block). Normal order of valve closure is reversed so that P2 sound occurs before delayed A2 sound. Therefore on inspiration, P2 closes later and moves closer to A2, thereby "paradoxically" eliminating the split.	Expiration Inspiration	| | | S1 P2 A2 | ||

Auscultation of the heart

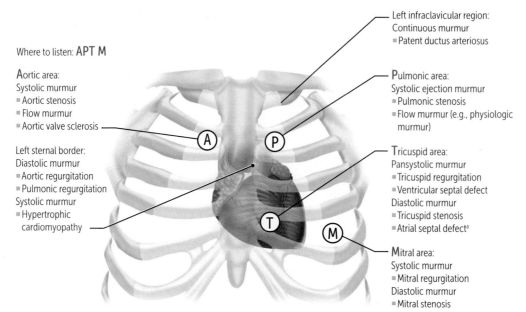

Where to listen: **APT M**

Aortic area:
Systolic murmur
- Aortic stenosis
- Flow murmur
- Aortic valve sclerosis

Left sternal border:
Diastolic murmur
- Aortic regurgitation
- Pulmonic regurgitation
Systolic murmur
- Hypertrophic cardiomyopathy

Left infraclavicular region:
Continuous murmur
- Patent ductus arteriosus

Pulmonic area:
Systolic ejection murmur
- Pulmonic stenosis
- Flow murmur (e.g., physiologic murmur)

Tricuspid area:
Pansystolic murmur
- Tricuspid regurgitation
- Ventricular septal defect
Diastolic murmur
- Tricuspid stenosis
- Atrial septal defect[a]

Mitral area:
Systolic murmur
- Mitral regurgitation
Diastolic murmur
- Mitral stenosis

[a] ASD commonly presents with a pulmonary flow murmur (↑ flow through pulmonary valve) and a diastolic rumble (↑ flow across tricuspid); blood flow across the actual ASD does not cause a murmur because there is no significant pressure gradient. The murmur later progresses to a louder diastolic murmur of pulmonic regurgitation from dilatation of the pulmonary artery.　℞

BEDSIDE MANEUVER	EFFECT
Inspiration (↑ venous return to right atrium)	↑ intensity of right heart sounds
Hand grip (↑ afterload)	↑ intensity of MR, AR, VSD murmurs ↓ hypertrophic cardiomyopathy murmurs MVP: later onset of click/murmur
Valsalva (phase II), standing up (↓ preload)	↓ intensity of most murmurs (including AS) ↑ intensity of hypertrophic cardiomyopathy murmur MVP: earlier onset of click/murmur
Rapid squatting (↑ venous return, ↑ preload	↓ intensity of hypertrophic cardiomyopathy murmur ↑ intensity of AS murmur MVP: later onset of click/murmur

Systolic heart sounds include aortic/pulmonic stenosis, mitral/tricuspid regurgitation, VSD, MVP.
Diastolic heart sounds include aortic/pulmonic regurgitation, mitral/tricuspid stenosis.

Heart murmurs

Systolic

Aortic stenosis (AS)

S1   S2

Crescendo-decrescendo systolic ejection murmur. LV >> aortic pressure during systole. Loudest at heart base; radiates to carotids. "Pulsus parvus et tardus"—pulses are weak with a delayed peak. Can lead to Syncope, Angina, and Dyspnea on exertion (**SAD**). Often due to age-related calcification or early-onset calcification of bicuspid aortic valve.

Mitral/tricuspid regurgitation (MR/TR)

S1   S2

Holosystolic, high-pitched "blowing murmur."
Mitral—loudest at apex and radiates toward axilla. MR is often due to ischemic heart disease (post-MI), MVP, LV dilatation.
Tricuspid—loudest at tricuspid area and radiates to right sternal border. TR commonly caused by RV dilatation.
Rheumatic fever and infective endocarditis can cause either MR or TR.

Mitral valve prolapse (MVP)

S1   MC   S2

Late systolic crescendo murmur with midsystolic click (MC; due to sudden tensing of chordae tendineae). Most frequent valvular lesion. Best heard over apex. Loudest just before S2. Usually benign. Can predispose to infective endocarditis. Can be caused by myxomatous degeneration (1° or 2° to connective tissue disease such as Marfan or Ehlers-Danlos syndrome), rheumatic fever, chordae rupture.

VSD

S1   S2

Holosystolic, harsh-sounding murmur. Loudest at tricuspid area.

Diastolic

Aortic regurgitation (AR)

S1   S2

High-pitched "blowing" early diastolic decrescendo murmur. Long diastolic murmur and signs of hyperdynamic pulse when severe and chronic. Often due to aortic root dilation, bicuspid aortic valve, endocarditis, rheumatic fever. Progresses to left HF.

Mitral stenosis (MS)

S1   S2 OS

Follows opening snap (OS; due to abrupt halt in leaflet motion in diastole, after rapid opening due to fusion at leaflet tips). Delayed rumbling late diastolic murmur (↓ interval between S2 and OS correlates with ↑ severity). LA >> LV pressure during diastole. Often occurs 2° to rheumatic fever. Chronic MS can result in LA dilatation.

Continuous

PDA

S1   S2

Continuous machine-like murmur. Loudest at S2. Often due to congenital rubella or prematurity. Best heard at left infraclavicular area.

Myocardial action potential

Also occurs in bundle of His and Purkinje fibers.

Phase 0 = rapid upstroke and depolarization—voltage-gated Na^+ channels open.

Phase 1 = initial repolarization—inactivation of voltage-gated Na^+ channels. Voltage-gated K^+ channels begin to open.

Phase 2 = plateau—Ca^{2+} influx through voltage-gated Ca^{2+} channels balances K^+ efflux. Ca^{2+} influx triggers Ca^{2+} release from sarcoplasmic reticulum and myocyte contraction.

Phase 3 = rapid repolarization—massive K^+ efflux due to opening of voltage-gated slow K^+ channels and closure of voltage-gated Ca^{2+} channels.

Phase 4 = resting potential—high K^+ permeability through K^+ channels.

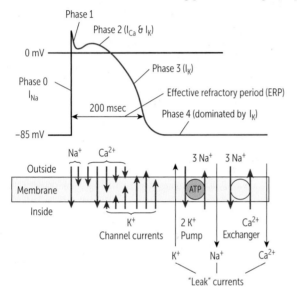

In contrast to skeletal muscle:
- Cardiac muscle action potential has a plateau, which is due to Ca^{2+} influx and K^+ efflux; myocyte contraction occurs due to Ca^{2+}-induced Ca^{2+} release from the sarcoplasmic reticulum.
- Cardiac nodal cells spontaneously depolarize during diastole, resulting in automaticity due to I_f channels ("funny current" channels responsible for a slow, mixed Na^+/K^+ inward current).
- Cardiac myocytes are electrically coupled to each other by gap junctions.

Pacemaker action potential

Occurs in the SA and AV nodes. Key differences from the ventricular action potential include:

Phase 0 = upstroke—opening of voltage-gated Ca^{2+} channels. Fast voltage-gated Na^+ channels are permanently inactivated because of the less negative resting voltage of these cells. Results in a slow conduction velocity that is used by the AV node to prolong transmission from the atria to ventricles.

Phases 1 and 2 are absent.

Phase 3 = inactivation of the Ca^{2+} channels and ↑ activation of K^+ channels → ↑ K^+ efflux.

Phase 4 = slow spontaneous diastolic depolarization as Na^+ conductance ↑ (I_f different from I_{Na} in phase 0 of ventricular action potential). Accounts for automaticity of SA and AV nodes. The slope of phase 4 in the SA node determines HR. ACh/adenosine ↓ the rate of diastolic depolarization and ↓ HR, while catecholamines ↑ depolarization and ↑ HR. Sympathetic stimulation ↑ the chance that I_f channels are open and thus ↑ HR.

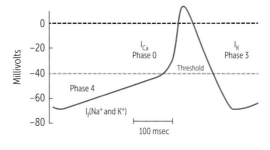

Electrocardiogram

P wave—atrial depolarization. Atrial repolarization is masked by QRS complex.

PR interval—time from start of atrial depolarization to start of ventricular depolarization (normally < 200 msec).

QRS complex—ventricular depolarization (normally < 120 msec).

QT interval—ventricular depolarization, mechanical contraction of the ventricles, ventricular repolarization.

T wave—ventricular repolarization. T-wave inversion may indicate recent MI.

J point—junction between end of QRS complex and start of ST segment.

ST segment—isoelectric, ventricles depolarized.

U wave—caused by hypokalemia, bradycardia.

Speed of conduction—Purkinje > atria > ventricles > AV node.

Pacemakers—SA > AV > bundle of His/ Purkinje/ventricles.

Conduction pathway—SA node → atria → AV node → common bundle → bundle branches → fascicles → Purkinje fibers → ventricles.

SA node "pacemaker" inherent dominance with slow phase of upstroke.

AV node—located in posteroinferior part of interatrial septum. Blood supply usually from RCA. 100-msec delay allows time for ventricular filling.

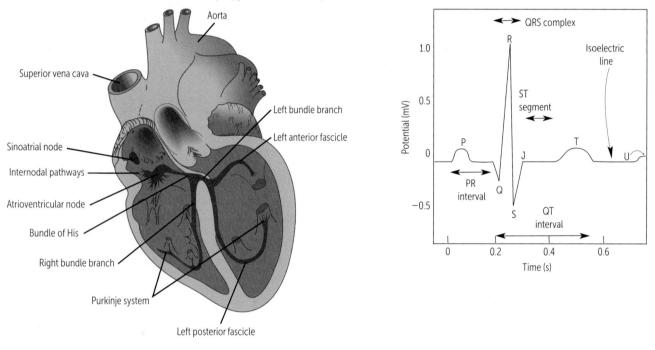

Torsades de pointes	Polymorphic ventricular tachycardia, characterized by shifting sinusoidal waveforms on ECG; can progress to ventricular fibrillation. Long QT interval predisposes to torsades de pointes. Caused by drugs, ↓ K^+, ↓ Mg^{2+}, other abnormalities. Treatment includes magnesium sulfate.	Drug-induced long QT (**ABCDE**): Anti**A**rrhythmics (class IA, III) Anti**B**iotics (e.g., macrolides) Anti"**C**"ychotics (e.g., haloperidol) Anti**D**epressants (e.g., TCAs) Anti**E**metics (e.g., ondansetron)
Congenital long QT syndrome	Inherited disorder of myocardial repolarization, typically due to ion channel defects; ↑ risk of sudden cardiac death (SCD) due to torsades de pointes. Includes: ▪ Romano-Ward syndrome—autosomal dominant, pure cardiac phenotype (no deafness). ▪ Jervell and Lange-Nielsen syndrome—autosomal recessive, sensorineural deafness.	
Brugada syndrome	Autosomal dominant disorder most common in Asian males. ECG pattern of pseudo-right bundle branch block and ST elevations in V1-V3. ↑ risk of ventricular tachyarrhythmias and SCD. Prevent SCD with implantable cardioverter-defibrillator (ICD).	
Wolff-Parkinson-White syndrome	Most common type of ventricular pre-excitation syndrome. Abnormal fast accessory conduction pathway from atria to ventricle (bundle of Kent) bypasses the rate-slowing AV node → ventricles begin to partially depolarize earlier → characteristic delta wave with widened QRS complex and shortened PR interval on ECG. May result in reentry circuit → supraventricular tachycardia.	Delta wave PR interval Shortened PR interval Normal PR interval

ECG tracings

Atrial fibrillation

Chaotic and erratic baseline (irregularly irregular) with no discrete P waves in between irregularly spaced QRS complexes. Associated with hypertension, coronary artery disease (CAD), rheumatic heart disease, binge drinking ("holiday heart"), HF, valvular disease, hyperthyroidism. Can result in atrial stasis and lead to cardioembolic events. Treatment includes antithrombotic therapy (e.g., warfarin), rate control (β-blocker, non-dihydropyridine Ca^{2+} channel blocker, digoxin), rhythm control (class IC or III antiarrhythmics), and/or cardioversion (pharmacological or electrical).

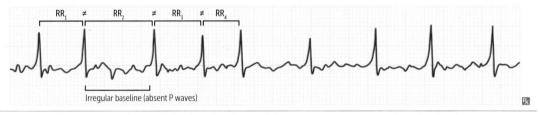

Atrial flutter

A rapid succession of identical, back-to-back atrial depolarization waves. The identical appearance accounts for the "sawtooth" appearance of the flutter waves. Management similar to atrial fibrillation (rate control, anticoagulation, cardioversion). Definitive treatment is catheter ablation.

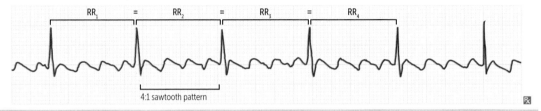

Ventricular fibrillation

A completely erratic rhythm with no identifiable waves. Fatal arrhythmia without immediate CPR and defibrillation.

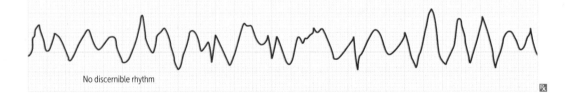

AV block

1st degree

The PR interval is prolonged (> 200 msec). Benign and asymptomatic. No treatment required.

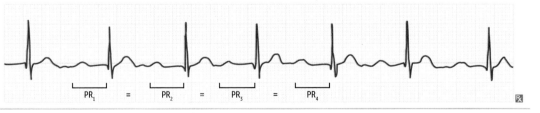

2nd degree

Mobitz type I (Wenckebach)

Progressive lengthening of PR interval until a beat is "dropped" (a P wave not followed by a QRS complex). Usually asymptomatic. Variable RR interval with a pattern (regularly irregular).

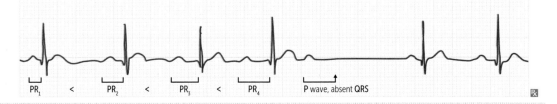

ECG tracings *(continued)*

Mobitz type II	Dropped beats that are not preceded by a change in the length of the PR interval (as in type I). May progress to 3rd-degree block. Often treated with pacemaker.

PR₁ = PR₂ = PR₃   P wave, absent QRS

3rd degree (complete)	The atria and ventricles beat independently of each other. Both P waves and QRS complexes are present, although the P waves bear no relation to the QRS complexes. Atrial rate is faster than ventricular rate. Usually treated with pacemaker. Lyme disease can result in 3rd-degree heart block.

RR₁ = RR₂   P wave on QRS complex   P wave on T wave

PP₁ = PP₂ = PP₃ = PP₄

Atrial natriuretic peptide	Released from **atrial myocytes** in response to ↑ blood volume and atrial pressure. Acts via cGMP. Causes vasodilation and ↓ Na^+ reabsorption at the renal collecting tubule. Dilates afferent renal arterioles and constricts efferent arterioles, promoting diuresis and contributing to "aldosterone escape" mechanism.

B-type (brain) natriuretic peptide	Released from **ventricular myocytes** in response to ↑ tension. Similar physiologic action to ANP, with longer half-life. BNP blood test used for diagnosing HF (very good negative predictive value). Available in recombinant form (nesiritide) for treatment of HF.

Baroreceptors and chemoreceptors

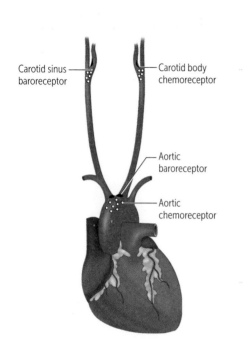

Carotid sinus baroreceptor

Carotid body chemoreceptor

Aortic baroreceptor

Aortic chemoreceptor

Receptors:

- Aortic arch transmits via vagus nerve to solitary nucleus of medulla (responds to ↓ and ↑ in BP).
- Carotid sinus (dilated region at carotid bifurcation) transmits via glossopharyngeal nerve to solitary nucleus of medulla (responds to ↓ and ↑ in BP).

Baroreceptors:

- Hypotension—↓ arterial pressure → ↓ stretch → ↓ afferent baroreceptor firing → ↑ efferent sympathetic firing and ↓ efferent parasympathetic stimulation → vasoconstriction, ↑ HR, ↑ contractility, ↑ BP. Important in the response to severe hemorrhage.
- Carotid massage—↑ pressure on carotid sinus → ↑ stretch → ↑ afferent baroreceptor firing → ↑ AV node refractory period → ↓ HR.
- Contributes to Cushing reaction (triad of hypertension, bradycardia, and respiratory depression)—↑ intracranial pressure constricts arterioles → cerebral ischemia → ↑ pCO_2 and ↓ pH → central reflex sympathetic ↑ in perfusion pressure (hypertension) → ↑ stretch → peripheral reflex baroreceptor induced–bradycardia.

Chemoreceptors:

- Peripheral—carotid and aortic bodies are stimulated by ↓ Po_2 (< 60 mmHg), ↑ Pco_2, and ↓ pH of blood.
- Central—are stimulated by changes in pH and Pco_2 of brain interstitial fluid, which in turn are influenced by arterial CO_2. Do not directly respond to Po_2.

Normal pressures

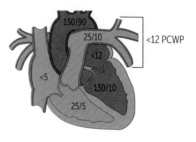

130/90

25/10

<12

<5

130/10

25/5

<12 PCWP

PCWP—pulmonary capillary wedge pressure (in mmHg) is a good approximation of left atrial pressure. In mitral stenosis, PCWP > LV diastolic pressure.

Measured with pulmonary artery catheter (Swan-Ganz catheter).

Autoregulation	How blood flow to an organ remains constant over a wide range of perfusion pressures.

ORGAN	FACTORS DETERMINING AUTOREGULATION	
Heart	Local metabolites (vasodilatory): adenosine, NO, CO_2, ↓ O_2	Note: the pulmonary vasculature is unique in that hypoxia causes vasoconstriction so that only well-ventilated areas are perfused. In other organs, hypoxia causes vasodilation.
Brain	Local metabolites (vasodilatory): CO_2 (pH)	
Kidneys	Myogenic and tubuloglomerular feedback	
Lungs	Hypoxia causes vasoconstriction	
Skeletal muscle	Local metabolites during exercise: lactate, adenosine, K^+, H^+, CO_2 At rest: sympathetic tone	
Skin	Sympathetic stimulation most important mechanism: temperature control	

Capillary fluid exchange

Interstitial fluid

Capillary

Starling forces determine fluid movement through capillary membranes:
- P_c = capillary pressure—pushes fluid out of capillary
- P_i = interstitial fluid pressure—pushes fluid into capillary
- π_c = plasma colloid osmotic pressure—pulls fluid into capillary
- π_i = interstitial fluid colloid osmotic pressure—pulls fluid out of capillary

J_v = net fluid flow = $K_f [(P_c - P_i) - \varsigma(\pi_c - \pi_i)]$

K_f = permeability of capillary to fluid

ς = permeability of capillary to protein

Edema—excess fluid outflow into interstitium commonly caused by:
- ↑ capillary pressure (↑ P_c; e.g., HF)
- ↓ plasma proteins (↓ π_c; e.g., nephrotic syndrome, liver failure)
- ↑ capillary permeability (↑ K_f; e.g., toxins, infections, burns)
- ↑ interstitial fluid colloid osmotic pressure (↑ π_i; e.g., lymphatic blockage)

▶ CARDIOVASCULAR—PATHOLOGY

Congenital heart diseases

RIGHT-TO-LEFT SHUNTS	Early cyanosis—"blue babies." Often diagnosed prenatally or become evident immediately after birth. Usually require urgent surgical correction and/or maintenance of a PDA.	The 5 Ts: 1. Truncus arteriosus (1 vessel) 2. Transposition (2 switched vessels) 3. Tricuspid atresia (3 = Tri) 4. Tetralogy of Fallot (4 = Tetra) 5. TAPVR (5 letters in the name)
Persistent truncus arteriosus	Truncus arteriosus fails to divide into pulmonary trunk and aorta due to lack of aorticopulmonary septum formation; most patients have accompanying VSD.	
D-transposition of great vessels	Aorta leaves RV (anterior) and pulmonary trunk leaves LV (posterior) → separation of systemic and pulmonary circulations. Not compatible with life unless a shunt is present to allow mixing of blood (e.g., VSD, PDA, or patent foramen ovale). Due to failure of the aorticopulmonary septum to spiral. Without surgical intervention, most infants die within the first few months of life.	
Tricuspid atresia	Absence of tricuspid valve and hypoplastic RV; requires both ASD and VSD for viability.	
Tetralogy of Fallot	Caused by anterosuperior displacement of the infundibular septum. Most common cause of early childhood cyanosis. ❶ Pulmonary infundibular stenosis (most important determinant for prognosis) ❷ Right ventricular hypertrophy (RVH)—boot-shaped heart on CXR [A] ❸ Overriding aorta ❹ VSD Pulmonary stenosis forces right-to-left flow across VSD → early cyanotic "tet spells," RVH.	PROVe. Squatting: ↑ SVR, ↓ right-to-left shunt, improves cyanosis. Treatment: early surgical correction.
Total anomalous pulmonary venous return (TAPVR)	Pulmonary veins drain into right heart circulation (SVC, coronary sinus, etc.); associated with ASD and sometimes PDA to allow for right-to-left shunting to maintain CO.	

Congenital heart diseases *(continued)*

LEFT-TO-RIGHT SHUNTS	Late cyanosis—"blue kids." Frequency: VSD > ASD > PDA.	Right-to-Left shunts: ea**RL**y cyanosis. Left-to-**R**ight shunts: "Late**R**" cyanosis.
Ventricular septal defect	Most common congenital cardiac defect. Asymptomatic at birth, may manifest weeks later or remain asymptomatic throughout life. Most self resolve; larger lesions may lead to LV overload and HF.	
Atrial septal defect 	Defect in interatrial septum ; loud S1; wide, fixed split S2. Ostium secundum defects most common and usually occur as isolated findings; ostium primum defects rarer yet usually occur with other cardiac anomalies. Symptoms range from none to HF. Distinct from patent foramen ovale in that septa are missing tissue rather than unfused.	
Patent ductus arteriosus — Aorta — Ductus arteriosus (patent) — Pulmonary artery	In fetal period, shunt is right to left (normal). In neonatal period, ↓ lung resistance → shunt becomes left to right → progressive RVH and/or LVH and HF. Associated with a continuous, "machine-like" murmur. Patency is maintained by PGE synthesis and low O$_2$ tension. Uncorrected PDA can eventually result in late cyanosis in the lower extremities (differential cyanosis).	"**End**omethacin" (indomethacin) **ends** patency of PDA; PGE k**EE**ps it open (may be necessary to sustain life in conditions such as transposition of the great vessels). PDA is normal in utero and normally closes only after birth.
Eisenmenger syndrome 	Uncorrected left-to-right shunt (VSD, ASD, PDA) → ↑ pulmonary blood flow → pathologic remodeling of vasculature → pulmonary arterial hypertension. RVH occurs to compensate → shunt becomes right to left. Causes late cyanosis, clubbing , and polycythemia. Age of onset varies.	
OTHER ANOMALIES		
Coarctation of the aorta	Aortic narrowing near insertion of ductus arteriosus ("juxtaductal"). Associated with bicuspid aortic valve, other heart defects, and Turner syndrome. Hypertension in upper extremities and weak, delayed pulse in lower extremities (brachial-femoral delay). With age, collateral arteries erode ribs (notched appearance on CXR).	

Congenital cardiac defect associations

DISORDER	DEFECT
Alcohol exposure in utero (fetal alcohol syndrome)	VSD, PDA, ASD, tetralogy of Fallot
Congenital rubella	Septal defects, PDA, pulmonary artery stenosis
Down syndrome	AV septal defect (endocardial cushion defect), VSD, ASD
Infant of diabetic mother	Transposition of great vessels
Marfan syndrome	MVP, thoracic aortic aneurysm and dissection, aortic regurgitation
Prenatal lithium exposure	Ebstein anomaly
Turner syndrome	Bicuspid aortic valve, coarctation of aorta
Williams syndrome	Supravalvular aortic stenosis
22q11 syndromes	Truncus arteriosus, tetralogy of Fallot

Hypertension

Defined as persistent systolic BP ≥ 140 mmHg and/or diastolic BP ≥ 90 mmHg

RISK FACTORS

↑ age, obesity, diabetes, physical inactivity, excess salt intake, excess alcohol intake, family history; black > white > Asian.

FEATURES

90% of hypertension is 1° (essential) and related to ↑ CO or ↑ TPR; remaining 10% mostly 2° to renal/renovascular disease (e.g., fibromuscular dysplasia 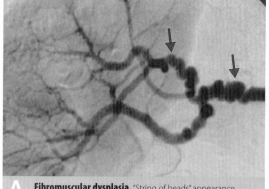, usually found in younger women) and 1° hyperaldosteronism.

Hypertensive urgency—severe (≥ 180/≥ 120 mmHg) hypertension without acute end-organ damage.

Hypertensive emergency—severe hypertension with evidence of acute end-organ damage (e.g., encephalopathy, stroke, retinal hemorrhages and exudates, papilledema, MI, HF, aortic dissection, kidney injury, microangiopathic hemolytic anemia, eclampsia).

PREDISPOSES TO

CAD, LVH, HF, atrial fibrillation; aortic dissection, aortic aneurysm; stroke; chronic kidney disease (hypertensive nephropathy) 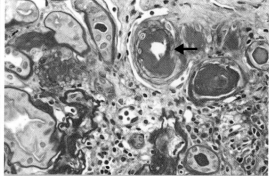; retinopathy.

A **Fibromuscular dysplasia.** "String of beads" appearance (arrows) of the renal artery in fibromuscular dysplasia. ✷

B **Hypertensive nephropathy.** Renal arterial hyalinosis (arrow) on PAS stain. ✷

Hyperlipidemia signs

Xanthomas	Plaques or nodules composed of lipid-laden histiocytes in skin **A**, especially the eyelids (xanthelasma **B**).
Tendinous xanthoma	Lipid deposit in tendon **C**, especially Achilles.
Corneal arcus	Lipid deposit in cornea. Common in elderly (arcus senilis **D**), but appears earlier in life in hypercholesterolemia.

Arteriosclerosis	Hardening of arteries, with arterial wall thickening and loss of elasticity.
Arteriolosclerosis	Common. Affects small arteries and arterioles. Two types: hyaline (thickening of vessel walls in essential hypertension or diabetes mellitus **A**) and hyperplastic ("onion skinning" in severe hypertension **B** with proliferation of smooth muscle cells).
Mönckeberg (medial calcific sclerosis)	Uncommon. Affects medium-sized arteries. Calcification of elastic lamina of arteries → vascular stiffening without obstruction. "Pipestem" appearance on x-ray **C**. Does not obstruct blood flow; intima not involved.

Atherosclerosis

Very common. Disease of elastic arteries and large- and medium-sized muscular arteries; a form of arteriosclerosis caused by buildup of cholesterol plaques.

RISK FACTORS	Modifiable: smoking, hypertension, hyperlipidemia, diabetes. Nonmodifiable: age, sex (↑ in men and postmenopausal women), family history.
PROGRESSION	Inflammation important in pathogenesis: endothelial cell dysfunction → macrophage and LDL accumulation → foam cell formation → fatty streaks → smooth muscle cell migration (involves PDGF and FGF), proliferation, and extracellular matrix deposition → fibrous plaque → complex atheromas **A**.
COMPLICATIONS	Aneurysms, ischemia, infarcts, peripheral vascular disease, thrombus, emboli.
LOCATION	Abdominal aorta > coronary artery > popliteal artery > carotid artery **B**.
SYMPTOMS	Angina, claudication, but can be asymptomatic.

Atherosclerosis. Atherosclerotic plaque in LAD coronary artery. Note the cholesterol crystals (arrow). ℞

Aortic aneurysm

Localized pathologic dilatation of the aorta. May cause abdominal and/or back pain, which is a sign of leaking, dissection, or imminent rupture.

Abdominal aortic aneurysm	Associated with atherosclerosis. Risk factors include history of tobacco use, ↑ age, male sex, family history. May present as palpable pulsatile abdominal mass **A**.
Thoracic aortic aneurysm	Associated with cystic medial degeneration. Risk factors include hypertension, bicuspid aortic valve, connective tissue disease (e.g., Marfan syndrome). Also historically associated with 3° syphilis (obliterative endarteritis of the vasa vasorum).

Abdominal aortic aneurysm. CT shows large suprarenal aneurysm with eccentric mural thrombus (arrows). ℞

Aortic dissection	Longitudinal intimal tear forming a false lumen 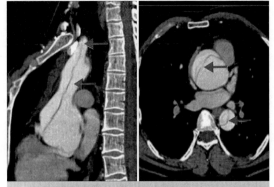. Associated with hypertension, bicuspid aortic valve, inherited connective tissue disorders (e.g., Marfan syndrome). Can present with tearing chest pain, of sudden onset, radiating to the back +/– markedly unequal BP in arms. CXR shows mediastinal widening. Can result in rupture, pericardial tamponade, death. Two types:

- Stanford type **A** (proximal): involves Ascending aorta. May extend to aortic arch or descending aorta. Treatment is surgery.
- Stanford type **B** (distal): involves descending aorta and/or aortic arch. No ascending aorta involvement. Treat medically with β-blockers, then vasodilators.

Aortic dissection. CT shows intraluminal tear (arrows) forming a "flap" separating true and false lumen, involving the ascending (Stanford Type A) and descending aorta. ✦

Ischemic heart disease manifestations

Angina	Chest pain due to ischemic myocardium 2° to coronary artery narrowing or spasm; no myocyte necrosis.

- **Stable**—usually 2° to atherosclerosis; exertional chest pain in classic distribution (usually with ST depression on ECG), resolving with rest or nitroglycerin.
- **Variant (Prinzmetal)**—occurs at rest 2° to coronary artery spasm; transient ST elevation on ECG. Known triggers include tobacco, cocaine, and triptans, but trigger is often unknown. Treat with Ca^{2+} channel blockers, nitrates, and smoking cessation (if applicable).
- **Unstable**—thrombosis with incomplete coronary artery occlusion; +/– ST depression and/or T-wave inversion on ECG but no cardiac biomarker elevation (unlike NSTEMI); ↑ in frequency or intensity of chest pain or any chest pain at rest.

Coronary steal syndrome	Distal to coronary stenosis, vessels are maximally dilated at baseline. Administration of vasodilators (e.g., dipyridamole, regadenoson) dilates normal vessels and shunts blood toward well-perfused areas → ↓ flow and ischemia in poststenotic region. Principle behind pharmacologic stress tests.
Myocardial infarction	Most often acute thrombosis due to rupture of coronary artery atherosclerotic plaque. If transmural, ECG may show ST elevations (STEMI); if subendocardial, ECG may show ST depressions (NSTEMI). Cardiac biomarkers are diagnostic.
Sudden cardiac death	Death from cardiac causes within 1 hour of onset of symptoms, most commonly due to a lethal arrhythmia (e.g., ventricular fibrillation). Associated with CAD (up to 70% of cases), cardiomyopathy (hypertrophic, dilated), and hereditary ion channelopathies (e.g., long QT syndrome, Brugada syndrome).
Chronic ischemic heart disease	Progressive onset of HF over many years due to chronic ischemic myocardial damage.

Evolution of MI

Commonly occluded coronary arteries: LAD > RCA > circumflex.
Symptoms: diaphoresis, nausea, vomiting, severe retrosternal pain, pain in left arm and/or jaw, shortness of breath, fatigue.

TIME	GROSS	LIGHT MICROSCOPE	COMPLICATIONS
0–4 hr	None	None	Arrhythmia, HF, cardiogenic shock.
4–24 hr	Occluded artery; Infarct; Dark mottling; pale with tetrazolium stain	Early coagulative necrosis, release of necrotic cell contents into blood; edema, hemorrhage, wavy fibers. Neutrophils appear. Reperfusion injury may cause contraction bands (due to free radical damage).	Arrhythmia, HF, cardiogenic shock.
1–3 days	Hyperemia	Extensive coagulative necrosis. Tissue surrounding infarct shows acute inflammation with neutrophils.	Postinfarction fibrinous pericarditis.
3–14 days	Hyperemic border; central yellow-brown softening— maximally yellow and soft by 10 days	Macrophages, then granulation tissue at margins.	Free wall rupture A → tamponade; papillary muscle rupture → mitral regurgitation; interventricular septal rupture due to macrophage-mediated structural degradation. LV pseudoaneurysm (risk of rupture).
2 weeks to several months	Recanalized artery; Gray-white	Contracted scar complete.	Dressler syndrome, HF, arrhythmias, true ventricular aneurysm (risk of mural thrombus).

Diagnosis of MI

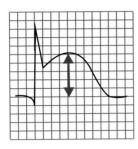

In the first 6 hours, ECG is the gold standard.

Cardiac troponin I rises after 4 hours and is ↑ for 7–10 days; more specific than other protein markers.

CK-MB rises after 6–12 hours and is predominantly found in myocardium but can also be released from skeletal muscle. Useful in diagnosing reinfarction following acute MI because levels return to normal after 48 hours.

ECG changes can include ST elevation (STEMI, transmural infarct), ST depression (NSTEMI, subendocardial infarct), hyperacute (peaked) T waves, T-wave inversion, new left bundle branch block, and pathologic Q waves or poor R wave progression (evolving or old transmural infarct).

Types of infarcts

Transmural infarcts	Subendocardial infarcts
↑ necrosis	Due to ischemic necrosis of < 50% of ventricle wall
Affects entire wall	Subendocardium especially vulnerable to ischemia
ST elevation on ECG, Q waves	ST depression on ECG

ECG localization of STEMI

INFARCT LOCATION	LEADS WITH ST ELEVATIONS OR Q WAVES
Anteroseptal (LAD)	V1–V2
Anteroapical (distal LAD)	V3–V4
Anterolateral (LAD or LCX)	V5–V6
Lateral (LCX)	I, aVL
InFerior (RCA)	II, III, aVF

MI complications

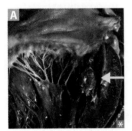

Cardiac arrhythmia—important cause of death before reaching hospital; common in first few days.

LV failure and pulmonary edema.

Cardiogenic shock (large infarct → high risk of mortality).

Ventricular free wall rupture → cardiac tamponade; papillary muscle rupture **A** → severe mitral regurgitation; and interventricular septum rupture → VSD. Greatest risk 3–14 days post-MI.

Ventricular pseudoaneurysm formation (contained free wall rupture)—↓ CO, risk of arrhythmia, embolus from mural thrombus; greatest risk approximately 3–14 days post-MI (as with rupture).

True ventricular aneurysm—outward bulge during contraction ("dyskinesia"), associated with fibrosis; arises 2 weeks to several months after MI.

Postinfarction fibrinous pericarditis—friction rub (1–3 days post-MI).

Dressler syndrome—autoimmune phenomenon resulting in fibrinous pericarditis (several weeks post-MI).

Acute coronary syndrome treatments

Unstable angina/NSTEMI—Anticoagulation (e.g., heparin), antiplatelet therapy (e.g., aspirin + clopidogrel), β-blockers, ACE inhibitors, statins. Symptom control with nitroglycerin and morphine.

STEMI—In addition to above, reperfusion therapy most important (percutaneous coronary intervention preferred over fibrinolysis).

Cardiomyopathies

Dilated cardiomyopathy	Most common cardiomyopathy (90% of cases). Often idiopathic or familial. Other etiologies include chronic **A**lcohol abuse, wet **B**eriberi, **C**oxsackie B virus myocarditis, chronic **C**ocaine use, **C**hagas disease, **D**oxorubicin toxicity, hemochromatosis, sarcoidosis, peripartum cardiomyopathy. Findings: HF, S3, systolic regurgitant murmur, dilated heart on echocardiogram, balloon appearance of heart on CXR. Treatment: Na⁺ restriction, ACE inhibitors, β-blockers, diuretics, digoxin, ICD, heart transplant.	Systolic dysfunction ensues. Eccentric hypertrophy **A** (sarcomeres added in series). **ABCCCD.**
Hypertrophic cardiomyopathy	60–70% of cases are familial, autosomal dominant (commonly a β-myosin heavy-chain mutation). Can be associated with Friedreich ataxia. Causes syncope during exercise and may lead to sudden death in young athletes due to ventricular arrhythmia. Findings: S4, systolic murmur. May see mitral regurgitation due to impaired mitral valve closure. Treatment: cessation of high-intensity athletics, use of β-blocker or non-dihydropyridine Ca²⁺ channel blockers (e.g., verapamil). ICD if patient is high risk.	Diastolic dysfunction ensues. Marked ventricular hypertrophy **B**, often septal predominance. Myofibrillar disarray and fibrosis. Obstructive hypertrophic cardiomyopathy (subset)—asymmetric septal hypertrophy and systolic anterior motion of mitral valve → outflow obstruction → dyspnea, possible syncope.
Restrictive/infiltrative cardiomyopathy	Major causes include sarcoidosis, amyloidosis, postradiation fibrosis, endocardial fibroelastosis (thick fibroelastic tissue in endocardium of young children), Löffler syndrome (endomyocardial fibrosis with a prominent eosinophilic infiltrate), and hemochromatosis (dilated cardiomyopathy can also occur).	Diastolic dysfunction ensues. Can have low-voltage ECG despite thick myocardium (especially amyloid).

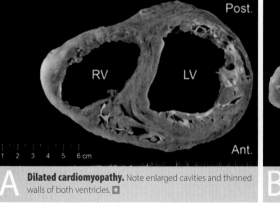

A **Dilated cardiomyopathy.** Note enlarged cavities and thinned walls of both ventricles.

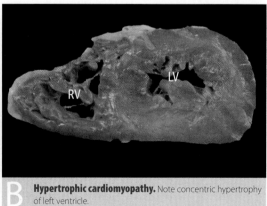

B **Hypertrophic cardiomyopathy.** Note concentric hypertrophy of left ventricle.

Heart failure

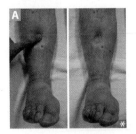

Clinical syndrome of cardiac pump dysfunction → congestion and low perfusion. Symptoms include dyspnea, orthopnea, fatigue; signs include rales, JVD, pitting edema **A**.

Systolic dysfunction—reduced EF, ↑ EDV; ↓ contractility often 2° to ischemia/MI or dilated cardiomyopathy.

Diastolic dysfunction—preserved EF, normal EDV; ↓ compliance often 2° to myocardial hypertrophy.

Right HF most often results from left HF. Isolated right HF is usually due to cor pulmonale.

ACE inhibitors or angiotensin II receptor blockers, β-blockers (except in acute decompensated HF), and spironolactone ↓ mortality. Thiazide or loop diuretics are used mainly for symptomatic relief. Hydralazine with nitrate therapy improves both symptoms and mortality in select patients.

Left heart failure

Orthopnea	Shortness of breath when supine: ↑ venous return from redistribution of blood (immediate gravity effect) exacerbates pulmonary vascular congestion.
Paroxysmal nocturnal dyspnea	Breathless awakening from sleep: ↑ venous return from redistribution of blood, reabsorption of edema, etc.
Pulmonary edema	↑ pulmonary venous pressure → pulmonary venous distention and transudation of fluid. Presence of hemosiderin-laden macrophages ("HF" cells) in lungs.

Right heart failure

Hepatomegaly (nutmeg liver)	↑ central venous pressure → ↑ resistance to portal flow. Rarely, leads to "cardiac cirrhosis."
Jugular venous distention	↑ venous pressure.
Peripheral edema	↑ venous pressure → fluid transudation.

Flow diagram:
↓ LV contractility → Pulmonary venous congestion → Pulmonary edema; ↓ Cardiac output → ↑ Renin-angiotensin-aldosterone → ↑ Renal Na⁺ and H₂O reabsorption; ↓ RV output → ↑ Systemic venous pressure → Peripheral edema; ↑ Preload, ↑ cardiac output (compensation) ← ↑ LV contractility ← ↑ Sympathetic activity

Shock

	CAUSED BY	SKIN	CVP (PRELOAD)	CO	SVR (AFTERLOAD)	TREATMENT
Hypovolemic	Hemorrhage, dehydration, burns	Cold, clammy	↓↓	↓	↑	IV fluids
Cardiogenic	Acute MI, HF, valvular dysfunction, arrhythmia	Cold, clammy	↑	↓↓	↑	Inotropes, diuresis
Obstructive	Cardiac tamponade, PE					Relieve obstruction
Distributive	Sepsis, CNS injury, anaphylaxis	Warm, dry	↓	↑	↓↓	Pressors, IV fluids

↓↓ = primary insult.

Systemic inflammatory response syndrome (≥ 2: fever/hypothermia, tachycardia, tachypnea, leukocytosis/leukopenia). First sign of shock is tachycardia. Multiple organ dysfunction syndrome (MODS) is the end result of shock.

Bacterial endocarditis

Fever (most common symptom), new murmur, Roth spots (round white spots on retina surrounded by hemorrhage), Osler nodes (tender raised lesions on finger or toe pads), Janeway lesions (small, painless, erythematous lesions on palm or sole) 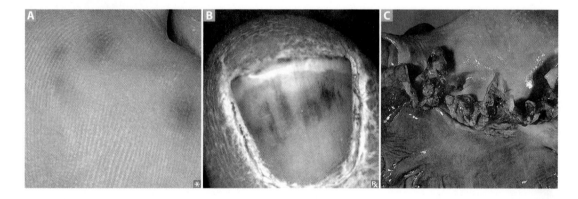, glomerulonephritis, septic arterial or pulmonary emboli, splinter hemorrhages **B** on nail bed. Multiple blood cultures necessary for diagnosis.

- Acute—*S. aureus* (high virulence). Large vegetations on previously normal valves **C**. Rapid onset.
- Subacute—viridans streptococci (low virulence). Smaller vegetations on congenitally abnormal or diseased valves. Sequela of dental procedures. Gradual onset.

S. bovis (*gallolyticus*) is present in colon cancer, *S. epidermidis* on prosthetic valves.

Endocarditis may also be nonbacterial (marantic/thrombotic) 2° to malignancy, hypercoagulable state, or lupus.

Mitral valve is most frequently involved.

Tricuspid valve endocarditis is associated with IV **drug** abuse (don't "**tri**" drugs). Associated with *S. aureus*, *Pseudomonas*, and *Candida*.

Culture ⊖—most likely *Coxiella burnetii*, *Bartonella* spp., HACEK (*Haemophilus*, *Actinobacillus*, *Cardiobacterium*, *Eikenella*, *Kingella*)

♥ Bacteria **FROM JANE** ♥:

Fever
Roth spots
Osler nodes
Murmur
Janeway lesions
Anemia
Nail-bed hemorrhage
Emboli

Rheumatic fever

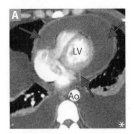

A consequence of pharyngeal infection with group A β-hemolytic streptococci. Late sequelae include rheumatic heart disease, which affects heart valves—mitral > aortic >> tricuspid (high-pressure valves affected most). Early lesion is mitral valve regurgitation; late lesion is mitral stenosis. Associated with Aschoff bodies (granuloma with giant cells [blue arrows in Ⓐ]), Anitschkow cells (enlarged macrophages with ovoid, wavy, rod-like nucleus [red arrow in Ⓐ]), ↑ anti-streptolysin O (ASO) titers.

Immune mediated (type II hypersensitivity); not a direct effect of bacteria. Antibodies to M protein cross-react with self antigens (molecular mimicry).

Treatment/prophylaxis: penicillin.

J♥NES (major criteria):
Joint (migratory polyarthritis)
♥ (carditis)
Nodules in skin (subcutaneous)
Erythema marginatum
Sydenham chorea

Acute pericarditis

Commonly presents with sharp pain, aggravated by inspiration, and relieved by sitting up and leaning forward. Presents with friction rub. ECG changes include widespread ST-segment elevation and/or PR depression.

Causes include idiopathic (most common; presumed viral), confirmed infection (e.g., Coxsackievirus), neoplasia, autoimmune (e.g., SLE, rheumatoid arthritis), uremia, cardiovascular (acute STEMI or Dressler syndrome), radiation therapy.

Cardiac tamponade

Compression of heart by fluid (e.g., blood, effusions) in pericardial space Ⓐ → ↓ CO.
Equilibration of diastolic pressures in all 4 chambers.
Findings: Beck triad (hypotension, distended neck veins, distant heart sounds), ↑ HR, pulsus paradoxus. ECG shows low-voltage QRS and electrical alternans (due to "swinging" movement of heart in large effusion).

Pulsus paradoxus—↓ in amplitude of systolic BP by > 10 mmHg during inspiration. Seen in cardiac tamponade, asthma, obstructive sleep apnea, pericarditis, croup.

Syphilitic heart disease

3° syphilis disrupts the vasa vasorum of the aorta with consequent atrophy of vessel wall and dilatation of aorta and valve ring.
May see calcification of aortic root and ascending aortic arch. Leads to "tree bark" appearance of aorta.

Can result in aneurysm of ascending aorta or aortic arch, aortic insufficiency.

Cardiac tumors	Most common heart tumor is a metastasis.
Myxomas	Most common 1° cardiac tumor in adults A. 90% occur in the atria (mostly left atrium). Myxomas are usually described as a "ball valve" obstruction in the left atrium (associated with multiple syncopal episodes). May hear early diastolic "tumor plop" sound.
Rhabdomyomas	Most frequent 1° cardiac tumor in children (associated with tuberous sclerosis).

Myxoma. MRI shows myxoma in left atrium (arrow).

Kussmaul sign	↑ in JVP on inspiration instead of a normal ↓. Inspiration → negative intrathoracic pressure not transmitted to heart → impaired filling of right ventricle → blood backs up into venae cavae → JVD. May be seen with constrictive pericarditis, restrictive cardiomyopathies, right atrial or ventricular tumors.

Vascular tumors

Angiosarcoma	Rare blood vessel malignancy typically occurring in the head, neck, and breast areas. Usually in elderly, on sun-exposed areas. Associated with radiation therapy and chronic postmastectomy lymphedema. Hepatic angiosarcoma associated with vinyl chloride and arsenic exposures. Very aggressive and difficult to resect due to delay in diagnosis.
Bacillary angiomatosis	Benign capillary skin papules **A** found in AIDS patients. Caused by *Bartonella henselae* infections. Frequently mistaken for Kaposi sarcoma, but has neutrophilic infiltrate.
Cherry hemangioma	Benign capillary hemangioma of the elderly **B**. Does not regress. Frequency ↑ with age.
Cystic hygroma	Cavernous lymphangioma of the neck **C**. Associated with Turner syndrome.
Glomus tumor	Benign, painful, red-blue tumor under fingernails. Arises from modified smooth muscle cells of the thermoregulatory glomus body.
Kaposi sarcoma	Endothelial malignancy most commonly of the skin, but also mouth, GI tract, and respiratory tract. Associated with HHV-8 and HIV. Frequently mistaken for bacillary angiomatosis, but has lymphocytic infiltrate.
Pyogenic granuloma	Polypoid capillary hemangioma **D** that can ulcerate and bleed. Associated with trauma and pregnancy.
Strawberry hemangioma	Benign capillary hemangioma of infancy **E**. Appears in first few weeks of life (1/200 births); grows rapidly and regresses spontaneously by 5–8 years old.

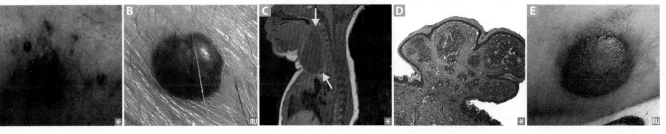

Raynaud phenomenon	↓ blood flow to the skin due to arteriolar (small vessel) vasospasm in response to cold or stress: color change from white (ischemia) to blue (hypoxia) to red (reperfusion). Most often in the fingers **A** and toes. Called **Raynaud disease** when 1° (idiopathic), **Raynaud syndrome** when 2° to a disease process such as mixed connective tissue disease, SLE, or CREST (limited form of systemic sclerosis) syndrome. Treat with Ca²⁺ channel blockers.

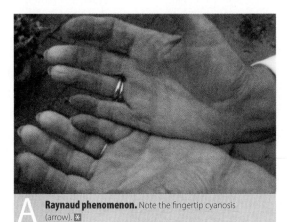

Raynaud phenomenon. Note the fingertip cyanosis (arrow).

Vasculitides

	EPIDEMIOLOGY/PRESENTATION	PATHOLOGY/LABS
Large-vessel vasculitis		
Temporal (giant cell) arteritis	Usually elderly females. Unilateral headache (temporal artery), jaw claudication. May lead to irreversible blindness due to ophthalmic artery occlusion. Associated with polymyalgia rheumatica.	Most commonly affects branches of carotid artery. Focal granulomatous inflammation A. ↑ ESR. Treat with high-dose corticosteroids prior to temporal artery biopsy to prevent blindness.
Takayasu arteritis	Usually Asian females < 40 years old. "Pulseless disease" (weak upper extremity pulses), fever, night sweats, arthritis, myalgias, skin nodules, ocular disturbances.	Granulomatous thickening and narrowing of aortic arch B and proximal great vessels. ↑ ESR. Treat with corticosteroids.
Medium-vessel vasculitis		
Polyarteritis nodosa	Young adults. Hepatitis B seropositivity in 30% of patients. Fever, weight loss, malaise, headache. GI: abdominal pain, melena. Hypertension, neurologic dysfunction, cutaneous eruptions, renal damage.	Typically involves renal and visceral vessels, not pulmonary arteries. Immune complex mediated. Transmural inflammation of the arterial wall with fibrinoid necrosis. Innumerable renal microaneurysms C and spasms on arteriogram. Treat with corticosteroids, cyclophosphamide.
Kawasaki disease	Asian children < 4 years old. Mucocutaneous lymph node syndrome: Conjunctival injection, **R**ash (polymorphous → desquamating), **A**denopathy (cervical), **S**trawberry tongue (oral mucositis) D, **H**and-foot changes (edema, erythema), **fever**.	**CRASH** and **burn**. May develop coronary artery aneurysms E; thrombosis or rupture can cause death. Treat with IV immunoglobulin and aspirin.
Buerger disease (thromboangiitis obliterans)	Heavy smokers, males < 40 years old. Intermittent claudication may lead to gangrene F, autoamputation of digits, superficial nodular phlebitis. Raynaud phenomenon is often present.	Segmental thrombosing vasculitis. Treat with smoking cessation.
Small-vessel vasculitis		
Granulomatosis with polyangiitis (Wegener)	Upper respiratory tract: perforation of nasal septum, chronic sinusitis, otitis media, mastoiditis. Lower respiratory tract: hemoptysis, cough, dyspnea. Renal: hematuria, red cell casts.	Triad: ▪ Focal necrotizing vasculitis ▪ Necrotizing granulomas in the lung and upper airway ▪ Necrotizing glomerulonephritis PR3-ANCA/c-ANCA G (anti-proteinase 3). CXR: large nodular densities. Treat with cyclophosphamide, corticosteroids.
Microscopic polyangiitis	Necrotizing vasculitis commonly involving lung, kidneys, and skin with pauci-immune glomerulonephritis and palpable purpura. Presentation similar to granulomatosis with polyangiitis but without nasopharyngeal involvement.	No granulomas. MPO-ANCA/p-ANCA H (anti-myeloperoxidase). Treat with cyclophosphamide, corticosteroids.

Vasculitides *(continued)*

	EPIDEMIOLOGY/PRESENTATION	PATHOLOGY/LABS
Small-vessel vasculitis *(continued)*		
Eosinophilic granulomatosis with polyangiitis (Churg-Strauss)	Asthma, sinusitis, skin nodules or purpura, peripheral neuropathy (e.g., wrist/foot drop). Can also involve heart, GI, kidneys (pauci-immune glomerulonephritis).	Granulomatous, necrotizing vasculitis with eosinophilia 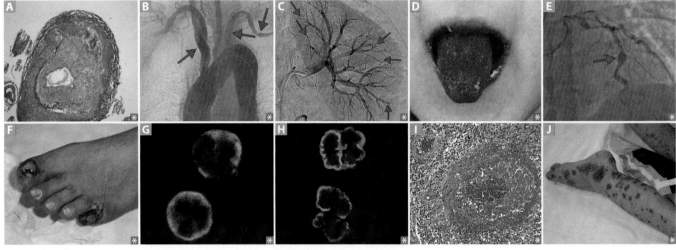. MPO-ANCA/p-ANCA, ↑ IgE level.
Henoch-Schönlein purpura	Most common childhood systemic vasculitis. Often follows URI. Classic triad: ▪ Skin: palpable purpura on buttocks/legs **J** ▪ Arthralgias ▪ GI: abdominal pain	Vasculitis 2° to IgA immune complex deposition. Associated with IgA nephropathy (Berger disease).

▶ CARDIOVASCULAR—PHARMACOLOGY

Antihypertensive therapy

Primary (essential) hypertension	Thiazide diuretics, ACE inhibitors, angiotensin II receptor blockers (ARBs), dihydropyridine Ca^{2+} channel blockers.	See the Renal chapter for more details about diuretics and ACE inhibitors/ARBs.
Hypertension with heart failure	Diuretics, ACE inhibitors/ARBs, β-blockers (compensated HF), aldosterone antagonists.	β-blockers must be used cautiously in decompensated HF and are contraindicated in cardiogenic shock.
Hypertension with diabetes mellitus	ACE inhibitors/ARBs, Ca^{2+} channel blockers, thiazide diuretics, β-blockers.	ACE inhibitors/ARBs are protective against diabetic nephropathy.
Hypertension in pregnancy	Hydralazine, labetalol, methyldopa, nifedipine.	

Calcium channel blockers

Amlodipine, clevidipine, nicardipine, nifedipine, nimodipine (dihydropyridines, act on vascular smooth muscle); diltiazem, verapamil (non-dihydropyridines, act on heart).

MECHANISM	Block voltage-dependent L-type calcium channels of cardiac and smooth muscle → ↓ muscle contractility. Vascular smooth muscle—amlodipine = nifedipine > diltiazem > verapamil. Heart—verapamil > diltiazem > amlodipine = nifedipine (verapamil = ventricle).
CLINICAL USE	Dihydropyridines (except nimodipine): hypertension, angina (including Prinzmetal), Raynaud phenomenon. Nimodipine: subarachnoid hemorrhage (prevents cerebral vasospasm). Clevidipine: hypertensive urgency or emergency. Non-dihydropyridines: hypertension, angina, atrial fibrillation/flutter.
TOXICITY	Cardiac depression, AV block (non-dihydropyridines), peripheral edema, flushing, dizziness, hyperprolactinemia (verapamil), constipation, gingival hyperplasia.

Hydralazine

MECHANISM	↑ cGMP → smooth muscle relaxation. Vasodilates arterioles > veins; afterload reduction.
CLINICAL USE	Severe hypertension (particularly acute), HF (with organic nitrate). Safe to use during pregnancy. Frequently coadministered with a β-blocker to prevent reflex tachycardia.
TOXICITY	Compensatory tachycardia (contraindicated in angina/CAD), fluid retention, headache, angina. Lupus-like syndrome.

Hypertensive emergency

Drugs include clevidipine, fenoldopam, labetalol, nicardipine, nitroprusside.

Nitroprusside	Short acting; ↑ cGMP via direct release of NO. Can cause cyanide toxicity (releases cyanide).
Fenoldopam	Dopamine D_1 receptor agonist—coronary, peripheral, renal, and splanchnic vasodilation. ↓ BP, ↑ natriuresis.

Nitrates	Nitroglycerin, isosorbide dinitrate, isosorbide mononitrate.
MECHANISM	Vasodilate by ↑ NO in vascular smooth muscle → ↑ in cGMP and smooth muscle relaxation. Dilate veins >> arteries. ↓ preload.
CLINICAL USE	Angina, acute coronary syndrome, pulmonary edema.
TOXICITY	Reflex tachycardia (treat with β-blockers), hypotension, flushing, headache, "Monday disease" in industrial exposure: development of tolerance for the vasodilating action during the work week and loss of tolerance over the weekend → tachycardia, dizziness, headache upon reexposure.

Antianginal therapy Goal is reduction of myocardial O_2 consumption (MVO_2) by ↓ 1 or more of the determinants of MVO_2: end-diastolic volume, BP, HR, contractility.

COMPONENT	NITRATES	β-BLOCKERS	NITRATES + β-BLOCKERS
End-diastolic volume	↓	No effect or ↓	No effect or ↓
Blood pressure	↓	↓	↓
Contractility	No effect	↓	Little/no effect
Heart rate	↑ (reflex response)	↓	No effect or ↓
Ejection time	↓	↑	Little/no effect
MVO_2	↓	↓	↓↓

Verapamil is similar to β-blockers in effect.
Pindolol and acebutolol—partial β-agonists contraindicated in angina.

Lipid-lowering agents

DRUG	LDL Δ	HDL Δ	TRIGLYCERIDES Δ	MECHANISMS OF ACTION	SIDE EFFECTS/PROBLEMS
HMG-CoA reductase inhibitors (lovastatin, pravastatin, simvastatin, atorvastatin, rosuvastatin)	↓↓↓	↑	↓	Inhibit conversion of HMG-CoA to mevalonate, a cholesterol precursor; ↓ mortality in CAD patients	Hepatotoxicity (↑ LFTs), myopathy (esp. when used with fibrates or niacin)
Bile acid resins (cholestyramine, colestipol, colesevelam)	↓↓	Slightly ↑	Slightly ↑	Prevent intestinal reabsorption of bile acids; liver must use cholesterol to make more	GI upset, ↓ absorption of other drugs and fat-soluble vitamins
Ezetimibe	↓↓	—	—	Prevent cholesterol absorption at small intestine brush border	Rare ↑ LFTs, diarrhea
Fibrates (gemfibrozil, clofibrate, bezafibrate, fenofibrate)	↓	↑	↓↓↓	Upregulate LPL → ↑ TG clearance. Activates PPAR-α to induce HDL synthesis	Myopathy (↑ risk with statins), cholesterol gallstones
Niacin (vitamin B$_3$)	↓↓	↑↑	↓	Inhibits lipolysis (hormone-sensitive lipase) in adipose tissue; reduces hepatic VLDL synthesis	Red, flushed face, which is ↓ by NSAIDs or long-term use. Hyperglycemia. Hyperuricemia

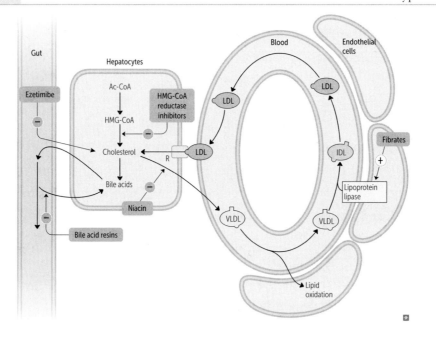

Cardiac glycosides	Digoxin.
MECHANISM	Direct inhibition of Na^+/K^+ ATPase → indirect inhibition of Na^+/Ca^{2+} exchanger. ↑ $[Ca^{2+}]_i$ → positive inotropy. Stimulates vagus nerve → ↓ HR.
CLINICAL USE	HF (↑ contractility); atrial fibrillation (↓ conduction at AV node and depression of SA node).
TOXICITY	Cholinergic—nausea, vomiting, diarrhea, blurry yellow vision (think van Gogh), arrhythmias, AV block. Can lead to hyperkalemia, which indicates poor prognosis. Factors predisposing to toxicity: renal failure (↓ excretion), hypokalemia (permissive for digoxin binding at K^+-binding site on Na^+/K^+ ATPase), verapamil, amiodarone, quinidine (↓ digoxin clearance; displaces digoxin from tissue-binding sites).
ANTIDOTE	Slowly normalize K^+, cardiac pacer, anti-digoxin Fab fragments, Mg^{2+}.

Antiarrhythmics—sodium channel blockers (class I)	Slow or block (↓) conduction (especially in depolarized cells). ↓ slope of phase 0 depolarization. Are state dependent (selectively depress tissue that is frequently depolarized [e.g., tachycardia]).	
Class IA	Quinidine, Procainamide, Disopyramide. "The Queen Proclaims Diso's pyramid."	Class IA
MECHANISM	↑ AP duration, ↑ effective refractory period (ERP) in ventricular action potential, ↑ QT interval.	
CLINICAL USE	Both atrial and ventricular arrhythmias, especially re-entrant and ectopic SVT and VT.	
TOXICITY	Cinchonism (headache, tinnitus with quinidine), reversible SLE-like syndrome (procainamide), heart failure (disopyramide), thrombocytopenia, torsades de pointes due to ↑ QT interval.	
Class IB	Lidocaine, MexileTine. "I'd Buy Liddy's Mexican Tacos."	Class IB
MECHANISM	↓ AP duration. Preferentially affect ischemic or depolarized Purkinje and ventricular tissue. Phenytoin can also fall into the IB category.	
CLINICAL USE	Acute ventricular arrhythmias (especially post-MI), digitalis-induced arrhythmias. IB is Best post-MI.	
TOXICITY	CNS stimulation/depression, cardiovascular depression.	
Class IC	Flecainide, Propafenone. "Can I have Fries, Please."	Class IC
MECHANISM	Significantly prolongs ERP in AV node and accessory bypass tracts. No effect on ERP in Purkinje and ventricular tissue. Minimal effect on AP duration.	
CLINICAL USE	SVTs, including atrial fibrillation. Only as a last resort in refractory VT.	
TOXICITY	Proarrhythmic, especially post-MI (contraindicated). IC is Contraindicated in structural and ischemic heart disease.	

Antiarrhythmics— β-blockers (class II)	Metoprolol, propranolol, esmolol, atenolol, timolol, carvedilol.	
MECHANISM	Decrease SA and AV nodal activity by ↓ cAMP, ↓ Ca^{2+} currents. Suppress abnormal pacemakers by ↓ slope of phase 4. AV node particularly sensitive—↑ PR interval. Esmolol very short acting.	
CLINICAL USE	SVT, ventricular rate control for atrial fibrillation and atrial flutter.	
TOXICITY	Impotence, exacerbation of COPD and asthma, cardiovascular effects (bradycardia, AV block, HF), CNS effects (sedation, sleep alterations). May mask the signs of hypoglycemia. Metoprolol can cause dyslipidemia. Propranolol can exacerbate vasospasm in Prinzmetal angina. β-blockers cause unopposed $α_1$-agonism if given alone for pheochromocytoma or cocaine toxicity. Treat β-blocker overdose with saline, atropine, glucagon.	

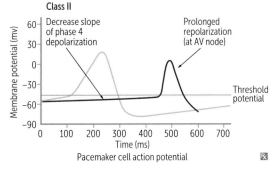

Class II

Pacemaker cell action potential

Antiarrhythmics— potassium channel blockers (class III)	Amiodarone, Ibutilide, Dofetilide, Sotalol.	AIDS.
MECHANISM	↑ AP duration, ↑ ERP, ↑ QT interval.	
CLINICAL USE	Atrial fibrillation, atrial flutter; ventricular tachycardia (amiodarone, sotalol).	
TOXICITY	Sotalol—torsades de pointes, excessive β blockade. Ibutilide—torsades de pointes. Amiodarone—pulmonary fibrosis, hepatotoxicity, hypothyroidism/ hyperthyroidism (amiodarone is 40% iodine by weight), acts as hapten (corneal deposits, blue/ gray skin deposits resulting in photodermatitis), neurologic effects, constipation, cardiovascular effects (bradycardia, heart block, HF).	Remember to check PFTs, LFTs, and TFTs when using amiodarone. Amiodarone is lipophilic and has class I, II, III, and IV effects.

Class III

Cell action potential

Antiarrhythmics—calcium channel blockers (class IV)	Verapamil, diltiazem.
MECHANISM	↓ conduction velocity, ↑ ERP, ↑ PR interval.
CLINICAL USE	Prevention of nodal arrhythmias (e.g., SVT), rate control in atrial fibrillation.
TOXICITY	Constipation, flushing, edema, cardiovascular effects (HF, AV block, sinus node depression).

Class IV

Slow rise of action potential
Prolonged repolarization (at AV node)
Threshold potential

Membrane potential (mv)
Time (ms)

Other antiarrhythmics

Adenosine	↑ K⁺ out of cells → hyperpolarizing the cell and ↓ I$_{Ca}$. Drug of choice in diagnosing/abolishing supraventricular tachycardia. Very short acting (~ 15 sec). Effects blunted by theophylline and caffeine (both are adenosine receptor antagonists). Adverse effects include flushing, hypotension, chest pain, sense of impending doom, bronchospasm.
Mg²⁺	Effective in torsades de pointes and digoxin toxicity.

Endocrine

"We have learned that there is an endocrinology of elation and despair, a chemistry of mystical insight, and, in relation to the autonomic nervous system, a meteorology and even . . . an astro-physics of changing moods."
—Aldous (Leonard) Huxley

"Chocolate causes certain endocrine glands to secrete hormones that affect your feelings and behavior by making you happy."
—Elaine Sherman, Book of Divine Indulgences

▶ ENDOCRINE—EMBRYOLOGY

Thyroid development

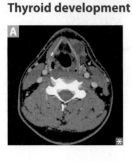

Thyroid diverticulum arises from floor of primitive pharynx and descends into neck. Connected to tongue by thyroglossal duct, which normally disappears but may persist as pyramidal lobe of thyroid. Foramen cecum is normal remnant of thyroglossal duct. Most common ectopic thyroid tissue site is the tongue.

Thyroglossal duct cyst A presents as an anterior midline neck mass that moves with swallowing or protrusion of the tongue (vs. persistent cervical sinus leading to branchial cleft cyst in lateral neck).

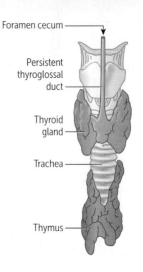

Foramen cecum

Persistent thyroglossal duct

Thyroid gland

Trachea

Thymus

▶ ENDOCRINE—ANATOMY

Adrenal cortex and medulla

Adrenal cortex (derived from mesoderm) and medulla (derived from neural crest).

	ANATOMY			PRIMARY REGULATORY CONTROL	SECRETORY PRODUCTS
	Zona **G**lomerulosa			Renin-angiotensin	Aldosterone
CORTEX	Zona **F**asciculata			ACTH, CRH	Cortisol, sex hormones
	Zona **R**eticularis			ACTH, CRH	Sex hormones (e.g., androgens)
MEDULLA	Chromaffin cells			Preganglionic sympathetic fibers	Catecholamines (epinephrine, norepinephrine)

GFR corresponds with **S**alt (Na+), **S**ugar (glucocorticoids), and **S**ex (androgens).
  "The deeper you go, **the sweeter it gets**."
Pheochromocytoma—most common tumor of the adrenal medulla in adults.
  Episodic hypertension.
Neuroblastoma—most common tumor of the adrenal medulla in children.
  Rarely causes hypertension.

Pituitary gland

Anterior pituitary (adenohypophysis)	Secretes FSH, LH, ACTH, TSH, prolactin, GH. Melanotropin (MSH) secreted from intermediate lobe of pituitary. Derived from oral ectoderm (Rathke pouch). <ul><li>α subunit—hormone subunit common to TSH, LH, FSH, and hCG.</li><li>β subunit—determines hormone specificity.</li></ul>	Acidophils—GH, prolactin. **B-FLAT:** Basophils—FSH, LH, ACTH, TSH. **FLAT PiG:** FSH, LH, ACTH, TSH, Prolactin, GH.
Posterior pituitary (neurohypophysis)	Secretes vasopressin (antidiuretic hormone, or ADH) and oxytocin, made in the hypothalamus (supraoptic and paraventricular nuclei, respectively) and transported to posterior pituitary via neurophysins (carrier proteins). Derived from neuroectoderm.	
Endocrine pancreas cell types	Islets of Langerhans are collections of α, β, and δ endocrine cells. Islets arise from pancreatic buds. <ul><li>α = glucagon (peripheral)</li><li>β = insulin (central)</li><li>δ = somatostatin (interspersed)</li></ul>	Insulin (β cells) inside.

▶ ENDOCRINE—PHYSIOLOGY

Insulin

SYNTHESIS	Preproinsulin (synthesized in RER) → cleavage of "presignal" → proinsulin (stored in secretory granules) → cleavage of proinsulin → exocytosis of insulin and C-peptide equally. Insulin and C-peptide are ↑ in insulinoma and sulfonylurea use, whereas exogenous insulin lacks C-peptide.
SOURCE	Released from pancreatic β cells.

FUNCTION

Binds insulin receptors (tyrosine kinase activity **❶**), inducing glucose uptake (carrier-mediated transport) into insulin-dependent tissue **❷** and gene transcription. Anabolic effects of insulin:
- ↑ glucose transport in skeletal muscle and adipose tissue
- ↑ glycogen synthesis and storage
- ↑ triglyceride synthesis
- ↑ Na^+ retention (kidneys)
- ↑ protein synthesis (muscles)
- ↑ cellular uptake of K^+ and amino acids
- ↓ glucagon release

Unlike glucose, insulin does not cross placenta.

Insulin-dependent glucose transporters:
- GLUT-4: adipose tissue, striated muscle (exercise can also increase GLUT-4 expression)

Insulin-independent transporters:
- GLUT-1: RBCs, brain, cornea
- GLUT-2 (bidirectional): β islet cells, liver, kidney, small intestine
- GLUT-3: brain
- GLUT-5 (fructose): spermatocytes, GI tract

Brain utilizes glucose for metabolism normally and ketone bodies during starvation. RBCs always utilize glucose because they lack mitochondria for aerobic metabolism.

BRICK L (insulin-independent glucose uptake): Brain, RBCs, Intestine, Cornea, Kidney, Liver.

REGULATION

Glucose is a major regulator of insulin release. GH (causes insulin resistance → ↑ insulin release) and $β_2$-agonists → ↑ insulin.

Glucose enters β cells **❸** → ↑ ATP generated from glucose metabolism **❹** closes K^+ channels (target of sulfonylureas) **❺** and depolarizes β cell membrane **❻**. Voltage-gated Ca^{2+} channels open → Ca^{2+} influx **❼** and stimulation of insulin exocytosis **❽**.

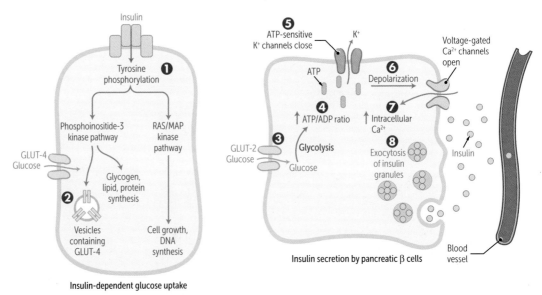

Insulin-dependent glucose uptake

Insulin secretion by pancreatic β cells

Glucagon

SOURCE	Made by α cells of pancreas.
FUNCTION	Catabolic effects of glucagon: ▪ Glycogenolysis, gluconeogenesis ▪ Lipolysis and ketone production
REGULATION	Secreted in response to hypoglycemia. Inhibited by insulin, hyperglycemia, and somatostatin.

Hypothalamic-pituitary hormones

HORMONE	FUNCTION	CLINICAL NOTES
CRH	↑ ACTH, MSH, β-endorphin	↓ in chronic exogenous steroid use
Dopamine	↓ prolactin	Dopamine antagonists (e.g., antipsychotics) can cause galactorrhea due to hyperprolactinemia
GHRH	↑ GH	Analog (tesamorelin) used to treat HIV-associated lipodystrophy
GnRH	↑ FSH, LH	Regulated by prolactin Tonic GnRH suppresses HPA axis Pulsatile GnRH leads to puberty, fertility
Prolactin	↓ GnRH	Pituitary prolactinoma → amenorrhea, osteoporosis, hypogonadism, galactorrhea
Somatostatin	↓ GH, TSH	Analogs used to treat acromegaly
TRH	↑ TSH, prolactin	

Prolactin

SOURCE	Secreted mainly by anterior pituitary.	
FUNCTION	Stimulates milk production in breast; inhibits ovulation in females and spermatogenesis in males by inhibiting GnRH synthesis and release.	Excessive amounts of prolactin associated with ↓ libido.
REGULATION	Prolactin secretion from anterior pituitary is tonically inhibited by dopamine from hypothalamus. Prolactin in turn inhibits its own secretion by ↑ dopamine synthesis and secretion from hypothalamus. TRH ↑ prolactin secretion (e.g., in 1° or 2° hypothyroidism).	Dopamine agonists (e.g., bromocriptine) inhibit prolactin secretion and can be used in treatment of prolactinoma. Dopamine antagonists (e.g., most antipsychotics) and estrogens (e.g., OCPs, pregnancy) stimulate prolactin secretion.

Growth hormone (somatotropin)

SOURCE	Secreted by anterior pituitary.	
FUNCTION	Stimulates linear growth and muscle mass through IGF-1 (somatomedin C) secretion. ↑ insulin resistance (diabetogenic).	
REGULATION	Released in pulses in response to growth hormone–releasing hormone (GHRH). Secretion ↑ during exercise and sleep. Secretion inhibited by glucose and somatostatin release via negative feedback by somatomedin.	Excess secretion of GH (e.g., pituitary adenoma) may cause acromegaly (adults) or gigantism (children).

Appetite regulation

Ghrelin	Stimulates hunger (orexigenic effect) and GH release (via GH secretagog receptor). Produced by stomach. ↑ with sleep loss and Prader-Willi syndrome.	Ghrelin make you hunghre.
Leptin	Satiety hormone. Produced by adipose tissue. ↓ during starvation. Mutation of leptin gene → congenital obesity. Sleep deprivation → ↓ leptin production.	Leptin keeps you thin.
Endocannabinoids	Stimulate cortical reward centers → ↑ desire for high-fat foods.	The munchies.

Antidiuretic hormone

SOURCE	Synthesized in hypothalamus (supraoptic nuclei), released by posterior pituitary.	
FUNCTION	Regulates serum osmolarity (V_2-receptors) and blood pressure (V_1-receptors). Primary function is serum osmolarity regulation (ADH ↓ serum osmolarity, ↑ urine osmolarity) via regulation of aquaporin channel insertion in principal cells of renal collecting duct.	ADH level is ↓ in central diabetes insipidus (DI), normal or ↑ in nephrogenic DI. Nephrogenic DI can be caused by mutation in V_2-receptor. Desmopressin acetate (ADH analog) is a treatment for central DI.
REGULATION	Osmoreceptors in hypothalamus (1°); hypovolemia (2°).	

Adrenal steroids and congenital adrenal hyperplasias

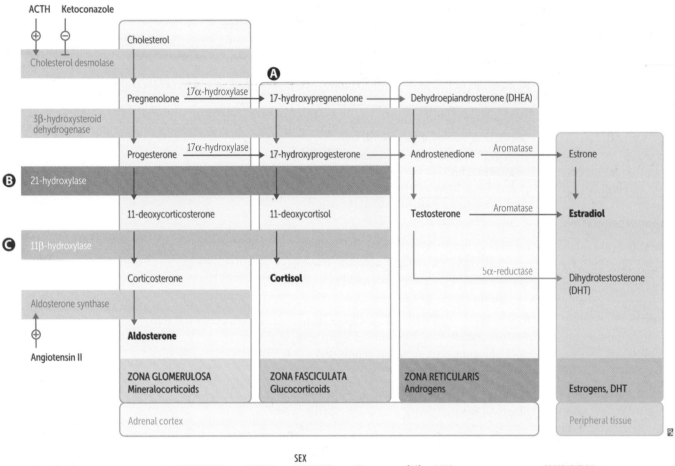

ENZYME DEFICIENCY	MINERALOCORTICOIDS	CORTISOL	SEX HORMONES	BP	[K⁺]	LABS	PRESENTATION
Ⓐ 17α-hydroxylase[a]	↑	↓	↓	↑	↓	↓ androstenedione	XY: pseudo-hermaphroditism (ambiguous genitalia, undescended testes) XX: lack secondary sexual development
Ⓑ 21-hydroxylase[a]	↓	↓	↑	↓	↑	↑ renin activity ↑ 17-hydroxy-progesterone	Most common Presents in infancy (salt wasting) or childhood (precocious puberty) XX: virilization
Ⓒ 11β-hydroxylase[a]	↓ aldosterone ↑ 11-deoxycorti-costerone (results in ↑ BP)	↓	↑	↑	↓	↓ renin activity	XX: virilization

[a]All congenital adrenal enzyme deficiencies are characterized by an enlargement of both adrenal glands due to ↑ ACTH stimulation (due to ↓ cortisol).

Cortisol

SOURCE	Adrenal zona fasciculata.	Bound to corticosteroid-binding globulin.

FUNCTION	↑ Blood pressure:
	  ▪ Upregulates α_1-receptors on arterioles → ↑ sensitivity to norepinephrine and epinephrine
	  ▪ At high concentrations, can bind to mineralocorticoid (aldosterone) receptors
	↑ Insulin resistance (diabetogenic)
	↑ Gluconeogenesis, lipolysis, and proteolysis
	↓ Fibroblast activity (causes striae)
	↓ Inflammatory and Immune responses:
	  ▪ Inhibits production of leukotrienes and prostaglandins
	  ▪ Inhibits WBC adhesion → neutrophilia
	  ▪ Blocks histamine release from mast cells
	  ▪ Reduces eosinophils
	  ▪ Blocks IL-2 production
	↓ Bone formation (↓ osteoblast activity)
		Cortisol is a **BIG FIB**.
		Exogenous corticosteroids can cause reactivation of TB and candidiasis (blocks IL-2 production).

REGULATION	CRH (hypothalamus) stimulates ACTH release (pituitary) → cortisol production in adrenal zona fasciculata. Excess cortisol ↓ CRH, ACTH, and cortisol secretion.	Chronic stress induces prolonged secretion.

Calcium homeostasis	Plasma Ca^{2+} exists in three forms:
	  ▪ Ionized (~ 45%)
	  ▪ Bound to albumin (~ 40%)
	  ▪ Bound to anions (~ 15%)
		↑ in pH → ↑ affinity of albumin (↑ negative charge) to bind Ca^{2+} → hypocalcemia (cramps, pain, paresthesias, carpopedal spasm).

Vitamin D (cholecalciferol)

SOURCE	D_3 from sun exposure in skin. D_2 ingested from plants. Both converted to 25-OH in liver and to 1,25-$(OH)_2$ (active form) in kidney.	Deficiency → rickets in kids, osteomalacia in adults. Caused by malabsorption, ↓ sunlight, poor diet, chronic kidney failure.
FUNCTION	↑ absorption of dietary Ca^{2+} and PO_4^{3-}. ↑ bone resorption → ↑ Ca^{2+} and PO_4^{3-}.	24,25-$(OH)_2$ D_3 is an inactive form of vitamin D. PTH leads to ↑ Ca^{2+} reabsorption and ↓ PO_4^{3-} reabsorption in the kidney, whereas 1,25-$(OH)_2$ D_3 leads to ↑ absorption of both Ca^{2+} and PO_4^{3-} in the gut.
REGULATION	↑ PTH, ↓ $[Ca^{2+}]$, ↓ PO_4^{3-} → ↑ 1,25-$(OH)_2$ production. 1,25-$(OH)_2$ feedback inhibits its own production.	

Parathyroid hormone

SOURCE	Chief cells of parathyroid.

FUNCTION

↑ bone resorption of Ca^{2+} and PO_4^{3-}.

↑ kidney reabsorption of Ca^{2+} in distal convoluted tubule.

↓ reabsorption of PO_4^{3-} in proximal convoluted tubule.

↑ 1,25-$(OH)_2$ D_3 (calcitriol) production by stimulating kidney 1α-hydroxylase in proximal convoluted tubule.

PTH ↑ serum Ca^{2+}, ↓ serum (PO_4^{3-}), ↑ urine (PO_4^{3-}).

↑ production of macrophage colony-stimulating factor and RANK-L (receptor activator of NF-κB ligand). RANK-L (ligand) secreted by osteoblasts and osteocytes binds RANK (receptor) on osteoclasts and their precursors to stimulate osteoclasts and ↑ Ca^{2+}.

Intermittent PTH release can stimulate bone formation.

PTH = Phosphate Trashing Hormone.

PTH-related peptide (PTHrP) functions like PTH and is commonly increased in malignancies.

REGULATION

↓ serum Ca^{2+} → ↑ PTH secretion.

↑ serum PO_4^{3-} → ↑ PTH secretion.

↓ serum Mg^{2+} → ↑ PTH secretion.

↓↓ serum Mg^{2+} → ↓ PTH secretion.

Common causes of ↓ Mg^{2+} include diarrhea, aminoglycosides, diuretics, alcohol abuse.

Low ionized calcium

(+)

Four parathyroid glands

(−) Feedback inhibition of PTH synthesis

(−) Feedback inhibition of PTH secretion

PTH (1-84) released into circulation

Renal tubular cells

Bone

• Stimulates reabsorption of calcium
• Inhibits phosphate reabsorption
• Stimulates production of 1,25-$(OH)_2$ D_3

• Stimulates calcium release from bone mineral compartment
• Stimulates osteoblastic cells
• Stimulates bone resorption via indirect effect on osteoclasts
• Enhances bone matrix degradation

• Increases intestinal calcium absorption → Increases serum calcium

Calcium homeostasis

Low serum phosphorus → ↑ Conversion 25-(OH) D_3 → 1,25-$(OH)_2$ D_3

• Releases phosphate from matrix

• Increases intestinal phosphate reabsorption

Phosphate homeostasis

Calcitonin

SOURCE	Parafollicular cells (C cells) of thyroid.	Calcitonin opposes actions of PTH. Not important in normal Ca^{2+} homeostasis. Calcitonin tones down Ca^{2+} levels.
FUNCTION	↓ bone resorption of Ca^{2+}.	
REGULATION	↑ serum Ca^{2+} → calcitonin secretion.	

Signaling pathways of endocrine hormones

cAMP	FSH, LH, ACTH, TSH, CRH, hCG, ADH (V_2-receptor), MSH, PTH, calcitonin, GHRH, glucagon	FLAT ChAMP
cGMP	ANP, BNP, NO (EDRF)	Think vasodilators
IP$_3$	GnRH, Oxytocin, ADH (V_1-receptor), TRH, Histamine (H_1-receptor), Angiotensin II, Gastrin	GOAT HAG
Intracellular receptor	Vitamin D, Estrogen, Testosterone, T_3/T_4, Cortisol, Aldosterone, Progesterone	VETTT CAP
Intrinsic tyrosine kinase	Insulin, IGF-1, FGF, PDGF, EGF	MAP kinase pathway Think growth factors
Receptor-associated tyrosine kinase	Prolactin, Immunomodulators (e.g., cytokines IL-2, IL-6, IFN), GH, G-CSF, Erythropoietin, Thrombopoietin	JAK/STAT pathway Think acidophils and cytokines PIGGLET

Signaling pathway of steroid hormones

Steroid hormones are lipophilic and therefore must circulate bound to specific binding globulins, which ↑ their solubility.

In men, ↑ sex hormone–binding globulin (SHBG) lowers free testosterone → gynecomastia.

In women, ↓ SHBG raises free testosterone → hirsutism.

OCPs, pregnancy ↑ SHBG (free estrogen levels remain unchanged).

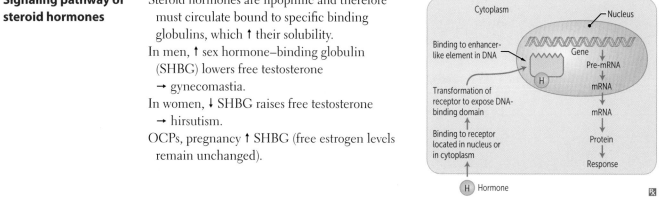

Thyroid hormones (T₃/T₄)

Iodine-containing hormones that control the body's metabolic rate.

SOURCE	Follicles of thyroid. Most T_3 formed in target tissues.
FUNCTION	Bone growth (synergism with GH) CNS maturation ↑ β_1 receptors in heart = ↑ CO, HR, SV, contractility ↑ basal metabolic rate via ↑ Na^+/K^+-ATPase activity → ↑ O_2 consumption, RR, body temperature ↑ glycogenolysis, gluconeogenesis, lipolysis
REGULATION	TRH (hypothalamus) stimulates TSH (pituitary), which stimulates follicular cells. Negative feedback by free T_3, T_4 to anterior pituitary ↓ sensitivity to TRH. Thyroid-stimulating immunoglobulins (e.g., TSH) stimulate follicular cells (e.g., Graves disease). Wolff-Chaikoff effect—excess iodine temporarily inhibits thyroid peroxidase → ↓ iodine organification → ↓ T_3/T_4 production.

T_3 functions—**4 B's:**
  Brain maturation
  Bone growth
  β-adrenergic effects
  Basal metabolic rate ↑
Thyroxine-binding globulin (TBG) binds most T_3/T_4 in blood; only free hormone is active.
  ↓ TBG in hepatic failure, steroids; ↑ TBG in pregnancy or OCP use (estrogen ↑ TBG).
T_4 is major thyroid product; converted to T_3 in peripheral tissue by 5'-deiodinase.
T_3 binds nuclear receptor with greater affinity than T_4.
Peroxidase is the enzyme responsible for oxidation and organification of iodide as well as coupling of monoiodotyrosine (MIT) and di-iodotyrosine (DIT).
Propylthiouracil inhibits both peroxidase and 5'-deiodinase. Methimazole inhibits peroxidase only.

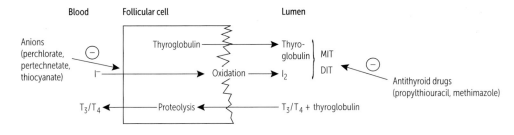

▸ ENDOCRINE—PATHOLOGY

Cushing syndrome

ETIOLOGY	↑ cortisol due to a variety of causes:
	▪ Exogenous corticosteroids—result in ↓ ACTH, bilateral adrenal atrophy. Most common cause.
	▪ Primary adrenal adenoma, hyperplasia, or carcinoma—result in ↓ ACTH, atrophy of uninvolved adrenal gland. Can also present with pseudohyperaldosteronism.
	▪ ACTH-secreting pituitary adenoma (Cushing disease); paraneoplastic ACTH secretion (e.g., small cell lung cancer, bronchial carcinoids)—result in ↑ ACTH, bilateral adrenal hyperplasia. Cushing disease is responsible for the majority of endogenous cases of Cushing syndrome.
FINDINGS	Hypertension, weight gain, moon facies, truncal obesity , buffalo hump, skin changes (thinning, striae), osteoporosis, hyperglycemia (insulin resistance), amenorrhea, immunosuppression.
DIAGNOSIS	Screening tests include: ↑ free cortisol on 24-hr urinalysis, ↑ midnight salivary cortisol, and no suppression with overnight low-dose dexamethasone test. Measure serum ACTH. If ↓, suspect adrenal tumor. If ↑, distinguish between Cushing disease and ectopic ACTH secretion with a high-dose (8 mg) dexamethasone suppression test and CRH stimulation test. Ectopic secretion will not decrease with dexamethasone because the source is resistant to negative feedback; ectopic secretion will not increase with CRH because pituitary ACTH is suppressed.

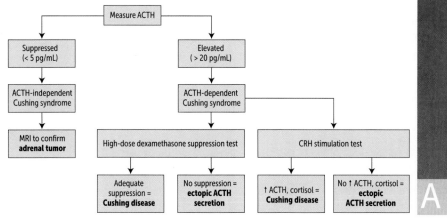

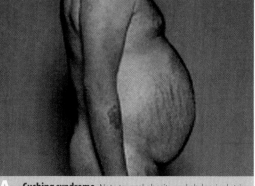

A **Cushing syndrome.** Note truncal obesity and abdominal striae.

Adrenal insufficiency	Inability of adrenal glands to generate enough glucocorticoids +/− mineralocorticoids for the body's needs. Symptoms include weakness, fatigue, orthostatic hypotension, muscle aches, weight loss, GI disturbances, sugar and/or salt cravings.	Diagnosis involves measurement of serum electrolytes, morning/random serum cortisol and ACTH, and response to ACTH stimulation test. Alternatively, can use metyrapone stimulation test: metyrapone blocks last step of cortisol synthesis (11-deoxycortisol → cortisol). Normal response is ↓ cortisol and compensatory ↑ ACTH. In adrenal insufficiency, ACTH remains ↓ after test.
Primary	Deficiency of aldosterone and cortisol production due to loss of gland function → hypotension (hyponatremic volume contraction), hyperkalemia, metabolic acidosis, skin and mucosal hyperpigmentation **A** (due to MSH, a byproduct of ↑ ACTH production from pro-opiomelanocortin). ▪ **Acute**—sudden onset (e.g., due to massive hemorrhage). May present with shock in acute adrenal crisis. ▪ **Chronic**—aka **Addison disease**. Due to adrenal atrophy or destruction by disease (e.g., autoimmune, TB, metastasis).	**Primary** **P**igments the skin/mucosa. Autoimmunity most common cause of 1° chronic adrenal insufficiency in Western world. Associated with autoimmune polyglandular syndromes. **Waterhouse-Friderichsen syndrome**—acute 1° adrenal insufficiency due to adrenal hemorrhage associated with septicemia (usually *Neisseria meningitidis*), DIC, endotoxic shock.
Secondary	Seen with ↓ pituitary ACTH production. No skin/mucosal hyperpigmentation, no hyperkalemia (aldosterone synthesis preserved).	**Secondary** **S**pares the skin/mucosa.
Tertiary	Seen in patients with chronic exogenous steroid use, precipitated by abrupt withdrawal. Aldosterone synthesis unaffected.	**Tertiary** from **T**reatment.

Neuroblastoma

Most common tumor of the adrenal medulla in **children**, usually < 4 years old. Originates from neural crest cells; Homer-Wright rosettes 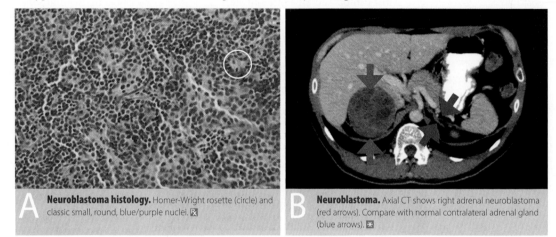 characteristic. Occurs anywhere along the sympathetic chain. Most common presentation is abdominal distension and a firm, irregular mass **B** that can cross the midline (vs. Wilms tumor, which is smooth and unilateral). Can also present with opsoclonus-myoclonus syndrome ("dancing eyes-dancing feet"). Homovanillic acid (HVA; a breakdown product of dopamine) and vanillylmandelic acid (VMA; a breakdown product of norepinephrine) ↑ in urine. Bombesin and neuron-specific enolase ⊕. Less likely to develop hypertension. Associated with overexpression of N-*myc* oncogene.

A **Neuroblastoma histology.** Homer-Wright rosette (circle) and classic small, round, blue/purple nuclei.

B **Neuroblastoma.** Axial CT shows right adrenal neuroblastoma (red arrows). Compare with normal contralateral adrenal gland (blue arrows).

Pheochromocytoma

ETIOLOGY	Most common tumor of the adrenal medulla in **adults** 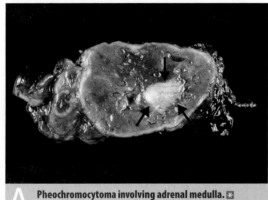. Derived from chromaffin cells (arise from neural crest) B.	Rule of 10's: 10% malignant 10% bilateral 10% extra-adrenal 10% calcify 10% kids
SYMPTOMS	Most tumors secrete epinephrine, norepinephrine, and dopamine, which can cause episodic hypertension. Associated with neurofibromatosis type 1, von Hippel-Lindau disease, MEN 2A and 2B. Symptoms occur in "spells"—relapse and remit.	Episodic hyperadrenergic symptoms (5 P's): Pressure (↑ BP) Pain (headache) Perspiration Palpitations (tachycardia) Pallor
FINDINGS	↑ catecholamines and metanephrines in urine and plasma.	
TREATMENT	Irreversible α-antagonists (e.g., phenoxybenzamine) followed by β-blockers prior to tumor resection. α-blockade must be achieved before giving β-blockers to avoid a hypertensive crisis.	

A **Pheochromocytoma involving adrenal medulla.** ✴

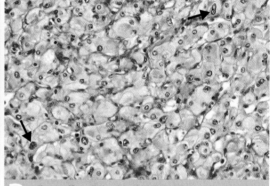

B **Chromaffin cells in pheochromocytoma.** Note enlarged pleomorphic nuclei (arrows) typical of malignancy. ✴

Hypothyroidism vs. hyperthyroidism

	Hypothyroidism	Hyperthyroidism
SIGNS/SYMPTOMS	Cold intolerance (↓ heat production)	Heat intolerance (↑ heat production)
	Weight gain, ↓ appetite	Weight loss, ↑ appetite
	Hypoactivity, lethargy, fatigue, weakness	Hyperactivity
	Constipation	Diarrhea
	↓ reflexes	↑ reflexes
	Myxedema (facial/periorbital)	Pretibial myxedema (Graves disease), periorbital edema
	Dry, cool skin; coarse, brittle hair	Warm, moist skin; fine hair
	Bradycardia, dyspnea on exertion	Chest pain, palpitations, arrhythmias, ↑ number and sensitivity of β-adrenergic receptors
LAB FINDINGS	↑ TSH (sensitive test for 1° hypothyroidism)	↓ TSH (if 1°)
	↓ free T_3 and T_4	↑ free or total T_3 and T_4
	Hypercholesterolemia (due to ↓ LDL receptor expression)	Hypocholesterolemia (due to ↑ LDL receptor expression)

Hypothyroidism

Hashimoto thyroiditis	Most common cause of hypothyroidism in iodine-sufficient regions; an autoimmune disorder (anti-thyroid peroxidase, antimicrosomal and antithyroglobulin antibodies). Associated with HLA-DR5. ↑ risk of non-Hodgkin lymphoma. May be hyperthyroid early in course due to thyrotoxicosis during follicular rupture. Histologic findings: Hürthle cells, lymphoid aggregate with germinal centers 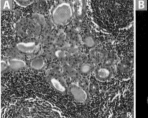. Findings: moderately enlarged, **nontender** thyroid.
Congenital hypothyroidism (cretinism)	Severe fetal hypothyroidism due to maternal hypothyroidism, thyroid agenesis, thyroid dysgenesis (most common cause in U.S.), iodine deficiency, dyshormonogenetic goiter. Findings: Pot-bellied, Pale, Puffy-faced child with Protruding umbilicus, Protuberant tongue, and Poor brain development: the 6 P's 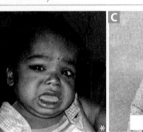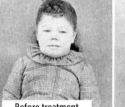.
Subacute thyroiditis (de Quervain)	Self-limited disease often following a flu-like illness. May be hyperthyroid early in course, followed by hypothyroidism. Histology: granulomatous inflammation. Findings: ↑ ESR, jaw pain, early inflammation, very **tender** thyroid. (de Quervain is associated with **pain**.)
Riedel thyroiditis	Thyroid replaced by fibrous tissue (hypothyroid). Fibrosis may extend to local structures (e.g., airway), mimicking anaplastic carcinoma. Considered a manifestation of IgG$_4$-related systemic disease (e.g., autoimmune pancreatitis, retroperitoneal fibrosis, noninfectious aortitis). Findings: fixed, hard (rock-like), **painless** goiter.
Other causes	Iodine deficiency 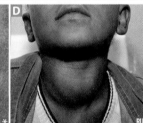, goitrogens, Wolff-Chaikoff effect (thyroid gland downregulation in response to ↑ iodide).

Before treatment   After treatment

Hyperthyroidism

Graves disease	Most common cause of hyperthyroidism. Autoantibodies (IgG) stimulate TSH receptors on thyroid (hyperthyroidism, diffuse goiter), retro-orbital fibroblasts (exophthalmos: proptosis, extraocular muscle swelling 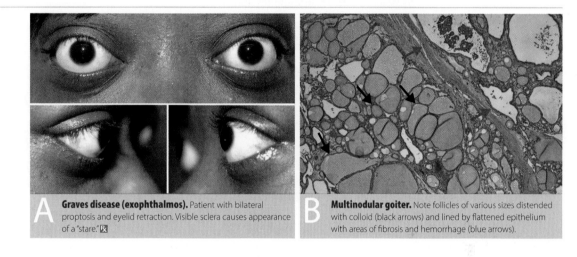), and dermal fibroblasts (pretibial myxedema). Often presents during stress (e.g., childbirth).
Toxic multinodular goiter	Focal patches of hyperfunctioning follicular cells **B** working independently of TSH due to mutation in TSH receptor. ↑ release of T_3 and T_4. Hot nodules are rarely malignant.
Thyroid storm	Stress-induced catecholamine surge seen as a serious complication of thyrotoxicosis due to disease and other hyperthyroid disorders. Presents with agitation, delirium, fever, diarrhea, coma, and tachyarrhythmia (cause of death). May see increased ALP due to ↑ bone turnover. Treat with the 3 P's: β-blockers (e.g., **P**ropranolol), **P**ropylthiouracil, corticosteroids (e.g., **P**rednisolone).
Jod-Basedow phenomenon	Thyrotoxicosis if a patient with iodine deficiency goiter is made iodine replete.

A **Graves disease (exophthalmos).** Patient with bilateral proptosis and eyelid retraction. Visible sclera causes appearance of a "stare." ℞

B **Multinodular goiter.** Note follicles of various sizes distended with colloid (black arrows) and lined by flattened epithelium with areas of fibrosis and hemorrhage (blue arrows).

Thyroid cancer	Thyroidectomy is an option for thyroid cancers and hyperthyroidism. Complications of surgery include hoarseness (due to recurrent laryngeal nerve damage), hypocalcemia (due to removal of parathyroid glands), and transection of recurrent and superior laryngeal nerves (during ligation of inferior thyroid artery and superior laryngeal artery, respectively).
Papillary carcinoma	Most common, excellent prognosis. Empty-appearing nuclei with central clearing ("Orphan Annie" eyes) **A**, psammoma bodies, nuclear grooves. Lymphatic invasion common. ↑ risk with *RET* and *BRAF* mutations, childhood irradiation.
Follicular carcinoma	Good prognosis, invades thyroid capsule (unlike follicular adenoma), uniform follicles.
Medullary carcinoma	From parafollicular "C cells"; produces calcitonin, sheets of cells in an amyloid stroma **B**, hematogenous spread common. Associated with MEN 2A and 2B (*RET* mutations).
Undifferentiated/ anaplastic carcinoma	Older patients; invades local structures, very poor prognosis.
Lymphoma	Associated with Hashimoto thyroiditis.

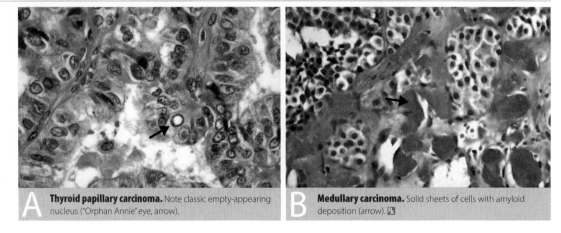

A | **Thyroid papillary carcinoma.** Note classic empty-appearing nucleus ("Orphan Annie" eye, arrow).

B | **Medullary carcinoma.** Solid sheets of cells with amyloid deposition (arrow). ℞

Hypoparathyroidism   Due to accidental surgical excision of
parathyroid glands, autoimmune destruction,
or DiGeorge syndrome. Findings:
hypocalcemia, tetany.

Chvostek sign—tapping of facial nerve (tap the
Cheek) → contraction of facial muscles.

Trousseau sign—occlusion of brachial artery
with BP cuff (cuff the Triceps) → carpal
spasm.

Pseudohypoparathyroidism (Albright
hereditary osteodystrophy)—unresponsiveness
of kidney to PTH. Hypocalcemia, shortened
4th/5th digits, short stature. Autosomal
dominant.

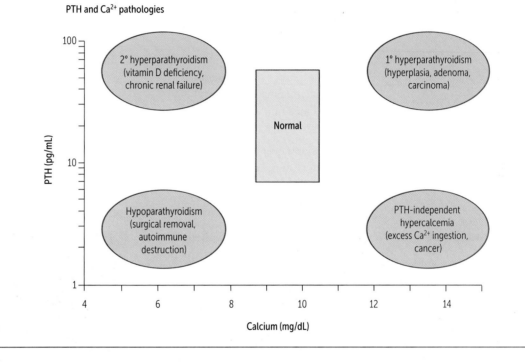

PTH and Ca²⁺ pathologies

Familial hypocalciuric   Defective Ca^{2+}-sensing receptor on parathyroid cells.
hypercalcemia   PTH cannot be suppressed by an increase in Ca^{2+} level → mild hypercalcemia with normal to
↑ PTH levels.

Hyperparathyroidism

Primary		
	Usually due to parathyroid adenoma or hyperplasia. **Hypercalcemia**, hypercalciuria (renal **stones**), hypophosphatemia, ↑ PTH, ↑ ALP, ↑ cAMP in urine. Most often asymptomatic. May present with weakness and constipation ("**groans**"), abdominal/flank pain (kidney stones, acute pancreatitis), depression ("**psychiatric overtones**").	**Osteitis fibrosa cystica**—cystic bone spaces filled with brown fibrous tissue **A** ("brown tumor" consisting of deposited hemosiderin from hemorrhages; causes bone pain). "**Stones, bones, groans, and psychiatric overtones.**"

Secondary		
	2° hyperplasia due to ↓ Ca^{2+} absorption and/or ↑ PO_4^{3-}, most often in chronic renal disease (causes hypovitaminosis D → ↓ Ca^{2+} absorption). **Hypocalcemia**, hyperphosphatemia in chronic renal failure (vs. hypophosphatemia with most other causes), ↑ ALP, ↑ PTH.	**Renal osteodystrophy**—bone lesions due to 2° or 3° hyperparathyroidism due in turn to renal disease.

Tertiary	
	Refractory (autonomous) hyperparathyroidism resulting from chronic renal disease. ↑↑ PTH, ↑ Ca^{2+}.

Pituitary adenoma	
Most commonly prolactinoma (benign). Adenoma **A** may be functional (hormone producing) or nonfunctional (silent). Nonfunctional tumors present with mass effect (bitemporal hemianopia, hypopituitarism, headache). Functional tumor presentation is based on the hormone produced (e.g., prolactinoma: amenorrhea, galactorrhea, low libido, infertility; somatotropic adenoma: acromegaly). Treatment for prolactinoma: dopamine agonists (bromocriptine or cabergoline), transsphenoidal resection.	 **Pituitary adenoma.** Coronal (left) and sagittal (right) MRI shows large lobulated mass (arrow).

Acromegaly | Excess GH in adults. Typically caused by pituitary adenoma.

FINDINGS	Large tongue with deep furrows, deep voice, large hands and feet, coarse facial features **A**, impaired glucose tolerance (insulin resistance). ↑ risk of colorectal polyps and cancer.	↑ GH in children → gigantism (↑ linear bone growth). HF most common cause of death.
DIAGNOSIS	↑ serum IGF-1; failure to suppress serum GH following oral glucose tolerance test; pituitary mass seen on brain MRI.	
TREATMENT	Pituitary adenoma resection. If not cured, treat with octreotide (somatostatin analog) or pegvisomant (growth hormone receptor antagonist).	

A **Acromegaly.** Note marked coarsening of facial features over time. RU

Diabetes insipidus | Characterized by intense thirst and polyuria with inability to concentrate urine due to lack of ADH (central) or failure of response to circulating ADH (nephrogenic).

	Central DI	**Nephrogenic DI**
ETIOLOGY	Pituitary tumor, autoimmune, trauma, surgery, ischemic encephalopathy, idiopathic	Hereditary (ADH receptor mutation), 2° to hypercalcemia, lithium, demeclocycline (ADH antagonist)
FINDINGS	↓ ADH Urine specific gravity < 1.006 Serum osmolality > 290 mOsm/kg Hyperosmotic volume contraction	Normal ADH levels Urine specific gravity < 1.006 Serum osmolality > 290 mOsm/kg Hyperosmotic volume contraction
WATER DEPRIVATION TEST[a]	> 50% ↑ in urine osmolality only after administration of ADH analog	Minimal change in urine osmolality, even after administration of ADH analog
TREATMENT	Intranasal desmopressin acetate Hydration	HCTZ, indomethacin, amiloride Hydration

[a]No water intake for 2–3 hr followed by hourly measurements of urine volume and osmolarity and plasma Na$^+$ concentration and osmolarity. ADH analog (desmopressin acetate) is administered if normal values are not clearly reached.

SIADH | Syndrome of inappropriate antidiuretic hormone secretion:
- Excessive free water retention
- Euvolemic hyponatremia with continued urinary Na$^+$ excretion
- Urine osmolality > serum osmolality

Body responds to water retention with ↓ aldosterone (hyponatremia) to maintain near-normal volume status. Very low serum Na$^+$ levels can lead to cerebral edema, seizures. Correct slowly to prevent osmotic demyelination syndrome (formerly known as central pontine myelinolysis).

Causes include:
- Ectopic ADH (e.g., small cell lung cancer)
- CNS disorders/head trauma
- Pulmonary disease
- Drugs (e.g., cyclophosphamide)

Treatment: fluid restriction, IV hypertonic saline, conivaptan, tolvaptan, demeclocycline.

Hypopituitarism

Undersecretion of pituitary hormones due to:
- Nonsecreting pituitary adenoma, craniopharyngioma
- Sheehan syndrome—ischemic infarct of pituitary following postpartum bleeding; usually presents with failure to lactate, absent menstruation, cold intolerance
- Empty sella syndrome—atrophy or compression of pituitary, often idiopathic, common in obese women
- Pituitary apoplexy—sudden hemorrhage of pituitary gland, often in the presence of an existing pituitary adenoma
- Brain injury
- Radiation

Treatment: hormone replacement therapy (corticosteroids, thyroxine, sex steroids, human growth hormone).

Diabetes mellitus

ACUTE MANIFESTATIONS

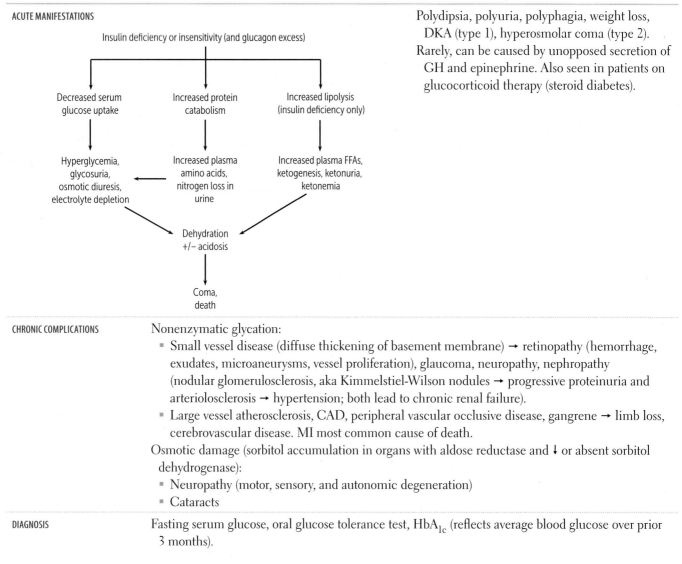

Polydipsia, polyuria, polyphagia, weight loss, DKA (type 1), hyperosmolar coma (type 2). Rarely, can be caused by unopposed secretion of GH and epinephrine. Also seen in patients on glucocorticoid therapy (steroid diabetes).

CHRONIC COMPLICATIONS

Nonenzymatic glycation:
- Small vessel disease (diffuse thickening of basement membrane) → retinopathy (hemorrhage, exudates, microaneurysms, vessel proliferation), glaucoma, neuropathy, nephropathy (nodular glomerulosclerosis, aka Kimmelstiel-Wilson nodules → progressive proteinuria and arteriolosclerosis → hypertension; both lead to chronic renal failure).
- Large vessel atherosclerosis, CAD, peripheral vascular occlusive disease, gangrene → limb loss, cerebrovascular disease. MI most common cause of death.

Osmotic damage (sorbitol accumulation in organs with aldose reductase and ↓ or absent sorbitol dehydrogenase):
- Neuropathy (motor, sensory, and autonomic degeneration)
- Cataracts

DIAGNOSIS

Fasting serum glucose, oral glucose tolerance test, HbA_{1c} (reflects average blood glucose over prior 3 months).

Type 1 vs. type 2 diabetes mellitus

Variable	Type 1	Type 2
1° DEFECT	Autoimmune destruction of β cells	↑ resistance to insulin, progressive pancreatic β-cell failure
INSULIN NECESSARY IN TREATMENT	Always	Sometimes
AGE (EXCEPTIONS COMMONLY OCCUR)	< 30 yr	> 40 yr
ASSOCIATION WITH OBESITY	No	Yes
GENETIC PREDISPOSITION	Relatively weak (50% concordance in identical twins), polygenic	Relatively strong (90% concordance in identical twins), polygenic
ASSOCIATION WITH HLA SYSTEM	Yes (HLA-DR3 and -DR4)	No
GLUCOSE INTOLERANCE	Severe	Mild to moderate
INSULIN SENSITIVITY	High	Low
KETOACIDOSIS	Common	Rare
β-CELL NUMBERS IN THE ISLETS	↓	Variable (with amyloid deposits)
SERUM INSULIN LEVEL	↓	Variable
CLASSIC SYMPTOMS OF POLYURIA, POLYDIPSIA, POLYPHAGIA, WEIGHT LOSS	Common	Sometimes
HISTOLOGY	Islet leukocytic infiltrate	Islet amyloid polypeptide (IAPP) deposits

Diabetic ketoacidosis

One of the most feared complications of diabetes. Usually due to ↑ insulin requirements from ↑ stress (e.g., infection). Excess fat breakdown and ↑ ketogenesis from ↑ free fatty acids, which are then made into ketone bodies (β-hydroxybutyrate > acetoacetate). Usually occurs in type 1 diabetes, as endogenous insulin in type 2 diabetes usually prevents lipolysis.

SIGNS/SYMPTOMS	Kussmaul respirations (rapid/deep breathing), nausea/vomiting, abdominal pain, psychosis/delirium, dehydration. Fruity breath odor (due to exhaled acetone).
LABS	Hyperglycemia, ↑ H$^+$, ↓ HCO$_3^-$ (↑ anion gap metabolic acidosis), ↑ blood ketone levels, leukocytosis. Hyperkalemia, but depleted intracellular K$^+$ due to transcellular shift from ↓ insulin (therefore total body K$^+$ is depleted).
COMPLICATIONS	Life-threatening mucormycosis (usually caused by *Rhizopus* infection), cerebral edema, cardiac arrhythmias, heart failure.
TREATMENT	IV fluids, IV insulin, and K$^+$ (to replete intracellular stores); glucose if necessary to prevent hypoglycemia.

Glucagonoma

Tumor of pancreatic α cells → overproduction of glucagon. Presents with dermatitis (necrolytic migratory erythema), diabetes (hyperglycemia), DVT, and depression.

Insulinoma	Tumor of pancreatic β cells → overproduction of insulin → hypoglycemia. May see Whipple triad: low blood glucose, symptoms of hypoglycemia (e.g., lethargy, syncope, diplopia), and resolution of symptoms after normalization of glucose levels. Symptomatic patients have ↓ blood glucose and ↑ C-peptide levels (vs. exogenous insulin use). Treatment: surgical resection.

Carcinoid syndrome

Rare syndrome caused by carcinoid tumors (neuroendocrine cells 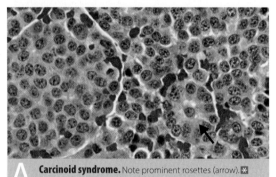), especially metastatic small bowel tumors, which secrete high levels of serotonin (5-HT). Not seen if tumor is limited to GI tract (5-HT undergoes first-pass metabolism in liver). Results in recurrent diarrhea, cutaneous flushing, asthmatic wheezing, right-sided valvular disease. ↑ 5-hydroxyindoleacetic acid (5-HIAA) in urine, niacin deficiency (pellagra).
Treatment: surgical resection, somatostatin analog (e.g., octreotide).

Rule of 1/3s:
1/3 metastasize
1/3 present with 2nd malignancy
1/3 are multiple
Most common malignancy in the small intestine.

Carcinoid syndrome. Note prominent rosettes (arrow).

Zollinger-Ellison syndrome

Gastrin-secreting tumor (gastrinoma) of pancreas or duodenum. Acid hypersecretion causes recurrent ulcers in duodenum and jejunum. Presents with abdominal pain (peptic ulcer disease, distal ulcers), diarrhea (malabsorption). Positive secretin stimulation test: gastrin levels remain elevated after administration of secretin, which normally inhibits gastrin release. May be associated with MEN 1.

Multiple endocrine neoplasias	All **MEN** syndromes have autosomal **dominant** inheritance. "All **MEN** are **dominant**" (or so they think).	
SUBTYPE	CHARACTERISTICS	COMMENTS
MEN 1	Parathyroid tumors Pituitary tumors (prolactin or GH) Pancreatic endocrine tumors—Zollinger-Ellison syndrome, insulinomas, VIPomas, glucagonomas (rare) Associated with mutation of *MEN1* gene (menin, a tumor suppressor)	MEN 1 = 3 P's: Pituitary, Parathyroid, and Pancreas; remember by drawing a diamond.
MEN 2A	Parathyroid hyperplasia Pheochromocytoma Medullary thyroid carcinoma (secretes calcitonin) Associated with marfanoid habitus; mutation in *RET* gene (codes for receptor tyrosine kinase)	MEN 2A = 2 P's: Parathyroids and Pheochromocytoma; remember by drawing a square.
MEN 2B	Pheochromocytoma Medullary thyroid carcinoma (secretes calcitonin) Oral/intestinal ganglioneuromatosis (mucosal neuromas) Associated with marfanoid habitus; mutation in *RET* gene	MEN 2B = 1 P: Pheochromocytoma; remember by drawing a triangle.

▸ ENDOCRINE—PHARMACOLOGY

Diabetes mellitus drugs	Treatment strategies:
	Type 1 DM—low-carbohydrate diet, insulin replacement
	Type 2 DM—dietary modification and exercise for weight loss; oral agents, non-insulin injectables, insulin replacement
	Gestational DM (GDM)—dietary modifications, exercise, insulin replacement if lifestyle modification fails

DRUG CLASSES	ACTION	CLINICAL USE	TOXICITIES
Insulin preparations			
Insulin, rapid acting Aspart, Glulisine, Lispro	Binds insulin receptor (tyrosine kinase activity). Liver: ↑ glucose stored as glycogen. Muscle: ↑ glycogen, protein synthesis; ↑ K^+ uptake. Fat: ↑ TG storage.	Type 1 DM, type 2 DM, GDM (postprandial glucose control).	Hypoglycemia, rare hypersensitivity reactions.
Insulin, short acting Regular		Type 1 DM, type 2 DM, GDM, DKA (IV), hyperkalemia (+ glucose), stress hyperglycemia.	
Insulin, intermediate acting NPH		Type 1 DM, type 2 DM, GDM.	
Insulin, long acting Detemir, Glargine		Type 1 DM, type 2 DM, GDM (basal glucose control).	
Oral hypoglycemic drugs			
Biguanides Metformin	Exact mechanism unknown. ↓ gluconeogenesis, ↑ glycolysis, ↑ peripheral glucose uptake (↑ insulin sensitivity).	Oral. First-line therapy in type 2 DM, causes modest weight loss. Can be used in patients without islet function.	GI upset; most serious adverse effect is lactic acidosis (thus contraindicated in renal insufficiency).
Sulfonylureas First generation: Chlorpropamide, Tolbutamide Second generation: Glimepiride, Glipizide, Glyburide	Close K^+ channel in β-cell membrane → cell depolarizes → insulin release via ↑ Ca^{2+} influx.	Stimulate release of endogenous insulin in type 2 DM. Require some islet function, so useless in type 1 DM.	Risk of hypoglycemia ↑ in renal failure. First generation: disulfiram-like effects. Second generation: hypoglycemia.
Glitazones/ thiazolidinediones Pioglitazone, Rosiglitazone	↑ insulin sensitivity in peripheral tissue. Binds to PPAR-γ nuclear transcription regulator.[a]	Used as monotherapy in type 2 DM or combined with above agents.	Weight gain, edema. Hepatotoxicity, HF, ↑ risk of fractures.

Diabetes mellitus drugs (continued)

DRUG CLASSES	ACTION	CLINICAL USE	TOXICITIES
Oral hypoglycemic drugs (continued)			
GLP-1 analogs Exenatide, Liraglutide	↑ insulin, ↓ glucagon release.	Type 2 DM.	Nausea, vomiting; pancreatitis.
DPP-4 inhibitors Linagliptin, Saxagliptin, Sitagliptin	↑ insulin, ↓ glucagon release.	Type 2 DM.	Mild urinary or respiratory infections.
Amylin analogs Pramlintide	↓ gastric emptying, ↓ glucagon.	Type 1 DM, type 2 DM.	Hypoglycemia, nausea, diarrhea.
SGLT-2 inhibitors Canagliflozin	Block reabsorption of glucose in PCT.	Type 2 DM.	Glucosuria, UTIs, vaginal yeast infections.
α-glucosidase inhibitors Acarbose, Miglitol	Inhibit intestinal brush-border α-glucosidases. Delayed carbohydrate hydrolysis and glucose absorption → ↓ postprandial hyperglycemia.	Used as monotherapy in type 2 DM or in combination with above agents.	GI disturbances.

[a]Genes activated by PPAR-γ regulate fatty acid storage and glucose metabolism. Activation of PPAR-γ ↑ insulin sensitivity and
levels of adiponectin.

Propylthiouracil, methimazole

MECHANISM	Block thyroid peroxidase, inhibiting the oxidation of iodide and the organification (coupling) of iodine → inhibition of thyroid hormone synthesis. Propylthiouracil also blocks 5'-deiodinase → ↓ peripheral conversion of T_4 to T_3.
CLINICAL USE	Hyperthyroidism. PTU blocks Peripheral conversion, used in Pregnancy.
TOXICITY	Skin rash, agranulocytosis (rare), aplastic anemia, hepatotoxicity (propylthiouracil). Methimazole is a possible teratogen (can cause aplasia cutis).

Levothyroxine (T_4), triiodothyronine (T_3)

MECHANISM	Thyroid hormone replacement.
CLINICAL USE	Hypothyroidism, myxedema. Used off-label as weight loss supplements.
TOXICITY	Tachycardia, heat intolerance, tremors, arrhythmias.

Hypothalamic/pituitary drugs

DRUG	CLINICAL USE
ADH antagonists (conivaptan, tolvaptan)	SIADH, block action of ADH at V_2-receptor.
Desmopressin acetate	Central (not nephrogenic) DI.
GH	GH deficiency, Turner syndrome.
Oxytocin	Stimulates labor, uterine contractions, milk let-down; controls uterine hemorrhage.
Somatostatin (octreotide)	Acromegaly, carcinoid syndrome, gastrinoma, glucagonoma, esophageal varices.

Demeclocycline

MECHANISM	ADH antagonist (member of tetracycline family).
CLINICAL USE	SIADH.
TOXICITY	Nephrogenic DI, photosensitivity, abnormalities of bone and teeth.

Glucocorticoids

	Beclomethasone, dexamethasone, fludrocortisone (mineralocorticoid and glucocorticoid activity), hydrocortisone, methylprednisolone, prednisone, triamcinolone.
MECHANISM	Metabolic, catabolic, anti-inflammatory, and immunosuppressive effects mediated by interactions with glucocorticoid response elements, inhibition of phospholipase A_2, and inhibition of transcription factors such as NF-κB.
CLINICAL USE	Addison disease, inflammation, immunosuppression, asthma.
TOXICITY	Iatrogenic Cushing syndrome (hypertension, weight gain, moon facies, truncal obesity, buffalo hump, thinning of skin, striae, osteoporosis, hyperglycemia, amenorrhea, immunosuppression), adrenocortical atrophy, peptic ulcers, steroid diabetes, steroid psychosis. Adrenal insufficiency when drug stopped abruptly after chronic use.

Cinacalcet

MECHANISM	Sensitizes Ca^{2+}-sensing receptor (CaSR) in parathyroid gland to circulating Ca^{2+} → ↓ PTH.
CLINICAL USE	Hypercalcemia due to 1° or 2° hyperparathyroidism.
TOXICITY	Hypocalcemia.

Gastrointestinal

"*A good set of bowels is worth more to a man than any quantity of brains.*"
—Josh Billings

"*Man should strive to have his intestines relaxed all the days of his life.*"
—Moses Maimonides

"*The colon is the playing field for all human emotions.*"
—Cyrus Kapadia, MD

▶ GASTROINTESTINAL—EMBRYOLOGY

GI embryology

Foregut—pharynx to duodenum.
Midgut—duodenum to proximal $2/3$ of transverse colon.
Hindgut—distal $1/3$ of transverse colon to anal canal above pectinate line.
Developmental defects of anterior abdominal wall due to failure of:
- Rostral fold closure—sternal defects
- Lateral fold closure—omphalocele, gastroschisis
- Caudal fold closure—bladder exstrophy

Duodenal atresia—failure to recanalize (trisomy 21).
Jejunal, ileal, colonic atresia—due to vascular accident (apple peel atresia).
Midgut development:
- 6th week—midgut herniates through umbilical ring
- 10th week—returns to abdominal cavity + rotates around superior mesenteric artery (SMA)

Pathology—malrotation of midgut, omphalocele, intestinal atresia or stenosis, volvulus.

Gastroschisis—extrusion of abdominal contents through abdominal folds; not covered by peritoneum.

Omphalocele—persistence of herniation of abdominal contents into umbilical cord, sealed by peritoneum **A**.

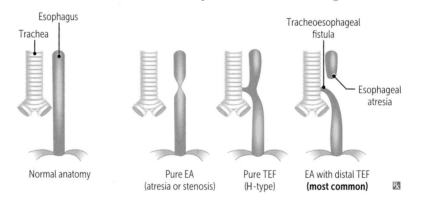

A   **Omphalocele.** Note protruding intestine covered in peritoneum. ℞

Tracheoesophageal anomalies

Esophageal atresia (EA) with distal tracheoesophageal fistula (TEF) is the most common (85%). Results in drooling, choking, and vomiting with first feeding. TEF allows air to enter stomach (visible on CXR). Cyanosis is 2° to laryngospasm (to avoid reflux-related aspiration). Clinical test: failure to pass nasogastric tube into stomach.
In **H**-type, the fistula resembles the letter **H**. In pure EA the CXR shows gasless abdomen.

Esophagus
Trachea
Tracheoesophageal fistula
Esophageal atresia

Normal anatomy   Pure EA (atresia or stenosis)   Pure TEF (H-type)   EA with distal TEF **(most common)**   ℞

Congenital pyloric stenosis

Hypertrophy of the pylorus causes obstruction. Palpable "olive" mass in epigastric region and nonbilious projectile vomiting at ≈ 2–6 weeks old. Occurs in 1/600 live births, more often in firstborn males. Results in hypokalemic hypochloremic metabolic alkalosis (2° to vomiting of gastric acid and subsequent volume contraction). Treatment is surgical incision (pyloromyotomy).

Pancreas and spleen embryology

Pancreas—derived from foregut. Ventral pancreatic buds contribute to uncinate process and main pancreatic duct. The dorsal pancreatic bud alone becomes the body, tail, isthmus, and accessory pancreatic duct. Both the ventral and dorsal buds contribute to the pancreatic head.

Annular pancreas—ventral pancreatic bud abnormally encircles 2nd part of duodenum; forms a ring of pancreatic tissue that may cause duodenal narrowing **A**.

Pancreas divisum—ventral and dorsal parts fail to fuse at 8 weeks. Common anomaly; mostly asymptomatic, but may cause chronic abdominal pain and/or pancreatitis.

Spleen—arises in mesentery of stomach (hence is mesodermal) but is supplied by foregut (celiac artery).

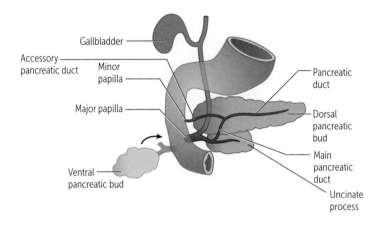

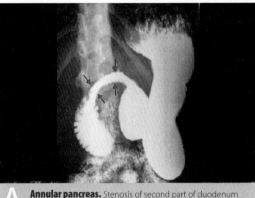

A **Annular pancreas.** Stenosis of second part of duodenum (arrows) caused by circumferential ectopic pancreatic tissue. ✳

▶ GASTROINTESTINAL—ANATOMY

Retroperitoneal structures

Retroperitoneal structures include GI structures that lack a mesentery and non-GI structures. Injuries to retroperitoneal structures can cause blood or gas accumulation in retroperitoneal space.

SAD PUCKER:
Suprarenal (adrenal) glands [not shown]
Aorta and IVC
Duodenum (2nd through 4th parts)
Pancreas (except tail)
Ureters [not shown]
Colon (descending and ascending)
Kidneys
Esophagus (thoracic portion) [not shown]
Rectum (partially) [not shown]

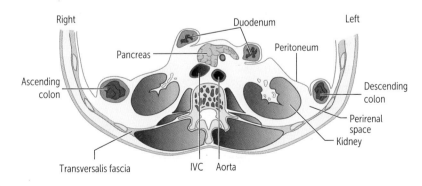

Important GI ligaments

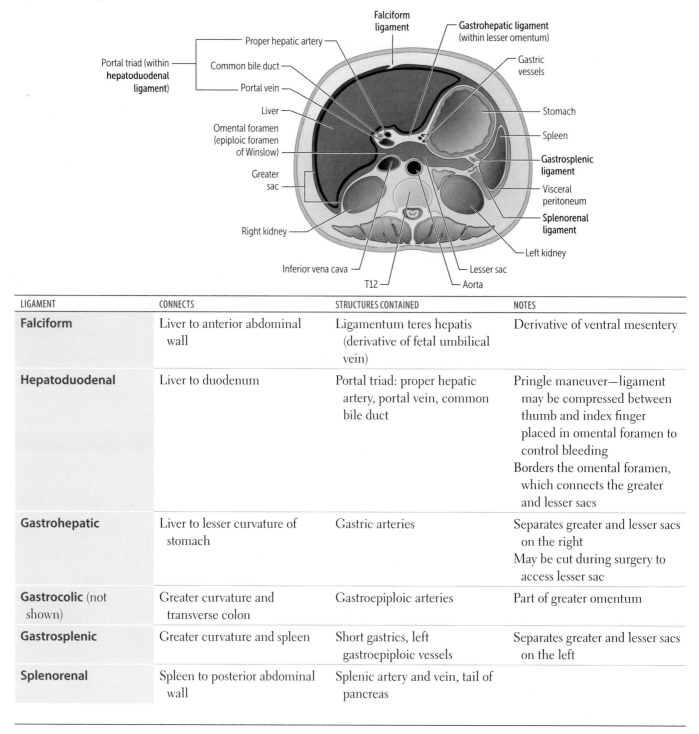

LIGAMENT	CONNECTS	STRUCTURES CONTAINED	NOTES
Falciform	Liver to anterior abdominal wall	Ligamentum teres hepatis (derivative of fetal umbilical vein)	Derivative of ventral mesentery
Hepatoduodenal	Liver to duodenum	Portal triad: proper hepatic artery, portal vein, common bile duct	Pringle maneuver—ligament may be compressed between thumb and index finger placed in omental foramen to control bleeding Borders the omental foramen, which connects the greater and lesser sacs
Gastrohepatic	Liver to lesser curvature of stomach	Gastric arteries	Separates greater and lesser sacs on the right May be cut during surgery to access lesser sac
Gastrocolic (not shown)	Greater curvature and transverse colon	Gastroepiploic arteries	Part of greater omentum
Gastrosplenic	Greater curvature and spleen	Short gastrics, left gastroepiploic vessels	Separates greater and lesser sacs on the left
Splenorenal	Spleen to posterior abdominal wall	Splenic artery and vein, tail of pancreas	

Digestive tract anatomy

Layers of gut wall (inside to outside—**MSMS**):
- **M**ucosa—epithelium, lamina propria, muscularis mucosa
- **S**ubmucosa—includes **S**ubmucosal nerve plexus (Meissner), **S**ecretes fluid
- **M**uscularis externa—includes **M**yenteric nerve plexus (Auerbach), **M**otility
- **S**erosa (when intraperitoneal), adventitia (when retroperitoneal)

Ulcers can extend into submucosa, inner or outer muscular layer. Erosions are in the mucosa only.

Frequencies of basal electric rhythm (slow waves):
- Stomach—3 waves/min
- Duodenum—12 waves/min
- Ileum—8–9 waves/min

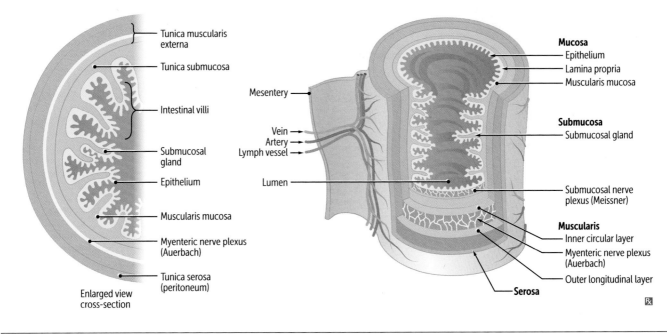

Enlarged view cross-section

Digestive tract histology

Esophagus	Nonkeratinized stratified squamous epithelium.
Stomach	Gastric glands.
Duodenum	Villi and microvilli ↑ absorptive surface. Brunner glands (HCO_3^--secreting cells of submucosa) and crypts of Lieberkühn.
Jejunum	Plicae circulares and crypts of Lieberkühn.
Ileum	Peyer patches (lymphoid aggregates in lamina propria, submucosa), plicae circulares (proximal ileum), and crypts of Lieberkühn. Largest number of goblet cells in the small intestine.
Colon	Colon has crypts of Lieberkühn but no villi; abundant goblet cells.

Abdominal aorta and branches

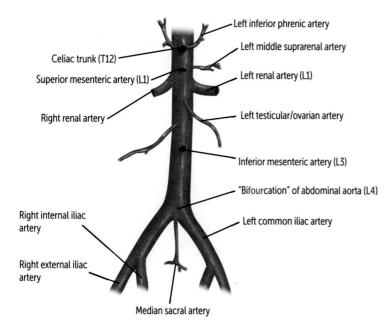

- Left inferior phrenic artery
- Left middle suprarenal artery
- Celiac trunk (T12)
- Left renal artery (L1)
- Superior mesenteric artery (L1)
- Right renal artery
- Left testicular/ovarian artery
- Inferior mesenteric artery (L3)
- "Bifourcation" of abdominal aorta (L4)
- Right internal iliac artery
- Left common iliac artery
- Right external iliac artery
- Median sacral artery

Arteries supplying GI structures branch **anteriorly**. Arteries supplying non-GI structures branch **laterally**.

Superior mesenteric artery (SMA) syndrome occurs when the transverse portion (third part) of the duodenum is entrapped between SMA and aorta, causing intestinal obstruction.

GI blood supply and innervation

EMBRYONIC GUT REGION	ARTERY	PARASYMPATHETIC INNERVATION	VERTEBRAL LEVEL	STRUCTURES SUPPLIED
Foregut	Celiac	Vagus	T12/L1	Pharynx (vagus nerve only) and lower esophagus (celiac artery only) to proximal duodenum; liver, gallbladder, pancreas, spleen (mesoderm)
Midgut	SMA	Vagus	L1	Distal duodenum to proximal $^2/_3$ of transverse colon
Hindgut	IMA	Pelvic	L3	Distal $^1/_3$ of transverse colon to upper portion of rectum; splenic flexure is a watershed region between SMA and IMA

Celiac trunk

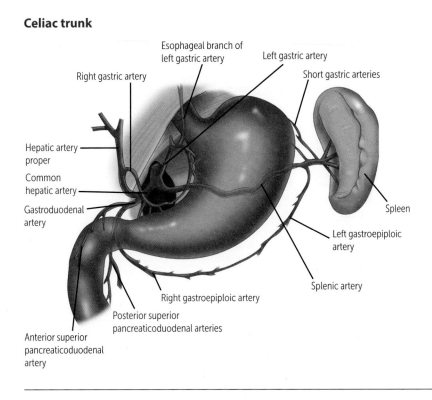

Right gastric artery

Esophageal branch of
left gastric artery

Left gastric artery

Short gastric arteries

Hepatic artery
proper

Common
hepatic artery

Gastroduodenal
artery

Spleen

Left gastroepiploic
artery

Splenic artery

Right gastroepiploic artery

Posterior superior
pancreaticoduodenal arteries

Anterior superior
pancreaticoduodenal
artery

Branches of celiac trunk: common hepatic, splenic, and left gastric. These constitute the main blood supply of the stomach.

Short gastrics have poor anastomoses if splenic artery is blocked.

Strong anastomoses exist between:

- Left and right gastroepiploics
- Left and right gastrics

Portosystemic anastomoses

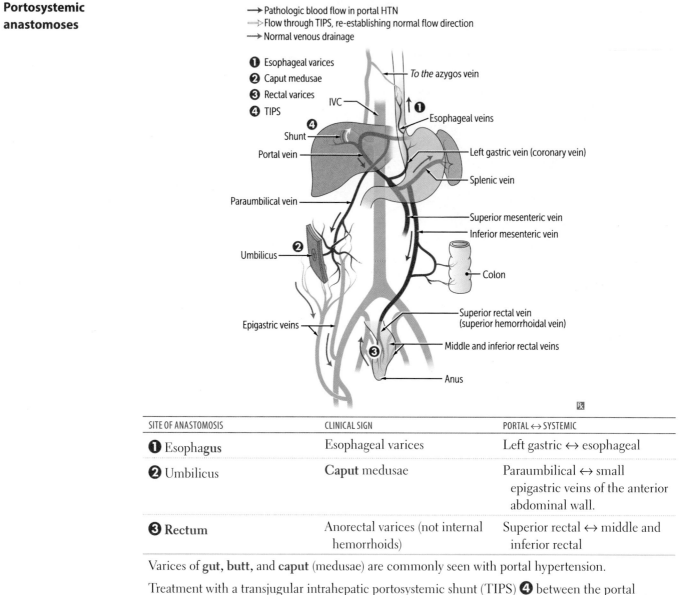

→ Pathologic blood flow in portal HTN
⇒ Flow through TIPS, re-establishing normal flow direction
→ Normal venous drainage

❶ Esophageal varices
❷ Caput medusae
❸ Rectal varices
❹ TIPS

SITE OF ANASTOMOSIS	CLINICAL SIGN	PORTAL ↔ SYSTEMIC
❶ **Esophagus**	Esophageal varices	Left gastric ↔ esophageal
❷ **Umbilicus**	**Caput** medusae	Paraumbilical ↔ small epigastric veins of the anterior abdominal wall.
❸ **Rectum**	Anorectal varices (not internal hemorrhoids)	Superior rectal ↔ middle and inferior rectal

Varices of **gut, butt,** and **caput** (medusae) are commonly seen with portal hypertension.

Treatment with a transjugular intrahepatic portosystemic shunt (TIPS) ❹ between the portal vein and hepatic vein relieves portal hypertension by shunting blood to the systemic circulation, bypassing the liver.

Pectinate (dentate) line

Formed where endoderm (hindgut) meets ectoderm.

Above pectinate line—internal hemorrhoids, adenocarcinoma.

Arterial supply from superior rectal artery (branch of IMA).

Venous drainage: superior rectal vein → inferior mesenteric vein → portal system.

Internal hemorrhoids receive visceral innervation and are therefore **not painful**. Lymphatic drainage to internal iliac lymph nodes.

Below pectinate line—external hemorrhoids, anal fissures, squamous cell carcinoma.

Arterial supply from inferior rectal artery (branch of internal pudendal artery).

Venous drainage: inferior rectal vein → internal pudendal vein → internal iliac vein → common iliac vein → IVC.

External hemorrhoids receive somatic innervation (inferior rectal branch of pudendal nerve) and are therefore **painful** if thrombosed. Lymphatic drainage to superficial inguinal nodes.

Anal fissure—tear in the anal mucosa below the Pectinate line. **P**ain while **P**ooping; blood on "toilet" **P**aper. Located **P**osteriorly since this area is **P**oorly **P**erfused.

Internal hemorrhoids
External hemorrhoid
Pectinate line

Liver anatomy

Apical surface of hepatocytes faces bile canaliculi. Basolateral surface faces sinusoids.

Zone I—periportal zone:
- Affected 1st by viral hepatitis
- Ingested toxins (e.g., cocaine)

Zone II—intermediate zone:
- Yellow fever

Zone III—pericentral vein (centrilobular) zone:
- Affected 1st by ischemia
- Contains cytochrome P-450 system
- Most sensitive to metabolic toxins
- Site of alcoholic hepatitis

Sinusoids draining to central vein
Bile canaliculus
Bile ductule
Branch of portal vein
Branch of hepatic artery
Portal triad
Liver cell plates
Kupffer cell **A**
Space of Disse (lymphatic drainage)
Central vein (to hepatic veins and systemic circulation)
Blood flow
Bile flow
Zone I *Zone II* *Zone III*

A **Kupffer cells.** Trichrome stain shows Kupffer cells (specialized macrophages; black arrows) in resolving liver injury. Yellow arrow, hepatic venule. ✱

Biliary structures

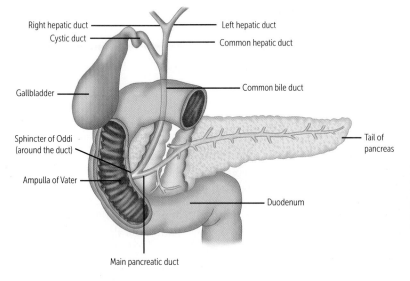

Gallstones 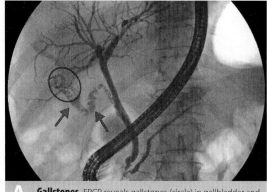 that reach the confluence of the common bile and pancreatic ducts at the ampulla of Vater can block both the common bile and pancreatic ducts (double duct sign), causing both cholangitis and pancreatitis, respectively.

Tumors that arise in head of pancreas can cause obstruction of common bile duct alone → painless jaundice.

A **Gallstones.** ERCP reveals gallstones (circle) in gallbladder and cystic duct (arrows). ✱

Femoral region

ORGANIZATION	Lateral to medial: Nerve-Artery-Vein-Empty space-Lymphatics.	You go from **lateral to medial** to find your **NAVEL**.
Femoral triangle	Contains femoral vein, artery, nerve.	**V**enous near the **pen**is.
Femoral sheath	Fascial tube 3–4 cm below inguinal ligament. Contains femoral vein, artery, and canal (deep inguinal lymph nodes) but not femoral nerve.	

Inguinal canal

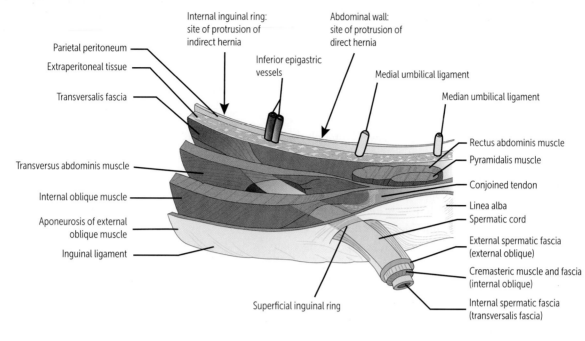

Internal inguinal ring:
site of protrusion of
indirect hernia

Abdominal wall:
site of protrusion of
direct hernia

Parietal peritoneum

Extraperitoneal tissue

Inferior epigastric
vessels

Medial umbilical ligament

Median umbilical ligament

Transversalis fascia

Rectus abdominis muscle

Pyramidalis muscle

Transversus abdominis muscle

Conjoined tendon

Internal oblique muscle

Linea alba

Aponeurosis of external
oblique muscle

Spermatic cord

External spermatic fascia
(external oblique)

Inguinal ligament

Cremasteric muscle and fascia
(internal oblique)

Superficial inguinal ring

Internal spermatic fascia
(transversalis fascia)

Hernias

A protrusion of peritoneum through an opening, usually a site of weakness.

Diaphragmatic hernia	Abdominal structures enter the thorax; may occur due to congenital defect of pleuroperitoneal membrane, or as a result of trauma. Commonly occurs on left side due to relative protection of right hemidiaphragm by liver. Most commonly a hiatal hernia, in which stomach herniates upward through the esophageal hiatus of the diaphragm.	Sliding hiatal hernia is most common. Gastroesophageal junction is displaced upward; "hourglass stomach." Paraesophageal hernia—gastroesophageal junction is usually normal. Fundus protrudes into the thorax.
Indirect inguinal hernia	Goes through the internal (deep) inguinal ring, external (superficial) inguinal ring, and into the scrotum. Enters internal inguinal ring lateral to inferior epigastric artery. Occurs in infants owing to failure of processus vaginalis to close (can form hydrocele). Much more common in males.	An indirect inguinal hernia follows the path of descent of the testes. Covered by all 3 layers of spermatic fascia.

Direct inguinal hernia	Protrudes through the inguinal (Hesselbach) triangle. Bulges directly through abdominal wall medial to inferior epigastric artery. Goes through the external (superficial) inguinal ring only. Covered by external spermatic fascia. Usually in older men.	MDs don't LIe:
		    Medial to inferior epigastric artery = Direct hernia.
		    Lateral to inferior epigastric artery = Indirect hernia.

Femoral hernia	Protrudes below inguinal ligament through femoral canal below and lateral to pubic tubercle. More common in females.	Leading cause of bowel incarceration.

Hesselbach triangle:
- Inferior epigastric vessels
- Lateral border of rectus abdominis
- Inguinal ligament

▶ GASTROINTESTINAL—PHYSIOLOGY

GI regulatory substances

REGULATORY SUBSTANCE	SOURCE	ACTION	REGULATION	NOTES
Gastrin	G cells (antrum of stomach, duodenum)	↑ gastric H⁺ secretion ↑ growth of gastric mucosa ↑ gastric motility	↑ by stomach distention/ alkalinization, amino acids, peptides, vagal stimulation ↓ by pH < 1.5	↑ in chronic atrophic gastritis (e.g., *H. pylori*). ↑↑ in Zollinger-Ellison syndrome. ↑ by chronic PPI use.
Somatostatin	D cells (pancreatic islets, GI mucosa)	↓ gastric acid and pepsinogen secretion ↓ pancreatic and small intestine fluid secretion ↓ gallbladder contraction ↓ insulin and glucagon release	↑ by acid ↓ by vagal stimulation	Inhibits secretion of GH, insulin, and other hormones (encourages **somato-stasis**). Octreotide is an analog used to treat acromegaly, insulinoma, carcinoid syndrome, and variceal bleeding.
Cholecystokinin	I cells (duodenum, jejunum)	↑ pancreatic secretion ↑ gallbladder contraction ↓ gastric emptying ↑ sphincter of Oddi relaxation	↑ by fatty acids, amino acids	CCK acts on neural muscarinic pathways to cause pancreatic secretion.
Secretin	S cells (duodenum)	↑ pancreatic HCO₃⁻ secretion ↓ gastric acid secretion ↑ bile secretion	↑ by acid, fatty acids in lumen of duodenum	↑ HCO₃⁻ neutralizes gastric acid in duodenum, allowing pancreatic enzymes to function.
Glucose-dependent insulinotropic peptide (GIP)	K cells (duodenum, jejunum)	Exocrine: ↓ gastric H⁺ secretion Endocrine: ↑ insulin release	↑ by fatty acids, amino acids, oral glucose	Also known as gastric inhibitory peptide. Oral glucose load leads to ↑ insulin compared to IV equivalent due to GIP secretion.
Motilin	Small intestine	Produces migrating motor complexes (MMCs)	↑ in fasting state	Motilin receptor agonists (e.g., erythromycin) are used to stimulate intestinal peristalsis.
Vasoactive intestinal polypeptide (VIP)	Parasympathetic ganglia in sphincters, gallbladder, small intestine	↑ intestinal water and electrolyte secretion ↑ relaxation of intestinal smooth muscle and sphincters	↑ by distention and vagal stimulation ↓ by adrenergic input	VIPoma—non-α, non-β islet cell pancreatic tumor that secretes VIP. Copious **W**atery **D**iarrhea, **H**ypokalemia, and **A**chlorhydria (**WDHA** syndrome).
Nitric oxide		↑ smooth muscle relaxation, including lower esophageal sphincter (LES)		Loss of NO secretion is implicated in ↑ LES tone of achalasia.

GI secretory products

PRODUCT	SOURCE	ACTION	REGULATION	NOTES
Intrinsic factor	Parietal cells (stomach)	Vitamin B_{12}–binding protein (required for B_{12} uptake in terminal ileum)		Autoimmune destruction of parietal cells → chronic gastritis and pernicious anemia.
Gastric acid	Parietal cells (stomach)	↓ stomach pH	↑ by histamine, ACh, gastrin ↓ by somatostatin, GIP, prostaglandin, secretin	Gastrinoma: gastrin-secreting tumor that causes high levels of acid and ulcers refractory to medical therapy (i.e., PPI).
Pepsin	Chief cells (stomach)	Protein digestion	↑ by vagal stimulation, local acid	Pepsinogen (inactive) is converted to pepsin (active) in the presence of H^+.
HCO_3^-	Mucosal cells (stomach, duodenum, salivary glands, pancreas) and Brunner glands (duodenum)	Neutralizes acid	↑ by pancreatic and biliary secretion with secretin	HCO_3^- is trapped in mucus that covers the gastric epithelium.

Locations of GI secretory cells

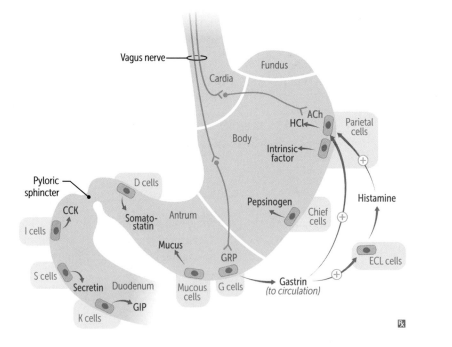

Gastrin ↑ acid secretion primarily through its effects on enterochromaffin-like (ECL) cells (leading to histamine release) rather than through its direct effect on parietal cells.

Gastric parietal cell

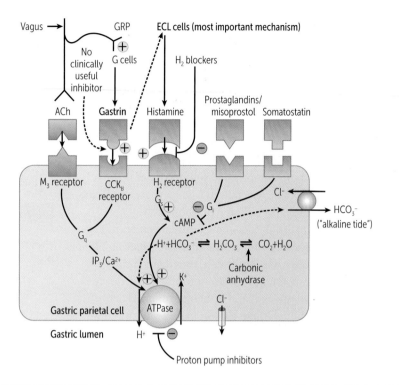

Pancreatic secretions	Isotonic fluid; low flow → high Cl^-, high flow → high HCO_3^-.	
ENZYME	ROLE	NOTES
α-amylase	Starch digestion	Secreted in active form
Lipases	Fat digestion	
Proteases	Protein digestion	Includes trypsin, chymotrypsin, elastase, carboxypeptidases Secreted as proenzymes also known as zymogens
Trypsinogen	Converted to active enzyme trypsin → activation of other proenzymes and cleaving of additional trypsinogen molecules into active trypsin (positive feedback loop)	Converted to trypsin by enterokinase/enteropeptidase, a brush-border enzyme on duodenal and jejunal mucosa

Carbohydrate absorption	Only monosaccharides (glucose, galactose, fructose) are absorbed by enterocytes. Glucose and galactose are taken up by SGLT1 (Na^+ dependent). Fructose is taken up by facilitated diffusion by GLUT-5. All are transported to blood by GLUT-2. D-xylose absorption test: distinguishes GI mucosal damage from other causes of malabsorption.

Vitamin/mineral absorption

Iron	Absorbed as Fe^{2+} in duodenum.	Iron Fist, Bro
Folate	Absorbed in small bowel.	Clinically relevant in patients with small bowel disease or after resection.
B$_{12}$	Absorbed in terminal ileum along with bile salts, requires intrinsic factor.	

Peyer patches	Unencapsulated lymphoid tissue A found in lamina propria and submucosa of ileum. Contain specialized M cells that sample and present antigens to immune cells. B cells stimulated in germinal centers of Peyer patches differentiate into IgA-secreting plasma cells, which ultimately reside in lamina propria. IgA receives protective secretory component and is then transported across the epithelium to the gut to deal with intraluminal antigen.	Think of **IgA**, the **I**ntra-gut **A**ntibody. And always say "secretory IgA."

Peyer patches. Seen in cross-section of ileum (oval). ✱

Bile	Composed of bile salts (bile acids conjugated to glycine or taurine, making them water soluble), phospholipids, cholesterol, bilirubin, water, and ions. Cholesterol 7α-hydroxylase catalyzes rate-limiting step of bile synthesis. Functions: ▪ Digestion and absorption of lipids and fat-soluble vitamins ▪ Cholesterol excretion (body's only means of eliminating cholesterol) ▪ Antimicrobial activity (via membrane disruption)

Bilirubin

Heme is metabolized by heme oxygenase to biliverdin, which is subsequently reduced to bilirubin. Unconjugated bilirubin is removed from blood by liver, conjugated with glucuronate, and excreted in bile.

Direct bilirubin—conjugated with glucuronic acid; water soluble.

Indirect bilirubin—unconjugated; water insoluble.

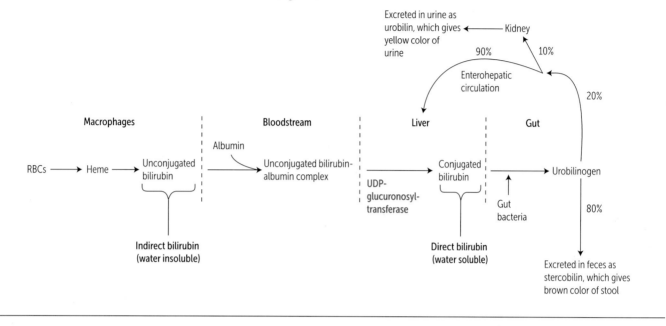

▶ GASTROINTESTINAL—PATHOLOGY

Salivary gland tumors

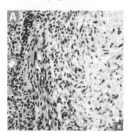

Generally benign and occur in parotid gland:

- Pleomorphic adenoma (benign mixed tumor)—most common salivary gland tumor **A**. Presents as painless, mobile mass. Composed of chondromyxoid stroma and epithelium and recurs if incompletely excised or ruptured intraoperatively.
- Mucoepidermoid carcinoma—most common malignant tumor, has mucinous and squamous components. Typically presents as painless, slow-growing mass.
- Warthin tumor (papillary cystadenoma lymphomatosum)—benign cystic tumor with germinal centers.

Achalasia

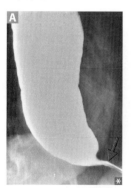

Failure of relaxation of LES due to loss of myenteric (Auerbach) plexus. High LES resting pressure and uncoordinated peristalsis → progressive dysphagia to solids and liquids (vs. obstruction—solids only). Barium swallow shows dilated esophagus with an area of distal stenosis. Associated with ↑ risk of esophageal squamous cell carcinoma.

A-chalasia = absence of relaxation.
"Bird's beak" on barium swallow **A**.
2° achalasia may arise from Chagas disease (*T. cruzi* infection) or malignancies (mass effect or paraneoplastic).

Esophageal pathologies

Boerhaave syndrome	Transmural, usually distal esophageal with pneumomediastinum (arrows) **A** due to violent retching; surgical emergency.
Eosinophilic esophagitis	Infiltration of eosinophils in the esophagus in atopic patients. Food allergens → dysphagia, heartburn, strictures. Unresponsive to GERD therapy.
Esophageal strictures	Associated with lye ingestion and acid reflux.
Esophageal varices	Dilated submucosal veins **B** **C** in lower ⅓ of esophagus 2° to portal hypertension. Common in alcoholics, may be source of upper GI bleeding.
Esophagitis	Associated with reflux, infection in immunocompromised (*Candida*: white pseudomembrane; HSV-1: punched-out ulcers; CMV: linear ulcers), or chemical ingestion.
Gastroesophageal reflux disease	Commonly presents as heartburn and regurgitation upon lying down. May also present with nocturnal cough and dyspnea, adult-onset asthma. Decrease in LES tone.
Mallory-Weiss syndrome	Mucosal lacerations at the gastroesophageal junction due to severe vomiting. Leads to hematemesis. Usually found in alcoholics and bulimics.
Plummer-Vinson syndrome	Triad of **D**ysphagia, **I**ron deficiency anemia, and **E**sophageal webs. May be associated with glossitis. Increased risk of esophageal squamous cell carcinoma ("**Plumbers**" DIE).
Sclerodermal esophageal dysmotility	Esophageal smooth muscle atrophy → ↓ LES pressure and dysmotility → acid reflux and dysphagia → stricture, Barrett esophagus, and aspiration. Part of CREST syndrome.

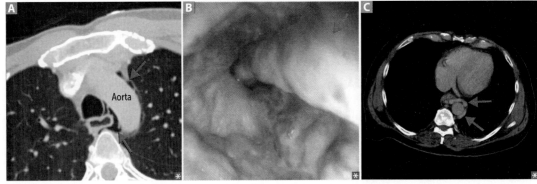

Aorta

Barrett esophagus   Glandular metaplasia—replacement of nonkeratinized stratified squamous epithelium with intestinal epithelium (nonciliated columnar with goblet cells) in distal esophagus **A**. Due to chronic acid reflux (GERD). Associated with esophagitis, esophageal ulcers, and ↑ risk of esophageal adenocarcinoma.

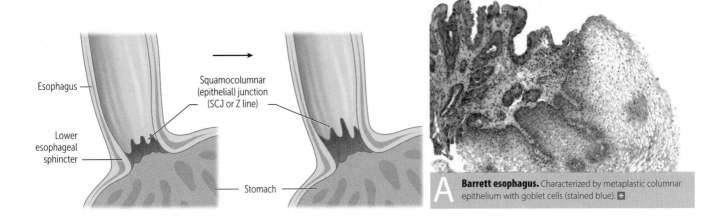

Esophagus

Squamocolumnar (epithelial) junction (SCJ or Z line)

Lower esophageal sphincter

Stomach

A **Barrett esophagus.** Characterized by metaplastic columnar epithelium with goblet cells (stained blue). ✱

Esophageal cancer

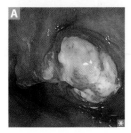

Can be squamous cell carcinoma A or adenocarcinoma. Typically presents with progressive dysphagia (first solids, then liquids) and weight loss; poor prognosis. Risk factors include:

- Achalasia
- Alcohol—squamous
- Barrett esophagus—adeno
- Cigarettes—both
- Diverticula (e.g., Zenker)—squamous
- Esophageal web—squamous
- Familial
- Fat (obesity)—adeno
- GERD—adeno
- Hot liquids—squamous

AABCDEFFGH.
Worldwide, squamous cell is more common.
Adenocarcinoma is most common type in America.
Squamous cell—upper $2/3$.
Adenocarcinoma—lower $1/3$.

Gastritis

Acute gastritis (erosive)	Disruption of mucosal barrier → inflammation. Can be caused by: - NSAIDs—↓ PGE_2 → ↓ gastric mucosa protection - Burns (Curling ulcer)—↓ plasma volume → sloughing of gastric mucosa - Brain injury (Cushing ulcer)—↑ vagal stimulation → ↑ ACh → ↑ H^+ production	Especially common among alcoholics and patients taking daily NSAIDs (e.g., patients with rheumatoid arthritis). **Burned** by the **Curling** iron. Always **Cushion** the **brain**.

Chronic gastritis (nonerosive)

Type A (fundus/body)	Autoimmune disorder characterized by Autoantibodies to parietal cells, pernicious Anemia, and Achlorhydria. Associated with other autoimmune disorders.	A comes before B: - Type **A**—**A**utoimmune; first part of the stomach (fundus/body). - Type **B**—*H. pylori* **B**acteria; second part of the stomach (antrum).
Type B (antrum)	Most common type. Caused by *H. pylori* infection. ↑ risk of MALT lymphoma.	

Ménétrier disease

Gastric hyperplasia of mucosa → hypertrophied rugae, excess mucus production with resultant protein loss and parietal cell atrophy with ↓ acid production. Precancerous. Rugae of stomach are so hypertrophied that they look like brain gyri A.

Ménétrier disease. Characteristic hypertrophied rugae (arrows).

Stomach cancer

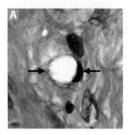

Commonly gastric adenocarcinoma; lymphoma; carcinoid (rare). Early aggressive local spread with node/liver metastases. Often presents with weight loss, early satiety, and in some cases acanthosis nigricans.

- **Intestinal**—associated with *H. pylori*, dietary nitrosamines (smoked foods), tobacco smoking, achlorhydria, chronic gastritis. Commonly on lesser curvature; looks like ulcer with raised margins.
- **Diffuse**—not associated with *H. pylori*; signet ring cells (mucin-filled cells with peripheral nuclei) A; stomach wall grossly thickened and leathery (linitis plastica).

Virchow node—involvement of left supraclavicular node by metastasis from stomach.

Krukenberg tumor—bilateral metastases to ovaries. Abundant mucin-secreting, signet ring cells.

Sister Mary Joseph nodule—subcutaneous periumbilical metastasis.

Peptic ulcer disease

	Gastric ulcer	Duodenal ulcer
PAIN	Can be Greater with meals—weight loss	Decreases with meals—weight gain
H. PYLORI INFECTION	In 70%	In almost 100%
MECHANISM	↓ mucosal protection against gastric acid	↓ mucosal protection or ↑ gastric acid secretion
OTHER CAUSES	NSAIDs	Zollinger-Ellison syndrome
RISK OF CARCINOMA	↑	Generally benign
OTHER	Biopsy margins to rule out malignancy	Hypertrophy of Brunner glands

Ulcer complications

Hemorrhage	Gastric, duodenal (posterior > anterior). Ruptured gastric ulcer on the lesser curvature of stomach → bleeding from left gastric artery. An ulcer on the posterior wall of duodenum → bleeding from gastroduodenal artery.
Perforation	Duodenal (anterior > posterior). May see free air under diaphragm A with referred pain to the shoulder via phrenic nerve.

A **Ulcer complications.** Upright chest radiograph shows free air under diaphragm (arrows). ✲

Malabsorption syndromes	Can cause diarrhea, steatorrhea, weight loss, weakness, vitamin and mineral deficiencies.	
Celiac disease	Autoimmune-mediated intolerance of gliadin (gluten protein found in wheat) → malabsorption and steatorrhea. Associated with HLA-DQ2, HLA-DQ8, northern European descent, dermatitis herpetiformis, ↓ bone density. Findings: anti-endomysial, anti-tissue transglutaminase, and anti-gliadin antibodies; blunting of villi; and lymphocytes in lamina propria **A**. Moderately ↑ risk of malignancy (e.g., T-cell lymphoma).	↓ mucosal absorption primarily affects distal duodenum and/or proximal jejunum. Treatment: gluten-free diet.
Disaccharidase deficiency	Most common is lactase deficiency → milk intolerance. Normal-appearing villi. Osmotic diarrhea. Since lactase is located at tips of intestinal villi, self-limited lactase deficiency can occur following injury (e.g., viral enteritis).	Lactose tolerance test: ⊕ for lactase deficiency if administration of lactose produces symptoms and serum glucose rises < 20 mg/dL.
Pancreatic insufficiency	Due to cystic fibrosis, obstructing cancer, chronic pancreatitis. Causes malabsorption of fat and fat-soluble vitamins (A, D, E, K) as well as vitamin B_{12}.	↑ neutral fat in stool. D-xylose absorption test: normal urinary excretion in pancreatic insufficiency; ↓ excretion with intestinal mucosa defects or bacterial overgrowth.
Tropical sprue	Similar findings as celiac sprue (affects small bowel), but responds to antibiotics. Cause is unknown, but seen in residents of or recent visitors to tropics.	
Whipple disease	Infection with *Tropheryma whipplei* (gram positive); PAS ⊕ **foamy** macrophages in intestinal lamina propria **B**, mesenteric nodes. Cardiac symptoms, Arthralgias, and Neurologic symptoms are common. Most often occurs in older men.	**Foamy Whipp**ed cream in a **CAN**.

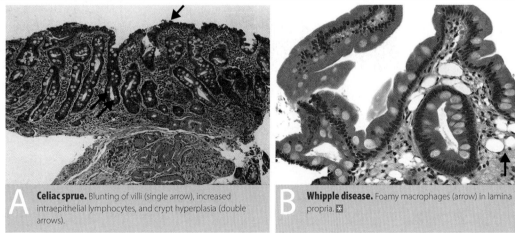

A **Celiac sprue.** Blunting of villi (single arrow), increased intraepithelial lymphocytes, and crypt hyperplasia (double arrows).

B **Whipple disease.** Foamy macrophages (arrow) in lamina propria.

Inflammatory bowel diseases

	Crohn disease	Ulcerative colitis
LOCATION	Any portion of the GI tract, usually the terminal ileum and colon. **Skip** lesions, **rectal** sparing.	Colitis = colon inflammation. Continuous colonic lesions, always with rectal involvement.
GROSS MORPHOLOGY	Transmural inflammation → fistulas. **Cobblestone** mucosa, creeping **fat**, bowel wall thickening ("string sign" on barium swallow x-ray 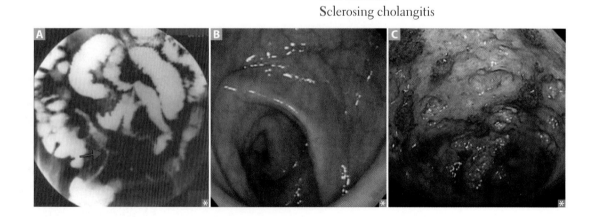), linear ulcers, fissures.	Mucosal and submucosal inflammation only. Friable mucosal pseudopolyps (compare normal B with diseased C) with freely hanging mesentery. Loss of haustra → "lead pipe" appearance on imaging.
MICROSCOPIC MORPHOLOGY	Noncaseating **gran**ulomas and lymphoid aggregates (Th1 mediated).	Crypt abscesses and ulcers, bleeding, no granulomas (Th2 mediated).
COMPLICATIONS	Strictures (leading to obstruction), fistulas (including enterovesical fistulae, which can cause recurrent polymicrobial UTIs), perianal disease, malabsorption, nutritional depletion, colorectal cancer, gallstones.	Malnutrition, sclerosing cholangitis, toxic megacolon, colorectal carcinoma (worse with right-sided colitis or pancolitis).
INTESTINAL MANIFESTATION	Diarrhea that may or may not be bloody.	Bloody diarrhea.
EXTRAINTESTINAL MANIFESTATIONS	Migratory polyarthritis, erythema nodosum, ankylosing spondylitis, pyoderma gangrenosum, aphthous ulcers, uveitis, kidney stones.	Pyoderma gangrenosum, erythema nodosum, 1° sclerosing cholangitis, ankylosing spondylitis, aphthous ulcers, uveitis.
TREATMENT	Corticosteroids, azathioprine, antibiotics (e.g., ciprofloxacin, metronidazole), infliximab, adalimumab.	5-aminosalicylic preparations (e.g., mesalamine), 6-mercaptopurine, infliximab, colectomy.
	For **Crohn**, think of a **fat gran**ny and an old **crone skip**ping down a **cobblestone** road away from the **wreck** (rectal sparing).	Ulcerative colitis causes **ULCCCERS**: Ulcers Large intestine Continuous, Colorectal carcinoma, Crypt abscesses Extends proximally Red diarrhea Sclerosing cholangitis

Irritable bowel syndrome

Recurrent abdominal pain associated with ≥ 2 of the following:

- Pain improves with defecation
- Change in stool frequency
- Change in appearance of stool

No structural abnormalities. Most common in middle-aged women. Chronic symptoms. May present with diarrhea, constipation, or alternating symptoms. Pathophysiology is multifaceted. Treat symptoms.

Appendicitis

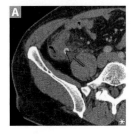

Acute inflammation of the appendix due to obstruction by fecalith **A** (in adults) or lymphoid hyperplasia (in children).

Initial diffuse periumbilical pain migrates to McBurney point (⅓ the distance from right anterior superior iliac spine to umbilicus). Nausea, fever; may perforate → peritonitis; may elicit psoas, obturator, Rovsing sign, guarding and rebound tenderness on exam.

Differential: diverticulitis (elderly), ectopic pregnancy (use β-hCG to rule out).

Treatment: appendectomy.

Diverticula of the GI tract

Diverticulum

Blind pouch **A** protruding from the alimentary tract that communicates with the lumen of the gut. Most diverticula (esophagus, stomach, duodenum, colon) are acquired and are termed "false" in that they lack or have an attenuated muscularis externa. Most often in sigmoid colon.

"True" diverticulum—all 3 gut wall layers outpouch (e.g., Meckel).

"False" diverticulum or pseudodiverticulum— only mucosa and submucosa outpouch. Occur especially where vasa recta perforate muscularis externa.

Diverticulosis

Many false diverticula of the colon, commonly sigmoid. Common (in ~ 50% of people > 60 years). Caused by ↑ intraluminal pressure and focal weakness in colonic wall. Associated with low-fiber diets.

Often asymptomatic or associated with vague discomfort. A common cause of hematochezia. Complications include diverticulitis, fistulas.

Diverticulitis

Inflammation of diverticula **B** classically causing LLQ pain, fever, leukocytosis. May perforate → peritonitis, abscess formation, or bowel stenosis. Give antibiotics.

May also cause colovesical fistula (fistula with bladder) → pneumaturia.

Sometimes called "left-sided appendicitis" due to overlapping clinical presentation.

B **Diverticulitis.** CT shows inflammation surrounding segment of colon (circled) in LLQ.

Zenker diverticulum

Pharyngoesophageal **false** diverticulum 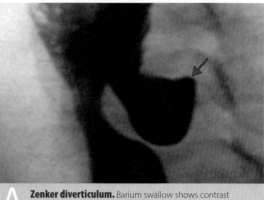. Herniation of mucosal tissue at Killian triangle between the thyropharyngeal and cricopharyngeal parts of the inferior pharyngeal constrictor. Presenting symptoms: dysphagia, obstruction, foul breath from trapped food particles (halitosis). Most common in elderly males.

A **Zenker diverticulum.** Barium swallow shows contrast filling false diverticulum (arrow) originating from posterior esophagus. ✦

Meckel diverticulum

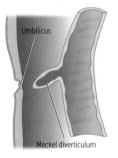

Umbilicus

Meckel diverticulum

True diverticulum. Persistence of the vitelline duct. May contain ectopic acid–secreting gastric mucosa and/or pancreatic tissue. Most common congenital anomaly of GI tract. Can cause melena, RLQ pain, intussusception, volvulus, or obstruction near terminal ileum. Contrast with omphalomesenteric cyst = cystic dilation of vitelline duct.

Diagnosis: pertechnetate study for uptake by ectopic gastric mucosa.

The **five 2's:**
2 inches long.
2 feet from the ileocecal valve.
2% of population.
Commonly presents in first **2** years of life.
May have **2** types of epithelia (gastric/ pancreatic).

Malrotation

Anomaly of midgut rotation during fetal development → improper positioning of bowel, formation of fibrous bands (Ladd bands). Can lead to volvulus, duodenal obstruction.

Volvulus

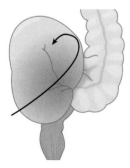

Twisting of portion of bowel around its mesentery; can lead to obstruction and infarction 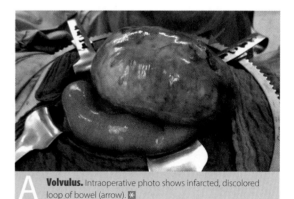. Can occur throughout the GI tract. Midgut volvulus more common in infants and children. Sigmoid volvulus more common in elderly.

A **Volvulus.** Intraoperative photo shows infarcted, discolored loop of bowel (arrow). ✦

Intussusception 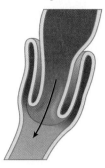	Telescoping of proximal bowel segment into distal segment **A**, commonly at ileocecal junction. Compromised blood supply → intermittent abdominal pain often with "currant jelly" stools. Unusual in adults (associated with intraluminal mass or tumor that acts as lead point that is pulled into the lumen). Majority of cases occur in children (usually idiopathic; may be associated with recent enteric or respiratory viral infection). Abdominal emergency in early childhood, with bull's-eye appearance on ultrasound.	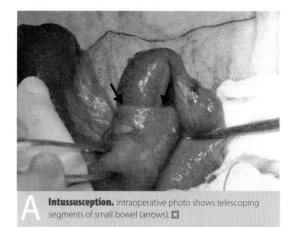 **A** **Intussusception.** Intraoperative photo shows telescoping segments of small bowel (arrows).

Hirschsprung disease	Congenital megacolon characterized by lack of ganglion cells/enteric nervous plexuses (Auerbach and Meissner plexuses) in segment of colon. Due to failure of neural crest cell migration. Associated with mutations in the *RET* gene. Presents with bilious emesis, abdominal distention, and failure to pass meconium → chronic constipation. Normal portion of the colon proximal to the aganglionic segment is dilated, resulting in a "transition zone." Involves rectum.	Think of Hirschsprung as a giant spring that has **sprung** in the colon. Risk ↑ with Down syndrome. Diagnosed by rectal suction biopsy. Treatment: resection.

Other intestinal disorders

Acute mesenteric ischemia	Critical blockage of intestinal blood flow (often embolic occlusion of SMA) → small bowel necrosis → abdominal pain out of proportion to physical findings. May see red "currant jelly" stools.
Adhesion	Fibrous band of scar tissue; commonly forms after surgery; most common cause of small bowel obstruction. Can have well-demarcated necrotic zones.
Angiodysplasia	Tortuous dilation of vessels → hematochezia. Most often found in cecum, terminal ileum, ascending colon. More common in older patients. Confirmed by angiography.
Duodenal atresia	Causes early bilious vomiting with proximal stomach distention ("double bubble" on X-ray) because of failure of small bowel recanalization. Associated with Down syndrome.
Ileus	Intestinal hypomotility without obstruction → constipation and ↓ flatus; distended/tympanic abdomen with ↓ bowel sounds. Associated with abdominal surgeries, opiates, hypokalemia, sepsis. Treatment: bowel rest, electrolyte correction, cholinergic drugs (stimulate intestinal motility).
Ischemic colitis	Reduction in intestinal blood flow causes ischemia. Pain after eating → weight loss. Commonly occurs at watershed areas (splenic flexure, distal colon). Typically affects elderly.
Meconium ileus	In cystic fibrosis, meconium plug obstructs intestine, preventing stool passage at birth.
Necrotizing enterocolitis	Seen in premature, formula-fed infants with immature immune system. Necrosis of intestinal mucosa (primarily colonic) with possible perforation, which can lead to pneumatosis intestinalis, free air in abdomen, portal venous gas.

Colonic polyps	Small growths of tissue within the colon 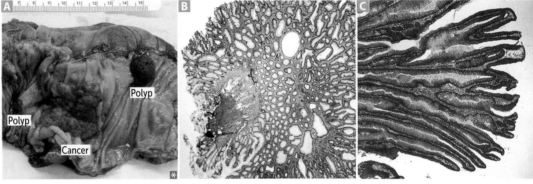. May be neoplastic or non-neoplastic. Grossly characterized as flat, sessile, or pedunculated (on a stalk) on the basis of protrusion into colonic lumen. Generally classified by histologic type.
HISTOLOGIC TYPE	**CHARACTERISTICS**
Hyperplastic	Non-neoplastic. Generally smaller and majority located in rectosigmoid area.
Hamartomatous	Non-neoplastic; solitary lesions do not have a significant risk of malignant transformation. Growths of normal colonic tissue with distorted architecture. Associated with Peutz-Jeghers syndrome and juvenile polyposis.
Adenomatous	Neoplastic, via chromosomal instability pathway with mutations in *APC* and *KRAS*. Tubular B histology has less malignant potential than villous C; tubulovillous has intermediate malignant potential.
Serrated	Premalignant, via CpG hypermethylation phenotype pathway with microsatellite instability and mutations in *BRAF*. "Saw-tooth" pattern of crypts on biopsy. Up to 20% of cases of sporadic CRC.

Polyposis syndromes

Familial adenomatous polyposis (FAP)	Autosomal dominant mutation of *APC* tumor suppressor gene on chromosome 5q. 2-hit hypothesis. 100% progress to CRC unless colon is resected. Thousands of polyps arise starting after puberty; pancolonic; always involves rectum.
Gardner syndrome	FAP + osseous and soft tissue tumors, congenital hypertrophy of retinal pigment epithelium, impacted/supernumerary teeth.
Turcot syndrome	FAP + malignant CNS tumor. **Turcot = Turban.**
Peutz-Jeghers syndrome	Autosomal dominant syndrome featuring numerous hamartomas throughout GI tract, along with hyperpigmented mouth, lips, hands, genitalia. Associated with ↑ risk of colorectal, breast, stomach, small bowel, and pancreatic cancers.
Juvenile polyposis syndrome	Autosomal dominant syndrome in children (typically < 5 years old) featuring numerous hamartomatous polyps in the colon, stomach, small bowel. Associated with ↑ risk of CRC.

Lynch syndrome	Previously known as hereditary nonpolyposis colorectal cancer (HNPCC). Autosomal dominant mutation of DNA mismatch repair genes with subsequent microsatellite instability. ~ 80% progress to CRC. Proximal colon is always involved. Associated with endometrial, ovarian, and skin cancers. Can be identified clinically in families using **3-2-1 rule: 3** relatives with Lynch syndrome–associated cancers across **2** generations, **1** of whom must be diagnosed before age 50 years.

Colorectal cancer

EPIDEMIOLOGY	Most patients are > 50 years old. ~ 25% have a family history.
RISK FACTORS	Adenomatous and serrated polyps, familial cancer syndromes, IBD, tobacco use, diet of processed meat with low fiber.
PRESENTATION	Rectosigmoid > ascending > descending. Ascending—exophytic mass, iron deficiency anemia, weight loss. Descending—infiltrating mass, partial obstruction, colicky pain, hematochezia. Rarely, presents with *Streptococcus bovis* bacteremia.
DIAGNOSIS	Iron deficiency anemia in males (especially > 50 years old) and postmenopausal females raises suspicion. Screen patients > 50 years old with colonoscopy, flexible sigmoidoscopy, or stool occult blood test. "Apple core" lesion seen on barium enema x-ray A. CEA tumor marker: good for monitoring recurrence, not useful for screening.

Right side bleeds; left side obstructs.

A **"Apple core" lesion.** Seen here in the sigmoid colon (arrow). ℞

Molecular pathogenesis of colorectal cancer

There are 2 molecular pathways that lead to CRC:

- Microsatellite instability pathway (~ 15%): DNA mismatch repair gene mutations → sporadic and Lynch syndrome. Mutations accumulate, but no defined morphologic correlates.
- APC/β-catenin (chromosomal instability) pathway (~ 85%) → sporadic cancer.

Order of gene events—AK-53.

	Loss of *APC* gene		*KRAS* mutation		Loss of tumor suppressor gene(s) (*p53*, DCC)	
Normal colon	→	Colon at risk	→	Adenoma	→	Carcinoma
	Decreased intercellular adhesion and increased proliferation		Unregulated intracellular signal transduction		Increased tumorigenesis	

Cirrhosis and portal hypertension

Cirrhosis—diffuse bridging fibrosis and nodular regeneration via stellate cells disrupts normal architecture of liver 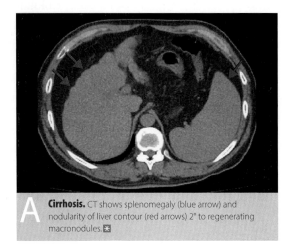; ↑ risk for hepatocellular carcinoma (HCC).

Etiologies: alcohol (60–70% of cases in the U.S.), chronic viral hepatitis, biliary disease, genetic/metabolic disorders.

Portosystemic shunts partially alleviate portal hypertension:

- Esophageal varices
- Caput medusae
- Anorectal varices

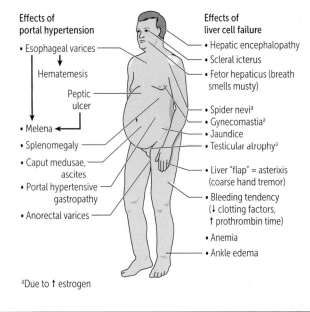

Effects of portal hypertension
- Esophageal varices
  ↓
  Hematemesis
  Peptic ulcer
  ↓
- Melena
- Splenomegaly
- Caput medusae, ascites
- Portal hypertensive gastropathy
- Anorectal varices

Effects of liver cell failure
- Hepatic encephalopathy
- Scleral icterus
- Fetor hepaticus (breath smells musty)
- Spider nevi[a]
- Gynecomastia[a]
- Jaundice
- Testicular atrophy[a]
- Liver "flap" = asterixis (coarse hand tremor)
- Bleeding tendency (↓ clotting factors, ↑ prothrombin time)
- Anemia
- Ankle edema

[a]Due to ↑ estrogen

A **Cirrhosis.** CT shows splenomegaly (blue arrow) and nodularity of liver contour (red arrows) 2° to regenerating macronodules. ✱

Serum markers of liver and pancreas pathology

SERUM MARKER	MAJOR DIAGNOSTIC USE
Alkaline phosphatase (ALP)	Cholestatic and obstructive hepatobiliary disease, HCC, infiltrative disorders, bone disease
Aminotransferases (AST and ALT) (often called "liver enzymes")	Viral hepatitis (ALT > AST) Alcoholic hepatitis (AST > ALT)
Amylase	Acute pancreatitis, mumps
Ceruloplasmin	↓ in Wilson disease
γ-glutamyl transpeptidase (GGT)	↑ in various liver and biliary diseases (just as ALP can), but **not** in bone disease; associated with alcohol use
Lipase	Acute pancreatitis (most specific)

Reye syndrome
Rare, often fatal childhood hepatic encephalopathy. Findings: mitochondrial abnormalities, fatty liver (microvesicular fatty change), hypoglycemia, vomiting, hepatomegaly, coma. Associated with viral infection (especially VZV and influenza B) that has been treated with aspirin. Mechanism: aspirin metabolites ↓ β-oxidation by reversible inhibition of mitochondrial enzymes. Avoid aspirin in children, except in those with Kawasaki disease.

Alcoholic liver disease

Hepatic steatosis	Macrovesicular fatty change **A** that may be reversible with alcohol cessation.	
Alcoholic hepatitis	Requires sustained, long-term consumption. Swollen and necrotic hepatocytes with neutrophilic infiltration. Mallory bodies **B** (intracytoplasmic eosinophilic inclusions of damaged keratin filaments).	Make a to**AST** with alcohol: AST > ALT (ratio usually > 1.5).
Alcoholic cirrhosis	Final and irreversible form. Micronodular, irregularly shrunken liver with "hobnail" appearance. Sclerosis (arrows in **C**) around central vein (zone III). Manifestations of chronic liver disease (e.g., jaundice, hypoalbuminemia).	

Non-alcoholic fatty liver disease	Metabolic syndrome (insulin resistance) → fatty infiltration of hepatocytes → cellular "ballooning" and eventual necrosis. May cause cirrhosis and HCC. Independent of alcohol use.	ALT > AST (Lipids)

Hepatic encephalopathy
Cirrhosis → portosystemic shunts → ↓ NH_3 metabolism → neuropsychiatric dysfunction. Spectrum from disorientation/asterixis (mild) to difficult arousal or coma (severe). Triggers:
  - ↑ NH_3 production and absorption (due to dietary protein, GI bleed, constipation, infection).
  - ↓ NH_3 removal (due to renal failure, diuretics, bypassed hepatic blood flow post-TIPS).
Treatment: lactulose (↑ NH_4^+ generation) and rifaximin.

Hepatocellular carcinoma/hepatoma	Most common 1° malignant tumor of liver in adults 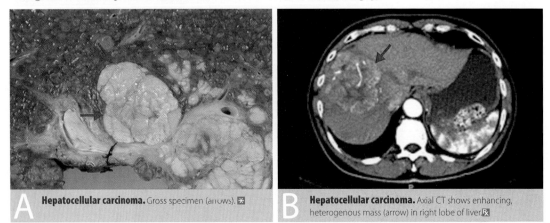A. Associated with HBV (+/− cirrhosis) and all other causes of cirrhosis (including HCV, alcoholic and non-alcoholic fatty liver disease, autoimmune disease, hemochromatosis, α_1-antitrypsin deficiency, Wilson disease) and specific carcinogens (e.g., aflatoxin from *Aspergillus*). May lead to Budd-Chiari syndrome. Findings: jaundice, tender hepatomegaly, ascites, polycythemia, anorexia. Spreads hematogenously. Diagnosis: ↑ α-fetoprotein; ultrasound or contrast CT/MRI B, biopsy.

Hepatocellular carcinoma. Gross specimen (arrows). ✱

Hepatocellular carcinoma. Axial CT shows enhancing, heterogenous mass (arrow) in right lobe of liver. ✱

Other liver tumors

Cavernous hemangioma	Common, benign liver tumor A; typically occurs at age 30–50 years. Biopsy contraindicated because of risk of hemorrhage.
Hepatic adenoma	Rare, benign liver tumor, often related to oral contraceptive or anabolic steroid use; may regress spontaneously or rupture (abdominal pain and shock).
Angiosarcoma	Malignant tumor of endothelial origin; associated with exposure to arsenic, vinyl chloride.
Metastases	GI malignancies, breast and lung cancer. Most common overall.

Cavernous liver hemangioma. Collection of dilated blood vessels. ✱

Budd-Chiari syndrome	Thrombosis or compression of hepatic veins with centrilobular congestion and necrosis → congestive liver disease (hepatomegaly, varices, abdominal pain, eventual liver failure). Absence of JVD. Associated with hypercoagulable states, polycythemia vera, postpartum state, HCC. May cause nutmeg liver (mottled appearance).

α₁-antitrypsin deficiency

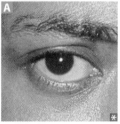

Misfolded gene product protein aggregates in hepatocellular ER → cirrhosis with PAS ⊕ globules **A** in liver. Codominant trait.

In lungs, ↓ α₁-antitrypsin → uninhibited elastase in alveoli → ↓ elastic tissue → panacinar emphysema.

Jaundice

Abnormal yellowing of the skin and/or sclera **A** due to bilirubin deposition. Occurs at high bilirubin levels (> 2.5 mg/dL) in blood 2° to ↑ production or defective metabolism.

Unconjugated (indirect) hyperbilirubinemia

Hemolytic, physiologic (newborns), Crigler-Najjar, Gilbert syndrome.

Conjugated (direct) hyperbilirubinemia

Biliary tract obstruction: gallstones, cholangiocarcinoma, pancreatic or liver cancer, liver fluke.
Biliary tract disease:
- 1° sclerosing cholangitis
- 1° biliary cirrhosis

Excretion defect: Dubin-Johnson syndrome, Rotor syndrome.

Mixed (direct and indirect) hyperbilirubinemia

Hepatitis, cirrhosis.

Physiologic neonatal jaundice

At birth, immature UDP-glucuronosyltransferase → unconjugated hyperbilirubinemia → jaundice/kernicterus (bilirubin deposition in brain, particularly basal ganglia).
Treatment: phototherapy (converts unconjugated bilirubin to water-soluble form).

Hereditary hyperbilirubinemias

❶ Gilbert syndrome	Mildly ↓ UDP-glucuronosyltransferase conjugation and impaired bilirubin uptake. Asymptomatic or mild jaundice. ↑ unconjugated bilirubin without overt hemolysis. Bilirubin ↑ with fasting and stress.	Very common. No clinical consequences.
❷ Crigler-Najjar syndrome, type I	Absent UDP-glucuronosyltransferase. Presents early in life; patients die within a few years. Findings: jaundice, kernicterus (bilirubin deposition in brain), ↑ unconjugated bilirubin. Treatment: plasmapheresis and phototherapy.	Type II is less severe and responds to phenobarbital, which ↑ liver enzyme synthesis.
❸ Dubin-Johnson syndrome	Conjugated hyperbilirubinemia due to defective liver excretion. Grossly black liver. Benign.	❹ Rotor syndrome is similar but even milder and does not cause black liver.

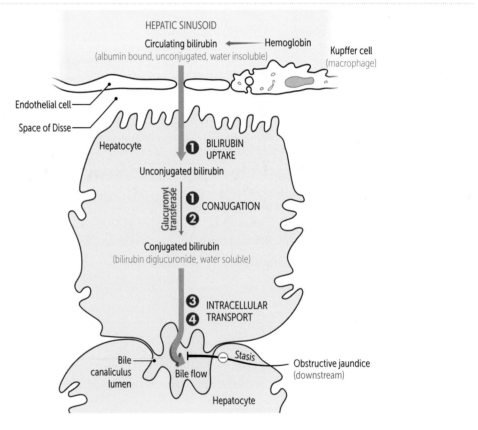

Wilson disease (hepatolenticular degeneration)

Inadequate hepatic copper excretion and failure of copper to enter circulation as ceruloplasmin. Leads to **copper** accumulation, especially in liver, brain, cornea, kidneys (Fanconi syndrome), and joints.

Autosomal recessive inheritance (chromosome 13). Copper is normally excreted into bile by hepatocyte copper transporting ATPase (*ATP7B* gene).

Treatment includes chelation with penicillamine or trientine, oral zinc.

Characterized by:
↓ Ceruloplasmin, Cirrhosis, Corneal deposits (Kayser-Fleischer rings) 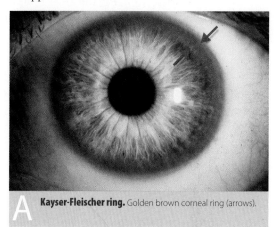, Copper accumulation, Carcinoma (hepatocellular)
Hemolytic anemia
Basal ganglia degeneration (parkinsonian symptoms)
Asterixis
Dementia, Dyskinesia, Dysarthria
"Copper is Hella **BAD**."

A **Kayser-Fleischer ring.** Golden brown corneal ring (arrows).

Hemochromatosis

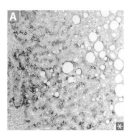

Hemosiderosis is the deposition of hemosiderin (iron), which stains blue **A**; hemochromatosis is the disease caused by this iron deposition. Classic triad of micronodular Cirrhosis, Diabetes mellitus, and skin pigmentation → "bronze" diabetes. Results in HF, testicular atrophy, and ↑ risk of HCC. Disease may be 1° (autosomal recessive) or 2° to chronic transfusion therapy (e.g., β-thalassemia major). ↑ ferritin, ↑ iron, ↓ TIBC → ↑ transferrin saturation. Can be identified on biopsy with Prussian blue stain.

Total body iron may reach 50 g, enough to set off metal detectors at airports.

Primary hemochromatosis due to C282Y or H63D mutation on *HFE* gene. Associated with HLA-A3.

Iron loss through menstruation slows progression in women.

Treatment of hereditary hemochromatosis: repeated phlebotomy, chelation with deferasirox, deferoxamine, deferiprone (oral).

Biliary tract disease	May present with pruritus, jaundice, dark urine, light-colored stool, hepatosplenomegaly. Typically with cholestatic pattern of LFTs (↑ conjugated bilirubin, ↑ cholesterol, ↑ ALP).		
	PATHOLOGY	EPIDEMIOLOGY	ADDITIONAL FEATURES
Secondary biliary cirrhosis	Extrahepatic biliary obstruction → ↑ pressure in intrahepatic ducts → injury/ fibrosis and bile stasis.	Patients with known obstructive lesions (gallstones, biliary strictures, pancreatic carcinoma).	May be complicated by ascending cholangitis.
Primary biliary cirrhosis	Autoimmune reaction → lymphocytic infiltrate + granulomas → destruction of intralobular bile ducts.	Classically in middle-aged women.	Anti-mitochondrial antibody ⊕, including IgM. Associated with other autoimmune conditions (e.g., CREST, Sjögren syndrome, rheumatoid arthritis, celiac disease).
Primary sclerosing cholangitis	Unknown cause of concentric "onion skin" bile duct fibrosis → alternating strictures and dilation with "beading" of intra- and extrahepatic bile ducts on ERCP, magnetic resonance cholangiopancreatography (MRCP).	Classically in young men with IBD.	Hypergammaglobulinemia (IgM). MPO-ANCA/p-ANCA ⊕. Associated with ulcerative colitis. Can lead to 2° biliary cirrhosis, cholangiocarcinoma.

Gallstones (cholelithiasis)

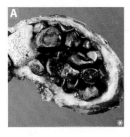

↑ cholesterol and/or bilirubin, ↓ bile salts, and gallbladder stasis all cause stones .

2 types of stones:

- Cholesterol stones (radiolucent with 10–20% opaque due to calcifications)—80% of stones. Associated with obesity, Crohn disease, advanced age, clofibrate, estrogen therapy, multiparity, rapid weight loss, Native American origin.
- Pigment stones (black = radiopaque, Ca^{2+} bilirubinate, hemolysis; brown = radiolucent, infection)—seen in patients with chronic hemolysis, alcoholic cirrhosis, advanced age, biliary infections, total parenteral nutrition (TPN).

Most often causes cholecystitis; also ascending cholangitis, acute pancreatitis, bile stasis.

Can also lead to biliary colic—neurohormonal activation (e.g., by CCK after a fatty meal) triggers contraction of gallbladder, forcing a stone into the cystic duct. May present without pain (e.g., in diabetics).

Can cause fistula between gallbladder and small intestine, leading to air in biliary tree and allowing the passage of gallstones into the intestinal tract. Gallstone may obstruct ileocecal valve → gallstone ileus.

Diagnose with ultrasound 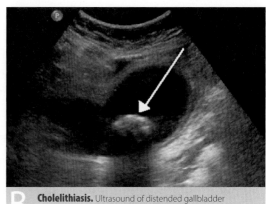. Treat with cholecystectomy if symptomatic.

Risk factors (**4 F's**):
1. Female
2. Fat
3. Fertile (pregnant)
4. Forty

Charcot triad of cholangitis:
- Jaundice
- Fever
- RUQ pain

B **Cholelithiasis.** Ultrasound of distended gallbladder containing large gallstone (arrow). ✴

Cholecystitis

Acute or chronic inflammation of gallbladder. Usually from cholelithiasis (gallstones 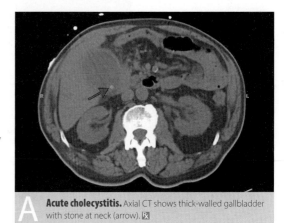); most commonly blocking the cystic duct → 2° infection; rarely ischemia or 1° infection (CMV). Murphy sign ⊕—inspiratory arrest on RUQ palpation due to pain. ↑ ALP if bile duct becomes involved (e.g., ascending cholangitis). Diagnose with ultrasound or cholescintigraphy (HIDA, or hepatobiliary iminodiacetic acid scan).

A **Acute cholecystitis.** Axial CT shows thick-walled gallbladder with stone at neck (arrow). ℞

Porcelain gallbladder

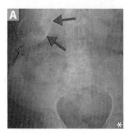

Calcified gallbladder due to chronic cholecystitis; usually found incidentally on imaging **A**. Treatment: prophylactic cholecystectomy due to high rates of gallbladder carcinoma.

Acute pancreatitis

Autodigestion of pancreas by pancreatic enzymes **A**.

Causes: idiopathic, **G**allstones, **E**thanol, **T**rauma, **S**teroids, **M**umps, **A**utoimmune disease, **S**corpion sting, **H**ypercalcemia/**H**ypertriglyceridemia (> 1000 mg/dL), **E**RCP, **D**rugs (e.g., sulfa drugs, NRTIs, protease inhibitors). **GET SMASHED**.

Clinical presentation: epigastric abdominal pain radiating to back, anorexia, nausea.

Labs: ↑ amylase, lipase (higher specificity).

Can lead to DIC, ARDS, diffuse fat necrosis, hypocalcemia (Ca^{2+} collects in pancreatic Ca^{2+} soap deposits), pseudocyst formation **B**, hemorrhage, infection, multiorgan failure.

Complication: pancreatic pseudocyst (lined by granulation tissue, not epithelium; can rupture and hemorrhage).

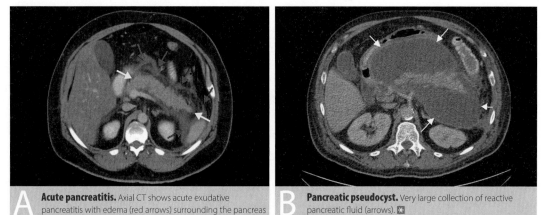

A **Acute pancreatitis.** Axial CT shows acute exudative pancreatitis with edema (red arrows) surrounding the pancreas (yellow arrows). ✱

B **Pancreatic pseudocyst.** Very large collection of reactive pancreatic fluid (arrows). ✱

Chronic pancreatitis

Chronic inflammation, atrophy, calcification of the pancreas **A**. Major causes are alcohol abuse and idiopathic. Mutations in *CFTR* (cystic fibrosis) can cause chronic pancreatic insufficiency.

Can lead to pancreatic insufficiency → steatorrhea, fat-soluble vitamin deficiency, diabetes mellitus.

Amylase and lipase may or may not be elevated (almost always elevated in acute pancreatitis).

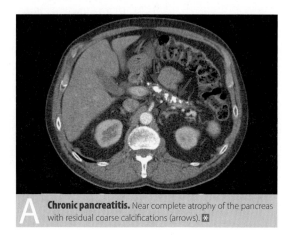

A **Chronic pancreatitis.** Near complete atrophy of the pancreas with residual coarse calcifications (arrows). ✱

Pancreatic adenocarcinoma

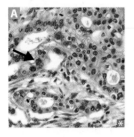

Average survival ~ 1 year after diagnosis. Very aggressive tumor arising from pancreatic ducts (disorganized glandular structure with cellular infiltration A); already metastasized at presentation; tumors more common in pancreatic head B (→ obstructive jaundice). Associated with CA 19-9 tumor marker (also CEA, less specific).

Risk factors:

- Tobacco use
- Chronic pancreatitis (especially > 20 years)
- Diabetes
- Age > 50 years
- Jewish and African-American males

Often presents with:

- Abdominal pain radiating to back
- Weight loss (due to malabsorption and anorexia)
- Migratory thrombophlebitis—redness and tenderness on palpation of extremities (Trousseau syndrome)
- Obstructive jaundice with palpable, nontender gallbladder (Courvoisier sign)

Treatment: Whipple procedure, chemotherapy, radiation therapy.

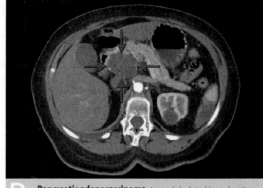

B **Pancreatic adenocarcinoma.** Large lobulated low-density mass in head of pancreas (arrows). ✳

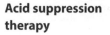

▶ GASTROINTESTINAL—PHARMACOLOGY

Acid suppression therapy

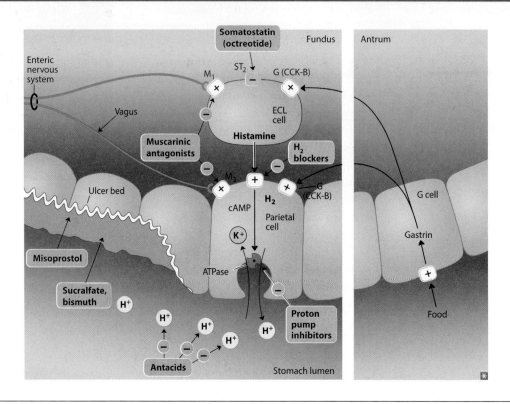

H₂ blockers	Cimetidine, ranitidine, famotidine, nizatidine.	Take H₂ blockers before you **dine**. Think "table for 2" to remember H₂.
MECHANISM	Reversible block of histamine H₂-receptors → ↓ H⁺ secretion by parietal cells.	
CLINICAL USE	Peptic ulcer, gastritis, mild esophageal reflux.	
TOXICITY	Cimetidine is a potent inhibitor of cytochrome P-450 (multiple drug interactions); it also has antiandrogenic effects (prolactin release, gynecomastia, impotence, ↓ libido in males); can cross blood-brain barrier (confusion, dizziness, headaches) and placenta. Both cimetidine and ranitidine ↓ renal excretion of creatinine. Other H₂ blockers are relatively free of these effects.	

Proton pump inhibitors	Omeprazole, lansoprazole, esomeprazole, pantoprazole, dexlansoprazole.
MECHANISM	Irreversibly inhibit H⁺/K⁺ ATPase in stomach parietal cells.
CLINICAL USE	Peptic ulcer, gastritis, esophageal reflux, Zollinger-Ellison syndrome.
TOXICITY	Increased risk of *C. difficile* infection, pneumonia. ↓ serum Mg²⁺ with long-term use.

Bismuth, sucralfate	
MECHANISM	Bind to ulcer base, providing physical protection and allowing HCO₃⁻ secretion to reestablish pH gradient in the mucous layer.
CLINICAL USE	↑ ulcer healing, travelers' diarrhea.

Misoprostol

MECHANISM	A PGE_1 analog. ↑ production and secretion of gastric mucous barrier, ↓ acid production.
CLINICAL USE	Prevention of NSAID-induced peptic ulcers (NSAIDs block PGE_1 production); maintenance of a PDA. Also used off-label for induction of labor (ripens cervix).
TOXICITY	Diarrhea. Contraindicated in women of childbearing potential (abortifacient).

Octreotide

MECHANISM	Long-acting somatostatin analog; inhibits actions of many splanchnic vasoconstriction hormones.
CLINICAL USE	Acute variceal bleeds, acromegaly, VIPoma, carcinoid tumors.
TOXICITY	Nausea, cramps, steatorrhea.

Antacid use

Can affect absorption, bioavailability, or urinary excretion of other drugs by altering gastric and urinary pH or by delaying gastric emptying.
All can cause hypokalemia.
Overuse can also cause the following problems.

Aluminum hydroxide	Constipation and hypophosphatemia; proximal muscle weakness, osteodystrophy, seizures	**Alu**minimum amount of feces.
Calcium carbonate	Hypercalcemia, rebound acid ↑	Can chelate and ↓ effectiveness of other drugs (e.g., tetracycline).
Magnesium hydroxide	Diarrhea, hyporeflexia, hypotension, cardiac arrest	**Mg** = **M**ust go to the bathroom.

Osmotic laxatives

Magnesium hydroxide, magnesium citrate, polyethylene glycol, lactulose.

MECHANISM	Provide osmotic load to draw water into the GI lumen.
CLINICAL USE	Constipation. Lactulose also treats hepatic encephalopathy since gut flora degrade it into metabolites (lactic acid and acetic acid) that promote nitrogen excretion as NH_4^+.
TOXICITY	Diarrhea, dehydration; may be abused by bulimics.

Sulfasalazine

MECHANISM	A combination of sulfapyridine (antibacterial) and 5-aminosalicylic acid (anti-inflammatory). Activated by colonic bacteria.
CLINICAL USE	Ulcerative colitis, Crohn disease (colitis component).
TOXICITY	Malaise, nausea, sulfonamide toxicity, reversible oligospermia.

Ondansetron

MECHANISM	5-HT$_3$ antagonist; ↓ vagal stimulation. Powerful central-acting antiemetic.	At a party but feeling queasy? Keep **on dancing** with **ondans**etron!
CLINICAL USE	Control vomiting postoperatively and in patients undergoing cancer chemotherapy.	
TOXICITY	Headache, constipation, QT interval prolongation.	

Metoclopramide

MECHANISM	D$_2$ receptor antagonist. ↑ resting tone, contractility, LES tone, motility. Does not influence colon transport time.
CLINICAL USE	Diabetic and postsurgery gastroparesis, antiemetic.
TOXICITY	↑ parkinsonian effects, tardive dyskinesia. Restlessness, drowsiness, fatigue, depression, diarrhea. Drug interaction with digoxin and diabetic agents. Contraindicated in patients with small bowel obstruction or Parkinson disease (due to D$_1$-receptor blockade).

Orlistat

MECHANISM	Inhibits gastric and pancreatic lipase → ↓ breakdown and absorption of dietary fats.
CLINICAL USE	Weight loss.
TOXICITY	Steatorrhea, ↓ absorption of fat-soluble vitamins.

Hematology and Oncology

"Of all that is written, I love only what a person has written with his own blood."

—Friedrich Nietzsche

"I used to get stressed out, but my cancer has put everything into perspective."

—Delta Goodrem

"The best blood will at some time get into a fool or a mosquito."

—Austin O'Malley

Study tip: When reviewing oncologic drugs, focus on mechanisms and side effects rather than details of clinical uses, which may be lower yield.

▶ HEMATOLOGY AND ONCOLOGY—ANATOMY

Erythrocyte

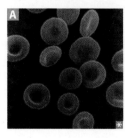

Carries O_2 to tissues and CO_2 to lungs. Anucleate and biconcave **A**, with large surface area-to-volume ratio for rapid gas exchange. Life span of 120 days. Source of energy is glucose (90% used in glycolysis, 10% used in HMP shunt). Membrane contains Cl^-/HCO_3^- antiporter, which allows RBCs to export HCO_3^- and transport CO_2 from the periphery to the lungs for elimination.

Eryth = red; *cyte* = cell.

Erythrocytosis = polycythemia = ↑ hematocrit.
Anisocytosis = varying sizes.
Poikilocytosis = varying shapes.

Reticulocyte = immature RBC; reflects erythroid proliferation.

Thrombocyte (platelet)

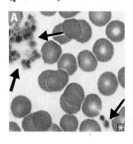

Involved in 1° hemostasis. Small cytoplasmic fragment **A** derived from megakaryocytes. Life span of 8–10 days. When activated by endothelial injury, aggregates with other platelets and interacts with fibrinogen to form platelet plug. Contains dense granules (ADP, Ca^{2+}) and α granules (vWF, fibrinogen). Approximately ⅓ of platelet pool is stored in the spleen.

Thrombocytopenia or ↓ platelet function results in petechiae.
vWF receptor: GpIb.
Fibrinogen receptor: GpIIb/IIIa.

Leukocyte

Divided into granulocytes (neutrophil, eosinophil, basophil) and mononuclear cells (monocytes, lymphocytes). Responsible for defense against infections. Normally 4000–10,000 cells/mm³.
WBC differential from highest to lowest (normal ranges per USMLE):
  Neutrophils (54–62%)
  Lymphocytes (25–33%)
  Monocytes (3–7%)
  Eosinophils (1–3%)
  Basophils (0–0.75%)

Leuk = white; *cyte* = cell.

Neutrophils Like Making Everything Better.

Neutrophil

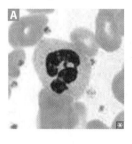

Acute inflammatory response cell. Increased in bacterial infections. Phagocytic. Multilobed nucleus **A**. Specific granules contain ALP, collagenase, lysozyme, and lactoferrin. Azurophilic granules (lysosomes) contain proteinases, acid phosphatase, myeloperoxidase, and β-glucuronidase.

Hypersegmented polys (5 or more lobes) are seen in vitamin B_{12}/folate deficiency.
↑ band cells (immature neutrophils) reflect states of ↑ myeloid proliferation (bacterial infections, CML).
Important neutrophil chemotactic agents: C5a, IL-8, LTB_4, kallikrein, platelet-activating factor.

Monocyte

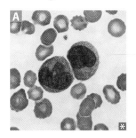

Differentiates into macrophage in tissues. Large, kidney-shaped nucleus **A**. Extensive "frosted glass" cytoplasm.

Mono = one (nucleus); *cyte* = cell.
Monocyte: in the blood.

Macrophage

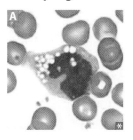

Phagocytoses bacteria, cellular debris, and senescent RBCs **A**. Long life in tissues. Macrophages differentiate from circulating blood monocytes. Activated by γ-interferon. Can function as antigen-presenting cell via MHC II.

Macro = large; *phage* = eater.
Macrophage: in the tissue.
Important component of granuloma formation (e.g., TB, sarcoidosis).
Lipid A from bacterial LPS binds CD14 on macrophages to initiate septic shock.

Eosinophil

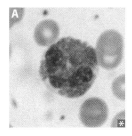

Defends against helminthic infections (major basic protein). Bilobate nucleus. Packed with large eosinophilic granules of uniform size **A**. Highly phagocytic for antigen-antibody complexes.
Produces histaminase and major basic protein (MBP, a helminthotoxin).

Eosin = pink dye; *philic* = loving.
Causes of eosinophilia = **NAACP**:
  Neoplasia
  Asthma
  Allergic processes
  Chronic adrenal insufficiency
  Parasites (invasive)

Basophil

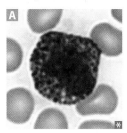

Mediates allergic reaction. Densely basophilic granules **A** contain heparin (anticoagulant) and histamine (vasodilator). Leukotrienes synthesized and released on demand.

Basophilic—staining readily with **basic** stains.
Basophilia is uncommon, but can be a sign of myeloproliferative disease, particularly CML.

Mast cell

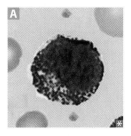

Mediates allergic reaction in local tissues. Mast cells contain basophilic granules and originate from the same precursor as basophils but are not the same cell type **A**. Can bind the Fc portion of IgE to membrane. IgE cross-links upon antigen binding, causing degranulation, which releases histamine, heparin, and eosinophil chemotactic factors.

Involved in type I hypersensitivity reactions. Cromolyn sodium prevents mast cell degranulation (used for asthma prophylaxis).

Dendritic cell

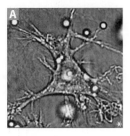

Highly phagocytic APC . Functions as link between innate and adaptive immune systems. Expresses MHC class II and Fc receptors on surface. Called Langerhans cell in the skin.

Lymphocyte

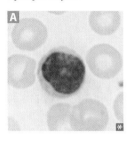

Refers to B cells, T cells, and NK cells. B cells and T cells mediate adaptive immunity. NK cells are part of the innate immune response. Round, densely staining nucleus with small amount of pale cytoplasm A.

B cell

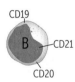

Part of humoral immune response. Originates from stem cells in bone marrow and matures in marrow. Migrates to peripheral lymphoid tissue (follicles of lymph nodes, white pulp of spleen, unencapsulated lymphoid tissue). When antigen is encountered, B cells differentiate into plasma cells (which produce antibodies) and memory cells. Can function as an APC via MHC II.

B = Bone marrow.

T cell

Mediates cellular immune response. Originates from stem cells in the bone marrow, but matures in the thymus. T cells differentiate into cytotoxic T cells (express CD8, recognize MHC I), helper T cells (express CD4, recognize MHC II), and regulatory T cells. CD28 (costimulatory signal) necessary for T-cell activation. The majority of circulating lymphocytes are T cells (80%).

T is for Thymus.
CD4+ helper T cells are the primary target of HIV.

$MHC \times CD = 8$ (e.g., MHC $2 \times CD4 = 8$, and MHC $1 \times CD8 = 8$).

Plasma cell

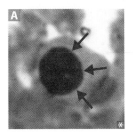

Produces large amounts of antibody specific to a particular antigen. "Clock-face" chromatin distribution Ⓐ, abundant RER, and well-developed Golgi apparatus.

Multiple myeloma is a plasma cell cancer.

▶ HEMATOLOGY AND ONCOLOGY—PHYSIOLOGY

Blood groups

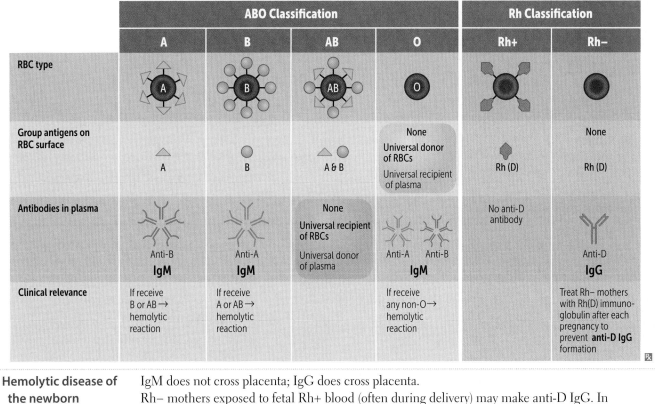

	ABO Classification				Rh Classification	
	A	**B**	**AB**	**O**	**Rh+**	**Rh−**
RBC type	A	B	AB	O		
Group antigens on RBC surface	A	B	A & B	**None** Universal donor of RBCs. Universal recipient of plasma	Rh (D)	**None** Rh (D)
Antibodies in plasma	Anti-B **IgM**	Anti-A **IgM**	**None** Universal recipient of RBCs. Universal donor of plasma	Anti-A Anti-B **IgM**	No anti-D antibody	Anti-D **IgG**
Clinical relevance	If receive B or AB → hemolytic reaction	If receive A or AB → hemolytic reaction		If receive any non-O → hemolytic reaction		Treat Rh− mothers with Rh(D) immuno-globulin after each pregnancy to prevent **anti-D IgG** formation

Hemolytic disease of the newborn

IgM does not cross placenta; IgG does cross placenta.

Rh− mothers exposed to fetal Rh+ blood (often during delivery) may make anti-D IgG. In subsequent pregnancies, anti-D IgG crosses the placenta → hemolytic disease of the newborn (erythroblastosis fetalis) in the next fetus that is Rh+. Prevented by administration of RhoGAM to Rh− pregnant women during third trimester, which prevents maternal anti-Rh IgG production. Rh− mothers have anti-D IgG only if previously exposed to Rh+ blood.

Coagulation and kinin pathways

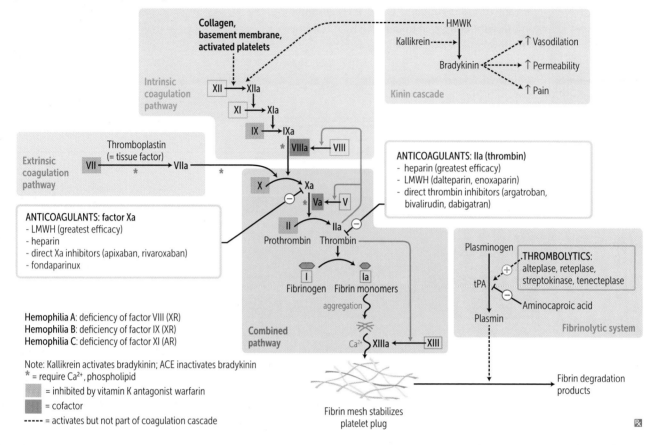

Hemophilia A: deficiency of factor VIII (XR)
Hemophilia B: deficiency of factor IX (XR)
Hemophilia C: deficiency of factor XI (AR)

Note: Kallikrein activates bradykinin; ACE inactivates bradykinin
* = require Ca^{2+}, phospholipid
▨ = inhibited by vitamin K antagonist warfarin
■ = cofactor
----- = activates but not part of coagulation cascade

ANTICOAGULANTS: factor Xa
- LMWH (greatest efficacy)
- heparin
- direct Xa inhibitors (apixaban, rivaroxaban)
- fondaparinux

ANTICOAGULANTS: IIa (thrombin)
- heparin (greatest efficacy)
- LMWH (dalteparin, enoxaparin)
- direct thrombin inhibitors (argatroban, bivalirudin, dabigatran)

THROMBOLYTICS:
alteplase, reteplase, streptokinase, tenecteplase

Coagulation cascade components

Procoagulation

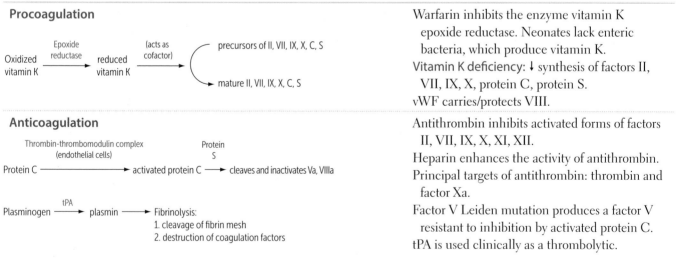

Warfarin inhibits the enzyme vitamin K
epoxide reductase. Neonates lack enteric
bacteria, which produce vitamin K.
Vitamin K deficiency: ↓ synthesis of factors II,
VII, IX, X, protein C, protein S.
vWF carries/protects VIII.

Anticoagulation

Antithrombin inhibits activated forms of factors
II, VII, IX, X, XI, XII.
Heparin enhances the activity of antithrombin.
Principal targets of antithrombin: thrombin and
factor Xa.
Factor V Leiden mutation produces a factor V
resistant to inhibition by activated protein C.
tPA is used clinically as a thrombolytic.

Platelet plug formation (primary hemostasis)

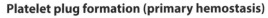

❶

INJURY
Endothelial damage → transient vasoconstriction via neural stimulation reflex and endothelin (released from damaged cell)

❷

EXPOSURE
vWF binds to exposed collagen
vWF is from Weibel-Palade bodies of endothelial cells and α-granules of platelets

❸

ADHESION
Platelets bind vWF via GpIb receptor at the site of injury only (specific) → platelets undergo conformational change

Platelets release ADP and Ca^{2+} (necessary for coagulation cascade), TXA_2[a]

ADP helps platelets adhere to endothelium

❹ᴬ

ACTIVATION
ADP binding to receptor induces GpIIb/IIIa expression at platelet surface

❹ᴮ

AGGREGATION
Fibrinogen binds GpIIb/IIIa receptors and links platelets

Balance between

Pro-aggregation factors:	Anti-aggregation factors:
TXA_2 (released by platelets)	PGI_2 and NO (released by endothelial cells)
↓ blood flow	↑ blood flow
↑ platelet aggregation	↓ platelet aggregation

Temporary plug stops bleeding; unstable, easily dislodged

2° hemostasis
Coagulation cascade

[a]Derivative of platelet cyclooxygenase.

Thrombogenesis

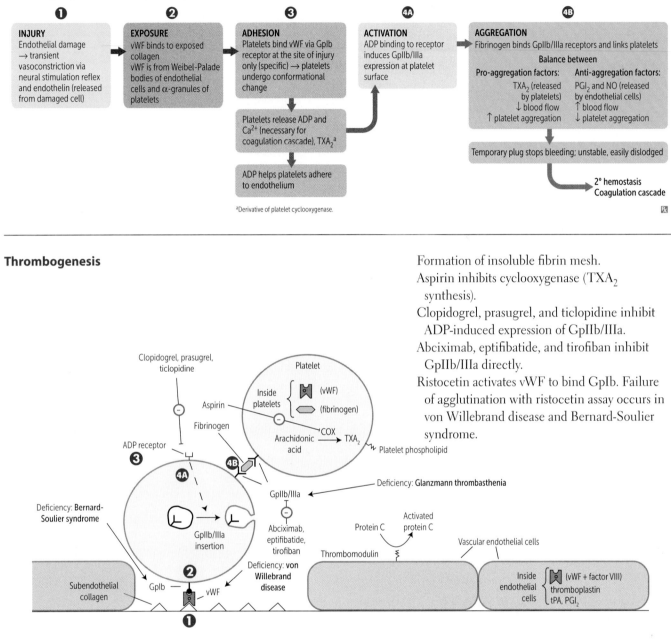

Formation of insoluble fibrin mesh.

Aspirin inhibits cyclooxygenase (TXA_2 synthesis).

Clopidogrel, prasugrel, and ticlopidine inhibit ADP-induced expression of GpIIb/IIIa.

Abciximab, eptifibatide, and tirofiban inhibit GpIIb/IIIa directly.

Ristocetin activates vWF to bind GpIb. Failure of agglutination with ristocetin assay occurs in von Willebrand disease and Bernard-Soulier syndrome.

▶ HEMATOLOGY AND ONCOLOGY—PATHOLOGY

Pathologic RBC forms

TYPE	EXAMPLE	ASSOCIATED PATHOLOGY	NOTES
Acanthocyte ("spur cell")		Liver disease, abetalipoproteinemia (states of cholesterol dysregulation).	*Acantho* = spiny.
Basophilic stippling		Lead poisoning.	
Degmacyte ("bite cell")		G6PD deficiency.	
Elliptocyte		Hereditary elliptocytosis.	
Macro-ovalocyte		Megaloblastic anemia (also hypersegmented PMNs), marrow failure.	
Ringed sideroblast		Sideroblastic anemia. Excess iron in mitochondria = pathologic.	
Schistocyte ("helmet cell")		DIC, TTP/HUS, HELLP syndrome, mechanical hemolysis (e.g., heart valve prosthesis).	

Pathologic RBC forms (continued)

TYPE	EXAMPLE	ASSOCIATED PATHOLOGY	NOTES
Sickle cell		Sickle cell anemia.	Sickling occurs with dehydration, deoxygenation, and at high altitude.
Spherocyte		Hereditary spherocytosis, drug- and infection-induced hemolytic anemia.	
Dacrocyte ("teardrop cell")		Bone marrow infiltration (e.g., myelofibrosis).	RBC "sheds a **tear**" because it's mechanically squeezed out of its home in the bone marrow.
Target cell		HbC disease, Asplenia, Liver disease, Thalassemia.	"**HALT**," said the hunter to his **target**.

Other RBC pathologies

TYPE	EXAMPLE	PROCESS	ASSOCIATED PATHOLOGY
Heinz bodies		Oxidation of Hb -SH groups to -S—S- → Hb precipitation (Heinz bodies A), with subsequent phagocytic damage to RBC membrane → bite cells.	Seen in G6PD deficiency; Heinz body–like inclusions seen in α-thalassemia.
Howell-Jolly bodies		Basophilic nuclear remnants B found in RBCs. Howell-Jolly bodies are normally removed from RBCs by splenic macrophages.	Seen in patients with functional hyposplenia or asplenia.

Anemias

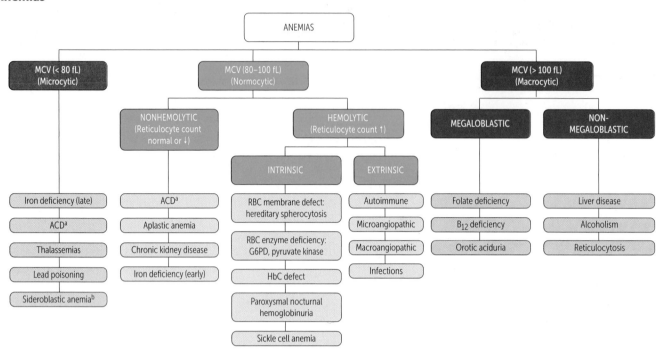

ANEMIAS

- MCV (< 80 fL) (Microcytic)
- MCV (80–100 fL) (Normocytic)
- MCV (> 100 fL) (Macrocytic)

MCV (< 80 fL) (Microcytic)
- Iron deficiency (late)
- ACD[a]
- Thalassemias
- Lead poisoning
- Sideroblastic anemia[b]

MCV (80–100 fL) (Normocytic)

NONHEMOLYTIC (Reticulocyte count normal or ↓)
- ACD[a]
- Aplastic anemia
- Chronic kidney disease
- Iron deficiency (early)

HEMOLYTIC (Reticulocyte count ↑)

INTRINSIC
- RBC membrane defect: hereditary spherocytosis
- RBC enzyme deficiency: G6PD, pyruvate kinase
- HbC defect
- Paroxysmal nocturnal hemoglobinuria
- Sickle cell anemia

EXTRINSIC
- Autoimmune
- Microangiopathic
- Macroangiopathic
- Infections

MCV (> 100 fL) (Macrocytic)

MEGALOBLASTIC
- Folate deficiency
- B$_{12}$ deficiency
- Orotic aciduria

NON-MEGALOBLASTIC
- Liver disease
- Alcoholism
- Reticulocytosis

[a]ACD and iron deficiency anemia may first present as a normocytic anemia and then progress to a microcytic anemia.
[b]Copper deficiency can cause a microcytic sideroblastic anemia.

Microcytic, hypochromic (MCV < 80 fL) anemia

	DESCRIPTION	FINDINGS
Iron deficiency	↓ iron due to chronic bleeding (e.g., GI loss, menorrhagia), malnutrition/absorption disorders, or ↑ demand (e.g., pregnancy) → ↓ final step in heme synthesis.	↓ iron, ↑ TIBC, ↓ ferritin. Fatigue, conjunctival pallor **A**, spoon nails (koilonychia). Microcytosis and hypochromia **B**. May manifest as **Plummer-Vinson syndrome** (triad of iron deficiency anemia, esophageal webs, and atrophic glossitis).

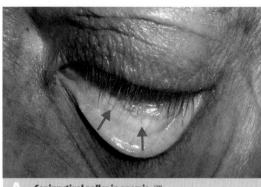

A Conjunctival pallor in anemia. [RU]

B **Iron deficiency.** Note microcytosis and hypochromia (central pallor, arrows).

α-thalassemia	Defect: α-globin gene deletions → ↓ α-globin synthesis. *cis* deletion prevalent in Asian populations; *trans* deletion prevalent in African populations.	4 allele deletion: No α-globin. Excess γ-globin forms γ$_4$ (Hb Barts). Incompatible with life (causes hydrops fetalis). 3 allele deletion: HbH disease. Very little α-globin. Excess β-globin forms β$_4$ (HbH). 1–2 allele deletion: less clinically severe anemia.

Microcytic, hypochromic (MCV < 80 fL) anemia *(continued)*

	DESCRIPTION	FINDINGS
β-thalassemia	Point mutations in splice sites and promoter sequences → ↓ β-globin synthesis. Prevalent in Mediterranean populations. **β-thalassemia major.** Note anisocytosis, poikilocytosis, target cells (arrows 1 and 2), microcytosis (arrow 3), and schistocytes (arrow 4). ℞	**β-thalassemia minor** (heterozygote): <ul><li>β chain is underproduced.</li><li>Usually asymptomatic.</li><li>Diagnosis confirmed by ↑ HbA_2 (> 3.5%) on electrophoresis.</li></ul> **β-thalassemia major** (homozygote): <ul><li>β chain is absent → severe anemia **C** requiring blood transfusion (2° hemochromatosis).</li><li>Marrow expansion ("crew cut" on skull x-ray) → skeletal deformities. "Chipmunk" facies.</li><li>Extramedullary hematopoiesis (leads to hepatosplenomegaly). ↑ risk of parvovirus B19–induced aplastic crisis.</li></ul> Major → ↑ HbF ($\alpha_2\gamma_2$). HbF is protective in the infant and disease becomes symptomatic only after 6 months. HbS/β-thalassemia heterozygote: mild to moderate sickle cell disease depending on amount of β-globin production.
Lead poisoning	Lead inhibits ferrochelatase and ALA dehydratase → ↓ heme synthesis and ↑ RBC protoporphyrin. Also inhibits rRNA degradation, causing RBCs to retain aggregates of rRNA (basophilic stippling). High risk in old houses with chipped paint.	**LEAD:** **L**ead **L**ines on gingivae (Burton lines) and on metaphyses of long bones **D** on x-ray. **E**ncephalopathy and **E**rythrocyte basophilic stippling. **A**bdominal colic and sideroblastic **A**nemia. **D**rops—wrist and foot drop. **D**imercaprol and EDTA are 1st line of treatment. **S**uccimer used for chelation for kids (It "**sucks**" to be a kid who eats lead).
Sideroblastic anemia	Defect in heme synthesis. Hereditary: X-linked defect in δ-ALA synthase gene. Causes: genetic, acquired (myelodysplastic syndromes), and reversible (alcohol is most common; also lead, vitamin B_6 deficiency, copper deficiency, isoniazid).	Ringed sideroblasts (with iron-laden, Prussian blue–stained mitochondria) seen in bone marrow **E**. ↑ iron, normal/↓ TIBC, ↑ ferritin. Treatment: pyridoxine (B_6, cofactor for δ-ALA synthase).

Macrocytic (MCV > 100 fL) anemia

	DESCRIPTION	FINDINGS
Megaloblastic anemia	Impaired DNA synthesis → maturation of nucleus of precursor cells in bone marrow delayed relative to maturation in cytoplasm.	RBC macrocytosis, hypersegmented neutrophils A, glossitis.
Folate deficiency	Causes: malnutrition (e.g., alcoholics), malabsorption, drugs (e.g., methotrexate, trimethoprim, phenytoin), ↑ requirement (e.g., hemolytic anemia, pregnancy).	↑ homocysteine, normal methylmalonic acid. **No neurologic symptoms** (vs. B_{12} deficiency).
B_{12} (cobalamin) deficiency	Causes: insufficient intake (e.g., veganism), malabsorption (e.g., Crohn disease), pernicious anemia, *Diphyllobothrium latum* (fish tapeworm), gastrectomy.	↑ homocysteine, ↑ methylmalonic acid. **Neurologic symptoms:** subacute combined degeneration (due to involvement of B_{12} in fatty acid pathways and myelin synthesis): spinocerebellar tract, lateral corticospinal tract, dorsal column dysfunction.
Orotic aciduria	Inability to convert orotic acid to UMP (de novo pyrimidine synthesis pathway) because of defect in UMP synthase. Autosomal recessive. Presents in children as failure to thrive, developmental delay, and megaloblastic anemia refractory to folate and B_{12}. No hyperammonemia (vs. ornithine transcarbamylase deficiency—↑ orotic acid with hyperammonemia).	Orotic acid in urine. Treatment: uridine monophosphate to bypass mutated enzyme.
Nonmegaloblastic macrocytic anemias	Macrocytic anemia in which DNA synthesis is unimpaired. Causes: alcoholism, liver disease, hypothyroidism, reticulocytosis.	RBC macrocytosis without hypersegmented neutrophils.

Normocytic, normochromic anemia	Normocytic, normochromic anemias are classified as nonhemolytic or hemolytic. The hemolytic anemias are further classified according to the cause of the hemolysis (intrinsic vs. extrinsic to the RBC) and by the location of the hemolysis (intravascular vs. extravascular).
Intravascular hemolysis	Findings: ↓ haptoglobin, ↑ LDH, schistocytes and ↑ reticulocytes on blood smear. Characteristic hemoglobinuria, hemosiderinuria, and urobilinogen in urine. Notable causes are mechanical hemolysis (e.g., prosthetic valve), paroxysmal nocturnal hemoglobinuria, microangiopathic hemolytic anemias.
Extravascular hemolysis	Findings: macrophages in spleen clear RBCs. Spherocytes in peripheral smear, ↑ LDH, no hemoglobinuria/hemosiderinuria, ↑ unconjugated bilirubin, which can cause jaundice.

Nonhemolytic, normocytic anemia

	DESCRIPTION	FINDINGS
Anemia of chronic disease	Inflammation → ↑ hepcidin (released by liver, binds ferroportin on intestinal mucosal cells and macrophages, thus inhibiting iron transport) → ↓ release of iron from macrophages. Associated with conditions such as rheumatoid arthritis, SLE, neoplastic disorders, and chronic kidney disease.	↓ iron, ↓ TIBC, ↑ ferritin. Normocytic, but can become microcytic. Treatment: EPO (chronic kidney disease only).
Aplastic anemia	Caused by failure or destruction of myeloid stem cells due to: ▪ Radiation and drugs (benzene, chloramphenicol, alkylating agents, antimetabolites) ▪ Viral agents (parvovirus B19, EBV, HIV, HCV) ▪ Fanconi anemia (DNA repair defect) ▪ Idiopathic (immune mediated, 1° stem cell defect); may follow acute hepatitis	Pancytopenia characterized by severe anemia, leukopenia, and thrombocytopenia. Normal cell morphology, but hypocellular bone marrow with fatty infiltration **A** (dry bone marrow tap). Symptoms: fatigue, malaise, pallor, purpura, mucosal bleeding, petechiae, infection. Treatment: withdrawal of offending agent, immunosuppressive regimens (e.g., antithymocyte globulin, cyclosporine), bone marrow allograft, RBC/platelet transfusion, bone marrow stimulation (e.g., GM-CSF).

Intrinsic hemolytic normocytic anemia   E = extravascular; I = intravascular.

	DESCRIPTION	FINDINGS
Hereditary spherocytosis (E)	Defect in proteins interacting with RBC membrane skeleton and plasma membrane (e.g., ankyrin, band 3, protein 4.2, spectrin). Results in small, round RBCs with less surface area and no central pallor (↑ MCHC, ↑ red cell distribution width) → premature removal by spleen.	Splenomegaly, aplastic crisis (parvovirus B19 infection). Labs: osmotic fragility test ⊕. Normal to ↓ MCV with abundance of cells. Treatment: splenectomy.
G6PD deficiency (I/E)	Most common enzymatic disorder of RBCs. X-linked recessive. Defect in G6PD → ↓ glutathione → ↑ RBC susceptibility to oxidant stress. Hemolytic anemia following oxidant stress (e.g., sulfa drugs, antimalarials, infections, **fava beans**).	Back pain, hemoglobinuria a few days after oxidant **stress**. Labs: blood smear shows RBCs with **Heinz** bodies and **bite** cells. "**Stress** makes me eat **bites** of **fava beans** with **Heinz** ketchup."
Pyruvate kinase deficiency (E)	Autosomal recessive. Defect in pyruvate kinase → ↓ ATP → rigid RBCs.	Hemolytic anemia in a newborn.
HbC defect (E)	Glutamic acid–to-lysine mutation in β-globin.	Patients with HbSC (1 of each mutant gene) have milder disease than HbSS patients.
Paroxysmal nocturnal hemoglobinuria (I)	↑ complement-mediated RBC lysis (impaired synthesis of GPI anchor for decay-accelerating factor that protects RBC membrane from complement). Acquired mutation in a hematopoietic stem cell. ↑ incidence of acute leukemias.	Triad: Coombs ⊖ hemolytic anemia, pancytopenia, and venous thrombosis. Labs: CD55/59 ⊖ RBCs on flow cytometry. Treatment: eculizumab (terminal complement inhibitor).
Sickle cell anemia (E)	HbS point mutation causes a single amino acid replacement in β chain (substitution of glutamic acid with valine). Pathogenesis: low O_2, high altitude, or acidosis precipitates sickling (deoxygenated HbS polymerizes) → anemia and vaso-occlusive disease. Newborns are initially asymptomatic because of ↑ HbF and ↓ HbS. Heterozygotes (sickle cell trait) also have resistance to malaria. 8% of African Americans carry an HbS allele. Sickle cells are crescent-shaped RBCs $\blacksquare$. "Crew cut" on skull x-ray due to marrow expansion from ↑ erythropoiesis (also seen in thalassemias).	Complications in sickle cell disease: • Aplastic crisis (due to parvovirus B19). • Autosplenectomy (Howell-Jolly bodies) → ↑ risk of infection by encapsulated organisms. • Splenic infarct/sequestration crisis. • *Salmonella* osteomyelitis. • Painful crises (vaso-occlusive): dactylitis (painful swelling of hands/feet), acute chest syndrome, avascular necrosis, stroke. • Renal papillary necrosis (↓ Po_2 in papilla) and microhematuria (medullary infarcts). Diagnosis: hemoglobin electrophoresis. Treatment: hydroxyurea (↑ HbF), hydration.

Extrinsic hemolytic normocytic anemia

	DESCRIPTION	FINDINGS
Autoimmune hemolytic anemia	Warm agglutinin (IgG)—chronic anemia seen in SLE and CLL and with certain drugs (e.g., α-methyldopa) ("**warm** weather is Great"). Cold agglutinin (IgM)—acute anemia triggered by cold; seen in CLL, *Mycoplasma pneumonia* infections, and infectious Mononucleosis ("**cold** weather is **MMM**iserable"). Many warm and cold AIHAs are idiopathic in etiology.	Autoimmune hemolytic anemias are usually Coombs ⊕. Direct Coombs test—anti-Ig antibody (Coombs reagent) added to patient's blood. RBCs agglutinate if RBCs are coated with Ig. Indirect Coombs test—normal RBCs added to patient's serum. If serum has anti-RBC surface Ig, RBCs agglutinate when Coombs reagent added.
Microangiopathic anemia	Pathogenesis: RBCs are damaged when passing through obstructed or narrowed vessel lumina. Seen in DIC, TTP/HUS, SLE, and malignant hypertension.	Schistocytes ("helmet cells") are seen on blood smear due to mechanical destruction of RBCs.
Macroangiopathic anemia	Prosthetic heart valves and aortic stenosis may also cause hemolytic anemia 2° to mechanical destruction.	Schistocytes on peripheral blood smear.
Infections	↑ destruction of RBCs (e.g., malaria, *Babesia*).	

Lab values in anemia

	Iron deficiency	Chronic disease	Hemo-chromatosis	Pregnancy/OCP use
Serum iron	↓ (1°)	↓	↑ (1°)	—
Transferrin or TIBC	↑	↓[a]	↓	↑ (1°)
Ferritin	↓	↑ (1°)	↑	—
% transferrin saturation (serum iron/TIBC)	↓↓	—	↑↑	↓

Transferrin—**trans**ports iron in blood.
TIBC—indirectly measures transferrin.
Ferritin—1° iron storage protein of body.
[a] Evolutionary reasoning—pathogens use circulating iron to thrive. The body has adapted a system in which iron is stored within the cells of the body and prevents pathogens from acquiring circulating iron.

Leukopenias

CELL TYPE	CELL COUNT	CAUSES
Neutropenia	Absolute neutrophil count < 1500 cells/mm^3	Sepsis/postinfection, drugs (including chemotherapy), aplastic anemia, SLE, radiation
Lymphopenia	Absolute lymphocyte count < 1500 cells/mm^3 (< 3000 cells/mm³ in children)	HIV, DiGeorge syndrome, SCID, SLE, corticosteroids,[a] radiation, sepsis, postoperative
Eosinopenia		Cushing syndrome, corticosteroids[a]

[a] Corticosteroids cause neutrophilia, despite causing eosinopenia and lymphopenia. Corticosteroids ↓ activation of neutrophil adhesion molecules, impairing migration out of the vasculature to sites of inflammation. In contrast, corticosteroids sequester eosinophils in lymph nodes and cause apoptosis of lymphocytes.

Heme synthesis, porphyrias, and lead poisoning

The porphyrias are hereditary or acquired conditions of defective heme synthesis that lead to the accumulation of heme precursors. Lead inhibits specific enzymes needed in heme synthesis, leading to a similar condition.

CONDITION	AFFECTED ENZYME	ACCUMULATED SUBSTRATE	PRESENTING SYMPTOMS
Lead poisoning 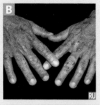	Ferrochelatase and ALA dehydratase	Protoporphyrin, δ-ALA (blood)	Microcytic anemia (basophilic stippling A), GI and kidney disease. Children—exposure to lead paint → mental deterioration. Adults—environmental exposure (e.g., batteries, ammunition) → headache, memory loss, demyelination.
Acute intermittent porphyria	Porphobilinogen deaminase	Porphobilinogen, δ-ALA, coporphobilinogen (urine)	Symptoms (**5 P's**): ▪ **P**ainful abdomen ▪ **P**ort wine–colored urine ▪ **P**olyneuropathy ▪ **P**sychological disturbances ▪ **P**recipitated by drugs (e.g., cytochrome P-450 inducers), alcohol, starvation Treatment: glucose and heme, which inhibit ALA synthase.
Porphyria cutanea tarda	Uroporphyrinogen decarboxylase	Uroporphyrin (tea-colored urine)	Blistering cutaneous photosensitivity B. Most common porphyria.

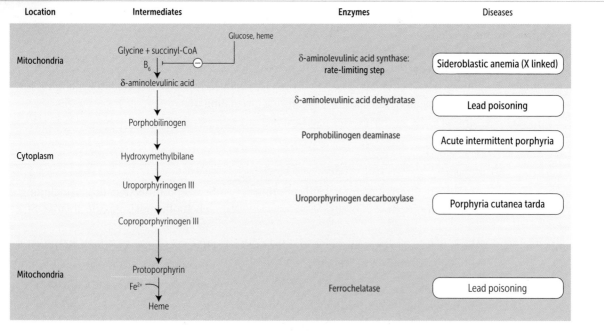

↓ heme → ↑ ALA synthase activity
↑ heme → ↓ ALA synthase activity

Iron poisoning	High mortality rate with accidental ingestion by children (adult iron tablets may look like candy).
MECHANISM	Cell death due to peroxidation of membrane lipids.
SYMPTOMS/SIGNS	Nausea, vomiting, gastric bleeding, lethargy, scarring leading to GI obstruction.
TREATMENT	Chelation (e.g., IV deferoxamine, oral deferasirox) and dialysis.

Coagulation disorders

PT—tests function of common and extrinsic pathway (factors I, II, V, VII, and X). Defect → ↑ PT.
PTT—tests function of common and intrinsic pathway (all factors except VII and XIII). Defect → ↑ PTT.

DISORDER	PT	PTT	MECHANISM AND COMMENTS
Hemophilia A, B, or C 	—	↑	Intrinsic pathway coagulation defect. ▪ A: deficiency of factor VIII → ↑ PTT; X-linked recessive. ▪ B: deficiency of factor IX → ↑ PTT; X-linked recessive. ▪ C: deficiency of factor XI → ↑ PTT; autosomal recessive. Macrohemorrhage in hemophilia—hemarthroses (bleeding into joints, such as knee **A**), easy bruising, bleeding after trauma or surgery (e.g., dental procedures). Treatment: desmopressin + factor VIII concentrate (A); factor IX concentrate (B); factor XI concentrate (C).
Vitamin K deficiency	↑	↑	General coagulation defect. Bleeding time normal. ↓ activation of factors II, VII, IX, X, protein C, protein S.

Platelet disorders

Defects in platelet plug formation → ↑ bleeding time (BT).
Platelet abnormalities → microhemorrhage: mucous membrane bleeding, epistaxis, petechiae, purpura, ↑ bleeding time, possibly decreased platelet count (PC).

DISORDER	PC	BT	MECHANISM AND COMMENTS
Bernard-Soulier syndrome	–/↓	↑	Defect in platelet plug formation. Large platelets. ↓ GpIb → defect in platelet-to-vWF adhesion. No agglutination on ristocetin cofactor assay.
Glanzmann thrombasthenia	–	↑	Defect in platelet plug formation. ↓ GpIIb/IIIa → defect in platelet-to-platelet aggregation. Labs: blood smear shows no platelet clumping. Agglutination with ristocetin cofactor assay.
Immune thrombocytopenia	↓	↑	Anti-GpIIb/IIIa antibodies → splenic macrophage consumption of platelet-antibody complex. Commonly due to viral illness. Labs: ↑ megakaryocytes on bone marrow biopsy. Treatment: steroids, intravenous immunoglobulin.
Thrombotic thrombocytopenic purpura	↓	↑	Inhibition or deficiency of ADAMTS 13 (vWF metalloprotease) → ↓ degradation of vWF multimers. Pathogenesis: ↑ large vWF multimers → ↑ platelet adhesion → ↑ platelet aggregation and thrombosis. Labs: schistocytes, ↑ LDH. Symptoms: pentad of neurologic and renal symptoms, fever, thrombocytopenia, and microangiopathic hemolytic anemia. Treatment: plasmapheresis, steroids.

Mixed platelet and coagulation disorders

DISORDER	PC	BT	PT	PTT	MECHANISM AND COMMENTS
von Willebrand disease	—	↑	—	↑[a]	Intrinsic pathway coagulation defect: ↓ vWF → ↑ PTT (vWF acts to carry/protect factor VIII). Defect in platelet plug formation: ↓ vWF → defect in platelet-to-vWF adhesion. Autosomal dominant. Mild but most common inherited bleeding disorder. Diagnosed in most cases by ristocetin cofactor assay (↓ agglutination is diagnostic). Treatment: desmopressin, which releases vWF stored in endothelium.
DIC	↓	↑	↑	↑	Widespread activation of clotting → deficiency in clotting factors → bleeding state. Causes: Sepsis (gram-negative), Trauma, Obstetric complications, acute Pancreatitis, Malignancy, Nephrotic syndrome, Transfusion (**STOP** Making New Thrombi). Labs: schistocytes, ↑ fibrin split products (D-dimers), ↓ fibrinogen, ↓ factors V and VIII.

[a]PTT may also be normal in von Willebrand disease.

Hereditary thrombosis syndromes leading to hypercoagulability

DISEASE	DESCRIPTION
Antithrombin deficiency	Inherited deficiency of antithrombin: has no direct effect on the PT, PTT, or thrombin time but diminishes the increase in PTT following heparin administration. Can also be acquired: renal failure/nephrotic syndrome → antithrombin loss in urine → ↓ inhibition of factors IIa and Xa.
Factor V Leiden	Production of mutant factor V that is resistant to degradation by activated protein C. Most common cause of inherited hypercoagulability in whites.
Protein C or S deficiency	↓ ability to inactivate factors Va and VIIIa. ↑ risk of thrombotic skin necrosis with hemorrhage following administration of warfarin. Skin and subcutaneous tissue necrosis after warfarin administration → think protein C deficiency. "Protein **C** **C**ancels **C**oagulation."
Prothrombin gene mutation	Mutation in 3′ untranslated region → ↑ production of prothrombin → ↑ plasma levels and venous clots.

Blood transfusion therapy

COMPONENT	DOSAGE EFFECT	CLINICAL USE
Packed RBCs	↑ Hb and O_2 carrying capacity	Acute blood loss, severe anemia
Platelets	↑ platelet count (↑ ~5000/mm³/unit)	Stop significant bleeding (thrombocytopenia, qualitative platelet defects)
Fresh frozen plasma	↑ coagulation factor levels	DIC, cirrhosis, immediate warfarin reversal
Cryoprecipitate	Contains fibrinogen, factor VIII, factor XIII, vWF, and fibronectin	Coagulation factor deficiencies involving fibrinogen and factor VIII

Blood transfusion risks include infection transmission (low), transfusion reactions, iron overload, hypocalcemia (citrate is a Ca^{2+} chelator), and hyperkalemia (RBCs may lyse in old blood units).

Leukemia vs. lymphoma

Leukemia	Lymphoid or myeloid neoplasm with widespread involvement of bone marrow. Tumor cells are usually found in peripheral blood.
Lymphoma	Discrete tumor mass arising from lymph nodes. Presentations often blur definitions.

Leukemoid reaction	Acute inflammatory response to infection. ↑ WBC count with ↑ neutrophils and neutrophil precursors such as band cells (left shift); ↑ leukocyte alkaline phosphatase (LAP). Contrast with CML (also ↑ WBC count with left shift, but ↓ LAP).

Hodgkin vs. non-Hodgkin lymphoma	Hodgkin	Non-Hodgkin
	Localized, single group of nodes; extranodal rare; contiguous spread (stage is strongest predictor of prognosis). Prognosis is much better than with non-Hodgkin lymphoma.	Multiple, peripheral nodes; extranodal involvement common; noncontiguous spread.
	Characterized by Reed-Sternberg cells.	Majority involve B cells (except those of lymphoblastic T-cell origin).
	Bimodal distribution–young adulthood and > 55 years; more common in men except for nodular sclerosing type.	Peak incidence for certain subtypes at 20–40 years old.
	Strongly associated with EBV.	May be associated with HIV and autoimmune diseases.
	Constitutional ("B") signs/symptoms: low-grade fever, night sweats, weight loss.	Fewer constitutional signs/symptoms.

Reed-Sternberg cells   Distinctive tumor giant cell seen in Hodgkin disease; binucleate or bilobed with the 2 halves as mirror images ("owl eyes" 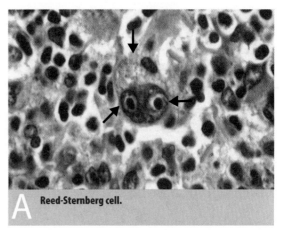). RS cells are CD15+ and CD30+ B-cell origin. Necessary but not sufficient for a diagnosis of Hodgkin disease. Better prognosis with strong stromal or lymphocytic reaction against RS cells. Nodular sclerosing form most common (affects women and men equally). Lymphocyte-rich form has best prognosis. Lymphocyte mixed or depleted forms have worse prognosis.

2 owl eyes × 15 = 30.

A   Reed-Sternberg cell.

Non-Hodgkin lymphoma

TYPE	OCCURS IN	GENETICS	COMMENTS
Neoplasms of mature B cells			
Burkitt lymphoma	Adolescents or young adults	t(8;14)—translocation of c-*myc* (8) and heavy-chain Ig (14)	"Starry sky" appearance **A**, sheets of lymphocytes with interspersed macrophages (arrows). Associated with EBV. Jaw lesion **B** in endemic form in Africa; pelvis or abdomen in sporadic form.
Diffuse large B-cell lymphoma	Usually older adults, but 20% in children		Most common type of non-Hodgkin lymphoma in adults.
Follicular lymphoma	Adults	t(14;18)—translocation of heavy-chain Ig (14) and *BCL*-2 (18)	Indolent course; Bcl-2 inhibits apoptosis. Presents with painless "waxing and waning" lymphadenopathy. Nodular, small cells; cleaved nuclei.
Mantle cell lymphoma	Older males	t(11;14)—translocation of cyclin D1 (11) and heavy-chain Ig (14)	CD5+.
Neoplasms of mature T cells			
Adult T-cell lymphoma	Adults	Caused by HTLV (associated with IV drug abuse)	Adults present with cutaneous lesions; especially affects populations in Japan, West Africa, and the Caribbean. Lytic bone lesions, hypercalcemia.
Mycosis fungoides/ Sézary syndrome	Adults	**C**	Mycosis fungoides presents with skin patches **C**/ plaques (cutaneous T-cell lymphoma), characterized by atypical CD4+ cells with "cerebriform" nuclei. May progress to Sézary syndrome (T-cell leukemia).

Multiple myeloma

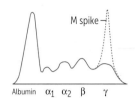

Monoclonal plasma cell ("fried egg" appearance) cancer that arises in the marrow and produces large amounts of IgG (55%) or IgA (25%). Most common 1° tumor arising within bone in people > 40–50 years old.
Associated with:

- ↑ susceptibility to infection
- Primary amyloidosis (AL)
- Punched-out lytic bone lesions on x-ray **A**
- M spike on serum protein electrophoresis
- Ig light chains in urine (Bence Jones protein)
- Rouleaux formation **B** (RBCs stacked like poker chips in blood smear)

Numerous plasma cells **C** with "clock-face" chromatin and intracytoplasmic inclusions containing immunoglobulin.

Monoclonal gammopathy of undetermined significance (MGUS)—monoclonal expansion of plasma cells, asymptomatic, may lead to multiple myeloma. No "**CRAB**" findings. Patients with MGUS develop multiple myeloma at a rate of 1–2% per year.

Think **CRAB**:
HyperCalcemia
Renal involvement
Anemia
Bone lytic lesions/Back pain
Multiple Myeloma: Monoclonal **M** protein spike
Distinguish from Waldenström macroglobulinemia → M spike = IgM → hyperviscosity syndrome (e.g., blurred vision, Raynaud phenomenon); no "**CRAB**" findings.

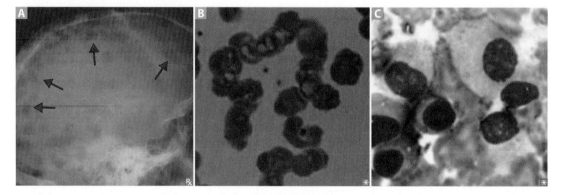

Myelodysplastic syndromes

Stem-cell disorders involving ineffective hematopoiesis → defects in cell maturation of all nonlymphoid lineages. Caused by de novo mutations or environmental exposure (e.g., radiation, benzene, chemotherapy). Risk of transformation to AML.

Pseudo–Pelger-Huet anomaly—neutrophils with bilobed nuclei. Typically seen after chemotherapy.

Leukemias	Unregulated growth and differentiation of WBCs in bone marrow → marrow failure → anemia (↓ RBCs), infections (↓ mature WBCs), and hemorrhage (↓ platelets). ↑ or ↓ number of circulating WBCs.	
	Leukemic cell infiltration of liver, spleen, lymph nodes, and skin (leukemia cutis) possible.	

TYPE	PERIPHERAL BLOOD SMEAR	COMMENTS
Lymphoid neoplasms		
Acute lymphoblastic leukemia/lymphoma (ALL)	Age: < 15 years. T-cell ALL can present as mediastinal mass (presenting as SVC-like syndrome). Associated with Down syndrome. Peripheral blood and bone marrow have ↑↑↑ lymphoblasts **A**. TdT+ (marker of pre-T and pre-B cells), CD10+ (pre-B cells only). Most responsive to therapy. May spread to CNS and testes. t(12;21) → better prognosis.	
Small lymphocytic lymphoma (SLL)/ chronic lymphocytic leukemia (CLL)	Age: > 60 years. Most common adult leukemia. CD20+, CD5+ B-cell neoplasm. Often asymptomatic, progresses slowly; smudge cells **B** in peripheral blood smear; autoimmune hemolytic anemia. SLL same as CLL except CLL has ↑ peripheral blood lymphocytosis or bone marrow involvement.	
Hairy cell leukemia	Age: Adults. Mature B-cell tumor in the elderly. Cells have filamentous, hair-like projections **C**. Causes marrow fibrosis → dry tap on aspiration. Stains TRAP (tartrate-resistant acid phosphatase ⊕). TRAP stain largely replaced with flow cytometry. Treatment: cladribine, pentostatin.	
Myeloid neoplasms		
Acute myelogenous leukemia (AML)	Age: median onset 65 years. Auer rods **D**; peroxidase ⊕ cytoplasmic inclusions seen mostly in M3 AML; ↑↑↑ circulating myeloblasts on peripheral smear; adults. Risk factors: prior exposure to alkylating chemotherapy, radiation, myeloproliferative disorders, Down syndrome. t(15;17) → M3 AML subtype responds to all-*trans* retinoic acid (vitamin A), inducing differentiation of myeloblasts; DIC is a common presentation.	
Chronic myelogenous leukemia (CML)	Age: peak incidence 45–85 years, median age at diagnosis 64 years. Defined by the Philadelphia chromosome (t[9;22], *BCR-ABL*); myeloid stem cell proliferation; presents with ↑ neutrophils, metamyelocytes, basophils **E**; splenomegaly; may accelerate and transform to AML or ALL ("blast crisis"). Very low LAP as a result of low activity in mature granulocytes (vs. leukemoid reaction, in which LAP is ↑). Responds to imatinib (a small-molecule inhibitor of the *bcr-abl* tyrosine kinase).	

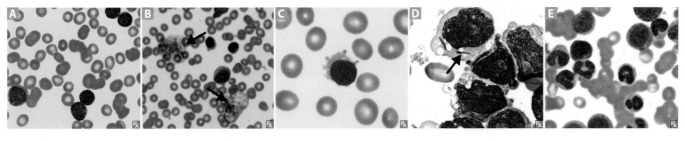

Chromosomal translocations

TRANSLOCATION	ASSOCIATED DISORDER	
t(8;14)	Burkitt lymphoma (c-*myc* activation)	
t(9;22) (**Philadelphia chromosome**)	CML (*BCR-ABL* hybrid)	Philadelphia CreaML cheese.
t(11;14)	Mantle cell lymphoma (cyclin D1 activation)	
t(14;18)	Follicular lymphoma (*BCL*-2 activation)	
t(15;17)	M3 type of AML	Responds to all-*trans* retinoic acid.

Langerhans cell histiocytosis

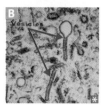

Collective group of proliferative disorders of dendritic (Langerhans) cells. Presents in a child as lytic bone lesions A and skin rash or as recurrent otitis media with a mass involving the mastoid bone. Cells are functionally immature and do not effectively stimulate primary T cells via antigen presentation. Cells express S-100 (mesodermal origin) and CD1a. Birbeck granules ("tennis rackets" or rod shaped on EM) are characteristic B.

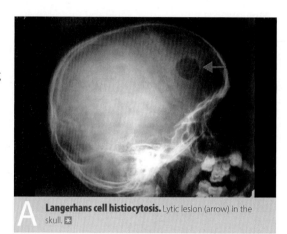

A **Langerhans cell histiocytosis.** Lytic lesion (arrow) in the skull. ✷

Chronic myeloproliferative disorders	The myeloproliferative disorders represent an often-overlapping spectrum, but the classic findings are described below. *JAK2* is involved in hematopoietic growth factor signaling. *JAK2* gene mutation is often found in chronic myeloproliferative disorders except CML (which has *BCR-ABL* translocation).
Polycythemia vera	Disorder of ↑ hematocrit, often associated with *JAK2* mutation. May present as intense itching after hot shower (due to ↑ basophils). Rare but classic symptom is erythromelalgia (severe, burning pain and red-blue coloration) due to episodic blood clots in vessels of the extremities **A**. 2° polycythemia is via natural or artificial ↑ in EPO levels.
Essential thrombocytosis	Similar to polycythemia vera, but specific for overproduction of abnormal platelets → bleeding, thrombosis. Bone marrow contains enlarged megakaryocytes **B**.
Myelofibrosis	Obliteration of bone marrow due to ↑ fibroblast activity in response to proliferation of monoclonal cell lines **C**. "Teardrop" RBCs and immature forms of the myeloid line. "Bone marrow is **crying** because it's fibrosed and is a dry tap." Often associated with massive splenomegaly.

	RBCs	WBCs	PLATELETS	PHILADELPHIA CHROMOSOME	*JAK2* MUTATIONS
Polycythemia vera	↑	↑	↑	⊖	⊕
Essential thrombocytosis	–	–	↑	⊖	⊕ (30–50%)
Myelofibrosis	↓	Variable	Variable	⊖	⊕ (30–50%)
CML	↓	↑	↑	⊕	⊖

Polycythemia

	PLASMA VOLUME	RBC MASS	O₂ SATURATION	EPO LEVELS	ASSOCIATIONS
Relative	↓	–	–	–	↓ plasma volume (dehydration, burns).
Appropriate absolute	–	↑	↓	↑	Lung disease, congenital heart disease, high altitude.
Inappropriate absolute	–	↑	–	↑	Renal cell carcinoma, hepatocellular carcinoma, hydronephrosis. Due to ectopic EPO.
Polycythemia vera	↑	↑↑	–	↓	EPO ↓ in PCV due to negative feedback suppressing renal EPO production.

▶ HEMATOLOGY AND ONCOLOGY—PHARMACOLOGY

Heparin

MECHANISM	Activator of antithrombin; ↓ thrombin and ↓ factor Xa. Short half-life.
CLINICAL USE	Immediate anticoagulation for pulmonary embolism (PE), acute coronary syndrome, MI, deep venous thrombosis (DVT). Used during pregnancy (does not cross placenta). Follow PTT.
TOXICITY	Bleeding, thrombocytopenia (HIT), osteoporosis, drug-drug interactions. For rapid reversal (antidote), use protamine sulfate (positively charged molecule that binds negatively charged heparin).
NOTES	Low-molecular-weight heparins (e.g., enoxaparin, dalteparin) and fondaparinux act more on factor Xa, have better bioavailability, and 2–4 times longer half-life; can be administered subcutaneously and without laboratory monitoring. Not easily reversible.
	Heparin-induced thrombocytopenia (HIT)—development of IgG antibodies against heparin-bound platelet factor 4 (PF4). Antibody-heparin-PF4 complex activates platelets → thrombosis and thrombocytopenia.

Argatroban, bivalirudin, dabigatran	Bivalirudin is related to hirudin, the anticoagulant used by leeches; inhibit thrombin directly. Alternatives to heparin for anticoagulating patients with HIT.

Warfarin

MECHANISM	Interferes with γ-carboxylation of vitamin K–dependent clotting factors II, VII, IX, and X, and proteins C and S. Metabolism affected by polymorphisms in the gene for vitamin K epoxide reductase complex (*VKORC1*). In laboratory assay, has effect on **EX**trinsic pathway and ↑ **PT**. Long half-life.	The **EX-PresidenT** went to **war**(farin).
CLINICAL USE	Chronic anticoagulation (e.g., venous thromboembolism prophylaxis, and prevention of stroke in atrial fibrillation). Not used in pregnant women (because warfarin, unlike heparin, crosses placenta). Follow PT/INR.	
TOXICITY	Bleeding, teratogenic, skin/tissue necrosis , drug-drug interactions. Proteins C and S have shorter half-lives than clotting factors II, VI, IX, and X, resulting in early transient hypercoagulability with warfarin use. Skin/tissue necrosis believed to be due to small vessel microthromboses.	For reversal of warfarin, give vitamin K. For rapid reversal, give fresh frozen plasma. Heparin "bridging": heparin frequently used when starting warfarin. Heparin's activation of antithrombin enables anticoagulation during initial, transient hypercoagulable state caused by warfarin. Initial heparin therapy reduces risk of recurrent venous thromboembolism and skin/tissue necrosis.

Heparin vs. warfarin

	Heparin	Warfarin
STRUCTURE	Large, anionic, acidic polymer	Small, amphipathic molecule
ROUTE OF ADMINISTRATION	Parenteral (IV, SC)	Oral
SITE OF ACTION	Blood	Liver
ONSET OF ACTION	Rapid (seconds)	Slow, limited by half-lives of normal clotting factors
MECHANISM OF ACTION	Activates antithrombin, which ↓ the action of IIa (thrombin) and factor Xa	Impairs activation of vitamin K–dependent clotting factors II, VII, IX, and X, and anti-clotting proteins C and S
DURATION OF ACTION	Acute (hours)	Chronic (days)
INHIBITS COAGULATION IN VITRO	Yes	No
AGENTS FOR REVERSAL	Protamine sulfate	Vitamin K, fresh frozen plasma
MONITORING	PTT (intrinsic pathway)	PT/INR (extrinsic pathway)
CROSSES PLACENTA	No	Yes (teratogenic)

Direct factor Xa inhibitors

Apixaban, rivaroxaban.

MECHANISM	Bind to and directly inhibit factor Xa.
CLINICAL USE	Treatment and prophylaxis for DVT and PE (rivaroxaban); stroke prophylaxis in patients with atrial fibrillation. Oral agents do not usually require coagulation monitoring.
TOXICITY	Bleeding (no reversal agent available).

Thrombolytics

Alteplase (tPA), reteplase (rPA), streptokinase, tenecteplase (TNK-tPA).

MECHANISM	Directly or indirectly aid conversion of plasminogen to plasmin, which cleaves thrombin and fibrin clots. ↑ PT, ↑ PTT, no change in platelet count.
CLINICAL USE	Early MI, early ischemic stroke, direct thrombolysis of severe PE.
TOXICITY	Bleeding. Contraindicated in patients with active bleeding, history of intracranial bleeding, recent surgery, known bleeding diatheses, or severe hypertension. Treat toxicity with aminocaproic acid, an inhibitor of fibrinolysis. Fresh frozen plasma and cryoprecipitate can also be used to correct factor deficiencies.

Aspirin

MECHANISM	Irreversibly inhibits cyclooxygenase (both COX-1 and COX-2) enzyme by covalent acetylation. Platelets cannot synthesize new enzyme, so effect lasts until new platelets are produced: ↑ bleeding time, ↓ TXA$_2$ and prostaglandins. No effect on PT or PTT.
CLINICAL USE	Antipyretic, analgesic, anti-inflammatory, antiplatelet (↓ aggregation).
TOXICITY	Gastric ulceration, tinnitus (CN VIII). Chronic use can lead to acute renal failure, interstitial nephritis, and upper GI bleeding. Reye syndrome in children with viral infection. Overdose initially causes hyperventilation and respiratory alkalosis, but transitions to mixed metabolic acidosis–respiratory alkalosis.

ADP receptor inhibitors

Clopidogrel, prasugrel, ticagrelor (reversible), ticlopidine.

MECHANISM	Inhibit platelet aggregation by irreversibly blocking ADP receptors. Prevent expression of glycoproteins IIb/IIIa on platelet surface.
CLINICAL USE	Acute coronary syndrome; coronary stenting. ↓ incidence or recurrence of thrombotic stroke.
TOXICITY	Neutropenia (ticlopidine). TTP may be seen.

Cilostazol, dipyridamole

MECHANISM	Phosphodiesterase III inhibitor; ↑ cAMP in platelets, resulting in inhibition of platelet aggregation; vasodilators.
CLINICAL USE	Intermittent claudication, coronary vasodilation, prevention of stroke or TIAs (combined with aspirin), angina prophylaxis.
TOXICITY	Nausea, headache, facial flushing, hypotension, abdominal pain.

GP IIb/IIIa inhibitors

Abciximab, eptifibatide, tirofiban.

MECHANISM	Bind to the glycoprotein receptor IIb/IIIa on activated platelets, preventing aggregation. Abciximab is made from monoclonal antibody Fab fragments.
CLINICAL USE	Unstable angina, percutaneous transluminal coronary angioplasty.
TOXICITY	Bleeding, thrombocytopenia.

Cancer drugs—cell cycle

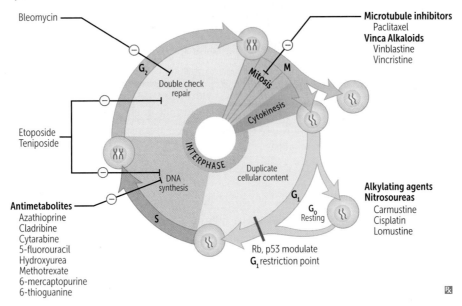

Bleomycin

Microtubule inhibitors
Paclitaxel
Vinca Alkaloids
Vinblastine
Vincristine

G₂

Double check repair

Mitosis

M

Cytokinesis

INTERPHASE

Etoposide
Teniposide

XX

Duplicate cellular content

G₁

Alkylating agents
Nitrosoureas
Carmustine
Cisplatin
Lomustine

DNA synthesis

Antimetabolites
Azathioprine
Cladribine
Cytarabine
5-fluorouracil
Hydroxyurea
Methotrexate
6-mercaptopurine
6-thioguanine

S

G₀
Resting

Rb, p53 modulate
G₁ restriction point

Antineoplastics

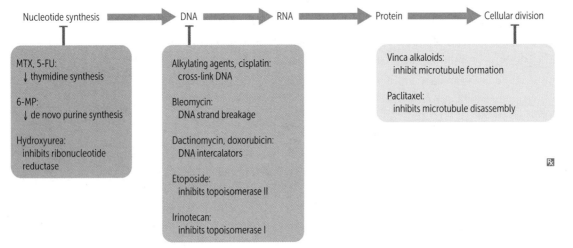

Nucleotide synthesis → DNA → RNA → Protein → Cellular division

MTX, 5-FU:
↓ thymidine synthesis

6-MP:
↓ de novo purine synthesis

Hydroxyurea:
inhibits ribonucleotide reductase

Alkylating agents, cisplatin:
cross-link DNA

Bleomycin:
DNA strand breakage

Dactinomycin, doxorubicin:
DNA intercalators

Etoposide:
inhibits topoisomerase II

Irinotecan:
inhibits topoisomerase I

Vinca alkaloids:
inhibit microtubule formation

Paclitaxel:
inhibits microtubule disassembly

Antimetabolites

DRUG	MECHANISM[a]	CLINICAL USE	TOXICITY
Azathioprine, 6-mercaptopurine (6-MP), 6-thioguanine (6-TG)	Purine (thiol) analogs → ↓ de novo purine synthesis. Activated by HGPRT. Azathioprine is metabolized into 6-MP.	Preventing organ rejection, rheumatoid arthritis, IBD, SLE; used to wean patients off steroids in chronic disease and to treat steroid-refractory chronic disease.	Myelosuppression, GI, liver. Azathioprine and 6-MP are metabolized by xanthine oxidase; thus both have ↑ toxicity with allopurinol or febuxostat.
Cladribine (2-CDA)	Purine analog → multiple mechanisms (e.g., inhibition of DNA polymerase, DNA strand breaks).	Hairy cell leukemia.	Myelosuppression, nephrotoxicity, and neurotoxicity.
Cytarabine (arabinofuranosyl cytidine)	Pyrimidine analog → inhibition of DNA polymerase.	Leukemias (AML), lymphomas.	Leukopenia, thrombocytopenia, megaloblastic anemia. CYTarabine causes panCYTopenia.
5-fluorouracil (5-FU)	Pyrimidine analog bioactivated to 5F-dUMP, which covalently complexes folic acid. This complex inhibits thymidylate synthase → ↓ dTMP → ↓ DNA synthesis.	Colon cancer, pancreatic cancer, basal cell carcinoma (topical).	Myelosuppression, which is not reversible with leucovorin (folinic acid).
Methotrexate (MTX)	Folic acid analog that competitively inhibits dihydrofolate reductase → ↓ dTMP → ↓ DNA synthesis.	Cancers: leukemias (ALL), lymphomas, choriocarcinoma, sarcomas. Non-neoplastic: ectopic pregnancy, medical abortion (with misoprostol), rheumatoid arthritis, psoriasis, IBD, vasculitis.	Myelosuppression, which is reversible with leucovorin "rescue." Hepatotoxicity. Mucositis (e.g., mouth ulcers). Pulmonary fibrosis.

[a]All are S-phase specific.

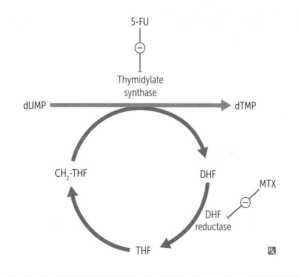

Antitumor antibiotics

DRUG	MECHANISM	CLINICAL USE	TOXICITY
Bleomycin	Induces free radical formation → breaks in DNA strands.	Testicular cancer, Hodgkin lymphoma.	Pulmonary fibrosis, skin hyperpigmentation, mucositis. Minimal myelosuppression.
Dactinomycin (actinomycin D)	Intercalates in DNA.	Wilms tumor, Ewing sarcoma, rhabdomyosarcoma. Used for childhood tumors ("children act out").	Myelosuppression.
Doxorubicin, daunorubicin	Generate free radicals. Intercalate in DNA → breaks in DNA → ↓ replication.	Solid tumors, leukemias, lymphomas.	Cardiotoxicity (dilated cardiomyopathy), myelosuppression, alopecia. Toxic to tissues following extravasation. Dexrazoxane (iron chelating agent), used to prevent cardiotoxicity.

Alkylating agents

DRUG	MECHANISM	CLINICAL USE	TOXICITY
Busulfan	Cross-links DNA.	CML. Also used to ablate patient's bone marrow before bone marrow transplantation.	Severe myelosuppression (in almost all cases), pulmonary fibrosis, hyperpigmentation.
Cyclophosphamide, ifosfamide	Cross-link DNA at guanine N-7. Require bioactivation by liver.	Solid tumors, leukemia, lymphomas.	Myelosuppression; hemorrhagic cystitis, partially prevented with mesna (thiol group of mesna binds toxic metabolites).
Nitrosoureas (carmustine, lomustine, semustine, streptozocin)	Require bioactivation. Cross blood-brain barrier → CNS. Cross-link DNA.	Brain tumors (including glioblastoma multiforme).	CNS toxicity (convulsions, dizziness, ataxia).

Microtubule inhibitors

DRUG	MECHANISM	CLINICAL USE	TOXICITY
Paclitaxel, other taxols	Hyperstabilize polymerized microtubules in M phase so that mitotic spindle cannot break down (anaphase cannot occur). "It is **taxing** to stay polymerized."	Ovarian and breast carcinomas.	Myelosuppression, alopecia, hypersensitivity.
Vincristine, vinblastine	Vinca alkaloids that bind β-tubulin and inhibit its polymerization into microtubules → prevent mitotic spindle formation (M-phase arrest).	Solid tumors, leukemias, Hodgkin (vinblastine) and non-Hodgkin (vincristine) lymphomas.	Vincristine: neurotoxicity (areflexia, peripheral neuritis), paralytic ileus. Vinblastine **blasts** bone marrow (suppression).

Cisplatin, carboplatin

MECHANISM	Cross-link DNA.
CLINICAL USE	Testicular, bladder, ovary, and lung carcinomas.
TOXICITY	Nephrotoxicity, ototoxicity. Prevent nephrotoxicity with amifostine (free radical scavenger) and chloride (saline) diuresis.

Etoposide, teniposide

MECHANISM	Etoposide inhibits **topoisomerase II** → ↑ DNA degradation.
CLINICAL USE	Solid tumors (particularly testicular and small cell lung cancer), leukemias, lymphomas.
TOXICITY	Myelosuppression, GI upset, alopecia.

Irinotecan, topotecan

MECHANISM	Inhibit topoisomerase I and prevent DNA unwinding and replication.
CLINICAL USE	Colon cancer (irinotecan); ovarian and small cell lung cancers (topotecan).
TOXICITY	Severe myelosuppression, diarrhea.

Hydroxyurea

MECHANISM	Inhibits ribonucleotide reductase → ↓ DNA Synthesis (**S**-phase specific).
CLINICAL USE	Melanoma, CML, sickle cell disease (↑ HbF).
TOXICITY	Severe myelosuppression, GI upset.

Prednisone, prednisolone

MECHANISM	Various; bind intracytoplasmic receptor; alter gene transcription.
CLINICAL USE	Most commonly used glucocorticoids in cancer chemotherapy. Used in CLL, non-Hodgkin lymphoma (part of combination chemotherapy regimen). Also used as immunosuppressants (e.g., in autoimmune diseases).
TOXICITY	Cushing-like symptoms; weight gain, central obesity, muscle breakdown, cataracts, acne, osteoporosis, hypertension, peptic ulcers, hyperglycemia, psychosis.

Bevacizumab

MECHANISM	Monoclonal antibody against VEGF. Inhibits angiogenesis.
CLINICAL USE	Solid tumors (colorectal cancer, renal cell carcinoma).
TOXICITY	Hemorrhage, blood clots, and impaired wound healing.

Erlotinib

MECHANISM	EGFR tyrosine kinase inhibitor.
CLINICAL USE	Non-small cell lung carcinoma.
TOXICITY	Rash.

Imatinib

MECHANISM	Tyrosine kinase inhibitor of *BCR-ABL* (Philadelphia chromosome fusion gene in CML) and c-*kit* (common in GI stromal tumors).
CLINICAL USE	CML, GI stromal tumors.
TOXICITY	Fluid retention.

Rituximab

MECHANISM	Monoclonal antibody against CD20, which is found on most B-cell neoplasms.
CLINICAL USE	Non-Hodgkin lymphoma, CLL, IBD, rheumatoid arthritis.
TOXICITY	↑ risk of progressive multifocal leukoencephalopathy.

Tamoxifen, raloxifene

MECHANISM	Selective estrogen receptor modulators (SERMs)—receptor antagonists in breast and agonists in bone. Block the binding of estrogen to ER ⊕ cells.
CLINICAL USE	Breast cancer treatment (tamoxifen only) and prevention. Raloxifene also useful to prevent osteoporosis.
TOXICITY	Tamoxifen—partial agonist in endometrium, which ↑ the risk of endometrial cancer; "hot flashes." Raloxifene—no ↑ in endometrial carcinoma because it is an estrogen receptor antagonist in endometrial tissue.

Trastuzumab (Herceptin)

MECHANISM	Monoclonal antibody against HER-2 (*c-erbB2*), a tyrosine kinase receptor. Helps kill cancer cells that overexpress HER-2, through inhibition of HER2-initiated cellular signaling and antibody-dependent cytotoxicity.
CLINICAL USE	HER-2 ⊕ breast cancer and gastric cancer (tras2zumab).
TOXICITY	Cardiotoxicity. "**Heart**ceptin" damages the **heart**.

Vemurafenib

MECHANISM	Small molecule inhibitor of *BRAF* oncogene ⊕ melanoma
CLINICAL USE	Metastatic melanoma.

Common chemotoxicities

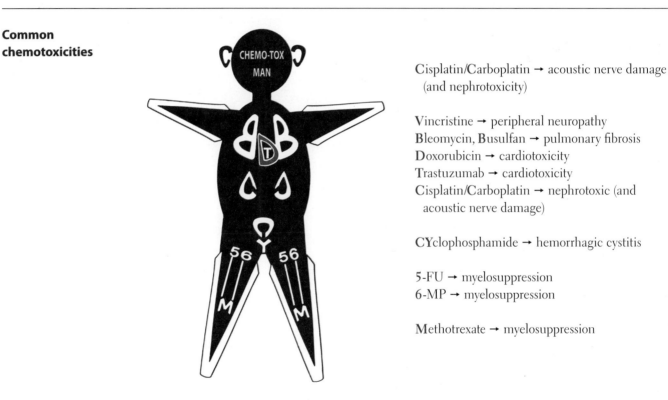

Cisplatin/Carboplatin → acoustic nerve damage (and nephrotoxicity)

Vincristine → peripheral neuropathy
Bleomycin, Busulfan → pulmonary fibrosis
Doxorubicin → cardiotoxicity
Trastuzumab → cardiotoxicity
Cisplatin/Carboplatin → nephrotoxic (and acoustic nerve damage)

CYclophosphamide → hemorrhagic cystitis

5-FU → myelosuppression
6-MP → myelosuppression

Methotrexate → myelosuppression

Musculoskeletal, Skin, and Connective Tissue

"Rigid, the skeleton of habit alone upholds the human frame."
—Virginia Woolf

"Beauty may be skin deep, but ugly goes clear to the bone."
—Redd Foxx

"The function of muscle is to pull and not to push, except in the case of the genitals and the tongue."
—Leonardo da Vinci

▶ **MUSCULOSKELETAL, SKIN, AND CONNECTIVE TISSUE—ANATOMY AND PHYSIOLOGY**

Knee exam

TEST	PROCEDURE	
Anterior drawer sign	With patient supine, bending knee at 90-degree angle, ↑ anterior gliding of tibia due to ACL injury.	"Anterior" and "posterior" in ACL and PCL refer to sites of tibial attachment.
Posterior drawer sign	With patient supine, bending knee at 90-degree angle, ↑ posterior gliding of tibia due to PCL injury.	
Abnormal passive abduction	With patient supine and knee either extended or at ~ 30-degree angle, lateral (valgus) force → medial space widening of tibia → MCL injury.	
Abnormal passive adduction	With patient supine and knee either extended or at ~ 30-degree angle, medial (varus) force → lateral space widening of tibia → LCL injury.	
McMurray test	With patient supine and knee internally and externally rotated during range of motion: ▪ Pain, "popping" on external rotation → medial meniscal tear ▪ Pain, "popping" on internal rotation → lateral meniscal tear	

Common knee conditions

"Unhappy triad"	Common injury in contact sports due to lateral force applied to a planted leg. Classically, consists of damage to the ACL, MCL, and medial meniscus (attached to MCL); however, lateral meniscus injury is more common. Presents with acute knee pain and signs of joint injury/instability.	
Prepatellar bursitis	"Housemaid's knee" (**A**, left). Can be caused by repeated trauma or pressure from extensive kneeling.	
Baker cyst	Popliteal fluid collection (**A**, right) commonly related to chronic joint disease.	

A **Common knee conditions.** Prepatellar bursitis (left) and Baker cyst (right). ▨, ▨

| **Rotator cuff muscles** | Shoulder muscles that form the rotator cuff:
▪ Supraspinatus (suprascapular nerve)—abducts arm initially (before the action of the deltoid); most common rotator cuff injury, assessed by "empty/full can" test.
▪ Infraspinatus (suprascapular nerve)—laterally rotates arm; pitching injury.
▪ teres minor (axillary nerve)—adducts and laterally rotates arm.
▪ Subscapularis (upper and lower subscapular nerves)—medially rotates and adducts arm.
Innervated primarily by C5-C6. | SItS (small t is for teres **minor**).
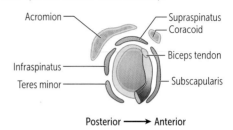 |

Overuse injuries of the elbow

Medial epicondylitis (golfer's elbow)	Repetitive flexion (forehand shots) or idiopathic → pain near medial epicondyle.
Lateral epicondylitis (tennis elbow)	Repetitive extension (backhand shots) or idiopathic → pain near lateral epicondyle.

Wrist bones	Scaphoid, Lunate, Triquetrum, Pisiform, Hamate, Capitate, Trapezoid, Trapezium ▣. (So Long To Pinky, Here Comes The Thumb). Scaphoid (palpated in anatomic snuff box) is the most commonly fractured carpal bone and is prone to avascular necrosis owing to retrograde blood supply. Dislocation of lunate may cause acute carpal tunnel syndrome. A fall on an outstretched hand that damages the hook of the hamate can cause ulnar nerve injury.	**A** Bones of wrist. ▣
Carpal tunnel syndrome	Entrapment of median nerve in carpal tunnel; nerve compression → paresthesia, pain, and numbness in distribution of median nerve. Associated with pregnancy, rheumatoid arthritis, hypothyroidism; may be associated with repetitive use.
Guyon canal syndrome	Compression of ulnar nerve at wrist or hand. Classically seen in cyclists due to pressure from handlebars.

Upper extremity nerves

NERVE	CAUSES OF INJURY	PRESENTATION
Axillary (C5-C6)	Fractured surgical neck of humerus; anterior dislocation of humerus	Flattened deltoid Loss of arm abduction at shoulder (> 15 degrees) Loss of sensation over deltoid muscle and lateral arm
Musculocutaneous (C5-C7)	Upper trunk compression	Loss of forearm flexion and supination Loss of sensation over lateral forearm
Radial (C5-T1)	Midshaft fracture of humerus; compression of axilla, e.g., due to crutches or sleeping with arm over chair ("Saturday night palsy")	Wrist drop: loss of elbow, wrist, and finger extension ↓ grip strength (wrist extension necessary for maximal action of flexors) Loss of sensation over posterior arm/forearm and dorsal hand
Median (C5-T1)	Supracondylar fracture of humerus (proximal lesion); carpal tunnel syndrome and wrist laceration (distal lesion)	"Ape hand" and "Pope's blessing" Loss of wrist flexion, flexion of lateral fingers, thumb opposition, lumbricals of 2nd and 3rd digits Loss of sensation over thenar eminence and dorsal and palmar aspects of lateral 3½ fingers with proximal lesion Tinel sign (tingling on percussion) in carpal tunnel syndrome
Ulnar (C8-T1)	Fracture of medial epicondyle of humerus "funny bone" (proximal lesion); fractured hook of hamate (distal lesion)	"Ulnar claw" on digit extension Radial deviation of wrist upon flexion (proximal lesion) Loss of wrist flexion, flexion of medial fingers, abduction and adduction of fingers (interossei), actions of medial 2 lumbrical muscles Loss of sensation over medial 1½ fingers including hypothenar eminence
Recurrent branch of median nerve (C5-T1)	Superficial laceration of palm	"Ape hand" Loss of thenar muscle group: opposition, abduction, and flexion of thumb No loss of sensation

Axillary nerve
Musculocutaneous nerve
Radial nerve in spiral groove
Radial nerve
Radial nerve
Recurrent branch of median nerve
Median nerve
Ulnar nerve
Median nerve
Ulnar nerve

Median nerve
Ulnar nerve
Radial nerve (superficial branch)
Palm of hand

Median nerve
Radial nerve (superficial branch)
Ulnar nerve
Dorsum of hand

Brachial plexus lesions

❶ Erb palsy ("waiter's tip")
❷ Claw hand (Klumpke palsy)
❸ Wrist drop
❹ Winged scapula
❺ Deltoid paralysis
❻ "Saturday night palsy" (wrist drop)
❼ Difficulty flexing elbow, variable sensory loss
❽ Decreased thumb function, "Pope's blessing"
❾ Intrinsic muscles of hand, claw hand

C5 C6 C7 C8 T1

Long thoracic — **R**oots ❹

Upper ❶ Middle Lower ❷ — **T**runks

— **D**ivisions

Lateral Posterior ❸ Medial — **C**ords

❺ ❻

Axillary Radial
(Extensors)

— **B**ranches

❼ ❽ ❾

Musculocutaneous Median Ulnar
(Flexors)

Randy
Travis
Drinks
Cold
Beer

CONDITION	INJURY	CAUSES	MUSCLE DEFICIT	FUNCTIONAL DEFICIT	PRESENTATION
Erb palsy ("waiter's tip")	Traction or tear of **upper** ("**Erb**-er") trunk: C5-C6 roots	Infants—lateral traction on neck during delivery Adults—trauma	Deltoid, supraspinatus	Abduction (arm hangs by side)	
			Infraspinatus	Lateral rotation (arm medially rotated)	
			Biceps brachii	Flexion, supination (arm extended and pronated)	
Klumpke palsy	Traction or tear of **lower** trunk: C8-T1 root	Infants—upward force on arm during delivery Adults—trauma (e.g., grabbing a tree branch to break a fall)	Intrinsic hand muscles: lumbricals, interossei, thenar, hypothenar	Total claw hand: lumbricals normally flex MCP joints and extend DIP and PIP joints	
Thoracic outlet syndrome	Compression of **lower** trunk and subclavian vessels	Cervical rib, Pancoast tumor	Same as Klumpke palsy	Atrophy of intrinsic hand muscles; ischemia, pain, and edema due to vascular compression	
Winged scapula	Lesion of long thoracic nerve	Axillary node dissection after mastectomy, stab wounds	Serratus anterior	Inability to anchor scapula to thoracic cage → cannot abduct arm above horizontal position	

Distortions of the hand   At rest, a balance exists between the extrinsic flexors and extensors of the hand, as well as the intrinsic muscles of the hand—particularly the lumbrical muscles (flexion of MCP, extension of DIP and PIP joints).

"Clawing"—seen best with **distal** lesions of median or ulnar nerves. Remaining extrinsic flexors of the digits exaggerate the loss of the lumbricals → fingers extend at MCP, flex at DIP and PIP joints.

Deficits less pronounced in **proximal** lesions; deficits present during voluntary flexion of the digits.

PRESENTATION				
CONTEXT	Extending fingers/at rest	Making a fist	Extending fingers/at rest	Making a fist
LOCATION OF LESION	Distal ulnar nerve	Proximal median nerve	Distal median nerve	Proximal ulnar nerve
SIGN	"Ulnar claw"	"Pope's blessing"	"Median claw"	"OK gesture" (with digits 1–3 flexed)

Note: Atrophy of the thenar eminence (unopposable thumb → "ape hand") can be seen in median nerve lesions, while atrophy of the hypothenar eminence can be seen in ulnar nerve lesions.

Hand muscles

Thenar eminence

Hypothenar eminence

Thenar (median)—Opponens pollicis, Abductor pollicis brevis, Flexor pollicis brevis, superficial head (deep head by ulnar nerve).

Hypothenar (ulnar)—Opponens digiti minimi, Abductor digiti minimi, Flexor digiti minimi brevis.

Dorsal interossei—abduct the fingers.
Palmar interossei—adduct the fingers.
Lumbricals—flex at the MCP joint, extend PIP and DIP joints.

Both groups perform the same functions: Oppose, Abduct, and Flex (**OAF**).

DAB = **D**orsals **AB**duct.
PAD = **P**almars **AD**duct.

Lower extremity nerves

NERVE	CAUSE OF INJURY	PRESENTATION
Obturator (L2–L4)	Pelvic surgery	↓ thigh sensation (medial) and ↓ adduction.
Femoral (L2–L4)	Pelvic fracture	↓ thigh flexion and leg extension.
Common peroneal (L4–S2)	Trauma or compression of lateral aspect of leg, fibular neck fracture	Foot drop—inverted and plantarflexed at rest, loss of eversion and dorsiflexion. "Steppage gait." Loss of sensation on dorsum of foot.
Tibial (L4–S3)	Knee trauma, Baker cyst (proximal lesion); tarsal tunnel syndrome (distal lesion)	Inability to curl toes and loss of sensation on sole of foot. In proximal lesions, foot everted at rest with loss of inversion and plantarflexion.
Superior gluteal (L4–S1)	Iatrogenic injury during intramuscular injection to upper medial gluteal region	Trendelenburg sign/gait—pelvis tilts because weight-bearing leg cannot maintain alignment of pelvis through hip abduction (superior nerve → medius and minimus). Lesion is contralateral to the side of the hip that drops, ipsilateral to extremity on which the patient stands.
Inferior gluteal (L5–S2)	Posterior hip dislocation	Difficulty climbing stairs, rising from seated position. Loss of hip extension (inferior nerve → maximus).

Superior gluteal nerve innervates gluteus medius and minimus. Inferior gluteal nerve innervates gluteus maximus.

PED = Peroneal Everts and Dorsiflexes; if injured, foot drop**PED**.

TIP = Tibial Inverts and Plantarflexes; if injured, can't stand on **TIP**toes.

Sciatic nerve (L4–S3) innervates posterior thigh, splits into common peroneal and tibial nerves.

Pudendal nerve (S2–S4) innervates perineum. Can be blocked with local anesthetic during childbirth using the ischial spine as a landmark for injection.

Signs of lumbosacral radiculopathy

Paresthesias and weakness in distribution of specific lumbar or sacral spinal nerves. Often due to intervertebral disc herniation in which the nerve association with the inferior vertebral body is impinged (e.g., herniation of L3–L4 disc affects the L4 spinal nerve).

Intervertebral discs generally herniate posterolaterally, due to the thin posterior longitudinal ligament and thicker anterior longitudinal ligament along the midline of the vertebral bodies.

DISC LEVEL	FINDINGS
L3–L4	Weakness of knee extension, ↓ patellar reflex
L4–L5	Weakness of dorsiflexion, difficulty in heel-walking
L5–S1	Weakness of plantarflexion, difficulty in toe-walking, ↓ Achilles reflex

Neurovascular pairing

Nerves and arteries are frequently named together by the bones/regions with which they are associated. The following are exceptions to this naming convention.

LOCATION	NERVE	ARTERY
Axilla/lateral thorax	Long thoracic	Lateral thoracic
Surgical neck of humerus	Axillary	Posterior circumflex
Midshaft of humerus	Radial	Deep brachial
Distal humerus/ cubital fossa	Median	Brachial
Popliteal fossa	Tibial	Popliteal
Posterior to medial malleolus	Tibial	Posterior tibial

Muscle conduction to contraction

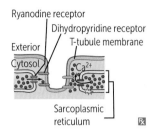

Ryanodine receptor
Dihydropyridine receptor
T-tubule membrane
Exterior
Cytosol
Ca²⁺
Sarcoplasmic reticulum

1. Action potential depolarization opens presynaptic voltage-gated Ca^{2+} channels, inducing neurotransmitter release.
2. Postsynaptic ligand binding leads to muscle cell depolarization in the motor end plate.
3. Depolarization travels along muscle cell and down the T-tubule.
4. Depolarization of the voltage-sensitive dihydropyridine receptor, mechanically coupled to the ryanodine receptor on the sarcoplasmic reticulum, induces a conformational change, causing Ca^{2+} release from sarcoplasmic reticulum.
5. Released Ca^{2+} binds to troponin C, causing a conformational change that moves tropomyosin out of the myosin-binding groove on actin filaments.
6. Myosin releases bound ADP and inorganic PO_4^{3-} → displacement of myosin on the actin filament (power stroke). Contraction results in shortening of **H** and **I** bands and between **Z** lines (**HIZ** shrinkage), but the A band remains the same length (**A** band is **A**lways the same length) 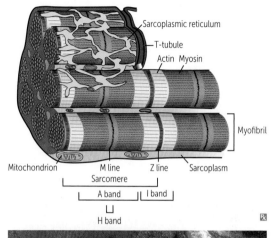.
7. Binding of a new ATP molecule causes detachment of myosin head from actin filament. Hydrolysis of bound ATP → ADP, myosin head adopts high-energy position ("cocked") for the next contraction cycle.

T-tubules (extensions of plasma membrane juxtaposed with terminal cisternae) are part of the sarcoplasmic reticulum.
In skeletal muscle, 1 T-tubule + 2 terminal cisternae = triad.
In cardiac muscle, 1 T-tubule + 1 terminal cisternae = diad.

Sarcoplasmic reticulum
T-tubule
Actin Myosin
Myofibril
Mitochondrion
M line
Sarcomere
Z line
Sarcoplasm
A band
I band
H band

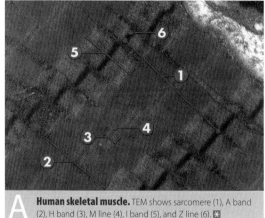

A **Human skeletal muscle.** TEM shows sarcomere (1), A band (2), H band (3), M line (4), I band (5), and Z line (6). ✷

Types of muscle fibers

Type 1 muscle	Slow twitch; **red** fibers resulting from ↑ mitochondria and myoglobin concentration (↑ **oxidative phosphorylation**) → sustained contraction.	Think "**1 slow red ox.**"
Type 2 muscle	Fast twitch; white fibers resulting from ↓ mitochondria and myoglobin concentration (↑ anaerobic glycolysis); weight training results in hypertrophy of fast-twitch muscle fibers.	

Smooth muscle contraction

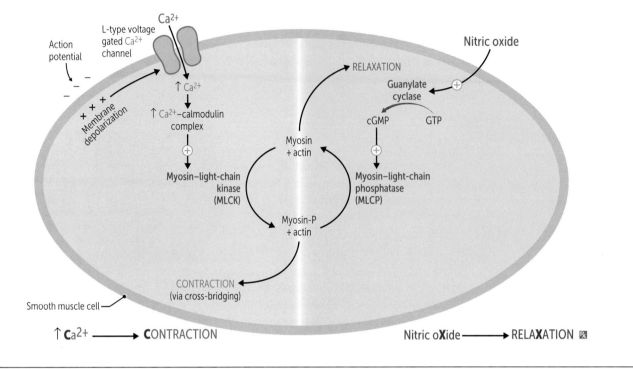

Bone formation

Endochondral ossification	Bones of axial and appendicular skeleton and base of skull. Cartilaginous model of bone is first made by chondrocytes. Osteoclasts and osteoblasts later replace with woven bone and then remodel to lamellar bone. In adults, woven bone occurs after fractures and in Paget disease.
Membranous ossification	Bones of calvarium and facial bones. Woven bone formed directly without cartilage. Later remodeled to lamellar bone.

Cell biology of bone

Osteoblasts	Build bone by secreting collagen and catalyzing mineralization. Differentiate from mesenchymal stem cells in periosteum.
Osteoclasts	Multinucleated cells that dissolve bone by secreting acid and collagenases. Differentiate from monocytes, macrophages.
Parathyroid hormone	At low, intermittent levels, exerts anabolic effects (building bone) on osteoblasts and osteoclasts (indirect). Chronically ↑ PTH levels (1° hyperparathyroidism) cause catabolic effects (osteitis fibrosa cystica).
Estrogen	Estrogen inhibits apoptosis in bone-forming osteoblasts and induces apoptosis in bone-resorbing osteoclasts. Estrogen deficiency (surgical or postmenopausal), excess cycles of remodeling, and bone resorption lead to osteoporosis.

▶ MUSCULOSKELETAL, SKIN, AND CONNECTIVE TISSUE—PATHOLOGY

Achondroplasia	Failure of longitudinal bone growth (endochondral ossification) → short limbs. Membranous ossification is not affected → large head relative to limbs. Constitutive activation of fibroblast growth factor receptor (FGFR3) actually inhibits chondrocyte proliferation. > 85% of mutations occur sporadically; autosomal dominant with full penetrance (homozygosity is lethal). Most common cause of dwarfism.

Primary osteoporosis	Trabecular (spongy) bone loses mass and interconnections despite normal bone mineralization and lab values (serum Ca^{2+} and PO_4^{3-}). Diagnosed by a bone mineral density test (DEXA) with a T-score of ≤ –2.5. Can be caused by long-term exogenous steroid use, anticonvulsants, anticoagulants, thyroid replacement therapy. Can lead to vertebral compression fractures—acute back pain, loss of height, kyphosis. Also can present with fractures of femoral neck, distal radius (Colles fracture).

Type I (post-menopausal)	↑ bone resorption due to ↓ estrogen levels.

Type II (senile)	Affects men and women > 70 years old. Mild compression fracture Normal vertebrae	Prophylaxis: regular weight-bearing exercise and adequate Ca^{2+} and vitamin D intake throughout adulthood. Treatment: bisphosphonates, PTH analogs, SERMs, rarely calcitonin; denosumab (monoclonal antibody against RANKL).

Osteopetrosis (marble bone disease)	Failure of normal bone resorption due to defective osteoclasts → thickened, dense bones that are prone to fracture. Bone fills marrow space → pancytopenia, extramedullary hematopoiesis. Mutations (e.g., carbonic anhydrase II) impair ability of osteoclast to generate acidic environment necessary for bone resorption. X-rays show bone-in-bone appearance **A**. Can result in cranial nerve impingement and palsies as a result of narrowed foramina. Bone marrow transplant is potentially curative as osteoclasts are derived from monocytes.	 **A** **Osteopetrosis.** Radiograph of pelvis shows diffusely dense bones.

Osteomalacia/rickets	Vitamin D deficiency → osteomalacia in adults; rickets in children. Due to defective mineralization/calcification of osteoid → soft bones that bow out. ↓ vitamin D → ↓ serum Ca^{2+} → ↑ PTH secretion → ↓ serum PO_4^{3-}. Hyperactivity of osteoblasts → ↑ ALP (osteoblasts require alkaline environment).

Paget disease of bone (osteitis deformans)

Common, localized disorder of bone remodeling caused by ↑ in both osteoblastic and osteoclastic activity. Serum Ca^{2+}, phosphorus, and PTH levels are normal. ↑ ALP. Mosaic pattern of woven and lamellar bone 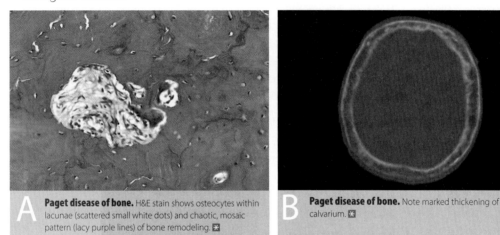; long bone chalk-stick fractures. ↑ blood flow from ↑ arteriovenous shunts may cause high-output heart failure. ↑ risk of osteogenic sarcoma.

Hat size can be increased **B**; hearing loss is common due to auditory foramen narrowing.
Stages of Paget disease:
- Lytic—osteoclasts
- Mixed—osteoclasts + osteoblasts
- Sclerotic—osteoblasts
- Quiescent—minimal osteoclast/osteoblast activity

A **Paget disease of bone.** H&E stain shows osteocytes within lacunae (scattered small white dots) and chaotic, mosaic pattern (lacy purple lines) of bone remodeling. ✱

B **Paget disease of bone.** Note marked thickening of calvarium. ✱

Osteonecrosis (avascular necrosis)

Infarction of bone and marrow, usually very painful. Most common site is femoral head **A** (due to insufficiency of medial circumflex femoral artery). Causes include Alcoholism, Sickle cell disease, Storage, Exogenous/Endogenous corticosteroids, Pancreatitis, Trauma, Idiopathic (Legg-Calvé-Perthes disease), Caisson ("the bends")—ASEPTIC.

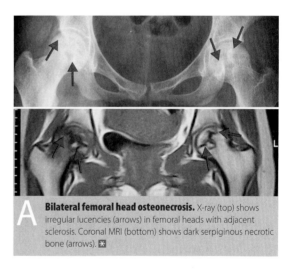

A **Bilateral femoral head osteonecrosis.** X-ray (top) shows irregular lucencies (arrows) in femoral heads with adjacent sclerosis. Coronal MRI (bottom) shows dark serpiginous necrotic bone (arrows). ✱

Lab values in bone disorders

DISORDER	SERUM Ca^{2+}	PO_4^{3-}	ALP	PTH	COMMENTS
Osteoporosis	—	—	—	—	↓ bone mass
Osteopetrosis	—/↓	—	—	—	Dense, brittle bones. Ca^{2+} ↓ in severe, malignant disease
Paget disease of bone	—	—	↑	—	Abnormal "mosaic" bone architecture
Osteomalacia/rickets	↓	↓	↑	↑	Soft bones
Hypervitaminosis D	↑	↑	—	↓	Caused by oversupplementation or granulomatous disease (e.g., sarcoidosis)
Osteitis fibrosa cystica					"Brown tumors" due to fibrous replacement of bone, subperiosteal thinning
1° hyperparathyroidism	↑	↓	↑	↑	Idiopathic or parathyroid hyperplasia, adenoma, carcinoma
2° hyperparathyroidism	↓	↑	↑	↑	Often as compensation for ESRD (↓ PO_4^{3-} excretion and production of activated vitamin D)

Primary bone tumors

TUMOR TYPE	EPIDEMIOLOGY/LOCATION	CHARACTERISTICS
Benign tumors		
Giant cell tumor	20–40 years old. Epiphyseal end of long bones. "Osteoclastoma."	Locally aggressive benign tumor often around knee. "Soap bubble" appearance on x-ray 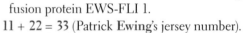. Multinucleated giant cells.
Osteochondroma	Most common benign tumor (an exostosis of the bone B). Males < 25 years old.	Mature bone with cartilaginous (**chondroid**) cap. Rarely transforms to chondrosarcoma.
Malignant tumors		
Osteosarcoma (osteogenic sarcoma)	2nd most common 1° malignant bone tumor (after multiple myeloma). Bimodal distribution: 10–20 years old (1°), > 65 (2°). Predisposing factors: Paget disease of bone, bone infarcts, radiation, familial retinoblastoma, Li-Fraumeni syndrome (germline $p53$ mutation). Metaphysis of long bones, often around knee C .	Codman triangle (from elevation of periosteum) or sunburst pattern on x-ray. Aggressive. Treat with surgical en bloc resection (with limb salvage) and chemotherapy.
Ewing sarcoma	Boys < 15 years old. Commonly appears in diaphysis of long bones, pelvis, scapula, ribs.	Anaplastic small blue cell malignant tumor D . Extremely aggressive with early metastases, but responsive to chemotherapy. "Onion skin" periosteal reaction in bone. Associated with t(**11;22**) translocation causing fusion protein EWS-FLI 1. **11** + **22** = **33** (Patrick **Ewing**'s jersey number).

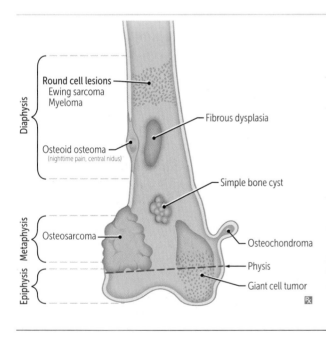

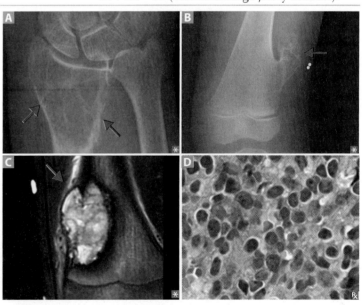

Osteoarthritis and rheumatoid arthritis

	Osteoarthritis	Rheumatoid arthritis
ETIOLOGY	Mechanical—joint wear and tear destroys articular cartilage.	Autoimmune—inflammatory destruction of synovial joints. Mediated by cytokines and type III and type IV hypersensitivity reactions.
JOINT FINDINGS	Subchondral cysts, sclerosis A, osteophytes (bone spurs), eburnation (polished, ivory-like appearance of bone), synovitis, Heberden nodes (DIP), Bouchard nodes (PIP). No MCP involvement.	Pannus (inflammatory granulation tissue) formation in joints (MCP, PIP), subcutaneous rheumatoid nodules (fibrinoid necrosis), ulnar deviation of fingers, subluxation B. Rare swan neck and boutonnière deformities. Rare DIP involvement.
PREDISPOSING FACTORS	Age, obesity, joint trauma.	Females > males. 80% have ⊕ rheumatoid factor (anti-IgG antibody); anti–cyclic citrullinated peptide antibody is more specific. Strong association with HLA-DR4.
CLASSIC PRESENTATION	Pain in weight-bearing joints after use (e.g., at the end of the day), improving with rest. Knee cartilage loss begins medially ("bowlegged"). Noninflammatory. No systemic symptoms.	Morning stiffness lasting > 30 minutes and improving with use, symmetric joint involvement, systemic symptoms (fever, fatigue, weight loss, pleuritis, pericarditis).
TREATMENT	Acetaminophen, NSAIDs, intra-articular glucocorticoids.	NSAIDs, glucocorticoids, disease-modifying agents (methotrexate, sulfasalazine), biologics (TNF-α inhibitors).

Normal | Osteoarthritis

Joint capsule and synovial lining
Synovial cavity
Cartilage

Thickened capsule
Slight synovial hypertrophy
Osteophyte
Ulcerated cartilage
Sclerotic bone
Joint space narrowing
Subchondral bone cyst

Normal | Rheumatoid arthritis

Joint capsule and synovial lining
Synovial cavity
Cartilage

Bone and cartilage erosion
Increased synovial fluid
Pannus formation

A **Osteoarthritis.** X-ray of hands shows joint space narrowing and sclerosis (arrows). ℞

B **Rheumatoid arthritis.** Note boutonnière deformities of PIP joints with ulnar deviation.

Sjögren syndrome

Autoimmune disorder characterized by destruction of exocrine glands (especially lacrimal and salivary) by lymphocytic infiltrates A. Predominantly affects females 40–60 years old.

Findings:

- Inflammatory joint pain
- Xerophthalmia (↓ tear production and subsequent corneal damage)
- Xerostomia (↓ saliva production)
- Presence of antinuclear antibodies: SS-A (anti-Ro) and/or SS-B (anti-La)
- Bilateral parotid enlargement

A common 1° disorder or a 2° syndrome associated with other autoimmune disorders (e.g., rheumatoid arthritis).

Complications: dental caries; mucosa-associated lymphoid tissue (MALT) lymphoma (may present as parotid enlargement).

Gout

FINDINGS	Acute inflammatory monoarthritis caused by precipitation of monosodium urate crystals in joints A. More common in males. Associated with hyperuricemia, which can be caused by: - Underexcretion of uric acid (90% of patients)—largely idiopathic; can be exacerbated by certain medications (e.g., thiazide diuretics). - Overproduction of uric acid (10% of patients)—Lesch-Nyhan syndrome, PRPP excess, ↑ cell turnover (e.g., tumor lysis syndrome), von Gierke disease. Crystals are needle shaped and ⊖ birefringent under polarized light (yellow under parallel light, blue under perpendicular light B).
SYMPTOMS	Asymmetric joint distribution. Joint is swollen, red, and painful. Classic manifestation is painful MTP joint of big toe (podagra). Tophus formation C (often on external ear, olecranon bursa, or Achilles tendon). Acute attack tends to occur after a large meal or alcohol consumption (alcohol metabolites compete for same excretion sites in kidney as uric acid → ↓ uric acid secretion and subsequent buildup in blood).
TREATMENT	Acute: NSAIDs (e.g., indomethacin), glucocorticoids, colchicine. Chronic (preventive): xanthine oxidase inhibitors (e.g., allopurinol, febuxostat).

Pseudogout

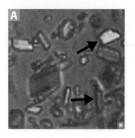

Presents with pain and effusion in a joint, caused by deposition of calcium pyrophosphate crystals within the joint space (chondrocalcinosis on x-ray). Forms basophilic, rhomboid crystals that are weakly birefringent under polarized light . Usually affects large joints (classically the knee). > 50 years old; both sexes affected equally. Diseases associated with pseudogout include hemochromatosis, hyperparathyroidism, osteoarthritis. Treatment includes NSAIDs for sudden, severe attacks; glucocorticoids; colchicine for prophylaxis.

Gout—crystals are yellow when parallel (∥) to the light.

Pseudogout—crystals are blue when parallel (∥) to the light.

Infectious arthritis

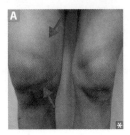

S. aureus, *Streptococcus*, and *Neisseria gonorrhoeae* are common causes. Gonococcal arthritis is an **STD** that presents as a migratory arthritis with an asymmetric pattern. Affected joint is swollen **A**, red, and painful. **STD** = **S**ynovitis (e.g., knee), **T**enosynovitis (e.g., hand), and **D**ermatitis (e.g., pustules).

Seronegative spondyloarthropathies

Arthritis without rheumatoid factor (no anti-IgG antibody). Strong association with HLA-B27 (gene that codes for MHC class I). Occurs more often in males. **PAIR**.

Psoriatic arthritis	Joint pain and stiffness associated with psoriasis. Asymmetric and patchy involvement **A**. Dactylitis ("sausage fingers"), "pencil-in-cup" deformity on x-ray **B**. Seen in fewer than ⅓ of patients with psoriasis.	
Ankylosing spondylitis	Chronic inflammatory disease of spine and sacroiliac joints → ankylosis (stiff spine due to fusion of joints), uveitis, aortic regurgitation.	Bamboo spine (vertebral fusion) **C**.
Inflammatory bowel disease	Crohn disease and ulcerative colitis are often accompanied by ankylosing spondylitis or peripheral arthritis.	
Reactive arthritis (Reiter syndrome)	Classic triad: <ul><li>Conjunctivitis and anterior uveitis</li><li>Urethritis</li><li>Arthritis</li></ul>	"Can't see, can't pee, can't bend my knee." Post-GI (*Shigella*, *Salmonella*, *Yersinia*, *Campylobacter*) or *Chlamydia* infections.

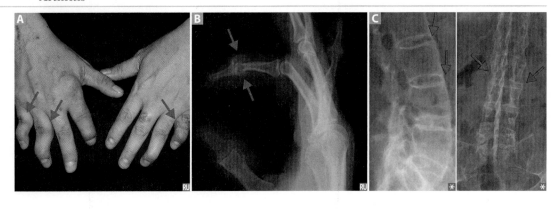

Systemic lupus erythematosus

SYMPTOMS	Classic presentation: rash, joint pain, and fever, most commonly in a female of reproductive age and African descent. Libman-Sacks endocarditis—nonbacterial, wart-like vegetations on both sides of valve. Lupus nephritis (type III hypersensitivity reaction): • Nephritic—diffuse proliferative glomerulonephritis • Nephrotic—membranous glomerulonephritis	**RASH OR PAIN:** **R**ash (malar A or discoid) **A**rthritis **S**oft tissues/serositis **H**ematologic disorders (e.g., cytopenias) **O**ral/nasopharyngeal ulcers **R**enal disease, **R**aynaud phenomenon **P**hotosensitivity, **P**ositive VDRL/RPR **A**ntinuclear antibodies **I**mmunosuppressants **N**eurologic disorders (e.g. seizures, psychosis) Common causes of death in SLE: • Cardiovascular disease • Infections • Renal disease
FINDINGS	Antinuclear antibodies (ANA)	Sensitive, not specific
	Anti-dsDNA antibodies	Specific, poor prognosis (renal disease)
	Anti-Smith antibodies	Specific, not prognostic (directed against snRNPs)
	Antihistone antibodies	Sensitive for drug-induced lupus
	↓ C3, C4, and CH_{50} due to immune complex formation.	
TREATMENT	NSAIDs, steroids, immunosuppressants, hydroxychloroquine.	

Antiphospholipid syndrome	1° or 2° autoimmune disorder (most commonly in SLE). Diagnose based on clinical criteria including history of thrombosis (arterial or venous) or spontaneous abortion along with laboratory findings of lupus anticoagulant, anticardiolipin, anti-β_2 glycoprotein antibodies. Treat with systemic anticoagulation.	Anticardiolipin antibodies and lupus anticoagulant can cause false-positive VDRL and prolonged PTT.

Sarcoidosis

Characterized by immune-mediated, widespread noncaseating granulomas A, elevated serum ACE levels, and elevated CD4+/CD8+ ratio. Common in black females. Often asymptomatic except for enlarged lymph nodes. Findings on CXR of bilateral adenopathy and coarse reticular opacities B; CT of the chest better demonstrates the extensive hilar and mediastinal adenopathy C.

Associated with restrictive lung disease (interstitial fibrosis), erythema nodosum, lupus pernio, Bell palsy, epithelioid granulomas containing microscopic Schaumann and asteroid bodies, uveitis, hypercalcemia (due to ↑ 1α-hydroxylase–mediated vitamin D activation in macrophages). Treatment: steroids.

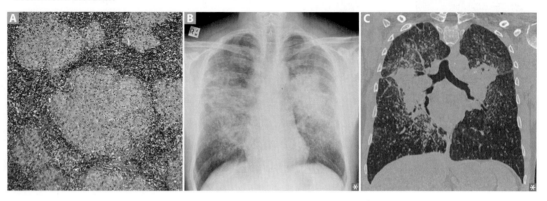

Polymyalgia rheumatica

SYMPTOMS	Pain and stiffness in shoulders and hips, often with fever, malaise, weight loss. Does not cause muscular weakness. More common in women > 50 years old; associated with temporal (giant cell) arteritis.
FINDINGS	↑ ESR, ↑ CRP, normal CK.
TREATMENT	Rapid response to low-dose corticosteroids.

Fibromyalgia

Most commonly seen in females 20–50 years old. Chronic, widespread musculoskeletal pain associated with stiffness, paresthesias, poor sleep, fatigue. Treat with regular exercise, antidepressants (TCAs, SNRIs), anticonvulsants.

Polymyositis/ dermatomyositis	↑ CK, ⊕ ANA, ⊕ anti-Jo-1, ⊕ anti-SRP, ⊕ anti-Mi-2 antibodies. Treatment: steroids followed by long-term immunosuppressant therapy (e.g., methotrexate).
Polymyositis	Progressive symmetric proximal muscle weakness, characterized by endomysial inflammation with CD8+ T cells. Most often involves shoulders.
Dermatomyositis	Similar to polymyositis, but also involves malar rash (similar to SLE), Gottron papules **A**, heliotrope (erythematous periorbital) rash **B**, "shawl and face" rash **C**, "mechanic's hands." ↑ risk of occult malignancy. Perimysial inflammation and atrophy with CD4+ T cells.

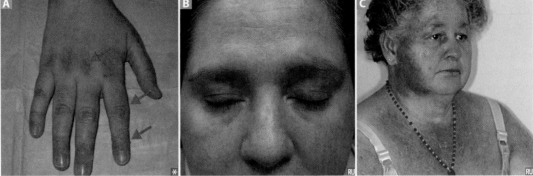

Neuromuscular junction diseases

	Myasthenia gravis	**Lambert-Eaton myasthenic syndrome**
FREQUENCY	Most common NMJ disorder	Uncommon
PATHOPHYSIOLOGY	Autoantibodies to postsynaptic ACh receptor	Autoantibodies to presynaptic Ca^{2+} channel → ↓ ACh release
CLINICAL	Ptosis, diplopia, weakness Worsens with muscle use	Proximal muscle weakness, autonomic symptoms (dry mouth, impotence) Improves with muscle use
ASSOCIATED WITH	Thymoma, thymic hyperplasia	Small cell lung cancer
AChE INHIBITOR ADMINISTRATION	Reversal of symptoms	Minimal effect

Myositis ossificans	Metaplasia of skeletal muscle into bone following muscular trauma **A**. Most often seen in upper or lower extremity. May present as suspicious "mass" at site of known trauma or as incidental finding on radiography.

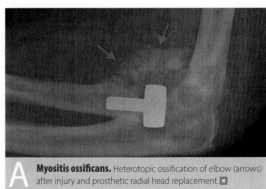

A **Myositis ossificans.** Heterotopic ossification of elbow (arrows) after injury and prosthetic radial head replacement. ✱

Scleroderma (systemic sclerosis)

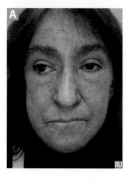

Triad of autoimmunity, noninflammatory vasculopathy, and collagen deposition with fibrosis. Commonly sclerosis of skin, manifesting as puffy, taut skin **A** without wrinkles, fingertip pitting **B**. Also sclerosis of renal, pulmonary (most common cause of death), cardiovascular, GI systems. 75% female. 2 major types:

- **Diffuse scleroderma**—widespread skin involvement, rapid progression, early visceral involvement. Associated with anti-Scl-70 antibody (anti-DNA topoisomerase I antibody).

- **Limited scleroderma**—limited skin involvement confined to fingers and face. Also with **CREST** involvement: Calcinosis, Raynaud phenomenon, Esophageal dysmotility, Sclerodactyly, and Telangiectasia. More benign clinical course. Associated with anti-centromere antibody.

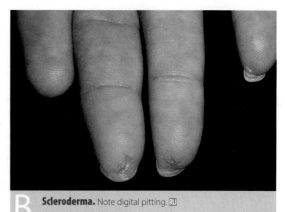

Scleroderma. Note digital pitting. RU

▶ MUSCULOSKELETAL, SKIN, AND CONNECTIVE TISSUE—DERMATOLOGY

Epidermis layers

Skin has 3 layers: epidermis, dermis, subcutaneous fat (hypodermis, subcutis). From surface to base:
- Stratum Corneum (keratin)
- Stratum Lucidum
- Stratum Granulosum
- Stratum Spinosum (desmosomes)
- Stratum Basale (stem cell site)

Californians Like Girls in String Bikinis.

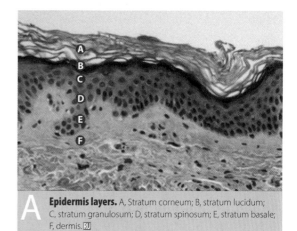

Epidermis layers. A, Stratum corneum; B, stratum lucidum; C, stratum granulosum; D, stratum spinosum; E, stratum basale; F, dermis. RU

Epithelial cell junctions

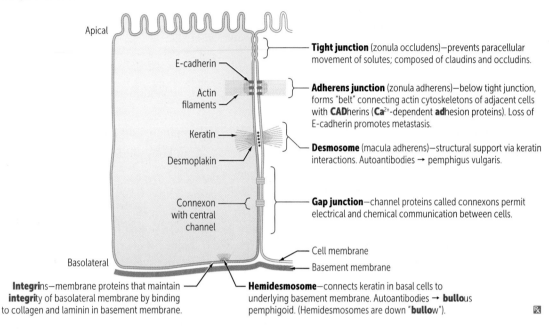

Apical

E-cadherin

Actin filaments

Keratin

Desmoplakin

Connexon with central channel

Basolateral

Cell membrane

Basement membrane

Tight junction (zonula occludens)—prevents paracellular movement of solutes; composed of claudins and occludins.

Adherens junction (zonula adherens)—below tight junction, forms "belt" connecting actin cytoskeletons of adjacent cells with **CAD**herins (**Ca**$^{2+}$-dependent **ad**hesion proteins). Loss of E-cadherin promotes metastasis.

Desmosome (macula adherens)—structural support via keratin interactions. Autoantibodies → pemphigus vulgaris.

Gap junction—channel proteins called connexons permit electrical and chemical communication between cells.

Integrins—membrane proteins that maintain **integri**ty of basolateral membrane by binding to collagen and laminin in basement membrane.

Hemidesmosome—connects keratin in basal cells to underlying basement membrane. Autoantibodies → **bullo**us pemphigoid. (Hemidesmosomes are down "**bullo**w"). ℞

Dermatologic macroscopic terms (morphology)

LESION	CHARACTERISTICS	EXAMPLES
Macule	Flat lesion with well-circumscribed change in skin color < 1 cm	Freckle, labial macule **A**
Patch	Macule > 1 cm	Large birthmark (congenital nevus) **B**
Papule	Elevated solid skin lesion < 1 cm	Mole (nevus) **C**, acne
Plaque	Papule > 1 cm	Psoriasis **D**
Vesicle	Small fluid-containing blister < 1 cm	Chickenpox (varicella), shingles (zoster) **E**
Bulla	Large fluid-containing blister > 1 cm	Bullous pemphigoid **F**
Pustule	Vesicle containing pus	Pustular psoriasis **G**
Wheal	Transient smooth papule or plaque	Hives (urticaria) **H**
Scale	Flaking off of stratum corneum	Eczema, psoriasis, SCC **I**
Crust	Dry exudate	Impetigo **J**

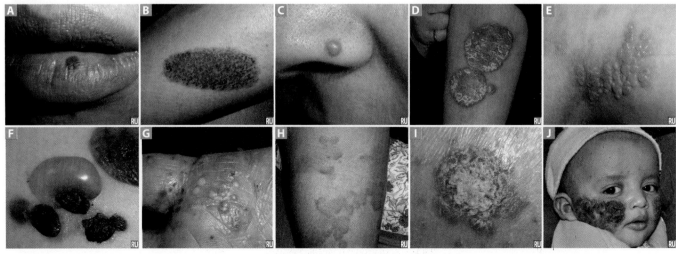

Dermatologic microscopic terms

LESION	CHARACTERISTICS	EXAMPLES
Hyperkeratosis	↑ thickness of stratum corneum	Psoriasis, calluses
Parakeratosis	Hyperkeratosis with retention of nuclei in stratum corneum	Psoriasis
Spongiosis	Epidermal accumulation of edematous fluid in intercellular spaces	Eczematous dermatitis
Acantholysis	Separation of epidermal cells	Pemphigus vulgaris
Acanthosis	Epidermal hyperplasia (↑ spinosum)	Acanthosis nigricans

Pigmented skin disorders

Albinism	Normal melanocyte number with ↓ melanin production A due to ↓ tyrosinase activity or defective tyrosine transport. Can also be caused by failure of neural crest cell migration during development. ↑ risk of skin cancer.	
Melasma (chloasma)	Hyperpigmentation associated with pregnancy ("mask of pregnancy" B) or OCP use.	
Vitiligo	Irregular areas of complete depigmentation C. Caused by autoimmune destruction of melanocytes.	

Common skin disorders

Acne	Obstructive and inflammatory disease of the pilosebaceous unit predominantly found on the face and trunk. Most common in adolescents but can occur at any age **A**.
Atopic dermatitis (eczema)	Pruritic eruption, commonly on skin flexures. Often associated with other atopic diseases (asthma, allergic rhinitis). Usually starts on the face in infancy **B** and often appears in antecubital fossae **C** thereafter.
Allergic contact dermatitis	Type IV hypersensitivity reaction that follows exposure to allergen. Lesions occur at site of contact (e.g., nickel **D**, poison ivy, neomycin **E**).
Melanocytic nevus	Common mole. Benign, but melanoma can arise in congenital or atypical moles. Intradermal nevi are papular **F**. Junctional nevi are flat macules **G**.
Psoriasis	Papules and plaques with silvery scaling **H**, especially on knees and elbows. Acanthosis with parakeratotic scaling (nuclei still in stratum corneum). ↑ stratum spinosum, ↓ stratum granulosum. Auspitz sign (arrow in **I**)—pinpoint bleeding spots from exposure of dermal papillae when scales are scraped off. Can be associated with nail pitting and psoriatic arthritis.
Rosacea	Inflammatory facial skin disorder characterized by erythematous papules and pustules **J**, but no comedones. May be associated with facial flushing in response to external stimuli (e.g., alcohol, heat). Chronic inflammatory changes may result in rhinophyma (bulbous deformation of nose).
Seborrheic keratosis	Flat, greasy, pigmented squamous epithelial proliferation with keratin-filled cysts (horn cysts) **K**. Looks "stuck on." Lesions occur on head, trunk, and extremities. Common benign neoplasm of older persons. Leser-Trélat sign **L**—sudden appearance of multiple seborrheic keratoses, indicating an underlying malignancy (e.g., GI, lymphoid).
Verrucae	Warts; caused by HPV. Soft, tan-colored, cauliflower-like papules **M**. Epidermal hyperplasia, hyperkeratosis, koilocytosis. Condyloma acuminatum on genitals **N**.
Urticaria	Hives. Pruritic wheals that form after mast cell degranulation **O**. Characterized by superficial dermal edema and lymphatic channel dilation.

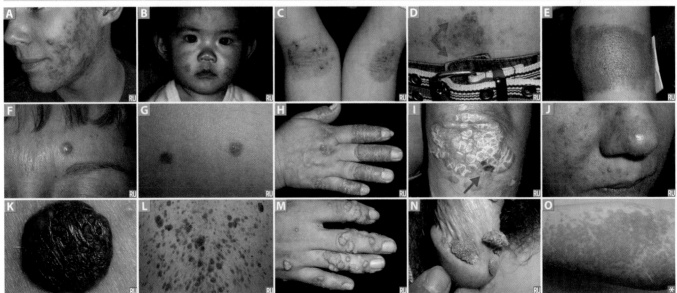

Skin infections

Bacterial infections	
Impetigo	Very superficial skin infection. Usually from S. *aureus* or S. *pyogenes*. Highly contagious. Honey-colored crusting A. Bullous impetigo B has bullae and is usually caused by S. *aureus*.
Cellulitis	Acute, painful, spreading infection of deeper dermis and subcutaneous tissues. Usually from S. *pyogenes* or S. *aureus*. Often starts with a break in skin from trauma or another infection C.
Erysipelas	Infection involving upper dermis and superficial lymphatics, usually from S. *pyogenes*. Presents with well-defined demarcation between infected and normal skin D.
Abscess	Collection of pus from a walled-off infection within deeper layers of skin E. Offending organism is almost always S. *aureus*, which is frequently methicillin resistant.
Necrotizing fasciitis	Deeper tissue injury, usually from anaerobic bacteria or S. *pyogenes*. Results in crepitus from methane and CO_2 production. "Flesh-eating bacteria." Causes bullae and a purple color to the skin F.
Staphylococcal scalded skin syndrome	Exotoxin destroys keratinocyte attachments in stratum granulosum only (vs. toxic epidermal necrolysis, which destroys epidermal-dermal junction). Characterized by fever and generalized erythematous rash with sloughing of the upper layers of the epidermis that heals completely. Seen in newborns and children, adults with renal insufficiency G.
Viral infections	
Herpes	Herpes virus infections (HSV1 and HSV2) of skin can occur anywhere from mucosal surfaces to normal skin. These include herpes labialis, herpes genitalis, herpetic whitlow (finger).
Molluscum contagiosum	Umbilicated papules caused by a poxvirus. While frequently seen in children, it may be sexually transmitted in adults.
Varicella zoster virus	Causes varicella (chickenpox) and zoster (shingles). Varicella presents with multiple crops of lesions in various stages from vesicles to crusts. Zoster is a reactivation of the virus in dermatomal distribution (unless it is disseminated).
Hairy leukoplakia	Irregular, white, painless plaques on tongue that cannot be scraped off H. EBV mediated. Occurs in HIV-positive patients, organ transplant recipients. Contrast with thrush (scrapable) and leukoplakia (precancerous).

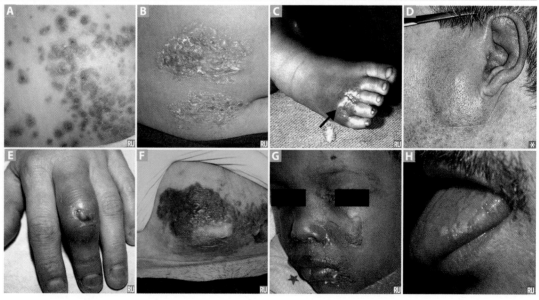

Blistering skin disorders

Pemphigus vulgaris	Potentially fatal autoimmune skin disorder with IgG antibody against desmoglein (component of desmosomes). Flaccid intraepidermal bullae **A** caused by acantholysis (keratinocytes in stratum spinosum are connected by desmosomes); oral mucosa also involved. Immunofluorescence reveals antibodies around epidermal cells in a reticular (net-like) pattern **B**. Nikolsky sign ⊕ (separation of epidermis upon manual stroking of skin).
Bullous pemphigoid	Less severe than pemphigus vulgaris. Involves IgG antibody against hemidesmosomes (epidermal basement membrane; antibodies are "**bullow**" the epidermis). Tense blisters **C** containing eosinophils affect skin but spare oral mucosa. Immunofluorescence reveals linear pattern at epidermal-dermal junction **D**. Nikolsky sign ⊖.
Dermatitis herpetiformis	Pruritic papules, vesicles, and bullae (often found on elbows) **E**. Deposits of IgA at tips of dermal papillae. Associated with celiac disease.
Erythema multiforme	Associated with infections (e.g., *Mycoplasma pneumoniae*, HSV), drugs (e.g., sulfa drugs, β-lactams, phenytoin), cancers, autoimmune disease. Presents with multiple types of lesions—macules, papules, vesicles, target lesions (look like targets with multiple rings and dusky center showing epithelial disruption) **F**.
Stevens-Johnson syndrome	Characterized by fever, bullae formation and necrosis, sloughing of skin, high mortality rate. Typically 2 mucous membranes are involved **G H**, and targetoid skin lesions may appear, as seen in erythema multiforme. Usually associated with adverse drug reaction. A more severe form of Stevens-Johnson syndrome (SJS) with > 30% of the body surface area involved is toxic epidermal necrolysis **I J** (TEN). 10–30% involvement denotes SJS-TEN.

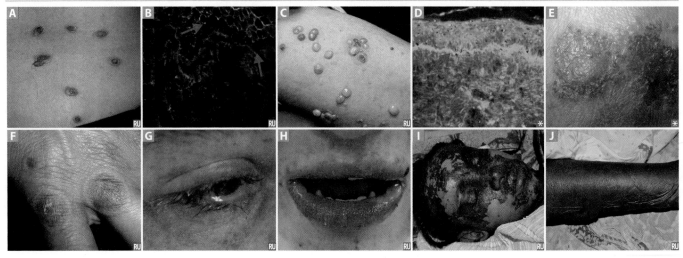

Miscellaneous skin disorders

Acanthosis nigricans	Epidermal hyperplasia causing symmetric, hyperpigmented thickening of skin, especially in axilla or on neck A B. Associated with hyperinsulinemia (e.g., diabetes, obesity, Cushing syndrome), visceral malignancy (e.g., gastric adenocarcinoma).
Actinic keratosis	Premalignant lesions caused by sun exposure. Small, rough, erythematous or brownish papules or plaques C D. Risk of squamous cell carcinoma is proportional to degree of epithelial dysplasia.
Erythema nodosum	Painful inflammatory lesions of subcutaneous fat, usually on anterior shins. Often idiopathic, but can be associated with sarcoidosis, coccidioidomycosis, histoplasmosis, TB, streptococcal infections E, leprosy F, Crohn disease.
Lichen Planus	Pruritic, Purple, Polygonal Planar Papules and Plaques are the 6 P's of lichen Planus G H. Mucosal involvement manifests as Wickham striae (reticular white lines). Sawtooth infiltrate of lymphocytes at dermal-epidermal junction. Associated with hepatitis C.
Pityriasis rosea	"Herald patch" I followed days later by other scaly erythematous plaques, often in a "Christmas tree" distribution J. Multiple plaques with collarette scale. Self-resolving in 6–8 weeks.
Sunburn	Acute cutaneous inflammatory reaction due to excessive UV irradiation. Causes DNA mutations, inducing apoptosis of keratinocytes. UVA is dominant in tanning and photoaging, UVB in sunburn. Can lead to impetigo, skin cancers (basal cell carcinoma, squamous cell carcinoma, melanoma).

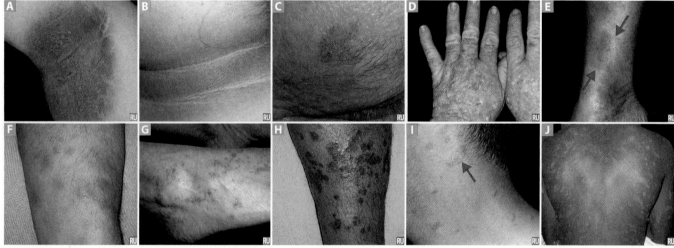

Skin cancer

Basal cell carcinoma	Most common skin cancer. Found in sun-exposed areas of body. Locally invasive, but rarely metastasizes. Pink, pearly nodules, commonly with telangiectasias, rolled borders, central crusting or ulceration **A**. BCCs also appear as nonhealing ulcers with infiltrating growth **B** or as a scaling plaque (superficial BCC) **C**. Basal cell tumors have "palisading" nuclei **D**.

Squamous cell carcinoma	Second most common skin cancer. Associated with excessive exposure to sunlight, immunosuppression, and occasionally arsenic exposure. Commonly appears on face **E**, lower lip **F**, ears, hands. Locally invasive, may spread to lymph nodes, and will rarely metastasize. Ulcerative red lesions with frequent scale. Associated with chronic draining sinuses. Histopathology: keratin "pearls" **G**. Actinic keratosis, a scaly plaque, is a precursor to squamous cell carcinoma. Keratoacanthoma is a variant that grows rapidly (4–6 weeks) and may regress spontaneously over months **H**.

Melanoma	Common tumor with significant risk of metastasis. S-100 tumor marker. Associated with sunlight exposure; fair-skinned persons are at ↑ risk. Depth of tumor correlates with risk of metastasis. Look for the ABCDEs: Asymmetry, Border irregularity, Color variation, Diameter > 6 mm, and Evolution over time. At least 4 different types of melanoma, including superficial spreading **I**, nodular **J**, lentigo maligna **K**, and acral lentiginous **L**. Often driven by activating mutation in BRAF kinase. Primary treatment is excision with appropriately wide margins. Metastatic or unresectable melanoma in patients with *BRAF* V600E mutation may benefit from vemurafenib, a BRAF kinase inhibitor.

▶ MUSCULOSKELETAL, SKIN, AND CONNECTIVE TISSUE—PHARMACOLOGY

Inflammatory mediators

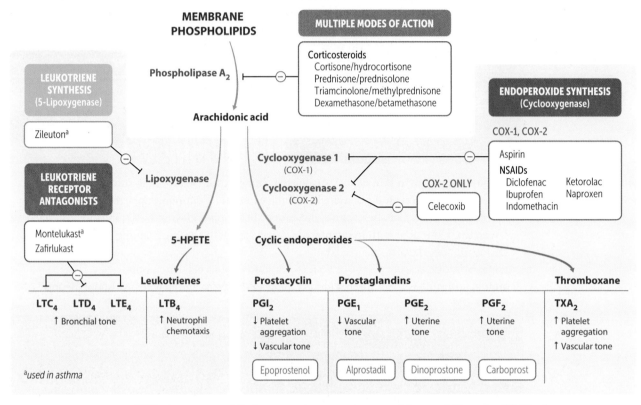

LTB$_4$ is a **neutrophil** chemotactic agent.
PGI$_2$ inhibits platelet aggregation and promotes vasodilation.

Neutrophils arrive "B4" others.
Platelet-**G**athering **I**nhibitor.

Acetaminophen

MECHANISM	Reversibly inhibits cyclooxygenase, mostly in CNS. Inactivated peripherally.
CLINICAL USE	Antipyretic, analgesic, but not anti-inflammatory. Used instead of aspirin to avoid Reye syndrome in children with viral infection.
TOXICITY	Overdose produces hepatic necrosis; acetaminophen metabolite (NAPQI) depletes glutathione and forms toxic tissue byproducts in liver. N-acetylcysteine is antidote—regenerates glutathione.

Aspirin

MECHANISM	Irreversibly inhibits cyclooxygenase (both COX-1 and COX-2) via acetylation, which ↓ synthesis of TXA_2 and prostaglandins. ↑ bleeding time. No effect on PT, PTT. A type of NSAID.
CLINICAL USE	Low dose (< 300 mg/day): ↓ platelet aggregation. Intermediate dose (300–2400 mg/day): antipyretic and analgesic. High dose (2400–4000 mg/day): anti-inflammatory.
TOXICITY	Gastric ulceration, tinnitus (CN VIII). Chronic use can lead to acute renal failure, interstitial nephritis, GI bleeding. Risk of Reye syndrome in children treated with aspirin for viral infection. Causes respiratory alkalosis early, but transitions to mixed metabolic acidosis-respiratory alkalosis.

Celecoxib

MECHANISM	Reversibly inhibits specifically the cyclooxygenase (COX) isoform 2, which is found in inflammatory cells and vascular endothelium and mediates inflammation and pain; spares COX-1, which helps maintain gastric mucosa. Thus, does not have the corrosive effects of other NSAIDs on the GI lining. Spares platelet function as TXA_2 production is dependent on COX-1.
CLINICAL USE	Rheumatoid arthritis, osteoarthritis.
TOXICITY	↑ risk of thrombosis. Sulfa allergy.

NSAIDs

	Ibuprofen, naproxen, indomethacin, ketorolac, diclofenac.
MECHANISM	Reversibly inhibit cyclooxygenase (both COX-1 and COX-2). Block prostaglandin synthesis.
CLINICAL USE	Antipyretic, analgesic, anti-inflammatory. Indomethacin is used to close a PDA.
TOXICITY	Interstitial nephritis, gastric ulcer (prostaglandins protect gastric mucosa), renal ischemia (prostaglandins vasodilate afferent arteriole).

Bisphosphonates

	Alendronate, other -dronates.
MECHANISM	Pyrophosphate analogs; bind hydroxyapatite in bone, inhibiting osteoclast activity.
CLINICAL USE	Osteoporosis, hypercalcemia, Paget disease of bone.
TOXICITY	Corrosive esophagitis (patients are advised to take with water and remain upright for 30 minutes), osteonecrosis of jaw.

Teriparatide

MECHANISM	Recombinant PTH analog given subcutaneously daily. ↑ osteoblastic activity.
CLINICAL USE	Osteoporosis. Causes ↑ bone growth compared to antiresorptive therapies (e.g., bisphosphonates).
TOXICITY	Transient hypercalcemia. May increase risk of osteosarcoma (seen in rodent studies).

Gout drugs

Chronic gout drugs (preventive)

Allopurinol	Inhibits xanthine oxidase after being converted to alloxanthine, ↓ conversion of xanthine to uric acid. Also used in lymphoma and leukemia to prevent tumor lysis–associated urate nephropathy. ↑ concentrations of azathioprine and 6-MP (both normally metabolized by xanthine oxidase).
Febuxostat	Inhibits xanthine oxidase.
Pegloticase	Recombinant uricase that catalyze metabolism of uric acid to allantoin (a more water-soluble product).
Probenecid	Inhibits reabsorption of uric acid in proximal convoluted tubule (also inhibits secretion of penicillin). Can precipitate uric acid calculi.

Acute gout drugs

NSAIDs	Naproxen, indomethacin.
Glucocorticoids	Oral or intra-articular.
Colchicine	Binds and stabilizes tubulin to inhibit microtubule polymerization, impairing neutrophil chemotaxis and degranulation. Acute and prophylactic value. GI side effects.
	Do not give salicylates; all but the highest doses depress uric acid clearance. Even high doses (5–6 g/day) have only minor uricosuric activity.

Diet → Purines ← Nucleic acids

Hypoxanthine

Xanthine oxidase — Allopurinol, febuxostat

Xanthine

Xanthine oxidase

Plasma uric acid → Urate crystals deposited in joints → Gout

Tubular reabsorption

Probenecid and high-dose salicylates

Tubular secretion

Diuretics and low-dose salicylates

Urine

TNF-α inhibitors	All TNF-α inhibitors predispose to infection, including reactivation of latent TB, since TNF is important in granuloma formation and stabilization.

DRUG	MECHANISM	CLINICAL USE
Etanercept	Fusion protein (receptor for TNF-α + IgG$_1$ Fc), produced by recombinant DNA. Etanercept is a TNF decoy receptor.	Rheumatoid arthritis, psoriasis, ankylosing spondylitis
Infliximab, adalimumab	Anti-TNF-α monoclonal antibody.	Inflammatory bowel disease, rheumatoid arthritis, ankylosing spondylitis, psoriasis

Neurology

"Estimated amount of glucose used by an adult human brain each day, expressed in M&Ms: 250."

—Harper's Index

"He has two neurons held together by a spirochete."

—Anonymous

"I never came upon any of my discoveries through the process of rational thinking."

—Albert Einstein

"I like nonsense; it wakes up the brain cells."

—Dr. Seuss

▶ **NEUROLOGY—EMBRYOLOGY**

Neural development

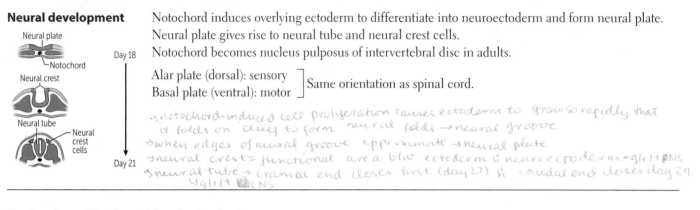

Neural plate
Notochord
Neural crest
Neural tube — Neural crest cells

Day 18

Day 21

Notochord induces overlying ectoderm to differentiate into neuroectoderm and form neural plate. Neural plate gives rise to neural tube and neural crest cells.

Notochord becomes nucleus pulposus of intervertebral disc in adults.

Alar plate (dorsal): sensory
Basal plate (ventral): motor] Same orientation as spinal cord.

→notochord-induced cell proliferation causes ectoderm to grow so rapidly that it folds on itself to form neural folds → neural groove
→when edges of neural groove approximate → neural plate
→neural crest = junctional area b/w ectoderm & neuroectoderm → glr/+PNS
→neural tube → cranial end closes first (day 27) & caudal end closes day 29
→glr/+ CNS

Regional specification of developing brain

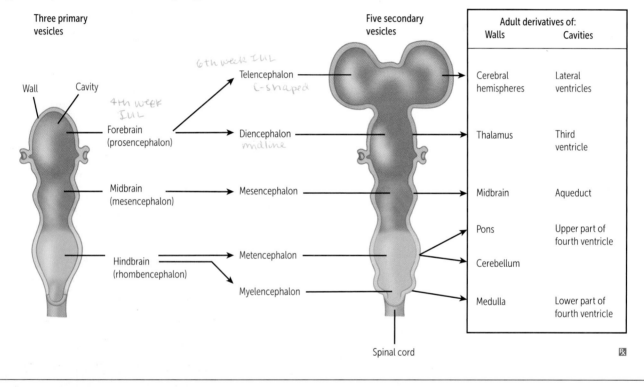

Three primary vesicles

Five secondary vesicles

Adult derivatives of:	
Walls	Cavities

Wall   Cavity

6th week IUL

4th week IUL

Telencephalon *L-shaped* → Cerebral hemispheres | Lateral ventricles

Forebrain (prosencephalon) → Diencephalon *midline* → Thalamus | Third ventricle

Midbrain (mesencephalon) → Mesencephalon → Midbrain | Aqueduct

Hindbrain (rhombencephalon) → Metencephalon → Pons | Upper part of fourth ventricle

Cerebellum

→ Myelencephalon → Medulla | Lower part of fourth ventricle

Spinal cord

CNS/PNS origins

Neuroectoderm—CNS neurons, ependymal cells (inner lining of ventricles, make CSF), oligodendroglia, astrocytes.
Neural crest—PNS neurons, Schwann cells.
Mesoderm—Microglia (like Macrophages, originate from Mesoderm).

Neural tube defects	Neuropores fail to fuse (4th week) → persistent connection between amniotic cavity and spinal canal. Associated with low folic acid intake before conception and during pregnancy. ↑ α-fetoprotein (AFP) in amniotic fluid and maternal serum. ↑ acetylcholinesterase (AChE) in amniotic fluid is a helpful confirmatory test (fetal AChE in CSF transudates across defect into amniotic fluid).
Spina bifida occulta	Failure of bony spinal canal to close, but no structural herniation. Usually seen at lower vertebral levels. Dura is intact. Associated with tuft of hair or skin dimple at level of bony defect. Normal AFP.
Meningocele	Meninges (but no neural tissue) herniate through bony defect.
Meningomyelocele	Meninges and neural tissue herniate through bony defect.

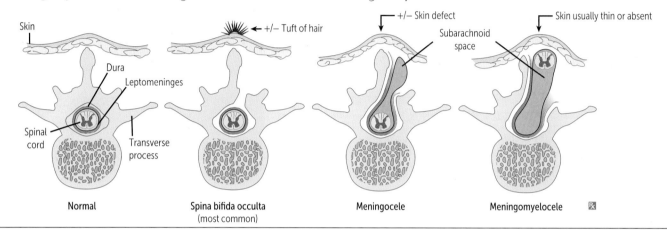

Forebrain anomalies	
Anencephaly	Malformation of anterior neural tube → no forebrain, open calvarium. Clinical findings: ↑ AFP; polyhydramnios (no swallowing center in brain). Associated with maternal type 1 diabetes. Maternal folate supplementation ↓ risk.
Holoprosencephaly	Failure of left and right hemispheres to separate; usually occurs during weeks 5–6. May be related to mutations in sonic hedgehog signaling pathway. Moderate form has cleft lip/palate, most severe form results in cyclopia. Seen in Patau syndrome and fetal alcohol syndrome.

Posterior fossa malformations

Chiari II	Significant herniation of cerebellar tonsils and vermis through foramen magnum with aqueductal stenosis and hydrocephalus. Often presents with lumbosacral meningomyelocele, paralysis below the defect.
Dandy-Walker	Agenesis of cerebellar vermis with cystic enlargement of 4th ventricle (fills the enlarged posterior fossa **A**). Associated with hydrocephalus, spina bifida.

A **Dandy-Walker malformation.** Midline sagittal MRI shows large cystic 4th ventricle (arrow).

Syringomyelia

Cystic cavity (syrinx) within spinal cord 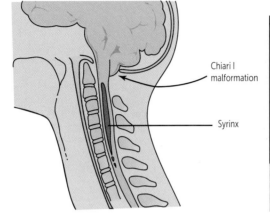 (if central canal → hydromyelia). Crossing anterior spinal commissural fibers are typically damaged first. Results in a "cape-like," bilateral loss of pain and temperature sensation in upper extremities (fine touch sensation is preserved). Associated with Chiari malformations, trauma, and tumors.

Syrinx = tube, as in syringe.
Most common at C8–T1.
Chiari I malformation— cerebellar tonsillar ectopia > 3–5 mm; congenital, usually asymptomatic in childhood, manifests with headaches and cerebellar symptoms.

Chiari I
malformation

Syrinx

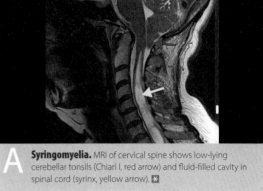

A **Syringomyelia.** MRI of cervical spine shows low-lying cerebellar tonsils (Chiari I, red arrow) and fluid-filled cavity in spinal cord (syrinx, yellow arrow). ✴

Tongue development

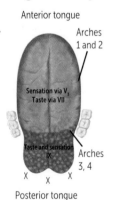

Anterior tongue

Arches 1 and 2

Sensation via V₃
Taste via VII

Taste and sensation IX

Arches 3, 4

X   X   X

Posterior tongue

1st and 2nd branchial arches form anterior ²/₃ (thus sensation via CN V₃, taste via CN VII).
3rd and 4th branchial arches form posterior ¹/₃ (thus sensation and taste mainly via CN IX, extreme posterior via CN X).
Motor innervation is via CN XII to hyoglossus (retracts and depresses tongue), genioglossus (protrudes tongue), and styloglossus (draws sides of tongue upward to create a trough for swallowing).
Motor innervation is via CN X to palatoglossus (elevates posterior tongue during swallowing).

Taste—CN VII, IX, X (solitary nucleus).
Pain—CN V₃, IX, X.
Motor—CN X, XII.

▶ NEUROLOGY—ANATOMY AND PHYSIOLOGY

Neurons

Signal-transmitting cells of the nervous system. Permanent cells—do not divide in adulthood. Signal-relaying cells with dendrites (receive input), cell bodies, and axons (send output). Cell bodies and dendrites can be seen on Nissle staining (stains RER). RER is not present in the axon. Injury to axon → Wallerian degeneration—degeneration distal to injury and axonal retraction proximally; allows for potential regeneration of axon (if in PNS).

Astrocytes

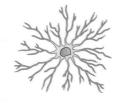

Physical support, repair, K⁺ metabolism, removal of excess neurotransmitter, component of blood-brain barrier, glycogen fuel reserve buffer. Reactive gliosis in response to neural injury. Astrocyte marker: GFAP. Derived from neuroectoderm.

Microglia

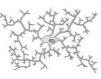

Phagocytic scavenger cells of CNS (mesodermal, mononuclear origin). Activated in response to tissue damage. Not readily discernible by Nissl stain.

HIV-infected microglia fuse to form multinucleated giant cells in CNS.

Myelin

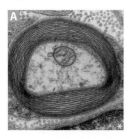

↑ conduction velocity of signals transmitted down axons → saltatory conduction of action potential at the nodes of Ranvier, where there are high concentrations of Na⁺ channels. CNS—oligodendrocytes; PNS—Schwann cells.

Wraps and insulates axons **A**: ↑ space constant and ↑ conduction velocity.

Schwann cells

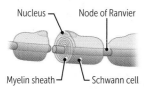

Nucleus — Node of Ranvier

Myelin sheath — Schwann cell

Each Schwann cell myelinates only 1 PNS axon. Also promote axonal regeneration. Derived from neural crest.
↑ conduction velocity via saltatory conduction at the nodes of Ranvier, where there is a high concentration of Na⁺ channels.

May be injured in Guillain-Barré syndrome. Acoustic neuroma—type of schwannoma. Typically located in internal acoustic meatus (CN VIII). If bilateral, strongly associated with neurofibromatosis type 2.

Oligodendroglia

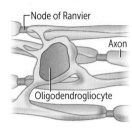

Node of Ranvier
Axon
Oligodendrogliocyte

Myelinates axons of neurons in CNS. Each oligodendrocyte can myelinate many axons (~ 30). Predominant type of glial cell in white matter.

Derived from neuroectoderm.
"Fried egg" appearance histologically.
Injured in multiple sclerosis, progressive multifocal leukoencephalopathy (PML), leukodystrophies.

Sensory receptors

RECEPTOR TYPE	DESCRIPTION	LOCATION	SENSES
Free nerve endings	C—slow, unmyelinated fibers Aδ—fast, myelinated fibers	All skin, epidermis, some viscera	Pain, temperature
Meissner corpuscles	Large, myelinated fibers; adapt quickly	Glabrous (hairless) skin	Dynamic, fine/light touch, position sense
Pacinian corpuscles	Large, myelinated fibers; adapt quickly	Deep skin layers, ligaments, joints	Vibration, pressure
Merkel discs	Large, myelinated fibers; adapt slowly	Finger tips, superficial skin	Pressure, deep static touch (e.g., shapes, edges), position sense
Ruffini corpuscles	Dendritic endings with capsule; adapt slowly	Finger tips, joints	Pressure, slippage of objects along surface of skin, joint angle change

Peripheral nerve

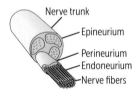

Nerve trunk
Epineurium
Perineurium
Endoneurium
Nerve fibers

Endoneurium—invests single nerve fiber layers (inflammatory infiltrate in Guillain-Barré syndrome).
Perineurium (Permeability barrier)—surrounds a fascicle of nerve fibers. Must be rejoined in microsurgery for limb reattachment.
Epineurium—dense connective tissue that surrounds entire nerve (fascicles and blood vessels).

Endo = inner.
Peri = around.
Epi = outer.

Neurotransmitters

TYPE	CHANGE IN DISEASE	LOCATIONS OF SYNTHESIS
Norepinephrine	↑ in anxiety ↓ in depression	Locus ceruleus (pons)[a]
Dopamine	↑ in Huntington disease ↓ in Parkinson disease ↓ in depression	Ventral tegmentum and substantia nigra pars compacta (midbrain)
5-HT	↓ in anxiety ↓ in depression	Raphe nuclei (pons, medulla, midbrain)
ACh	↑ in Parkinson disease ↓ in Alzheimer disease ↓ in Huntington disease	Basal nucleus of Meynert
GABA	↓ in anxiety ↓ in Huntington disease	Nucleus accumbens[b]

[a]Locus ceruleus—stress and panic.
[b]Nucleus accumbens and septal nucleus—reward center, pleasure, addiction, fear.

Blood-brain barrier

Prevents circulating blood substances (e.g., bacteria, drugs) from reaching the CSF/CNS. Formed by 3 structures:
- Tight junctions between nonfenestrated capillary endothelial cells
- Basement membrane
- Astrocyte foot processes

Glucose and amino acids cross slowly by carrier-mediated transport mechanisms.

Nonpolar/lipid-soluble substances cross rapidly via diffusion.

A few specialized brain regions with fenestrated capillaries and no blood-brain barrier allow molecules in blood to affect brain function (e.g., area postrema—vomiting after chemo; OVLT—osmotic sensing) or neurosecretory products to enter circulation (e.g., neurohypophysis—ADH release).

Infarction and/or neoplasm destroys endothelial cell tight junctions → vasogenic edema.

Other notable barriers include:
- Blood-testis barrier
- Maternal-fetal blood barrier of placenta

Hypothalamus	The hypothalamus wears **TAN HATS**—Thirst and water balance, Adenohypophysis control (regulates anterior pituitary), Neurohypophysis releases hormones produced in the hypothalamus, Hunger, Autonomic regulation, Temperature regulation, Sexual urges. Inputs (areas not protected by blood-brain barrier): OVLT (organum vasculosum of the lamina terminalis; senses change in osmolarity), area postrema (responds to emetics). Supraoptic nucleus primarily makes ADH. Paraventricular nucleus primarily makes oxytocin. ADH and oxytocin—made by hypothalamus but stored and released by posterior pituitary.	
Lateral area	Hunger. Destruction → anorexia, failure to thrive (infants). Inhibited by leptin.	If you zap your **lateral** nucleus, you shrink **laterally**.
Ventromedial area	Satiety. Destruction (e.g., craniopharyngioma) → hyperphagia. Stimulated by leptin.	If you zap your **ventromedial** nucleus, you grow **ventrally** and **medially**.
Anterior hypothalamus	Cooling, parasympathetic.	Anterior nucleus = cool off (**cooling**, p**A**rasympathetic). A/C = **anterior cooling**.
Posterior hypothalamus	Heating, sympathetic.	Posterior nucleus = get fired up (heating, sympathetic). If you zap your posterior hypothalamus, you become a poikilotherm (cold-blooded, like a snake).
Suprachiasmatic nucleus	Circadian rhythm.	You need **sleep** to be **charismatic** (chiasmatic).

Sleep physiology

Sleep cycle is regulated by the circadian rhythm, which is driven by suprachiasmatic nucleus (SCN) of hypothalamus. Circadian rhythm controls nocturnal release of ACTH, prolactin, melatonin, norepinephrine: SCN → norepinephrine release → pineal gland → melatonin. SCN is regulated by environment (e.g., light).

Two stages: rapid-eye movement (REM) and non-REM. Extraocular movements during REM sleep due to activity of PPRF (paramedian pontine reticular formation/conjugate gaze center). REM sleep occurs every 90 minutes, and duration ↑ through the night.

Alcohol, benzodiazepines, and barbiturates are associated with ↓ REM sleep and delta wave sleep; norepinephrine also ↓ REM sleep.

Treat bedwetting (sleep enuresis) with oral desmopressin (ADH analog); preferred over imipramine because of the latter's adverse effects.

Benzodiazepines are useful for night terrors and sleepwalking.

SLEEP STAGE (% OF TOTAL SLEEP TIME IN YOUNG ADULTS)	DESCRIPTION	EEG WAVEFORM
Awake (eyes open)	Alert, active mental concentration	Beta (highest frequency, lowest amplitude)
Awake (eyes closed)		Alpha
Non-REM sleep		
Stage N1 (5%)	Light sleep	Theta
Stage N2 (45%)	Deeper sleep; when bruxism occurs	Sleep spindles and K complexes
Stage N3 (25%)	Deepest non-REM sleep (slow-wave sleep); when sleepwalking, night terrors, and bedwetting occur	Delta (lowest frequency, highest amplitude)
REM sleep (25%)	Loss of motor tone, ↑ brain O_2 use, ↑ and variable pulse and blood pressure; when dreaming and penile/clitoral tumescence occur; may serve memory processing function	Beta At night, **BATS** Drink Blood

Thalamus   Major relay for all ascending sensory information except olfaction.

NUCLEUS	INPUT	INFO	DESTINATION	MNEMONIC
VPL	Spinothalamic and dorsal columns/medial lemniscus	Pain, temperature; pressure, touch, vibration, proprioception	1° somatosensory cortex	
VPM	Trigeminal and gustatory pathway	**Face** sensation, taste	1° somatosensory cortex	Makeup goes on the **face** (VPM)
LGN	CN II	Vision	Calcarine sulcus	Lateral = Light
MGN	Superior olive and inferior colliculus of tectum	Hearing	Auditory cortex of temporal lobe	Medial = Music
VL	Basal ganglia, cerebellum	Motor	Motor cortex	

Limbic system

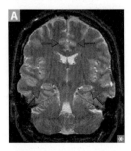

Collection of neural structures involved in emotion, long-term memory, olfaction, behavior modulation, ANS function. Structures include hippocampus (red arrows in), amygdala, fornix, mammillary bodies, cingulate gyrus (blue arrows in A). Responsible for Feeding, Fleeing, Fighting, Feeling, and Sex.

The famous 5 F's.

Osmotic demyelination syndrome (central pontine myelinolysis)

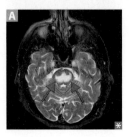

Acute paralysis, dysarthria, dysphagia, diplopia, loss of consciousness. Can cause "locked-in syndrome." Massive axonal demyelination in pontine white matter A 2° to osmotic changes. Commonly iatrogenic, caused by overly rapid correction of hyponatremia. In contrast, correcting hypernatremia too quickly results in cerebral edema/herniation.

Correcting serum Na^+ too fast:
- "From low to high, your pons will die" (osmotic demyelination syndrome)
- "From high to low, your brain will blow" (cerebral edema/herniation)

Cerebellum

Modulates movement; aids in coordination and balance.

Input:
- Contralateral cortex via middle cerebellar peduncle.
- Ipsilateral proprioceptive information via inferior cerebellar peduncle from spinal cord.

Output:
- Sends information to contralateral cortex to modulate movement. Output nerves = Purkinje cells → deep nuclei of cerebellum → contralateral cortex via superior cerebellar peduncle.
- Deep nuclei (lateral → medial)—Dentate, Emboliform, Globose, Fastigial ("Don't Eat Greasy Foods").

Lateral lesions—voluntary movement of extremities; when injured, propensity to fall toward injured (ipsilateral) side.

Medial lesions–lesions involving midline structures (vermal cortex, fastigial nuclei) and/or flocculonodular lobe → truncal ataxia (wide-based cerebellar gait), nystagmus, head tilting. Generally, midline lesions result in bilateral motor deficits affecting axial and proximal limb musculature.

Basal ganglia

Important in voluntary movements and making postural adjustments.

Receives cortical input, provides negative feedback to cortex to modulate movement.

Striatum = putamen (motor) + caudate (cognitive).

Lentiform = putamen + globus pallidus.

D_1-Receptor = D1Rect pathway.

Indirect = Inhibitory.

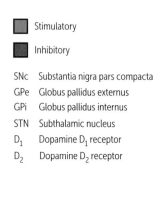

■ Stimulatory

■ Inhibitory

SNc   Substantia nigra pars compacta
GPe   Globus pallidus externus
GPi   Globus pallidus internus
STN   Subthalamic nucleus
D_1 Dopamine D_1 receptor
D_2 Dopamine D_2 receptor

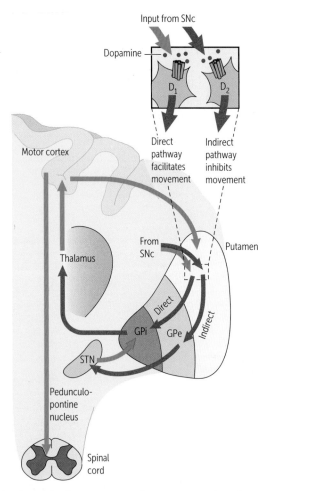

Excitatory pathway—cortical inputs stimulate the striatum, stimulating the release of GABA, which disinhibits the thalamus via the GPi/SNr (↑ motion).

Inhibitory pathway—cortical inputs stimulate the striatum, which disinhibits STN via GPe, and STN stimulates GPi/SNr to inhibit the thalamus (↓ motion).

Dopamine binds to D_1, stimulating the excitatory pathway, and to D_2, inhibiting the inhibitory pathway → ↑ motion.

Movement disorders

DISORDER	PRESENTATION	CHARACTERISTIC LESION	NOTES
Athetosis	Slow, writhing movements; especially seen in fingers	Basal ganglia (e.g., Huntington)	Writhing, snake-like movement.
Chorea	Sudden, jerky, purposeless movements	Basal ganglia (e.g., Huntington)	*Chorea* = dancing.
Dystonia	Sustained, involuntary muscle contractions		Writer's cramp; blepharospasm (sustained eyelid twitch).
Essential tremor	High-frequency tremor with sustained posture (e.g., outstretched arms), worsened with movement or when anxious		Often familial. Patients often self-medicate with EtOH, which ↓ tremor amplitude. Treatment: β-blockers, primidone.
Hemiballismus	Sudden, wild flailing of 1 arm +/− ipsilateral leg	Contralateral subthalamic nucleus (e.g., lacunar stroke)	Pronounce "**Half-of-body** ballistic." Contralateral lesion.
Intention tremor	Slow, zigzag motion when pointing/extending toward a target	Cerebellar dysfunction	
Myoclonus	Sudden, brief, uncontrolled muscle contraction		Jerks; hiccups; common in metabolic abnormalities such as renal and liver failure.
Resting tremor	Uncontrolled movement of distal appendages (most noticeable in hands); tremor alleviated by intentional movement	Parkinson disease	Occurs at rest; "pill-rolling tremor" of Parkinson disease.

Parkinson disease

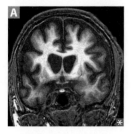

Degenerative disorder of CNS associated with Lewy bodies (composed of α-synuclein—intracellular eosinophilic inclusions) and loss of dopaminergic neurons (i.e., depigmentation) of substantia nigra pars compacta.

Parkinson **TRAPS** your body:
  Tremor (pill-rolling tremor at rest)
  Rigidity (cogwheel)
  Akinesia (or bradykinesia)
  Postural instability
  Shuffling gait

Huntington disease

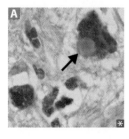

Autosomal dominant trinucleotide repeat disorder on chromosome 4. Symptoms manifest between ages 20 and 50; characterized by choreiform movements, aggression, depression, dementia (sometimes initially mistaken for substance abuse). ↑ dopamine, ↓ GABA, ↓ ACh in brain. Neuronal death via NMDA-R binding and glutamate toxicity. Atrophy of caudate nuclei with ex vacuo dilatation of frontal horns on MRI .

Expansion of **CAG** repeats (anticipation). Caudate loses ACh and GABA.

Cerebral cortex functions

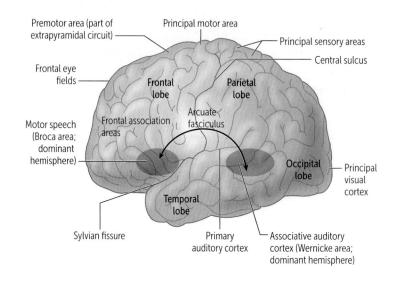

Aphasia	Aphasia = higher-order inability to speak (language deficit). Dysarthria = motor inability to speak (movement deficit).	
Broca	Nonfluent aphasia with intact comprehension and impaired repetition. Broca area—inferior frontal gyrus of frontal lobe.	**Broca** = **Broken Boca** (boca = mouth in Spanish).
Wernicke	Fluent aphasia with impaired comprehension and repetition. Wernicke area—superior temporal gyrus of temporal lobe.	Wernicke is Wordy but makes no sense. Wernicke = "What?"
Conduction	Poor repetition but fluent speech, intact comprehension. Can be caused by damage to arcuate fasciculus.	Can't repeat phrases such as, "No ifs, ands, or buts."
Global	Nonfluent aphasia with impaired comprehension.	Arcuate fasciculus, Broca and Wernicke areas affected.
Transcortical motor	Nonfluent aphasia with good comprehension and intact repetition.	
Transcortical sensory	Poor comprehension with fluent speech and intact repetition.	
Mixed transcortical	Nonfluent speech, poor comprehension, intact repetition.	Broca and Wernicke areas involved; arcuate fasciculus not involved.

Common brain lesions

AREA OF LESION	CONSEQUENCE	NOTES
Amygdala (bilateral)	Klüver-Bucy syndrome—disinhibited behavior (e.g., hyperphagia, hypersexuality, hyperorality).	Associated with HSV-1.
Frontal lobe	Disinhibition and deficits in concentration, orientation, judgment; may have reemergence of primitive reflexes.	
Nondominant parietal-temporal cortex	Hemispatial neglect syndrome (agnosia of the contralateral side of the world).	
Dominant parietal-temporal cortex	Agraphia, acalculia, finger agnosia, left-right disorientation.	Gerstmann syndrome.
Reticular activating system (midbrain)	Reduced levels of arousal and wakefulness (e.g., coma).	
Mammillary bodies (bilateral)	Wernicke-Korsakoff syndrome—confusion, ophthalmoplegia, ataxia; memory loss (anterograde and retrograde amnesia), confabulation, personality changes.	Associated with thiamine (B_1) deficiency and excessive EtOH use; can be precipitated by giving glucose without B_1 to a B_1-deficient patient. Wernicke problems come in a **CAN** of beer: Confusion, Ataxia, Nystagmus.
Basal ganglia	May result in tremor at rest, chorea, athetosis.	Parkinson disease, Huntington disease.
Cerebellar hemisphere	Intention tremor, limb ataxia, loss of balance; damage to cerebellum → ipsilateral deficits; fall toward side of lesion.	Cerebellar hemispheres are **lateral**ly located—affect **lateral** limbs.
Cerebellar vermis	Truncal ataxia, dysarthria.	Vermis is **central**ly located—affects **central** body.
Subthalamic nucleus	Contralateral hemiballismus.	
Hippocampus (bilateral)	Anterograde amnesia—inability to make new memories.	
Paramedian pontine reticular formation	Eyes look away from side of lesion.	
Frontal eye fields	Eyes look toward lesion.	

Cerebral arteries—cortical distribution

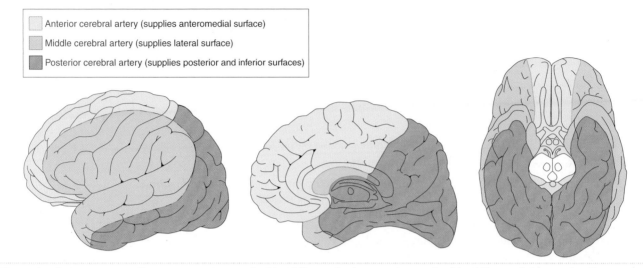

- Anterior cerebral artery (supplies anteromedial surface)
- Middle cerebral artery (supplies lateral surface)
- Posterior cerebral artery (supplies posterior and inferior surfaces)

Watershed zones	Between anterior cerebral/middle cerebral, posterior cerebral/middle cerebral arteries. Damage in severe hypotension → upper leg/upper arm weakness, defects in higher-order visual processing.

Circle of Willis	System of anastomoses between anterior and posterior blood supplies to brain.

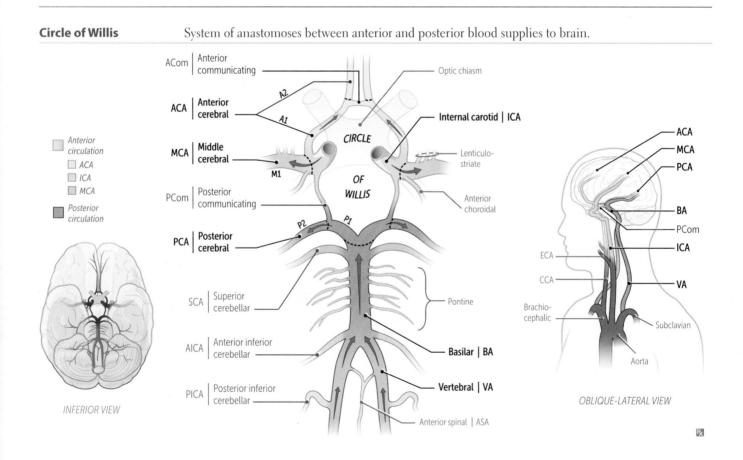

Anterior circulation
- ACA
- ICA
- MCA

Posterior circulation

ACom | Anterior communicating
ACA | Anterior cerebral
A2
A1
MCA | Middle cerebral
M1
PCom | Posterior communicating
PCA | Posterior cerebral
P2 P1
SCA | Superior cerebellar
AICA | Anterior inferior cerebellar
PICA | Posterior inferior cerebellar

CIRCLE OF WILLIS

Optic chiasm
Internal carotid | ICA
Lenticulo-striate
Anterior choroidal
Pontine
Basilar | BA
Vertebral | VA
Anterior spinal | ASA

INFERIOR VIEW

OBLIQUE-LATERAL VIEW

ACA
MCA
PCA
BA
PCom
ICA
VA

ECA
CCA
Brachio-cephalic
Subclavian
Aorta

Homunculus

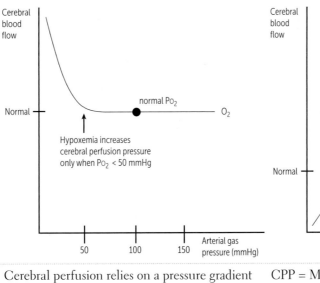

Topographic representation of motor (shown) and sensory areas in the cerebral cortex. Distorted appearance is due to certain body regions being more richly innervated and thus having ↑ cortical representation.

Regulation of cerebral perfusion

Brain perfusion relies on tight autoregulation. Cerebral perfusion is primarily driven by Pco_2 (Po_2 also modulates perfusion in severe hypoxia).

Therapeutic hyperventilation (↓ Pco_2) helps ↓ intracranial pressure (ICP) in cases of acute cerebral edema (stroke, trauma) via vasoconstriction. Fainting in panic attacks due to ↓ perfusion.

Cerebral perfusion and blood pressure

Cerebral perfusion relies on a pressure gradient between mean arterial pressure (MAP) and ICP. ↓ blood pressure or ↑ ICP → ↓ cerebral perfusion pressure (CPP).

CPP = MAP – ICP. If CPP = 0, there is no cerebral perfusion → brain death.

Effects of strokes

ARTERY	AREA OF LESION	SYMPTOMS	NOTES
Anterior circulation			
MCA	Motor cortex—upper limb and face.	Contralateral paralysis—upper limb and face.	
	Sensory cortex—upper limb and face.	Contralateral loss of sensation—upper limb and face.	
	Temporal lobe (Wernicke area); frontal lobe (Broca area).	Aphasia if in dominant (usually left) hemisphere. Hemineglect if lesion affects nondominant (usually right) side.	
ACA	Motor cortex—lower limb.	Contralateral paralysis—lower limb.	
	Sensory cortex—lower limb.	Contralateral loss of sensation—lower limb.	
Lenticulo-striate artery	Striatum, internal capsule.	Contralateral hemiparesis/hemiplegia.	Common location of lacunar infarcts, 2° to unmanaged hypertension.
Posterior circulation			
ASA	Lateral corticospinal tract.	Contralateral hemiparesis—upper and lower limbs.	Stroke commonly bilateral. Medial medullary syndrome—caused by infarct of paramedian branches of ASA and vertebral arteries.
	Medial lemniscus.	↓ contralateral proprioception.	
	Caudal medulla—hypoglossal nerve.	Ipsilateral hypoglossal dysfunction (tongue deviates ipsilaterally).	
PICA	Lateral medulla—vestibular nuclei, lateral spinothalamic tract, spinal trigeminal nucleus, nucleus ambiguus, sympathetic fibers, inferior cerebellar peduncle.	Vomiting, vertigo, nystagmus; ↓ pain and temperature sensation from ipsilateral face and contralateral body; **dysphagia, hoarseness**, ↓ gag reflex; ipsilateral Horner syndrome; ataxia, dysmetria.	Lateral medullary (Wallenberg) syndrome. Nucleus ambiguus effects are specific to PICA lesions. "Don't **pick a** (**PICA**) **horse** (hoarseness) that **can't eat** (dysphagia)."
AICA	Lateral pons—cranial nerve nuclei; vestibular nuclei, facial nucleus, spinal trigeminal nucleus, cochlear nuclei, sympathetic fibers.	Vomiting, vertigo, nystagmus. **Paralysis of face**, ↓ lacrimation, salivation, ↓ taste from anterior ⅔ of tongue. Ipsilateral ↓ pain and temperature of the face, contralateral ↓ pain and temperature of the body.	Lateral pontine syndrome. Facial nucleus effects are specific to AICA lesions. "**Facial droop** means AICA's **pooped**."
	Middle and inferior cerebellar peduncles.	Ataxia, dysmetria.	
PCA	Occipital cortex, visual cortex.	Contralateral hemianopia with macular sparing.	
Basilar artery	Pons, medulla, lower midbrain, corticospinal and corticobulbar tracts, ocular cranial nerve nuclei, paramedian pontine reticular formation.	Preserved consciousness and blinking, quadriplegia, loss of voluntary facial, mouth, and tongue movements.	"Locked-in syndrome."

Effects of strokes *(continued)*

ARTERY	AREA OF LESION	SYMPTOMS	NOTES
Communicating arteries			
ACom	Most common lesion is aneurysm. Can lead to stroke. Saccular (berry) aneurysm can impinge cranial nerves.	Visual field defects.	Lesions are typically aneurysms, not strokes.
PCom	Common site of saccular aneurysm.	CN III palsy—eye is "down and out" with ptosis and mydriasis.	Lesions are typically aneurysms, not strokes.

Aneurysms	In general, an abnormal dilation of artery due to weakening of vessel wall.

Saccular (berry) aneurysm	Occurs at bifurcations in the circle of Willis **A B**. Most common site is junction of anterior communicating artery and anterior cerebral artery. Rupture (most common complication) → subarachnoid hemorrhage ("worst headache of my life") or hemorrhagic stroke. Can also cause bitemporal hemianopia via compression of optic chiasm. Associated with ADPKD, Ehlers-Danlos syndrome. Other risk factors: advanced age, hypertension, smoking, race (↑ risk in blacks).	
Charcot-Bouchard microaneurysm	Associated with chronic hypertension; affects small vessels (e.g., in basal ganglia, thalamus).	

Berry aneurysm. Coronal (left) and sagittal (right) contrast CT shows berry aneurysm (arrows). ✴

Central post-stroke pain syndrome	Neuropathic pain due to thalamic lesions. Initial paresthesias followed in weeks to months by allodynia (ordinarily painless stimuli cause pain) and dysesthesia. Occurs in 10% of stroke patients.

Intracranial hemorrhage

Epidural hematoma

Rupture of middle meningeal artery (branch of maxillary artery), often 2° to fracture of temporal bone. Lucid interval. Rapid expansion under systemic arterial pressure → transtentorial herniation, CN III palsy.

CT shows biconvex (lentiform), hyperdense blood collection 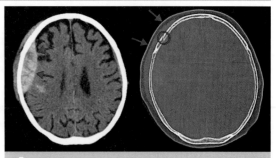 **not crossing suture lines. Can cross falx, tentorium.**

A **Epidural hematoma.** Axial CT of brain shows lens-shaped collection of epidural blood (left, arrows), with bone windows showing associated skull fracture (right, circle) and scalp hematoma (arrows). ✴, ✴

Subdural hematoma

Rupture of bridging veins. Slow venous bleeding (less pressure = hematoma develops over time). Seen in elderly individuals, alcoholics, blunt trauma, shaken baby (predisposing factors: brain atrophy, shaking, whiplash).

Crescent-shaped hemorrhage 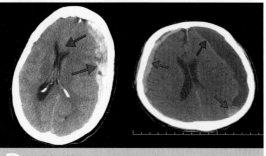 that **crosses suture lines. Midline shift. Cannot cross falx, tentorium.**

B **Subdural hematoma.** Axial CTs show crescent-shaped subdural blood collections. Left image shows acute bleed (red arrow) with midline shift (subfalcine herniation, blue arrow). ✴ Right image shows "acute on chronic" hemorrhage (red arrows, acute; blue arrow, chronic). ℞

Subarachnoid hemorrhage

Rupture of an aneurysm (such as a berry [saccular] aneurysm, as seen in Ehlers-Danlos syndrome, ADPKD) or arteriovenous malformation. Rapid time course. Patients complain of "worst headache of my life (WHOML)." Bloody or yellow (xanthochromic) spinal tap. 2–3 days afterward, risk of vasospasm due to blood breakdown (not visible on CT, treat with nimodipine) and rebleed (visible on CT) 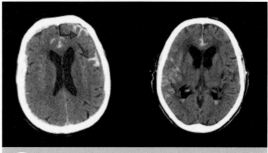.

C **Subarachnoid hemorrhage.** Axial CT of brain shows subarachnoid blood in sulci (left, arrows) and intraventricular blood (right, arrows) layering in posterior horn of lateral ventricles. ℞, ℞

Intraparenchymal (hypertensive) hemorrhage

Most commonly caused by systemic hypertension 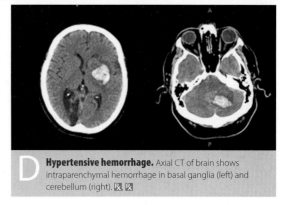. Also seen with amyloid angiopathy (recurrent lobar hemorrhagic stroke in elderly), vasculitis, neoplasm. Typically occurs in basal ganglia and internal capsule (Charcot-Bouchard aneurysm of lenticulostriate vessels), but can be lobar.

D **Hypertensive hemorrhage.** Axial CT of brain shows intraparenchymal hemorrhage in basal ganglia (left) and cerebellum (right). ℞, ℞

Ischemic brain disease/stroke

Irreversible damage begins after 5 minutes of hypoxia. Most vulnerable: hippocampus, neocortex, cerebellum, watershed areas. Irreversible neuronal injury.

Stroke imaging: Noncontrast CT to exclude hemorrhage (before tPA can be given). CT detects ischemic changes in 6–24 hr. Diffusion-weighted MRI can detect ischemia within 3–30 min.

Ischemic **hypo**xia—"**hypo**campus" is most vulnerable.

TIME SINCE ISCHEMIC EVENT	12–48 HOURS	24–72 HOURS	3–5 DAYS	1–2 WEEKS	> 2 WEEKS
Histologic features	Red neurons	Necrosis + neutrophils	Macrophages (microglia)	Reactive gliosis + vascular proliferation	Glial scar

Hemorrhagic stroke

Intracerebral bleeding, often due to hypertension, anticoagulation, cancer (abnormal vessels can bleed). May be 2° to ischemic stroke followed by reperfusion (↑ vessel fragility). Basal ganglia are most common site of intracerebral hemorrhage.

Ischemic stroke

Acute blockage of vessels → disruption of blood flow and subsequent ischemia → liquefactive necrosis.

3 types:

- Thrombotic—due to a clot forming directly at site of infarction (commonly the MCA **A**), usually over an atherosclerotic plaque.
- Embolic—embolus from another part of the body obstructs vessel. Can affect multiple vascular territories. Examples: atrial fibrillation; DVT with patent foramen ovale.
- Hypoxic—due to hypoperfusion or hypoxemia. Common during cardiovascular surgeries, tends to affect watershed areas.

Treatment: tPA (if within 3–4.5 hr of onset and no hemorrhage/risk of hemorrhage). Reduce risk with medical therapy (e.g., aspirin, clopidogrel); optimum control of blood pressure, blood sugars, lipids; and treat conditions that ↑ risk (e.g., atrial fibrillation).

Transient ischemic attack

Brief, reversible episode of focal neurologic dysfunction without acute infarction (⊖ MRI), with the majority resolving in < 15 minutes; deficits due to focal ischemia.

Dural venous sinuses

Large venous channels that run through the dura. Drain blood from cerebral veins and receive CSF from arachnoid granulations. Empty into internal jugular vein.

Superior sagittal sinus (*main location of CSF return via arachnoid granulations*)
Inferior sagittal sinus
Great cerebral vein of Galen
Straight sinus
Confluence of the sinuses
Occipital sinus
Transverse sinus
Superior ophthalmic vein
Sphenoparietal sinus
Cavernous sinus
Sigmoid sinus
Jugular foramen
Internal jugular vein

Ventricular system

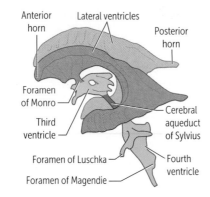

Lateral ventricle → 3rd ventricle via right and left interventricular foramina of Monro.

3rd ventricle → 4th ventricle via cerebral aqueduct (of Sylvius).

4th ventricle → subarachnoid space via:
- Foramina of **L**uschka = **L**ateral.
- Foramen of **M**agendie = **M**edial.

CSF is made by ependymal cells of choroid plexus; it is reabsorbed by arachnoid granulations and then drains into dural venous sinuses.

Idiopathic intracranial hypertension (pseudotumor cerebri)

↑ ICP with no apparent cause on imaging (i.e., hydrocephalus, obstruction of CSF outflow). Patients present with headaches, diplopia (usually from CN VI palsy), no mental status alterations. Papilledema seen on exam. Risk factors include being a woman of childbearing age, vitamin A excess, danazol. Lumbar puncture reveals ↑ opening pressure and provides headache relief. Treatment: weight loss, acetazolamide, topiramate, invasive procedures for refractory cases (e.g., repeat lumbar puncture, CSF shunt placement, optic nerve fenestration surgery).

Hydrocephalus

Communicating (nonobstructive)

Communicating hydrocephalus	↓ CSF absorption by arachnoid granulations → ↑ ICP, papilledema, herniation (e.g., arachnoid scarring post-meningitis).
Normal pressure hydrocephalus	Affects the elderly; idiopathic; CSF pressure elevated only episodically; does not result in increased subarachnoid space volume. Expansion of ventricles A distorts the fibers of the corona radiata → triad of **urinary incontinence**, **ataxia**, and **cognitive dysfunction** (sometimes reversible). "**Wet, wobbly, and wacky.**"

Noncommunicating (obstructive)

Noncommunicating hydrocephalus	Caused by structural blockage of CSF circulation within ventricular system (e.g., stenosis of aqueduct of Sylvius; colloid cyst blocking foramen of Monro).

Hydrocephalus mimics

Ex vacuo ventriculomegaly	Appearance of ↑ CSF on imaging, is actually due to decreased brain tissue (neuronal atrophy) (e.g., Alzheimer disease, advanced HIV, Pick disease). ICP is normal; triad is not seen.

Spinal nerves	There are 31 pairs of spinal nerves in total: 8 cervical, 12 thoracic, 5 lumbar, 5 sacral, 1 coccygeal. Nerves C1–C7 exit above the corresponding vertebra. C8 spinal nerve exits below C7 and above T1. All other nerves exit below (e.g., C3 exits above the 3rd cervical vertebra; L2 exits below the 2nd lumbar vertebra).	31, just like **31** flavors of Baskin-Robbins ice cream! **Vertebral disc herniation**—nucleus pulposus (soft central disc) herniates through annulus fibrosus (outer ring); usually occurs posterolaterally at L4–L5 or L5–S1.
Spinal cord—lower extent	In adults, spinal cord extends to lower border of L1–L2 vertebrae. Subarachnoid space (which contains the CSF) extends to lower border of S2 vertebra. Lumbar puncture is usually performed between L3–L4 or L4–L5 (level of cauda equina).	Goal of lumbar puncture is to obtain sample of CSF without damaging spinal cord. To **keep** the cord **alive,** keep the spinal needle between **L3** and **L5.**
Spinal cord and associated tracts	Legs (Lumbosacral) are Lateral in Lateral corticospinal, spinothalamic tracts 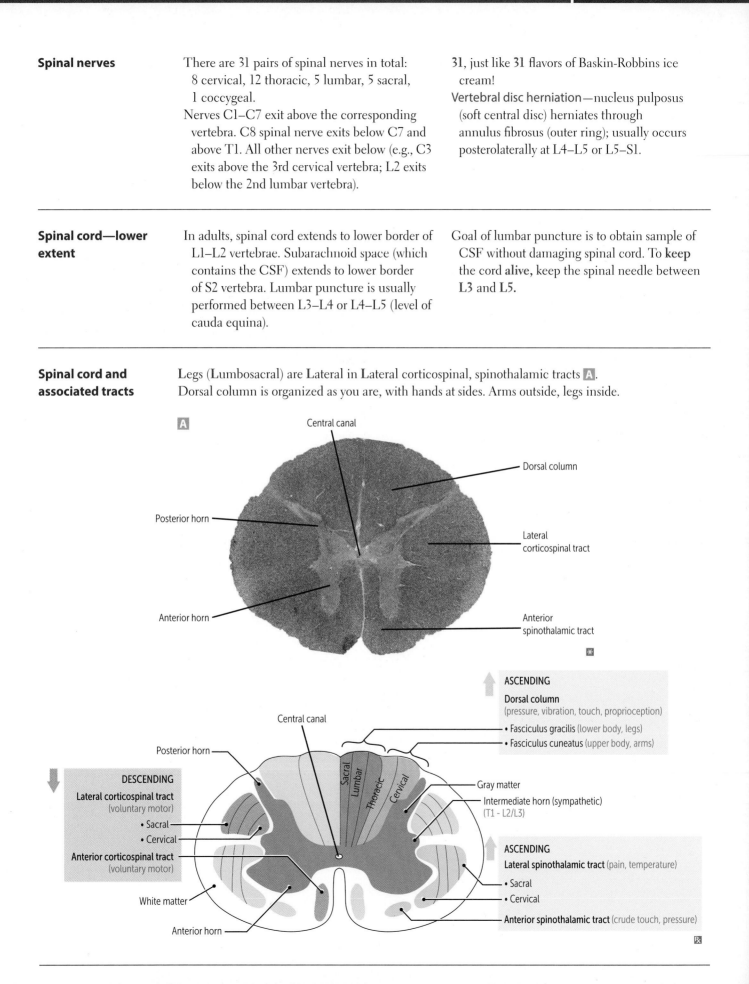. Dorsal column is organized as you are, with hands at sides. Arms outside, legs inside.	

A

Central canal

Dorsal column

Posterior horn

Lateral corticospinal tract

Anterior horn

Anterior spinothalamic tract

DESCENDING
Lateral corticospinal tract (voluntary motor)
• Sacral
• Cervical
Anterior corticospinal tract (voluntary motor)

Posterior horn

Central canal

White matter

Anterior horn

Sacral
Lumbar
Thoracic
Cervical

Gray matter

Intermediate horn (sympathetic) (T1 - L2/L3)

ASCENDING
Dorsal column (pressure, vibration, touch, proprioception)
• Fasciculus gracilis (lower body, legs)
• Fasciculus cuneatus (upper body, arms)

ASCENDING
Lateral spinothalamic tract (pain, temperature)
• Sacral
• Cervical
Anterior spinothalamic tract (crude touch, pressure)

Spinal tract anatomy and functions

Remember, ascending tracts synapse and then cross.

TRACT AND FUNCTION	1ST-ORDER NEURON	SYNAPSE 1	2ND-ORDER NEURON	SYNAPSE 2	3RD-ORDER NEURON
Dorsal column Ascending: pressure, vibration, fine touch, and proprioception	Sensory nerve ending → cell body in dorsal root ganglion → enters spinal cord, ascends ipsilaterally in dorsal column	Ipsilateral nucleus cuneatus or gracilis (medulla)	Decussates in medulla → ascends contralaterally in medial lemniscus	VPL (thalamus)	Sensory cortex
Spinothalamic tract Ascending Lateral: pain, temperature Anterior: crude touch, pressure	Sensory nerve ending (Aδ and C fibers) (cell body in dorsal root ganglion) → enters spinal cord	Ipsilateral gray matter (spinal cord)	Decussates at anterior white commissure → ascends contralaterally	VPL (thalamus)	Sensory cortex
Lateral corticospinal tract Descending: voluntary movement of contralateral limbs	UMN: cell body in 1° motor cortex → descends ipsilaterally (through internal capsule), most fibers decussate at caudal medulla (pyramidal decussation) → descends contralaterally	Cell body of anterior horn (spinal cord)	LMN: leaves spinal cord	NMJ	

Motor neuron signs

SIGN	UMN LESION	LMN LESION	COMMENTS
Weakness	+	+	**Lower** MN = everything **lowered** (less muscle mass, ↓ muscle tone, ↓ reflexes, downgoing toes).
Atrophy	–	+	
Fasciculations	–	+	**Upper** MN = everything **up** (tone, DTRs, toes).
Reflexes	↑	↓	
Tone	↑	↓	Fasciculations = muscle twitching.
Babinski	+	–	Positive Babinski is normal in infants.
Spastic paralysis	+	–	
Flaccid paralysis	–	+	
Clasp knife spasticity	+	–	

Spinal cord lesions

AREA AFFECTED	DISEASE	CHARACTERISTICS
	Poliomyelitis and spinal muscular atrophy (Werdnig-Hoffmann disease)	LMN lesions only, due to destruction of anterior horns; flaccid paralysis.
	Multiple sclerosis	Due to demyelination; mostly white matter of cervical region; random and asymmetric lesions, due to demyelination; scanning speech, intention tremor, nystagmus.
	Amyotrophic lateral sclerosis	Combined UMN and LMN deficits with no sensory or oculomotor deficits; both UMN and LMN signs. Can be caused by defect in superoxide dismutase 1. Commonly presents as fasciculations with eventual atrophy and weakness of hands; fatal. Riluzole treatment modestly ↑ survival by ↓ presynaptic glutamate release. Commonly known as Lou Gehrig disease. For **Lou** Gehrig disease, give ri**lou**zole (a glutamate antagonist).
Posterior spinal arteries / Anterior spinal artery	Complete occlusion of anterior spinal artery	Spares dorsal columns and Lissauer tract; upper thoracic ASA territory is watershed area, as artery of Adamkiewicz supplies ASA below ~ T8.
	Tabes dorsalis	Caused by 3° syphilis. Results from degeneration (demyelination) of dorsal columns and roots → impaired sensation and proprioception, progressive sensory ataxia (inability to sense or feel the legs → poor coordination). Associated with Charcot joints, shooting pain, Argyll Robertson pupils. Exam will demonstrate absence of DTRs and ⊕ Romberg sign.
	Syringomyelia	Syrinx expands and damages anterior white commissure of spinothalamic tract (2nd-order neurons) → bilateral loss of pain and temperature sensation (usually C8–T1); seen with Chiari I malformation; can expand and affect other tracts.
	Vitamin B$_{12}$ deficiency	Subacute combined degeneration—demyelination of dorsal columns, lateral corticospinal tracts, and spinocerebellar tracts; ataxic gait, paresthesia, impaired position and vibration sense.

Poliomyelitis	Caused by poliovirus (fecal-oral transmission). Replicates in oropharynx and small intestine before spreading via bloodstream to CNS. Infection causes destruction of cells in anterior horn of spinal cord (LMN death).
SYMPTOMS	LMN lesion signs: weakness, hypotonia, flaccid paralysis, fasciculations, hyporeflexia, muscle atrophy. Signs of infection: malaise, headache, fever, nausea, etc.
FINDINGS	CSF with ↑ WBCs and slight ↑ of protein (with no change in CSF glucose). Virus recovered from stool or throat.

Spinal muscular atrophy (Werdnig-Hoffmann disease)	Congenital degeneration of anterior horns of spinal cord → LMN lesion. "Floppy baby" with marked hypotonia and tongue fasciculations. Infantile type has median age of death of 7 months. Autosomal recessive inheritance.

Friedreich ataxia

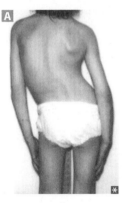

Autosomal recessive trinucleotide repeat disorder (GAA) on chromosome 9 in gene that encodes frataxin (iron binding protein). Leads to impairment in mitochondrial functioning. Degeneration of multiple spinal cord tracts → muscle weakness and loss of DTRs, vibratory sense, proprioception. **Staggering** gait, frequent **falling**, nystagmus, dysarthria, pes cavus, hammer toes, **diabetes mellitus**, **hypertrophic cardiomyopathy** (cause of death). Presents in childhood with kyphoscoliosis .

Friedreich is Fratastic (**frataxin**): he's your favorite **frat** brother, always **staggering** and **falling** but has a **sweet, big heart**.

Brown-Séquard syndrome

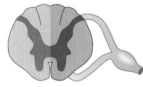

Lesion

Hemisection of spinal cord. Findings:
- Ipsilateral UMN signs below level of lesion (due to corticospinal tract damage)
- Ipsilateral loss of tactile, vibration, proprioception sense below level of lesion (due to dorsal column damage)
- Contralateral pain and temperature loss below level of lesion (due to spinothalamic tract damage)
- Ipsilateral loss of all sensation at level of lesion
- Ipsilateral LMN signs (e.g., flaccid paralysis) at level of lesion

If lesion occurs above T1, patient may present with Horner syndrome due to damage of oculosympathetic pathway.

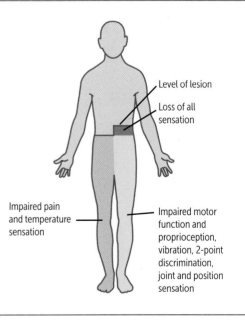

Level of lesion

Loss of all sensation

Impaired pain and temperature sensation

Impaired motor function and proprioception, vibration, 2-point discrimination, joint and position sensation

Landmark dermatomes

C2—posterior half of a skull "cap."
C3—high turtleneck shirt.
C4—low-collar shirt.
T4—at the nipple.
T7—at the xiphoid process.
T10—at the umbilicus (important for early appendicitis pain referral).
L1—at the inguinal ligament.
L4—includes the kneecaps.
S2, S3, S4—erection and sensation of penile and anal zones.

Diaphragm and gallbladder pain referred to the right shoulder via phrenic nerve.

T4 at the **teat pore**.

T10 at the belly but**ten**.

L1 is **IL** (Inguinal Ligament).
Down on **ALL 4's** (**L4**).
"**S2, 3, 4** keep the penis off the **floor**."

Clinical reflexes

Biceps = C5 nerve root.
Triceps = C7 nerve root.
Patella = L4 nerve root.
Achilles = S1 nerve root.

Reflexes count up in order:
  S1, 2—"buckle my shoe" (Achilles reflex)
  L3, 4—"kick the door" (patellar reflex)
  C5, 6—"pick up sticks" (biceps reflex)
  C7, 8—"lay them straight" (triceps reflex)
Additional reflexes:
  L1, L2—"testicles move" (cremaster reflex)
  S3, S4—"winks galore" (anal wink reflex)

Primitive reflexes

CNS reflexes that are present in a healthy infant, but are absent in a neurologically intact adult. Normally disappear within 1st year of life. These "primitive" reflexes are inhibited by a mature/developing frontal lobe. They may reemerge in adults following frontal lobe lesions → loss of inhibition of these reflexes.

Moro reflex	"Hang on for life" reflex—abduct/extend arms when startled, and then draw together
Rooting reflex	Movement of head toward one side if cheek or mouth is stroked (nipple seeking)
Sucking reflex	Sucking response when roof of mouth is touched
Palmar reflex	Curling of fingers if palm is stroked
Plantar reflex	Dorsiflexion of large toe and fanning of other toes with plantar stimulation Babinski sign—presence of this reflex in an adult, which may signify a UMN lesion
Galant reflex	Stroking along one side of the spine while newborn is in ventral suspension (face down) causes lateral flexion of lower body toward stimulated side

Brain stem—ventral view

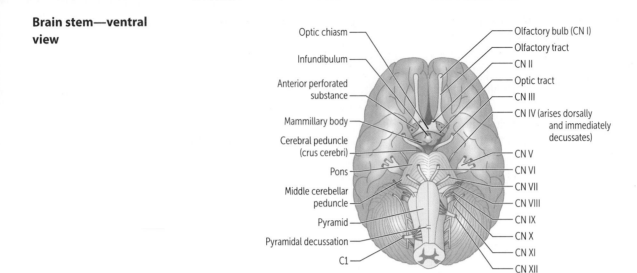

Optic chiasm
Infundibulum
Anterior perforated substance
Mammillary body
Cerebral peduncle (crus cerebri)
Pons
Middle cerebellar peduncle
Pyramid
Pyramidal decussation
C1

Olfactory bulb (CN I)
Olfactory tract
CN II
Optic tract
CN III
CN IV (arises dorsally and immediately decussates)
CN V
CN VI
CN VII
CN VIII
CN IX
CN X
CN XI
CN XII

CN nuclei that lie medially at brain stem: III, IV, VI, XII. "Factors of **12**, except 1 and 2."

Brain stem—dorsal view (cerebellum removed)

Pineal gland—melatonin secretion, circadian rhythms.

Superior colliculi—conjugate vertical gaze center.

Inferior colliculi—auditory.

Parinaud syndrome—paralysis of conjugate vertical gaze due to lesion in superior colliculi (e.g., stroke, hydrocephalus, pinealoma).

Your eyes are **above** your ears, and the superior colliculus (visual) is **above** the inferior colliculus (auditory).

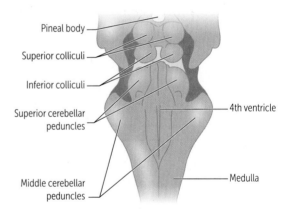

Pineal body
Superior colliculi
Inferior colliculi
Superior cerebellar peduncles
Middle cerebellar peduncles
4th ventricle
Medulla

Cranial nerve nuclei

Located in tegmentum portion of brain stem (between dorsal and ventral portions):
- Midbrain—nuclei of CN III, IV
- Pons—nuclei of CN V, VI, VII, VIII
- Medulla—nuclei of CN IX, X, XII
- Spinal cord—nucleus of CN XI

Lateral nuclei = sensory (aLar plate).
—Sulcus limitans—
Medial nuclei = Motor (basal plate).

Cranial nerve and vessel pathways

Cribriform plate (CN I).

Middle cranial fossa (CN II–VI)—through sphenoid bone:

- Optic canal (CN II, ophthalmic artery, central retinal vein)
- Superior orbital fissure (CN III, IV, V_1, VI, ophthalmic vein, sympathetic fibers)
- Foramen **R**otundum (CN V_2)
- Foramen **O**vale (CN V_3)
- Foramen spinosum (middle meningeal artery)

Posterior cranial fossa (CN VII–XII)—through temporal or occipital bone:

- Internal auditory meatus (CN VII, VIII)
- Jugular foramen (CN IX, X, XI, jugular vein)
- Hypoglossal canal (CN XII)
- Foramen magnum (spinal roots of CN XI, brain stem, vertebral arteries)

Divisions of CN V exit owing to **S**tanding **R**oom **O**nly.

Cranial nerves

NERVE	CN	FUNCTION	TYPE	MNEMONIC
Olfactory	I	Smell (only CN without thalamic relay to cortex)	Sensory	Some
Optic	II	Sight	Sensory	Say
Oculomotor	III	Eye movement (SR, IR, MR, IO), pupillary constriction (sphincter pupillae: Edinger-Westphal nucleus, muscarinic receptors), accommodation, eyelid opening (levator palpebrae)	Motor	Marry
Trochlear	IV	Eye movement (SO)	Motor	Money
Trigeminal	V	Mastication, facial sensation (ophthalmic, maxillary, mandibular divisions), somatosensation from anterior $^2/_3$ of tongue	Both	But
Abducens	VI	Eye movement (LR)	Motor	My
Facial	VII	Facial movement, taste from anterior $^2/_3$ of tongue, lacrimation, salivation (submandibular and sublingual glands), eyelid closing (orbicularis oculi), stapedius muscle in ear (note: nerve courses through the parotid gland, but does not innervate it)	Both	Brother
Vestibulocochlear	VIII	Hearing, balance	Sensory	Says
Glossopharyngeal	IX	Taste and somatosensation from posterior $^1/_3$ of tongue, swallowing, salivation (parotid gland), monitoring carotid body and sinus chemo- and baroreceptors, and stylopharyngeus (elevates pharynx, larynx)	Both	Big
Vagus	X	Taste from epiglottic region, swallowing, soft palate elevation, midline uvula, talking, coughing, thoracoabdominal viscera, monitoring aortic arch chemo- and baroreceptors	Both	Brains
Accessory	XI	Head turning, shoulder shrugging (SCM, trapezius)	Motor	Matter
Hypoglossal	XII	Tongue movement	Motor	Most

Vagal nuclei

Nucleus Solitarius	Visceral Sensory information (e.g., taste, baroreceptors, gut distention).	VII, IX, X.
Nucleus aMbiguus	Motor innervation of pharynx, larynx, upper esophagus (e.g., swallowing, palate elevation).	IX, X, XI (cranial portion).
Dorsal motor nucleus	Sends autonomic (parasympathetic) fibers to heart, lungs, upper GI.	X.

Cranial nerve reflexes

REFLEX	AFFERENT	EFFERENT
Corneal	V_1 ophthalmic (nasociliary branch)	VII (temporal branch: orbicularis oculi)
Lacrimation	V_1 (loss of reflex does not preclude emotional tears)	VII
Jaw jerk	V_3 (sensory—muscle spindle from masseter)	V_3 (motor—masseter)
Pupillary	II	III
Gag	IX	X

Common cranial nerve lesions

CN V motor lesion	Jaw deviates **toward** side of lesion due to unopposed force from the opposite pterygoid muscle.
CN X lesion	Uvula deviates **away** from side of lesion. Weak side collapses and uvula points away.
CN XI lesion	Weakness turning head to contralateral side of lesion (SCM). Shoulder droop on side of lesion (trapezius). The left SCM contracts to help turn the head to the right.
CN XII lesion (LMN)	Tongue deviates **toward** side of lesion ("lick your wounds") due to weakened tongue muscles on affected side.

Cavernous sinus   Collection of venous sinuses on either side of pituitary. Blood from eye and superficial cortex → cavernous sinus → internal jugular vein. CN III, IV, V_1, VI, and occasionally V_2 plus postganglionic sympathetic pupillary fibers en route to orbit all pass through cavernous sinus. Cavernous portion of internal carotid artery is also here.

Nerves that control extraocular muscles (plus V_1 and V_2) pass through the cavernous sinus. Cavernous sinus syndrome—presents with variable ophthalmoplegia, ↓ corneal sensation, Horner syndrome and occasional decreased maxillary sensation. 2° to pituitary tumor mass effect, carotid-cavernous fistula, or cavernous sinus thrombosis related to infection. CN VI is most susceptible to injury.

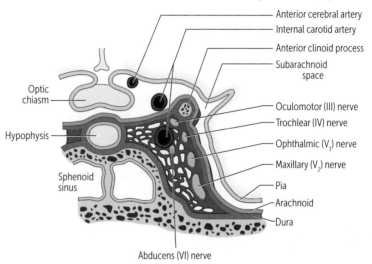

Auditory physiology

Outer ear	Visible portion of ear (pinna), includes auditory canal and eardrum. Transfers sound waves via vibration of eardrum.
Middle ear	Air-filled space with three bones called the ossicles (malleus, incus, stapes). Ossicles conduct and amplify sound from eardrum to inner ear.
Inner ear	Snail-shaped, fluid-filled cochlea. Contains basilar membrane that vibrates 2° to sound waves. Vibration transduced via specialized hair cells → auditory nerve signaling → brain stem. Each frequency leads to vibration at specific location on basilar membrane (tonotopy): ▪ Low frequency heard at apex near helicotrema (wide and flexible). ▪ High frequency heard best at base of cochlea (thin and rigid).

Hearing loss

	RINNE TEST	WEBER TEST
Conductive	Abnormal (bone > air)	Localizes to affected ear
Sensorineural	Normal (air > bone)	Localizes to unaffected ear
Noise-induced	Damage to stereociliated cells in organ of Corti; loss of high-frequency hearing 1st; sudden extremely loud noises can produce hearing loss due to tympanic membrane rupture.	

Cholesteatoma	Overgrowth of desquamated keratin debris within middle ear space A; may erode ossicles, mastoid air cells → conductive hearing loss.	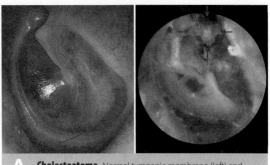 A **Cholesteatoma.** Normal tympanic membrane (left) and cholesteatoma (right).

Facial lesions

UMN lesion	Lesion of motor cortex or connection between cortex and facial nucleus. Contralateral paralysis of lower face; forehead spared due to bilateral UMN innervation.	
LMN lesion	Ipsilateral paralysis of upper **and** lower face.	
Facial nerve palsy	Complete destruction of the facial nucleus itself or its branchial efferent fibers (facial nerve proper). Peripheral ipsilateral facial paralysis (absent forehead creases and drooping smile A) with inability to close eye on involved side. Can occur idiopathically (called **Bell palsy**); gradual recovery in most cases. Associated with Lyme disease, herpes simplex and (less common) herpes zoster (Ramsay Hunt syndrome), sarcoidosis, tumors, diabetes. Treatment includes corticosteroids.	

Mastication muscles	3 muscles close jaw: Masseter, teMporalis, Medial pterygoid. 1 opens: lateral pterygoid. All are innervated by trigeminal nerve (V_3).	M's Munch. Lateral Lowers (when speaking of pterygoids with respect to jaw motion). "It takes more muscle to keep your mouth shut."

▶ NEUROLOGY—OPHTHALMOLOGY

Normal eye

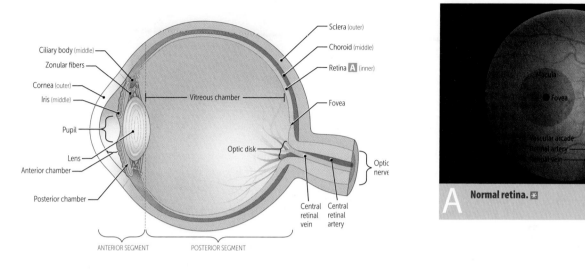

A **Normal retina.** ✱

Aqueous humor pathway

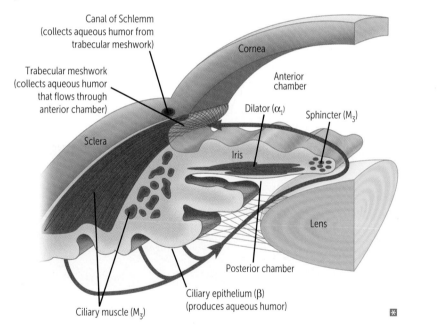

Refractive errors	Common cause of impaired vision, correctable with glasses.
Hyperopia	Eye too short for refractive power of cornea and lens → light focused behind retina.
Myopia	Eye too long for refractive power of cornea and lens → light focused in front of retina.
Astigmatism	Abnormal curvature of cornea → different refractive power at different axes.
Presbyopia	Age-related impaired accommodation (focusing on near objects), possibly due to decreased lens elasticity. Often necessitates "reading glasses."

Cataract	Painless, often bilateral, opacification of lens 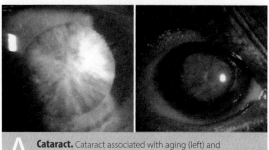 → ↓ in vision. Risk factors: ↑ age, smoking, EtOH, excessive sunlight, prolonged corticosteroid use, classic galactosemia, galactokinase deficiency, diabetes mellitus (sorbitol), trauma, infection.

A **Cataract.** Cataract associated with aging (left) and corticosteroid use (right). ✳ ✳

Glaucoma	Optic disc atrophy with characteristic cupping (thinning of outer rim of optic nerve head **B** versus normal **A**), usually with elevated intraocular pressure (IOP) and progressive peripheral visual field loss.
Open angle	Associated with ↑ age, African-American race, family history. Painless, more common in U.S. Primary—cause unclear. Secondary—blocked trabecular meshwork from WBCs (e.g., uveitis), RBCs (e.g., vitreous hemorrhage), retinal elements (e.g., retinal detachment).
Closed/narrow angle	Primary—enlargement or forward movement of lens against central iris (pupil margin) → obstruction of normal aqueous flow through pupil → fluid builds up behind iris, pushing peripheral iris against cornea **C** and impeding flow through trabecular meshwork. Secondary—hypoxia from retinal disease (e.g., diabetes mellitus, vein occlusion) induces vasoproliferation in iris that contracts angle. Chronic closure—often asymptomatic with damage to optic nerve and peripheral vision. Acute closure—true ophthalmic emergency. ↑ IOP pushes iris forward → angle closes abruptly. Very painful, red eye, sudden vision loss, halos around lights, rock-hard eye, frontal headache **D**. Do not give epinephrine because of its mydriatic effect.

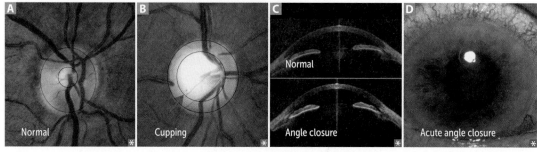

A — Normal | B — Cupping | C — Normal / Angle closure | D — Acute angle closure

Uveitis	Inflammation of uvea (e.g., iritis aka anterior uveitis, choroiditis aka posterior uveitis). May have hypopyon (accumulation of pus in anterior chamber **A**) or conjunctival redness. Associated with systemic inflammatory disorders (e.g., sarcoidosis, rheumatoid arthritis, juvenile idiopathic arthritis, HLA-B27–associated conditions).

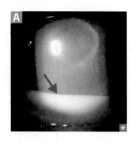

Age-related macular degeneration

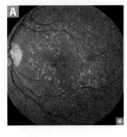

Degeneration of macula (central area of retina). Causes distortion (metamorphopsia) and eventual loss of central vision (scotomas).

- Dry (nonexudative, > 80%)—deposition of yellowish extracellular material in and beneath Bruch membrane and retinal pigment epithelium ("drusen") with gradual ↓ in vision. Prevent progression with multivitamin and antioxidant supplements.
- Wet (exudative, 10–15%)—rapid loss of vision due to bleeding 2° to choroidal neovascularization. Treat with anti-VEGF (vascular endothelial growth factor) injections (e.g., ranibizumab) or laser.

Diabetic retinopathy

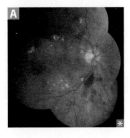

Retinal damage due to chronic hyperglycemia. Two types:

- Nonproliferative—damaged capillaries leak blood → lipids and fluid seep into retina → hemorrhages and macular edema . Treatment: blood sugar control, macular laser.
- Proliferative—chronic hypoxia results in new blood vessel formation with resultant traction on retina. Treatment: peripheral retinal photocoagulation, anti-VEGF (e.g., bevacizumab).

Retinal vein occlusion

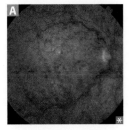

Blockage of central or branch retinal vein due to compression from nearby arterial atherosclerosis. Retinal hemorrhage and venous engorgement , edema in affected area.

Retinal detachment

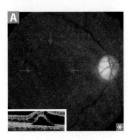

Separation of neurosensory layer of retina (photoreceptor layer with rods and cones) from outermost pigmented epithelium (normally shields excess light, supports retina) → degeneration of photoreceptors → vision loss. May be 2° to retinal breaks, diabetic traction, inflammatory effusions. Visualized on fundoscopy by the splaying and paucity of retinal vessels [blue arrows,]. Correlation with cross-sectional "optical ultrasound" shown on inset .

Breaks more common in patients with high myopia and are often preceded by posterior vitreous detachment ("flashes" and "floaters") and eventual monocular loss of vision like a "curtain drawn down." Surgical emergency.

Central retinal artery occlusion

Acute, painless monocular vision loss. Retina cloudy with attenuated vessels and "cherry-red" spot at fovea (center of macula) 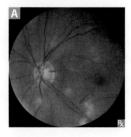.

Retinitis pigmentosa

Inherited retinal degeneration. Painless, progressive vision loss beginning with night blindness (rods affected first). Bone spicule–shaped deposits around macula 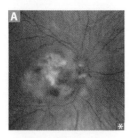.

Retinitis

Retinal edema and necrosis leading to scar A. Often viral (CMV, HSV, HZV). Associated with immunosuppression.

Papilledema

Optic disc swelling (usually bilateral) due to ↑ ICP (e.g., 2° to mass effect). Enlarged blind spot and elevated optic disc with blurred margins seen on fundoscopic exam 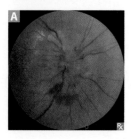.

Pupillary control

Miosis	Constriction, parasympathetic: ▪ 1st neuron: Edinger-Westphal nucleus to ciliary ganglion via CN III ▪ 2nd neuron: short ciliary nerves to pupillary sphincter muscles

Pupillary light reflex

Light in either retina sends a signal via CN II to pretectal nuclei (dashed lines in image) in midbrain that activates bilateral Edinger-Westphal nuclei; pupils contract bilaterally (consensual reflex).

Result: illumination of 1 eye results in bilateral pupillary constriction.

Mydriasis

Dilation, sympathetic:
▪ 1st neuron: hypothalamus to ciliospinal center of Budge (C8–T2)
▪ 2nd neuron: exit at T1 to superior cervical ganglion (travels along cervical sympathetic chain near lung apex, subclavian vessels)
▪ 3rd neuron: plexus along internal carotid, through cavernous sinus; enters orbit as long ciliary nerve to pupillary dilator muscles. Sympathetic fibers also innervate smooth muscle of eyelids (minor retractors) and sweat glands of forehead and face.

Marcus Gunn pupil

Afferent pupillary defect—due to optic nerve damage or severe retinal injury. ↓ bilateral pupillary constriction when light is shone in affected eye relative to unaffected eye. Tested with "swinging flashlight test."

Horner syndrome

Sympathetic denervation of face:
▪ Ptosis (slight drooping of eyelid: superior tarsal muscle)
▪ Anhidrosis (absence of sweating) and flushing (rubor) of affected side of face
▪ Miosis (pupil constriction)
Associated with lesion of spinal cord above T1 (e.g., Pancoast tumor, Brown-Séquard syndrome [cord hemisection], late-stage syringomyelia).
Any interruption results in Horner syndrome.

PAM is horny (Horner).
Ptosis, anhidrosis, and miosis (rhyming).

Ocular motility

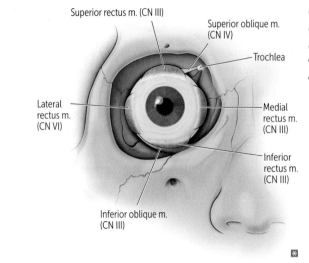

Superior rectus m. (CN III)

Superior oblique m. (CN IV)

Trochlea

Lateral rectus m. (CN VI)

Medial rectus m. (CN III)

Inferior rectus m. (CN III)

Inferior oblique m. (CN III)

CN **VI** innervates the Lateral Rectus.
CN **IV** innervates the Superior Oblique.
CN **III** innervates the Rest.
The "chemical formula" $LR_6SO_4R_3$.
The superior oblique abducts, intorts, and depresses while adducted.

To test function of each muscle, ask patient to follow a path from 1° position as diagramed (i.e., SO depression function best tested when eye is adducted).

Obliques go Opposite (left SO and IO tested with patient looking right).
IOU: **IO** tested looking **U**p.

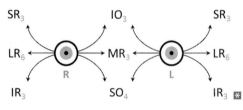

SR_3 IO_3 SR_3

LR_6 MR_3 LR_6

R   L

IR_3 SO_4 IR_3

CN III, IV, VI palsies

CN III damage

CN III has both motor (central) and parasympathetic (peripheral) components.

A **CN III damage.** Right CN III palsy in straight-ahead gaze (right eye "down-and-out" and pupil dilated). ✳

▶ Motor output to ocular muscles—affected primarily by vascular disease (e.g., diabetes mellitus: glucose → sorbitol) due to ↓ diffusion of oxygen and nutrients to the interior fibers from compromised vasculature that resides on outside of nerve. Signs: ptosis, "down and out" gaze **A**.

▶ Parasympathetic output—fibers on the periphery are 1st affected by compression (e.g., posterior communicating artery aneurysm, uncal herniation). Signs: diminished or absent pupillary light reflex, "blown pupil" often with "down-and-out" gaze.

CN III

CN IV damage

Eye moves upward, particularly with contralateral gaze **B** and head tilt toward the side of the lesion (problems going down stairs, may present with compensatory head tilt in the opposite direction).

B **CN IV damage.** Right CN IV palsy in left gaze (right hypertropia worse in left gaze). ✳

CN VI damage

Medially directed eye that cannot abduct **C**.

C **CN VI damage.** Right CN VI palsy in right gaze (right eye will not look right). ✳

Visual field defects

1. Right anopia
2. Bitemporal hemianopia
   (pituitary lesion, chiasm)
3. Left homonymous hemianopia
4. Left upper quadrantic anopia
   (right temporal lesion, MCA)
5. Left lower quadrantic anopia
   (right parietal lesion, MCA)
6. Left hemianopia with macular sparing
   (PCA infarct),
   macula → bilateral projection to occiput
7. Central scotoma (macular degeneration)

Meyer loop—inferior retina; loops around
   inferior horn of lateral ventricle.
Dorsal optic radiation—superior retina; takes
   shortest path via internal capsule.

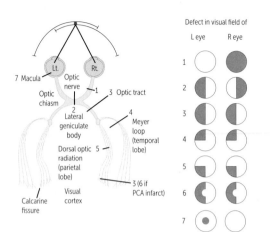

Note: When an image hits 1° visual cortex, it is upside
down and left-right reversed.

Internuclear ophthalmoplegia

Medial longitudinal fasciculus (MLF): pair of
tracts that allows for crosstalk between CN VI
and CN III nuclei. Coordinates both eyes to
move in same horizontal direction. Highly
myelinated (must communicate quickly so eyes
move at same time). Lesions may be unilateral
or bilateral (latter classically seen in multiple
sclerosis).

Lesion in MLF = internuclear ophthalmoplegia
(INO), a conjugate horizontal gaze palsy.
Lack of communication such that when
CN VI nucleus activates ipsilateral lateral
rectus, contralateral CN III nucleus does not
stimulate medial rectus to fire. Abducting eye
gets nystagmus (CN VI overfires to stimulate
CN III). Convergence normal.

MLF in MS.

When looking left, the left nucleus of CN VI
fires, which contracts the left lateral rectus and
stimulates the contralateral (right) nucleus of
CN III via the right MLF to contract the right
medial rectus.

Directional term (e.g., right INO, left INO)
refers to which eye is paralyzed.

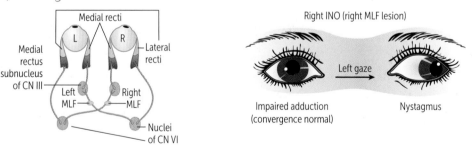

▶ NEUROLOGY—PATHOLOGY

Dementia   A ↓ in cognitive ability, memory, or function with intact consciousness.

DISEASE	DESCRIPTION	HISTOLOGIC/GROSS FINDINGS
Alzheimer disease 	Most common cause in elderly. Down syndrome patients have an ↑ risk of developing Alzheimer. Familial form (10%) associated with the following altered proteins: ▪ ApoE2: ↓ risk ▪ ApoE4: ↑ risk ▪ APP, presenilin-1, presenilin-2: ↑ risk of early onset	Widespread cortical atrophy. Narrowing of gyri and widening of sulci ↓ ACh Senile plaques **A** in gray matter: extracellular β-amyloid core; may cause amyloid angiopathy → intracranial hemorrhage; Aβ (amyloid-β) synthesized by cleaving amyloid precursor protein (APP) Neurofibrillary tangles: intracellular, hyperphosphorylated tau protein = insoluble cytoskeletal elements; number of tangles correlates with degree of dementia
Frontotemporal dementia 	Dementia, aphasia, parkinsonian aspects; change in personality. Spares parietal lobe and posterior ⅔ of superior temporal gyrus.	Also called Pick disease. Note the Pick bodies: silver-staining spherical tau protein aggregates **B** Frontotemporal atrophy
Lewy body dementia	Initially dementia and visual hallucinations ("ha**Lewy**cinations") followed by parkinsonian features.	α-synuclein defect (Lewy bodies, primarily cortical)
Creutzfeldt-Jakob disease	Rapidly progressive (weeks to months) dementia with myoclonus ("startle myoclonus").	Spongiform cortex Prions (PrP^c → PrP^{sc} sheet [β-pleated sheet resistant to proteases])
Other causes	Multi-infarct (aka vascular, 2nd most common cause of dementia in elderly); syphilis; HIV; vitamins B_1, B_3, or B_{12} deficiency; Wilson disease; normal pressure hydrocephalus.	

Multiple sclerosis	Autoimmune inflammation and demyelination of CNS (brain and spinal cord). Patients can present with optic neuritis (sudden loss of vision resulting in Marcus Gunn pupils), INO, hemiparesis, hemisensory symptoms, bladder/bowel incontinence. Relapsing and remitting course. Most often affects women in their 20s and 30s; more common in whites living further from equator.	Charcot classic triad of MS is a **SIN**: ▪ **S**canning speech ▪ **I**ntention tremor (also Incontinence and Internuclear ophthalmoplegia) ▪ **N**ystagmus

FINDINGS

↑ protein (IgG) in CSF. Oligoclonal bands are diagnostic. MRI is gold standard. Periventricular plaques **A** (areas of oligodendrocyte loss and reactive gliosis) with destruction of axons. Multiple white matter lesions separated in space and time.

TREATMENT

Slow progression with disease-modifying therapies (e.g., β-interferon, natalizumab). Treat acute flares with IV steroids. Symptomatic treatment for neurogenic bladder (catheterization, muscarinic antagonists), spasticity (baclofen, GABA$_B$ receptor agonists), pain (opioids).

Acute inflammatory demyelinating polyradiculopathy	Most common subtype of Guillain-Barré syndrome. Autoimmune condition that destroys Schwann cells → inflammation and demyelination of peripheral nerves and motor fibers. Results in symmetric ascending muscle weakness/paralysis beginning in lower extremities. Facial paralysis in 50% of cases. May see autonomic dysregulation (e.g., cardiac irregularities, hypertension, hypotension) or sensory abnormalities. Almost all patients survive; the majority recover completely after weeks to months. Findings: ↑ CSF protein with normal cell count (albuminocytologic dissociation). ↑ protein may cause papilledema.	Associated with infections (e.g., *Campylobacter jejuni*, viral) → autoimmune attack of peripheral myelin due to molecular mimicry, inoculations, and stress, but no definitive link to pathogens. Respiratory support is critical until recovery. Additional treatment: plasmapheresis, IV immunoglobulins.

Other demyelinating and dysmyelinating diseases

Acute disseminated (postinfectious) encephalomyelitis	Multifocal periventricular inflammation and demyelination after infection (commonly measles or VZV) or certain vaccinations (e.g., rabies, smallpox).
Charcot-Marie-Tooth disease	Also known as hereditary motor and sensory neuropathy (HMSN). Group of progressive hereditary nerve disorders related to the defective production of proteins involved in the structure and function of peripheral nerves or the myelin sheath. Typically autosomal dominant inheritance pattern and associated with scoliosis and foot deformities (high or flat arches).
Krabbe disease	Autosomal recessive lysosomal storage disease due to deficiency of galactocerebrosidase. Buildup of galactocerebroside and psychosine destroys myelin sheath. Findings: peripheral neuropathy, developmental delay, optic atrophy, globoid cells.
Metachromatic leukodystrophy	Autosomal recessive lysosomal storage disease, most commonly due to arylsulfatase A deficiency. Buildup of sulfatides → impaired production and destruction of myelin sheath. Findings: central and peripheral demyelination with ataxia, dementia.
Progressive multifocal leukoencephalopathy	Demyelination of CNS due to destruction of oligodendrocytes. Associated with JC virus. Seen in 2–4% of AIDS patients (reactivation of latent viral infection). Rapidly progressive, usually fatal. ↑ risk associated with natalizumab, rituximab.

Adrenoleukodystrophy	X-linked genetic disorder typically affecting males. Disrupts metabolism of very-long-chain fatty acids → excessive buildup in nervous system, adrenal gland, testes. Progressive disease that can lead to long-term coma/death and adrenal gland crisis.

Seizures	Characterized by synchronized, high-frequency neuronal firing. Variety of forms.	
Partial (focal) seizures	Affect single area of the brain. Most commonly originate in medial temporal lobe. Often preceded by seizure aura; can secondarily generalize. Types: ▪ Simple partial (consciousness intact)—motor, sensory, autonomic, psychic ▪ Complex partial (impaired consciousness)	Epilepsy—a disorder of recurrent seizures (febrile seizures are not epilepsy). Status epilepticus—continuous or recurring seizure(s) that may result in brain injury; variably defined as > 10–30 min. Causes of seizures by age: ▪ Children—genetic, infection (febrile), trauma, congenital, metabolic ▪ Adults—tumor, trauma, stroke, infection ▪ Elderly—stroke, tumor, trauma, metabolic, infection
Generalized seizures	Diffuse. Types: ▪ Absence (petit mal)—3 Hz, no postictal confusion, blank stare ▪ Myoclonic—quick, repetitive jerks ▪ Tonic-clonic (grand mal)—alternating stiffening and movement ▪ Tonic—stiffening ▪ Atonic—"drop" seizures (falls to floor); commonly mistaken for fainting	

Differentiating headaches   Pain due to irritation of structures such as the dura, cranial nerves, or extracranial structures.

CLASSIFICATION	LOCALIZATION	DURATION	DESCRIPTION	TREATMENT
Cluster[a]	Unilateral	15 min–3 hr; repetitive	Repetitive brief headaches. Excruciating periorbital pain with lacrimation and rhinorrhea. May induce Horner syndrome. More common in males.	100% O_2, sumatriptan
Tension	Bilateral	> 30 min (typically 4–6 hr); constant	Steady pain. No photophobia or phonophobia. No aura.	Analgesics, NSAIDs, acetaminophen; amitriptyline for chronic pain
Migraine	Unilateral	4–72 hr	Pulsating pain with nausea, photophobia, or phonophobia. May have "aura." Due to irritation of CN V, meninges, or blood vessels (release of substance P, calcitonin gene–related peptide, vasoactive peptides).	Abortive therapies (e.g., triptans, NSAIDs) and prophylaxis (e.g., propranolol, topiramate, Ca^{2+} channel blockers, amitriptyline). **POUND**–Pulsatile, One-day duration, Unilateral, Nausea, Disabling

Other causes of headache include subarachnoid hemorrhage ("worst headache of my life"), meningitis, hydrocephalus, neoplasia, arteritis.

[a]Compare with trigeminal neuralgia, which produces repetitive shooting pain in the distribution of CN V that lasts (typically) for < 1 minute.

Vertigo	Sensation of spinning while actually stationary. Subtype of "dizziness," but distinct from "lightheadedness."
Peripheral vertigo	More common. Inner ear etiology (e.g., semicircular canal debris, vestibular nerve infection, Ménière disease). Positional testing → delayed horizontal nystagmus.
Central vertigo	Brain stem or cerebellar lesion (e.g., stroke affecting vestibular nuclei or posterior fossa tumor). Findings: directional change of nystagmus, skew deviation, diplopia, dysmetria. Positional testing → immediate nystagmus in any direction; may change directions. Focal neurologic findings.

Neurocutaneous disorders

Sturge-Weber syndrome	Congenital, non-inherited (somatic), developmental anomaly of neural crest derivatives (mesoderm/ectoderm) due to activating mutation of *GNAQ* gene. Affects small (capillary-sized) blood vessels → port-wine stain of the face **A** (nevus flammeus, a non-neoplastic "birthmark" in CN V_1/V_2 distribution); ipsilateral leptomeningeal angioma **B** → seizures/epilepsy; intellectual disability; and episcleral hemangioma → ↑ IOP → early-onset glaucoma. **STURGE**-Weber: Sporadic, port-wine **S**tain; **T**ram track calcifications (opposing gyri); **U**nilateral; **R**etardation (intellectual disability); **G**laucoma; *GNAQ* gene; **E**pilepsy.
Tuberous sclerosis	**HAMARTOMAS**: **H**amartomas in CNS and skin; **A**ngiofibromas **C**; **M**itral regurgitation; **A**sh-leaf spots **D**; cardiac **R**habdomyoma; (**T**uberous sclerosis); autosomal d**O**minant; **M**ental retardation (intellectual disability); renal **A**ngiomyolipoma **E**; **S**eizures, **S**hagreen patches. ↑ incidence of subependymal astrocytomas and ungual fibromas.
Neurofibromatosis type I (von Recklinghausen disease)	Café-au-lait spots **F**, Lisch nodules (pigmented iris hamartomas **G**), cutaneous neurofibromas **H**, optic gliomas, pheochromocytomas. Mutated *NF1* tumor suppressor gene (neurofibromin, a negative regulator of *RAS*) on chromosome 17. Skin tumors of NF-1 are derived from neural crest cells.
von Hippel-Lindau disease	Hemangioblastomas (high vascularity with hyperchromatic nuclei **I**) in retina, brain stem, cerebellum, spine **J**; angiomatosis (e.g., cavernous hemangiomas in skin, mucosa, organs); bilateral renal cell carcinomas; pheochromocytomas.

Adult primary brain tumors

Glioblastoma multiforme (grade IV astrocytoma)	Common, highly malignant 1° brain tumor with ~ 1-year median survival. Found in cerebral hemispheres A. Can cross corpus callosum ("butterfly glioma"). Stain astrocytes for GFAP. Histology: "pseudopalisading" B pleomorphic tumor cells—border central areas of necrosis and hemorrhage.
Meningioma	Common, typically benign 1° brain tumor. Most often occurs in convexities of hemispheres (near surfaces of brain) and parasagittal region. Arises from arachnoid cells, is extra-axial (external to brain parenchyma), and may have a dural attachment ("tail" C). Often asymptomatic; may present with seizures or focal neurologic signs. Resection and/or radiosurgery. Histology: spindle cells concentrically arranged in a whorled pattern; psammoma bodies (laminated calcifications D).
Hemangioblastoma	Most often cerebellar E. Associated with von Hippel-Lindau syndrome when found with retinal angiomas. Can produce erythropoietin → 2° polycythemia. Histology: closely arranged, thin-walled capillaries with minimal intervening parenchyma F.
Schwannoma	Classically at the cerebellopontine angle, but can be along any peripheral nerve G. Schwann cell origin H, S-100 ⊕; often localized to CN VIII → vestibular schwannoma. Resectable or treated with stereotactic radiosurgery. Bilateral vestibular schwannomas found in NF-2.
Oligodendroglioma	Relatively rare, slow growing. Most often in frontal lobes I. "Chicken-wire" capillary pattern. Histology: oligodendrocytes = "fried egg" cells—round nuclei with clear cytoplasm J. Often calcified in oligodendroglioma.
Pituitary adenoma	Most commonly prolactinoma K. Bitemporal hemianopia (L shows normal visual field above, patient's perspective below) due to pressure on optic chiasm. Hyper- or hypopituitarism are sequelae.

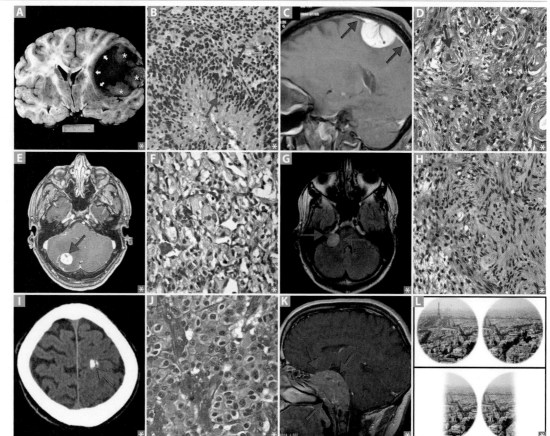

Childhood primary brain tumors

Pilocytic (low-grade) astrocytoma	Usually well circumscribed. In children, most often found in posterior fossa (e.g., cerebellum). May be supratentorial. GFAP ⊕. Benign; good prognosis.	Rosenthal fibers—eosinophilic, corkscrew fibers B. Cystic + solid (gross).
Medulloblastoma	Highly malignant cerebellar tumor C. A form of primitive neuroectodermal tumor. Can compress 4th ventricle, causing hydrocephalus. Can send "drop metastases" to spinal cord.	Homer-Wright rosettes. Solid (gross), small blue cells D (histology).
Ependymoma	Ependymal cell tumors most commonly found in 4th ventricle E. Can cause hydrocephalus. Poor prognosis.	Characteristic perivascular rosettes F. Rod-shaped blepharoplasts (basal ciliary bodies) found near nucleus.
Craniopharyngioma	Benign childhood tumor, may be confused with pituitary adenoma (both can cause bitemporal hemianopia). Most common childhood supratentorial tumor.	Derived from remnants of Rathke pouch. Calcification is common G, H (tooth enamel–like).

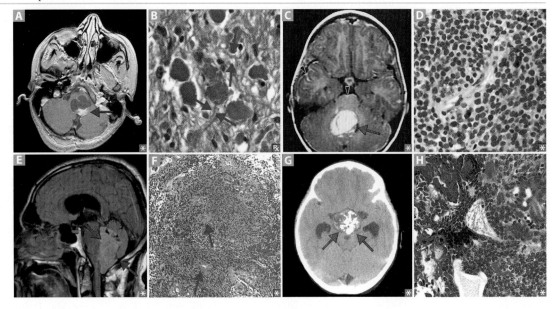

Herniation syndromes

	❶ Cingulate (subfalcine) herniation under falx cerebri	Can compress anterior cerebral artery.
	❷ Downward transtentorial (central) herniation	Caudal displacement of brain stem → rupture of paramedian basilar artery branches → Duret hemorrhages. Usually fatal.
	❸ Uncal herniation	Uncus = medial temporal lobe. Compresses ipsilateral CN III (blown pupil, "down-and-out" gaze), ipsilateral PCA (contralateral homonymous hemianopia), contralateral crus cerebri at the Kernohan notch (ipsilateral paresis; a "false localization" sign).
	❹ Cerebellar tonsillar herniation into the foramen magnum	Coma and death result when these herniations compress the brain stem.

Diagram labels: Falx cerebri, Lateral ventricles, Supratentorial mass, Uncus, Tentorium cerebelli, Kernohan notch, Duret hemorrhage

▶ **NEUROLOGY—PHARMACOLOGY**

Glaucoma drugs	↓ IOP via ↓ amount of aqueous humor (inhibit synthesis/secretion or ↑ drainage).	
DRUG	MECHANISM	SIDE EFFECTS
α-agonists		
Epinephrine ($α_1$) **Brimonidine ($α_2$)**	↓ aqueous humor synthesis via vasoconstriction ↓ aqueous humor synthesis	Mydriasis ($α_1$); do not use in closed-angle glaucoma Blurry vision, ocular hyperemia, foreign body sensation, ocular allergic reactions, ocular pruritus
β-blockers		
Timolol, betaxolol, carteolol	↓ aqueous humor synthesis	No pupillary or vision changes
Diuretics		
Acetazolamide	↓ aqueous humor synthesis via inhibition of carbonic anhydrase	No pupillary or vision changes
Cholinomimetics		
Direct (pilocarpine, carbachol) **Indirect (physostigmine, echothiophate)**	↑ outflow of aqueous humor via contraction of ciliary muscle and opening of trabecular meshwork Use pilocarpine in emergencies—very effective at opening meshwork into canal of Schlemm	Miosis and cyclospasm (contraction of ciliary muscle)
Prostaglandin		
Latanoprost ($PGF_{2α}$)	↑ outflow of aqueous humor	Darkens color of iris (browning)

Opioid analgesics	Morphine, fentanyl, codeine, loperamide, methadone, meperidine, dextromethorphan, diphenoxylate, pentazocine.
MECHANISM	Act as agonists at opioid receptors (μ = morphine, δ = enkephalin, κ = dynorphin) to modulate synaptic transmission—open K^+ channels, close Ca^{2+} channels → ↓ synaptic transmission. Inhibit release of ACh, norepinephrine, 5-HT, glutamate, substance P.
CLINICAL USE	Pain, cough suppression (dextromethorphan), diarrhea (loperamide, diphenoxylate), acute pulmonary edema, maintenance programs for heroin addicts (methadone, buprenorphine + naloxone).
TOXICITY	Addiction, respiratory depression, constipation, miosis (pinpoint pupils), additive CNS depression with other drugs. Tolerance does not develop to miosis and constipation. Toxicity treated with naloxone or naltrexone (opioid receptor antagonist).

Butorphanol

MECHANISM	κ-opioid receptor agonist and μ-opioid receptor partial agonist; produces analgesia.
CLINICAL USE	Severe pain (e.g., migraine, labor). Causes less respiratory depression than full opioid agonists.
TOXICITY	Can cause opioid withdrawal symptoms if patient is also taking full opioid agonist (competition for opioid receptors). Overdose not easily reversed with naloxone.

Tramadol

MECHANISM	Very weak opioid agonist; also inhibits 5-HT and norepinephrine reuptake (works on multiple neurotransmitters—"**tram it all**" in with **tramadol**).
CLINICAL USE	Chronic pain.
TOXICITY	Similar to opioids. Decreases seizure threshold. Serotonin syndrome.

Epilepsy drugs

	PARTIAL (FOCAL)		GENERALIZED			MECHANISM	SIDE EFFECTS	NOTES
	SIMPLE	COMPLEX	TONIC-CLONIC	ABSENCE	STATUS EPILEPTICUS			
Ethosuximide				* ✓		Blocks thalamic T-type Ca^{2+} channels	GI, fatigue, headache, urticaria, Stevens-Johnson syndrome. EFGHIJ—Ethosuximide causes Fatigue, GI distress, Headache, Itching, and Stevens-Johnson syndrome	Sucks to have Silent (absence) Seizures
Benzodiazepines (diazepam, lorazepam)					** ✓	↑ $GABA_A$ action	Sedation, tolerance, dependence, respiratory depression	Also for eclampsia seizures (1st line is $MgSO_4$)
Phenytoin	✓	✓	* ✓		*** ✓	↑ Na^+ channel inactivation; zero-order kinetics	Nystagmus, diplopia, ataxia, sedation, gingival hyperplasia, hirsutism, peripheral neuropathy, megaloblastic anemia, teratogenesis (fetal hydantoin syndrome), SLE-like syndrome, induction of cytochrome P-450, lymphadenopathy, Stevens-Johnson syndrome, osteopenia	Fosphenytoin for parenteral use
Carbamazepine	* ✓	* ✓	* ✓			↑ Na^+ channel inactivation	Diplopia, ataxia, blood dyscrasias (agranulocytosis, aplastic anemia), liver toxicity, teratogenesis, induction of cytochrome P-450, SIADH, Stevens-Johnson syndrome	1st line for trigeminal neuralgia
Valproic acid	✓	✓	* ✓	✓		↑ Na^+ channel inactivation, ↑ GABA concentration by inhibiting GABA transaminase	GI, distress, rare but fatal hepatotoxicity (measure LFTs), neural tube defects (e.g., spina bifida), tremor, weight gain, contraindicated in pregnancy	Also used for myoclonic seizures, bipolar disorder
Gabapentin	✓	✓				Primarily inhibits high-voltage-activated Ca^{2+} channels; designed as GABA analog	Sedation, ataxia	Also used for peripheral neuropathy, postherpetic neuralgia
Phenobarbital	✓	✓	✓			↑ $GABA_A$ action	Sedation, tolerance, dependence, induction of cytochrome P-450, cardiorespiratory depression	1st line in neonates
Topiramate	✓	✓	✓			Blocks Na^+ channels, ↑ GABA action	Sedation, mental dulling, kidney stones, weight loss	Also used for migraine prevention
Lamotrigine	✓	✓	✓	✓		Blocks voltage-gated Na^+ channels	Stevens-Johnson syndrome (must be titrated slowly)	
Levetiracetam	✓	✓	✓			Unknown; may modulate GABA and glutamate release		
Tiagabine	✓	✓				↑ GABA by inhibiting reuptake		
Vigabatrin	✓	✓				↑ GABA by irreversibly inhibiting GABA transaminase		
Stevens-Johnson syndrome	Prodrome of malaise and fever followed by rapid onset of erythematous/purpuric macules (oral, ocular, genital). Skin lesions progress to epidermal necrosis and sloughing.							

* = 1st line; ** = 1st line for acute; *** = 1st line for prophylaxis.

Barbiturates	Phenobarbital, pentobarbital, thiopental, secobarbital.	
MECHANISM	Facilitate GABA$_A$ action by ↑ **duration** of Cl⁻ channel opening, thus ↓ neuron firing (barbi**dur**ates ↑ **dur**ation). Contraindicated in porphyria.	
CLINICAL USE	Sedative for anxiety, seizures, insomnia, induction of anesthesia (thiopental).	
TOXICITY	Respiratory and cardiovascular depression (can be fatal); CNS depression (can be exacerbated by EtOH use); dependence; drug interactions (induces cytochrome P-450). Overdose treatment is supportive (assist respiration and maintain BP).	

Benzodiazepines	Diazepam, lorazepam, triazolam, temazepam, oxazepam, midazolam, chlordiazepoxide, alprazolam.	
MECHANISM	Facilitate GABA$_A$ action by ↑ **frequency** of Cl⁻ channel opening. ↓ REM sleep. Most have long half-lives and active metabolites (exceptions: **A**lprazolam, **T**riazolam, **O**xazepam, and **M**idazolam are short acting → higher addictive potential).	"Fren**z**odiazepines" ↑ **frequency**. Benzos, barbs, and EtOH all bind the GABA$_A$ receptor, which is a ligand-gated Cl⁻ channel. **ATOM**.
CLINICAL USE	Anxiety, spasticity, status epilepticus (lorazepam and diazepam), detoxification (especially alcohol withdrawal–DTs), night terrors, sleepwalking, general anesthetic (amnesia, muscle relaxation), hypnotic (insomnia).	
TOXICITY	Dependence, additive CNS depression effects with alcohol. Less risk of respiratory depression and coma than with barbiturates. Treat overdose with flumazenil (competitive antagonist at GABA benzodiazepine receptor).	

Nonbenzodiazepine hypnotics	**Z**olpidem, **Z**aleplon, es**Z**opiclone. "All **ZZZ**s put you to sleep."
MECHANISM	Act via the BZ1 subtype of the GABA receptor. Effects reversed by flumazenil.
CLINICAL USE	Insomnia.
TOXICITY	Ataxia, headaches, confusion. Short duration because of rapid metabolism by liver enzymes. Unlike older sedative-hypnotics, cause only modest day-after psychomotor depression and few amnestic effects. ↓ dependence risk than benzodiazepines.

Anesthetics—general principles	CNS drugs must be lipid soluble (cross the blood-brain barrier) or be actively transported. Drugs with ↓ solubility in blood = rapid induction and recovery times.
	Drugs with ↑ solubility in lipids = ↑ potency = $\dfrac{1}{\text{MAC}}$
	MAC = **M**inimal **A**lveolar **C**oncentration (of inhaled anesthetic) required to prevent 50% of subjects from moving in response to noxious stimulus (e.g., skin incision). Examples: nitrous oxide (N$_2$O) has ↓ blood and lipid solubility, and thus fast induction and low potency. Halothane, in contrast, has ↑ lipid and blood solubility, and thus high potency and slow induction.

Inhaled anesthetics	Halothane, enflurane, isoflurane, sevoflurane, methoxyflurane, N_2O.
MECHANISM	Mechanism unknown.
EFFECTS	Myocardial depression, respiratory depression, nausea/emesis, ↑ cerebral blood flow (↓ cerebral metabolic demand).
TOXICITY	Hepatotoxicity (halothane), nephrotoxicity (methoxyflurane), proconvulsant (enflurane), expansion of trapped gas in a body cavity (N_2O). Can cause malignant hyperthermia—rare, life-threatening hereditary condition in which inhaled anesthetics (except N_2O) and succinylcholine induce fever and severe muscle contractions. Treatment: dantrolene.

Intravenous anesthetics

Barbiturates	Thiopental—high potency, high lipid solubility, rapid entry into brain. Used for induction of anesthesia and short surgical procedures. Effect terminated by rapid redistribution into tissue (i.e., skeletal muscle) and fat. ↓ cerebral blood flow.	B. B. King on **OPIOIDS PROPO**ses **FOOL**ishly.
Benzodiazepines	Midazolam most common drug used for endoscopy; used adjunctively with gaseous anesthetics and narcotics. May cause severe postoperative respiratory depression, ↓ BP (treat overdose with flumazenil), anterograde amnesia.	
Arylcyclohexylamines (Ketamine)	PCP analogs that act as dissociative anesthetics. Block NMDA receptors. Cardiovascular stimulants. Cause disorientation, hallucination, bad dreams. ↑ cerebral blood flow.	
Opioids	Morphine, fentanyl used with other CNS depressants during general anesthesia.	
Propofol	Used for sedation in ICU, rapid anesthesia induction, short procedures. Less postoperative nausea than thiopental. Potentiates $GABA_A$.	

Local anesthetics	Esters—procaine, cocaine, tetracaine.
	Amides—lIdocaIne, mepIvacaIne, bupIvacaIne (amIdes have 2 I's in name).
MECHANISM	Block Na$^+$ channels by binding to specific receptors on inner portion of channel. Preferentially bind to activated Na$^+$ channels, so most effective in rapidly firing neurons. 3° amine local anesthetics penetrate membrane in uncharged form, then bind to ion channels as charged form.
PRINCIPLE	Can be given with vasoconstrictors (usually epinephrine) to enhance local action—↓ bleeding, ↑ anesthesia by ↓ systemic concentration.
	In infected (acidic) tissue, alkaline anesthetics are charged and cannot penetrate membrane effectively → need more anesthetic.
	Order of nerve blockade: small-diameter fibers > large diameter. Myelinated fibers > unmyelinated fibers. Overall, size factor predominates over myelination such that small myelinated fibers > small unmyelinated fibers > large myelinated fibers > large unmyelinated fibers.
	Order of loss: (1) pain, (2) temperature, (3) touch, (4) pressure.
CLINICAL USE	Minor surgical procedures, spinal anesthesia. If allergic to esters, give amides.
TOXICITY	CNS excitation, severe cardiovascular toxicity (bupivacaine), hypertension, hypotension, arrhythmias (cocaine), methemoglobinemia (benzocaine).

Neuromuscular blocking drugs	Muscle paralysis in surgery or mechanical ventilation. Selective for motor (vs. autonomic) nicotinic receptor.
Depolarizing	Succinylcholine—strong ACh receptor agonist; produces sustained depolarization and prevents muscle contraction.
	Reversal of blockade:
	▪ Phase I (prolonged depolarization)—no antidote. Block potentiated by cholinesterase inhibitors.
	▪ Phase II (repolarized but blocked; ACh receptors are available, but desensitized)—antidote is cholinesterase inhibitors.
	Complications include hypercalcemia, hyperkalemia, malignant hyperthermia.
Nondepolarizing	Tubocurarine, atracurium, mivacurium, pancuronium, vecuronium, rocuronium—competitive antagonists—compete with ACh for receptors.
	Reversal of blockade—neostigmine (must be given with atropine to prevent muscarinic effects such as bradycardia), edrophonium, and other cholinesterase inhibitors.

Dantrolene	
MECHANISM	Prevents release of Ca^{2+} from the sarcoplasmic reticulum of skeletal muscle.
CLINICAL USE	Malignant hyperthermia and neuroleptic malignant syndrome (a toxicity of antipsychotic drugs).

Baclofen	
MECHANISM	Inhibits GABA$_B$ receptors at spinal cord level, inducing skeletal muscle relaxation.
CLINICAL USE	Muscle spasms (e.g., acute low back pain).

Cyclobenzaprine	
MECHANISM	Centrally acting skeletal muscle relaxant. Structurally related to TCAs, similar anticholinergic side effects.
CLINICAL USE	Muscle spasms.

Parkinson disease drugs

Parkinsonism is due to loss of dopaminergic neurons and excess cholinergic activity.

STRATEGY	AGENTS	
Dopamine agonists	Ergot—Bromocriptine Non-ergot (preferred)—pramipexole, ropinirole	**BALSA:** Bromocriptine Amantadine Levodopa (with carbidopa) Selegiline (and COMT inhibitors) Antimuscarinics
↑ dopamine availability	Amantadine (↑ dopamine release and ↓ dopamine reuptake); also used as an antiviral against influenza A and rubella; toxicity = ataxia, livedo reticularis.	
↑ L-DOPA availability	Agents prevent peripheral (pre-BBB) L-dopa degradation → ↑ L-DOPA entering CNS → ↑ central L-DOPA available for conversion to dopamine. ■ Levodopa (L-dopa)/carbidopa—carbidopa blocks peripheral conversion of L-DOPA to dopamine by inhibiting DOPA decarboxylase. Also reduces side effects of peripheral L-dopa conversion into dopamine (e.g., nausea, vomiting). ■ Entacapone, tolcapone—prevent peripheral L-dopa degradation to 3-O-methyldopa (3-OMD) by inhibiting COMT.	
Prevent dopamine breakdown	Agents act centrally (post-BBB) to block breakdown of dopamine → ↑ available dopamine. ■ Selegiline—blocks conversion of dopamine into 3-MT by selectively inhibiting MAO-B. ■ Tolcapone—blocks conversion of dopamine to DOPAC by inhibiting central COMT.	
Curb excess cholinergic activity	**Benztropine** (Antimuscarinic; improves tremor and rigidity but has little effect on bradykinesia).	**Park** your Mercedes-**Benz**.

Handwritten note: ADR = GI disturbances, postural hypotension, sleep disturbances & orange discoloration of urine → can exacerbate dysphoria/nausea of levodopa ✦ Entacapone preferred b/c tolcapone a/w acute fatal hepatic failure

Parkinson disease drugs (continued)

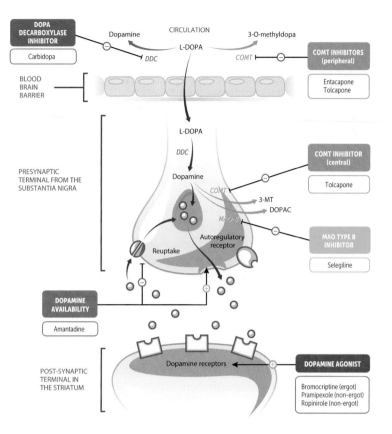

L-dopa (levodopa)/carbidopa

MECHANISM	↑ level of dopamine in brain. Unlike dopamine, L-dopa can cross blood-brain barrier and is converted by dopa decarboxylase in the CNS to dopamine. Carbidopa, a peripheral DOPA decarboxylase inhibitor, is given with L-dopa to ↑ the bioavailability of L-dopa in the brain and to limit peripheral side effects.
CLINICAL USE	Parkinson disease.
TOXICITY	Arrhythmias from ↑ peripheral formation of catecholamines. Long-term use can lead to dyskinesia following administration ("on-off" phenomenon), akinesia between doses.

Selegiline

MECHANISM	Selectively inhibits MAO-B, which preferentially metabolizes dopamine over norepinephrine and 5-HT, thereby ↑ the availability of dopamine.
CLINICAL USE	Adjunctive agent to L-dopa in treatment of Parkinson disease.
TOXICITY	May enhance adverse effects of L-dopa.

Alzheimer drugs

Memantine

MECHANISM	NMDA receptor antagonist; helps prevent excitotoxicity (mediated by Ca^{2+}).
TOXICITY	Dizziness, confusion, hallucinations.

Donepezil, galantamine, rivastigmine, tacrine

MECHANISM	AChE inhibitors.
TOXICITY	Nausea, dizziness, insomnia.

Huntington disease drugs

Neurotransmitter changes in Huntington disease: ↓ GABA, ↓ ACh, ↑ dopamine.
Treatments:
- Tetrabenazine and reserpine—inhibit vesicular monoamine transporter (VMAT); limit dopamine vesicle packaging and release.
- Haloperidol—D_2 receptor antagonist.

Triptans

Sumatriptan

MECHANISM	$5\text{-HT}_{1B/1D}$ agonists. Inhibit trigeminal nerve activation; prevent vasoactive peptide release; induce vasoconstriction.	A SUMo wrestler TRIPs ANd falls on your head.
CLINICAL USE	Acute migraine, cluster headache attacks.	
TOXICITY	Coronary vasospasm (contraindicated in patients with CAD or Prinzmetal angina), mild paresthesia.	

Psychiatry

"A Freudian slip is when you say one thing but mean your mother."
—Anonymous

"Men will always be mad, and those who think they can cure them are the maddest of all."
—Voltaire

"Anyone who goes to a psychiatrist ought to have his head examined."
—Samuel Goldwyn

The DSM-5 was released by the American Psychiatric Association in 2013, reclassifying several psychiatric conditions and updating diagnostic criteria. We have updated this chapter to reflect certain DSM-5 revisions.

▶ PSYCHIATRY—PSYCHOLOGY

Classical conditioning	Learning in which a natural response (salivation) is elicited by a conditioned, or learned, stimulus (bell) that previously was presented in conjunction with an unconditioned stimulus (food).	Usually deals with **involuntary** responses. Pavlov's classical experiments with dogs— ringing the bell provoked salivation.

Operant conditioning	Learning in which a particular action is elicited because it produces a punishment or reward. Usually deals with **voluntary** responses.
Positive reinforcement	Desired reward produces action (mouse presses button to get food).
Negative reinforcement	Target behavior (response) is followed by removal of aversive stimulus (mouse presses button to turn off continuous loud noise).
Punishment	Repeated application of aversive stimulus extinguishes unwanted behavior.
Extinction	Discontinuation of reinforcement (positive or negative) eventually eliminates behavior. Can occur in operant or classical conditioning.

Transference and countertransference

Transference	Patient projects feelings about formative or other important persons onto physician (e.g., psychiatrist is seen as parent).
Countertransference	Doctor projects feelings about formative or other important persons onto patient (e.g., patient reminds physician of younger sibling).

Ego defenses	Unconscious mental processes used to resolve conflict and prevent undesirable feelings (e.g., anxiety, depression).

IMMATURE DEFENSES	DESCRIPTION	EXAMPLE
Acting out	Expressing unacceptable feelings and thoughts through actions.	Tantrums.
Denial	Avoiding the awareness of some painful reality.	A common reaction in newly diagnosed AIDS and cancer patients.
Displacement	Transferring avoided ideas and feelings to a neutral person or object (vs. projection).	Mother yells at her child, because her husband yelled at her.
Dissociation	Temporary, drastic change in personality, memory, consciousness, or motor behavior to avoid emotional stress.	Extreme forms can result in dissociative identity disorder (multiple personality disorder).
Fixation	Partially remaining at a more childish level of development (vs. regression).	Adults fixating on video games.
Identification	Modeling behavior after another person who is more powerful (though not necessarily admired).	Abused child identifies with an abuser.
Isolation (of affect)	Separating feelings from ideas and events.	Describing murder in graphic detail with no emotional response.

Ego defenses *(continued)*

IMMATURE DEFENSES	DESCRIPTION	EXAMPLE
Passive aggression	Expressing negativity and performing below what is expected as an indirect show of opposition.	Disgruntled employee is repeatedly late to work.
Projection	Attributing an unacceptable internal impulse to an external source (vs. displacement).	A man who wants another woman thinks his wife is cheating on him.
Rationalization	Proclaiming logical reasons for actions actually performed for other reasons, usually to avoid self-blame.	After getting fired, claiming that the job was not important anyway.
Reaction formation	Replacing a warded-off idea or feeling by an (unconsciously derived) emphasis on its opposite (vs. sublimation).	A patient with libidinous thoughts enters a monastery.
Regression	Turning back the maturational clock and going back to earlier modes of dealing with the world (vs. fixation).	Seen in children under stress such as illness, punishment, or birth of a new sibling (e.g., bedwetting in a previously toilet-trained child when hospitalized).
Repression	Involuntarily withholding an idea or feeling from conscious awareness (vs. suppression).	A 20-year-old does not remember going to counseling during his parents' divorce 10 years earlier.
Splitting	Believing that people are either all good or all bad at different times due to intolerance of ambiguity. Commonly seen in borderline personality disorder.	A patient says that all the nurses are cold and insensitive but that the doctors are warm and friendly.

MATURE DEFENSES		
Altruism	Alleviating negative feelings via unsolicited generosity.	Mafia boss makes large donation to charity.
Humor	Appreciating the amusing nature of an anxiety-provoking or adverse situation.	Nervous medical student jokes about the boards.
Sublimation	Replacing an unacceptable wish with a course of action that is similar to the wish but does not conflict with one's value system (vs. reaction formation).	Teenager's aggression toward his father is redirected to perform well in sports.
Suppression	Intentionally withholding an idea or feeling from conscious awareness (vs. repression); temporary.	Choosing to not worry about the big game until it is time to play.

Mature adults wear a **SASH**: Sublimation, Altruism, Suppression, Humor.

▶ PSYCHIATRY—PATHOLOGY

| **Infant deprivation effects** | Long-term deprivation of affection results in: <ul><li>Failure to thrive</li><li>Poor language/socialization skills</li><li>Lack of basic trust</li><li>Anaclitic depression (infant withdrawn/unresponsive)</li></ul> | The **4 W's**: Weak, Wordless, Wanting (socially), Wary.
Deprivation for > 6 months can lead to irreversible changes.
Severe deprivation can result in infant death. |

Child abuse

	Physical abuse	**Sexual abuse**
EVIDENCE	Spiral fractures (or multiple fractures at different stages of healing), burns (e.g., cigarette, buttocks/thighs), subdural hematomas, posterior rib fractures, retinal detachment. During exam, children often avoid eye contact.	Genital, anal, or oral trauma; STDs; UTIs.
ABUSER	Usually biological mother.	Known to victim, usually male.
EPIDEMIOLOGY	40% of deaths in children < 1 year old.	Peak incidence 9–12 years old.

| **Child neglect** | Failure to provide a child with adequate food, shelter, supervision, education, and/or affection. Most common form of child maltreatment. Evidence: poor hygiene, malnutrition, withdrawal, impaired social/emotional development, failure to thrive.
As with child abuse, child neglect must be reported to local child protective services. |

Childhood and early-onset disorders

Attention-deficit hyperactivity disorder	Onset before age 12. Limited attention span and poor impulse control. Characterized by hyperactivity, impulsivity, and/or inattention in multiple settings (school, home, places of worship, etc.). Normal intelligence, but commonly coexists with difficulties in school. Continues into adulthood in as many as 50% of individuals. Associated with ↓ frontal lobe volume/metabolism. Treatment: stimulants (e.g., methylphenidate) +/– cognitive behavioral therapy (CBT); atomoxetine may be an alternative to stimulants in selected patients.
Conduct disorder	Repetitive and pervasive behavior violating the basic rights of others (e.g., physical aggression, destruction of property, theft). After age 18, many of these patients will meet criteria for diagnosis of antisocial personality disorder. Treatment for both: CBT.
Oppositional defiant disorder	Enduring pattern of hostile, defiant behavior toward authority figures in the absence of serious violations of social norms. Treatment: CBT.
Separation anxiety disorder	Common onset at 7–9 years. Overwhelming fear of separation from home or loss of attachment figure. May lead to factitious physical complaints to avoid going to or staying at school. Treatment: CBT, play therapy, family therapy.
Tourette syndrome	Onset before age 18. Characterized by sudden, rapid, recurrent, nonrhythmic, stereotyped motor and vocal tics that persist for > 1 year. Coprolalia (involuntary obscene speech) found in only 10–20% of patients. Associated with OCD and ADHD. Treatment: psychoeducation, behavioral therapy. For intractable tics, low-dose high-potency antipsychotics (e.g., fluphenazine, pimozide), tetrabenazine, and clonidine may be used.

Pervasive developmental disorders	Characterized by difficulties with language and failure to acquire or early loss of social skills.
Autism spectrum disorder	Characterized by poor social interactions, communication deficits, repetitive/ritualized behaviors, restricted interests. Must present in early childhood. May or may not be accompanied by intellectual disability; rarely accompanied by unusual abilities (savants). More common in boys.
Rett syndrome	X-linked disorder seen almost exclusively in girls (affected males die in utero or shortly after birth). Symptoms usually become apparent around ages 1–4, including regression characterized by loss of development, loss of verbal abilities, intellectual disability, ataxia, stereotyped hand-wringing.

Neurotransmitter changes with disease	DISORDER	NEUROTRANSMITTER CHANGES
	Alzheimer disease	↓ ACh ↑ glutamate
	Anxiety	↑ norepinephrine ↓ GABA, ↓ 5-HT
	Depression	↓ norepinephrine ↓ 5-HT, ↓ dopamine
	Huntington disease	↓ GABA, ↓ ACh ↑ dopamine
	Parkinson disease	↓ dopamine ↑ ACh
	Schizophrenia	↑ dopamine
	Understanding these changes can help guide pharmacologic treatment choice.	

Orientation	Patient's ability to know who he or she is, where he or she is, and the date and time. Common causes of loss of orientation: alcohol, drugs, fluid/electrolyte imbalance, head trauma, hypoglycemia, infection, nutritional deficiencies.	Order of loss: 1st—time; 2nd—place; last—person.

Amnesias	
Retrograde amnesia	Inability to remember things that occurred **before** a CNS insult.
Anterograde amnesia	Inability to remember things that occurred **after** a CNS insult (↓ acquisition of new memory).
Korsakoff syndrome	Amnesia (anterograde > retrograde) caused by vitamin B_1 deficiency and associated destruction of mammillary bodies. Seen in alcoholics. Confabulations are characteristic.
Dissociative amnesia	Inability to recall important personal information, usually subsequent to severe trauma or stress. May be accompanied by **dissociative fugue** (abrupt travel or wandering during a period of dissociative amnesia, associated with traumatic circumstances).

Delirium	"Waxing and waning" level of consciousness with acute onset; rapid ↓ in attention span and level of arousal. Characterized by disorganized thinking, hallucinations (often visual), illusions, misperceptions, disturbance in sleep-wake cycle, cognitive dysfunction. Usually 2° to other illness (e.g., CNS disease, infection, trauma, substance abuse/withdrawal, metabolic/electrolyte disturbances, hemorrhage, urinary/fecal retention). Most common presentation of altered mental status in inpatient setting. Abnormal EEG. Treatment is aimed at identifying and addressing underlying condition. Haloperidol may be used as needed. Use benzodiazepines for alcohol withdrawal.	Delirium = changes in sensorium. May be caused by medications (e.g., anticholinergics), especially in the elderly. Reversible. T-A-DA approach (Tolerate, Anticipate, Don't Agitate) helpful for management.
Dementia	↓ in intellectual function without affecting level of consciousness. Characterized by memory deficits, apraxia, aphasia, agnosia, loss of abstract thought, behavioral/personality changes, impaired judgment. A patient with dementia can develop delirium (e.g., patient with Alzheimer disease who develops pneumonia is at ↑ risk for delirium). Irreversible causes: Alzheimer disease, Lewy body dementia, Huntington disease, Pick disease, cerebral infarct, Creutzfeldt-Jakob disease, chronic substance abuse (due to neurotoxicity of drugs). Reversible causes: hypothyroidism, depression, vitamin B_{12} deficiency, normal pressure hydrocephalus. ↑ incidence with age. EEG usually normal.	"De**mem**tia" is characterized by **memory** loss. Usually irreversible. In elderly patients, depression and hypothyroidism may present like dementia (pseudodementia). Screen for depression and measure TSH, B_{12} levels.

Psychosis	A distorted perception of reality characterized by delusions, hallucinations, and/or disorganized thinking. Psychosis can occur in patients with medical illness, psychiatric illness, or both.
Hallucinations	Perceptions in the absence of external stimuli (e.g., seeing a light that is not actually present).
Delusions	Unique, false beliefs about oneself or others that persist despite the facts (e.g., thinking aliens are communicating with you).
Disorganized speech	Words and ideas are strung together based on sounds, puns, or "loose associations."

Hallucination types

Visual	More commonly a feature of medical illness (e.g., drug intoxication) than psychiatric illness.
Auditory	More commonly a feature of psychiatric illness (e.g., schizophrenia) than medical illness.
Olfactory	Often occur as an aura of psychomotor epilepsy and in brain tumors.
Gustatory	Rare, but seen in epilepsy.
Tactile	Common in alcohol withdrawal (e.g., formication—the sensation of bugs crawling on one's skin). Also seen in cocaine abusers ("cocaine crawlies").
Hypnagogic	Occurs while going to sleep. Sometimes seen in narcolepsy.
Hypnopompic	Occurs while waking from sleep ("**pomp**ous upon awakening"). Sometimes seen in narcolepsy.

Schizophrenia

Chronic mental disorder with periods of psychosis, disturbed behavior and thought, and decline in functioning **lasting > 6 months**. Associated with ↑ dopaminergic activity, ↓ dendritic branching.

Diagnosis requires 2 or more of the following (first 4 are "positive symptoms"):
- Delusions
- Hallucinations—often auditory
- Disorganized speech (loose associations)
- Disorganized or catatonic behavior
- "Negative symptoms"—flat affect, social withdrawal, lack of motivation, lack of speech or thought

Brief psychotic disorder—lasting < 1 month, usually stress related.

Schizophreniform disorder—lasting 1–6 months.

Schizoaffective disorder—lasting > 2 weeks; psychotic symptoms with episodic superimposed major depression or mania (or both). Psychosis is present with and without mood disorder, but mood disorder is present only with psychosis.

Genetics and environment contribute to the etiology of schizophrenia.

Frequent cannabis use is associated with psychosis/schizophrenia in teens.

Lifetime prevalence—1.5% (males = females, blacks = whites). Presents earlier in men (late teens to early 20s vs. late 20s to early 30s in women). Patients are at ↑ risk for suicide.

Treatment: atypical antipsychotics (e.g., risperidone) are first line.

Delusional disorder

Fixed, persistent, false belief system **lasting > 1 month**. Functioning otherwise not impaired. Example: a woman who genuinely believes she is married to a celebrity when, in fact, she is not.

Dissociative disorders

Dissociative identity disorder	Formerly known as multiple personality disorder. Presence of 2 or more distinct identities or personality states. More common in women. Associated with history of sexual abuse, PTSD, depression, substance abuse, borderline personality, somatoform conditions.
Depersonalization/ derealization disorder	Persistent feelings of detachment or estrangement from one's own body, thoughts, perceptions, and actions (depersonalization) or one's environment (derealization).

Mood disorder	Characterized by an abnormal range of moods or internal emotional states and loss of control over them. Severity of moods causes distress and impairment in social and occupational functioning. Includes major depressive disorder, bipolar disorder, dysthymic disorder, and cyclothymic disorder. Episodic superimposed psychotic features (delusions or hallucinations) may be present.

Manic episode	Distinct period of abnormally and persistently elevated, expansive, or irritable mood and abnormally and persistently ↑ activity or energy lasting at least 1 week. Often disturbing to patient. Diagnosis requires hospitalization or at least 3 of the following (manics **DIG FAST**): ■ Distractibility ■ Irresponsibility—seeks pleasure without regard to consequences (hedonistic) ■ Grandiosity—inflated self-esteem ■ Flight of ideas—racing thoughts ■ ↑ in goal-directed Activity/psychomotor Agitation ■ ↓ need for Sleep ■ Talkativeness or pressured speech

Hypomanic episode	Like manic episode except mood disturbance is not severe enough to cause marked impairment in social and/or occupational functioning or to necessitate hospitalization. No psychotic features. Lasts at least 4 consecutive days.

Bipolar disorder (manic depression)	Bipolar I defined by presence of at least 1 manic episode with or without a hypomanic or depressive episode. Bipolar II defined by presence of a hypomanic and a depressive episode. Patient's mood and functioning usually return to normal between episodes. Use of antidepressants can precipitate mania. High suicide risk. Treatment: mood stabilizers (e.g., lithium, valproic acid, carbamazepine), atypical antipsychotics. **Cyclothymic disorder**—dysthymia and hypomania; milder form of bipolar disorder lasting at least 2 years.

Major depressive disorder	May be self-limited disorder, with major depressive episodes usually **lasting 6–12 months**. Episodes characterized by at least 5 of the following 9 symptoms for 2 or more weeks (symptoms must include patient-reported depressed mood or anhedonia). Treatment: CBT and SSRIs are first line. SNRIs, mirtazapine, bupropion can also be considered. Electroconvulsive therapy (ECT) in select patients. **Persistent depressive disorder (dysthymia)**—depression, often milder, **lasting at least 2 years**.	SIG E CAPS: ▪ Sleep disturbance ▪ Loss of Interest (anhedonia) ▪ Guilt or feelings of worthlessness ▪ Energy loss and fatigue ▪ Concentration problems ▪ Appetite/weight changes ▪ Psychomotor retardation or agitation ▪ Suicidal ideations ▪ Depressed mood Patients with depression typically have the following changes in their sleep stages: ▪ ↓ slow-wave sleep ▪ ↓ REM latency ▪ ↑ REM early in sleep cycle ▪ ↑ total REM sleep ▪ Repeated nighttime awakenings ▪ Early-morning wakening (terminal insomnia)
Atypical depression	Differs from classical forms of depression. Characterized by mood reactivity (being able to experience improved mood in response to positive events, albeit briefly), "reversed" vegetative symptoms (hypersomnia, hyperphagia), leaden paralysis (heavy feeling in arms and legs), long-standing interpersonal rejection sensitivity. Most common subtype of depression. Treatment: CBT and SSRIs are first line. MAO inhibitors are effective but not first line because of their risk profile.	
Postpartum mood disturbances	Onset within 4 weeks of delivery.	
Maternal (postpartum) "blues"	50–85% incidence rate. Characterized by depressed affect, tearfulness, and fatigue starting 2–3 days after delivery. Usually resolves within 10 days. Treatment: supportive. Follow up to assess for possible postpartum depression.	
Postpartum depression	10–15% incidence rate. Characterized by depressed affect, anxiety, and poor concentration starting within 4 weeks after delivery. Treatment: CBT and SSRIs are first line.	
Postpartum psychosis	0.1–0.2% incidence rate. Characterized by mood-congruent delusions, hallucinations, and thoughts of harming the baby or self. Risk factors include history of bipolar or psychotic disorder, first pregnancy, family history, recent discontinuation of psychotropic medication. Treatment: hospitalization and initiation of atypical antipsychotic; if insufficient, ECT may be used.	

Pathologic grief	Normal bereavement characterized by shock, denial, guilt, and somatic symptoms. Duration varies widely. Pathologic grief lasts > 6 months, satisfies major depressive criteria (e.g., weight loss, anhedonia, passive death wish), and/or includes psychotic symptoms (e.g., delusions). Hallucinations (e.g., hearing the voice of a deceased loved one) in the absence of other psychotic symptoms are not considered pathologic.	
Electroconvulsive therapy	Used mainly for treatment-refractory depression, depression with psychotic symptoms, and acutely suicidal patients. Produces grand mal seizure in an anesthetized patient. Adverse effects include disorientation, temporary headache, partial anterograde/retrograde amnesia usually resolving in 6 months.	
Risk factors for suicide completion	**S**ex (male), **A**ge (teenager or elderly), **D**epression, **P**revious attempt, **E**thanol or drug use, loss of **R**ational thinking, **S**ickness (medical illness, 3 or more prescription medications), **O**rganized plan, **N**o spouse (divorced, widowed, or single, especially if childless), **S**ocial support lacking. Women try more often; men succeed more often.	**SAD PERSONS** are more likely to complete suicide.
Anxiety disorder	Inappropriate experience of fear/worry and its physical manifestations (anxiety) incongruent with the magnitude of the perceived stressor. Symptoms interfere with daily functioning. Includes panic disorder, phobias, generalized anxiety disorder, PTSD. Treatment: CBT, SSRIs, SNRIs.	

Panic disorder	Defined by recurrent panic attacks (periods of intense fear and discomfort peaking in 10 minutes with at least 4 of the following): **P**alpitations, **P**aresthesias, **A**bdominal distress, **N**ausea, **I**ntense fear of dying or losing control, l**I**ght-headedness, **C**hest pain, **C**hills, **C**hoking, dis**C**onnectedness, **S**weating, **S**haking, **S**hortness of breath. Strong genetic component. Treatment: CBT, SSRIs, and venlafaxine are first line. Benzodiazepines occasionally used in acute setting.	**PANICS**. Diagnosis requires attack followed by 1 month (or more) of 1 (or more) of the following:
		  ▪ Persistent concern of additional attacks
		  ▪ Worrying about consequences of attack
		  ▪ Behavioral change related to attacks
		Symptoms are the systemic manifestations of fear.

Specific phobia	Fear that is excessive or unreasonable and interferes with normal function. Cued by presence or anticipation of a specific object or situation. Person recognizes fear is excessive. Can treat with systematic desensitization.
	Social anxiety disorder—exaggerated fear of embarrassment in social situations (e.g., public speaking, using public restrooms). Treatment: CBT, SSRIs.
	Agoraphobia—exaggerated fear of open or enclosed places, using public transportation, being in line or in crowds, or leaving home alone. Treatment: CBT, SSRIs, MAO inhibitors.
Generalized anxiety disorder	Anxiety **lasting > 6 months** unrelated to a specific person, situation, or event. Associated with sleep disturbance, fatigue, GI disturbance, difficulty concentrating. Treatment: CBT, SSRIs, SNRIs are first line. Buspirone, TCAs, benzodiazepines are second line.
	Adjustment disorder—emotional symptoms (anxiety, depression) causing impairment following an identifiable psychosocial stressor (e.g., divorce, illness) and **lasting < 6 months** (> 6 months in presence of chronic stressor). Treatment: CBT, SSRIs.
Obsessive-compulsive disorder	Recurring intrusive thoughts, feelings, or sensations (obsessions) that cause severe distress; relieved in part by the performance of repetitive actions (compulsions). Ego-dystonic: behavior inconsistent with one's own beliefs and attitudes (vs. obsessive-compulsive personality disorder). Associated with Tourette syndrome. Treatment: CBT, SSRIs, and clomipramine are first line.
	Body dysmorphic disorder—preoccupation with minor or imagined defect in appearance → significant emotional distress or impaired functioning; patients often repeatedly seek cosmetic surgery. Treatment: CBT.
Post-traumatic stress disorder	Persistent reexperiencing of a previous traumatic event (e.g., war, rape, robbery, serious accident, fire). May involve nightmares or flashbacks, intense fear, helplessness, horror. Leads to avoidance of stimuli associated with the trauma and persistently ↑ arousal. Disturbance **lasts > 1 month** and impairs social-occupational functioning. Treatment: CBT, SSRIs, and venlafaxine are first line.
	Acute stress disorder—**lasts between 3 days and 1 month**. Treatment: CBT; pharmacotherapy is usually not indicated.

Malingering	Patient **consciously** fakes, profoundly exaggerates, or claims to have a disorder in order to attain a specific 2° **(external) gain** (e.g., avoiding work, obtaining compensation). Poor compliance with treatment or follow-up of diagnostic tests. Complaints cease after gain (vs. factitious disorder).

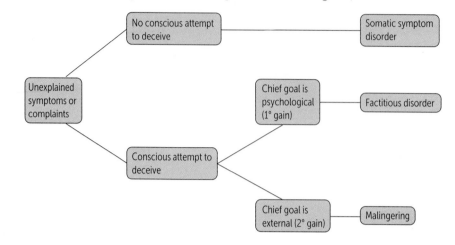

Factitious disorders	Patient **consciously** creates physical and/or psychological symptoms in order to assume "sick role" and to get medical attention (1° [**internal**] **gain**).
Munchausen syndrome	**Chronic** factitious disorder with predominantly physical signs and symptoms. Characterized by a history of multiple hospital admissions and willingness to undergo invasive procedures.
Munchausen syndrome by proxy	Illness in a child or elderly patient is caused or fabricated by the caregiver. Motivation is to assume a sick role by proxy. Form of child/elder abuse.

Somatic symptom and related disorders	Category of disorders characterized by physical symptoms with no identifiable physical cause. Both illness production and motivation are **unconscious** drives. Symptoms not intentionally produced or feigned. More common in women.
Conversion disorder	Loss of sensory or motor function (e.g., paralysis, blindness, mutism), often following an acute stressor; patient is aware of but sometimes indifferent toward symptoms ("la belle indifférence"); more common in females, adolescents, and young adults.
Illness anxiety disorder (hypochondriasis)	Preoccupation with and fear of having a serious illness despite medical evaluation and reassurance.
Somatic symptom disorder	Variety of complaints in one or more organ systems lasting for months to years. Associated with excessive, persistent thoughts and anxiety about symptoms. May co-occur with medical illness.

Personality	
Personality trait	An enduring, repetitive pattern of perceiving, relating to, and thinking about the environment and oneself.
Personality disorder	Inflexible, maladaptive, and rigidly pervasive pattern of behavior causing subjective distress and/or impaired functioning; person is usually not aware of problem. Usually presents by early adulthood. Three clusters, A, B, and C; remember as **Weird, Wild,** and **Worried** based on symptoms.

Cluster A personality disorders	Odd or eccentric; inability to develop meaningful social relationships. No psychosis; genetic association with schizophrenia.	"Weird" (Accusatory, Aloof, Awkward).
Paranoid	Pervasive distrust and suspiciousness; projection is the major defense mechanism.	
Schizoid	Voluntary social withdrawal, limited emotional expression, content with social isolation (vs. avoidant).	Schizoid = distant.
Schizotypal	Eccentric appearance, odd beliefs or magical thinking, interpersonal awkwardness.	Schizotypal = magical thinking.
Cluster B personality disorders	Dramatic, emotional, or erratic; genetic association with mood disorders and substance abuse.	"Wild" (Bad to the Bone).
Antisocial	Disregard for and violation of rights of others, criminality, impulsivity; males > females; must be ≥ 18 years old and have history of conduct disorder before age 15. Conduct disorder if < 18 years old.	Antisocial = sociopath.
Borderline	Unstable mood and interpersonal relationships, impulsivity, self-mutilation, boredom, sense of emptiness; females > males; splitting is a major defense mechanism.	Treatment: dialectical behavior therapy.
Histrionic	Excessive emotionality and excitability, attention seeking, sexually provocative, overly concerned with appearance.	
Narcissistic	Grandiosity, sense of entitlement; lacks empathy and requires excessive admiration; often demands the "best" and reacts to criticism with rage.	
Cluster C personality disorders	Anxious or fearful; genetic association with anxiety disorders.	"Worried" (Cowardly, Compulsive, Clingy).
Avoidant	Hypersensitive to rejection, socially inhibited, timid, feelings of inadequacy, desires relationships with others (vs. schizoid).	
Obsessive-compulsive	Preoccupation with order, perfectionism, and control; ego-syntonic: behavior consistent with one's own beliefs and attitudes (vs. OCD).	
Dependent	Submissive and clingy, excessive need to be taken care of, low self-confidence.	Patients often get stuck in abusive relationships.

Keeping "schizo-" straight	Schizoid	<	Schizotypal	<	Schizophrenic	<	Schizoaffective
			(schizoid + odd thinking)		(greater odd thinking than schizotypal)		(schizophrenic psychotic symptoms + bipolar or depressive mood disorder)

Schizophrenia time course:
  < 1 mo—brief psychotic disorder, usually stress related
  1–6 mo—schizophreniform disorder
  > 6 mo—schizophrenia

Eating disorders

Anorexia nervosa	Excessive dieting +/– purging; intense fear of gaining weight and body image distortion; BMI < 18.5. Associated with ↓ bone density, severe weight loss, metatarsal stress fractures, amenorrhea, lanugo, anemia, electrolyte disturbances. Seen primarily in adolescent girls. Commonly coexists with excessive exercise and/or depression. Psychotherapy and nutritional rehabilitation are first line. Refeeding syndrome (hypophosphatemia) can occur in significantly malnourished patients.
Bulimia nervosa	Binge eating with recurrent inappropriate compensatory behaviors (e.g., self-induced vomiting, using laxatives or diuretics, fasting, excessive exercise) occurring weekly for at least 3 months. Body weight often maintained within normal range. Associated with parotitis, enamel erosion, electrolyte disturbances, alkalosis, dorsal hand calluses from induced vomiting (Russell sign). Seen predominantly in adolescent girls.

Gender dysphoria	Strong, persistent cross-gender identification. Characterized by persistent discomfort with one's sex assigned at birth, causing significant distress and/or impaired functioning. Affected individuals are often referred to as transgender.
	Transsexualism—desire to live as the opposite **sex**, often through surgery or hormone treatment.
	Transvestism—paraphilia, not gender dysphoria. Wearing clothes (e.g., **vest**) of the opposite sex (cross-dressing).

Sexual dysfunction	Includes sexual desire disorders (hypoactive sexual desire or sexual aversion), sexual arousal disorders (erectile dysfunction), orgasmic disorders (anorgasmia, premature ejaculation), sexual pain disorders (dyspareunia, vaginismus). Differential diagnosis includes:
	▪ Drugs (e.g., antihypertensives, neuroleptics, SSRIs, ethanol)
	▪ Diseases (e.g., depression, diabetes, STIs)
	▪ Psychological (e.g., performance anxiety)

Sleep terror disorder	Periods of terror with screaming in the middle of the night; occurs during slow-wave sleep. Most common in children. Occurs during non-REM sleep (no memory of arousal) as opposed to nightmares that occur during REM sleep (memory of a scary dream). Cause unknown, but triggers include emotional stress, fever, or lack of sleep. Usually self limited.

Narcolepsy	Disordered regulation of sleep-wake cycles; 1° characteristic is excessive daytime sleepiness. Caused by ↓ hypocretin (orexin) production in lateral hypothalamus. Also associated with:	
	▪ Hypnagogic (just before sleep) or hypnopompic (just before awakening) hallucinations.	Hypnagogic—**going** to sleep
		Hypno**pompic**—"**pomp**ous upon awakening"
	▪ Nocturnal and narcoleptic sleep episodes that start with REM sleep.	
	▪ Cataplexy (loss of all muscle tone following strong emotional stimulus, such as laughter) in some patients.	
	Strong genetic component. Treatment: daytime stimulants (e.g., amphetamines, modafinil) and nighttime sodium oxybate (GHB).	

Substance use disorder	Maladaptive pattern of substance use defined as 2 or more of the following signs in 1 year:
	▪ Tolerance—need more to achieve same effect
	▪ Withdrawal
	▪ Substance taken in larger amounts, or over longer time, than desired
	▪ Persistent desire or unsuccessful attempts to cut down
	▪ Significant energy spent obtaining, using, or recovering from substance
	▪ Important social, occupational, or recreational activities reduced because of substance use
	▪ Continued use despite knowing substance causes physical and/or psychological problems
	▪ Craving
	▪ Recurrent use in physically dangerous situations
	▪ Failure to fulfill major obligations at work, school, or home due to use
	▪ Social or interpersonal conflicts related to substance use

Stages of change in overcoming substance addiction	1. **Precontemplation**—not yet acknowledging that there is a problem
	2. **Contemplation**—acknowledging that there is a problem, but not yet ready or willing to make a change
	3. **Preparation/determination**—getting ready to change behaviors
	4. **Action/willpower**—changing behaviors
	5. **Maintenance**—maintaining the behavior changes
	6. **Relapse**—returning to old behaviors and abandoning new changes

Psychoactive drug intoxication and withdrawal

DRUG	INTOXICATION	WITHDRAWAL
Depressants		
	Nonspecific: mood elevation, ↓ anxiety, sedation, behavioral disinhibition, respiratory depression.	Nonspecific: anxiety, tremor, seizures, insomnia.
Alcohol	Emotional lability, slurred speech, ataxia, coma, blackouts. Serum γ-glutamyltransferase (GGT)—sensitive indicator of alcohol use. AST value is twice ALT value.	Mild alcohol withdrawal: symptoms similar to other depressants. Severe alcohol withdrawal can cause autonomic hyperactivity and DTs (5–15% mortality rate). Treatment for DTs: benzodiazepines.
Opioids (e.g., morphine, heroin, methadone)	Euphoria, respiratory and CNS depression, ↓ gag reflex, pupillary constriction (pinpoint pupils), seizures (overdose). Treatment: naloxone, naltrexone.	Sweating, dilated pupils, piloerection ("cold turkey"), fever, rhinorrhea, yawning, nausea, stomach cramps, diarrhea ("flu-like" symptoms). Treatment: long-term support, methadone, buprenorphine.
Barbiturates	Low safety margin, marked respiratory depression. Treatment: symptom management (e.g., assist respiration, ↑ BP).	Delirium, life-threatening cardiovascular collapse.
Benzodiazepines	Greater safety margin. Ataxia, minor respiratory depression. Treatment: flumazenil (benzodiazepine receptor antagonist, but rarely used as it can precipitate seizures).	Sleep disturbance, depression, rebound anxiety, seizure.
Stimulants		
	Nonspecific: mood elevation, psychomotor agitation, insomnia, cardiac arrhythmias, tachycardia, anxiety.	Nonspecific: post-use "crash," including depression, lethargy, weight gain, headache.
Amphetamines	Euphoria, grandiosity, pupillary dilation, prolonged wakefulness and attention, hypertension, tachycardia, anorexia, paranoia, fever. Severe: cardiac arrest, seizure.	Anhedonia, ↑ appetite, hypersomnolence, existential crisis.
Cocaine	Impaired judgment, pupillary dilation, hallucinations (including tactile), paranoid ideations, angina, sudden cardiac death. Treatment: α-blockers, benzodiazepines. β-blockers not recommended.	Hypersomnolence, malaise, severe psychological craving, depression/suicidality.
Caffeine	Restlessness, ↑ diuresis, muscle twitching.	Lack of concentration, headache.
Nicotine	Restlessness.	Irritability, anxiety, craving. Treatment: nicotine patch, gum, or lozenges; bupropion/varenicline.

Psychoactive drug intoxication and withdrawal *(continued)*

DRUG	INTOXICATION	WITHDRAWAL
Hallucinogens		
PCP	Belligerence, impulsivity, fever, psychomotor agitation, analgesia, vertical and horizontal nystagmus, tachycardia, homicidality, psychosis, delirium, seizures. Treatment: benzodiazepines, rapid-acting antipsychotic.	Depression, anxiety, irritability, restlessness, anergia, disturbances of thought and sleep.
LSD	Perceptual distortion (visual, auditory), depersonalization, anxiety, paranoia, psychosis, possible flashbacks.	
Marijuana (cannabinoid)	Euphoria, anxiety, paranoid delusions, perception of slowed time, impaired judgment, social withdrawal, ↑ appetite, dry mouth, conjunctival injection, hallucinations. Pharmaceutical form is dronabinol (tetrahydrocannabinol isomer): used as antiemetic (chemotherapy) and appetite stimulant (in AIDS).	Irritability, depression, insomnia, nausea, anorexia. Most symptoms peak in 48 hours and last for 5–7 days. Generally detectable in urine for up to 1 month.

Heroin addiction	Users at ↑ risk for hepatitis, HIV, abscesses, bacteremia, right-heart endocarditis. Treatment is described below.	
Methadone	Long-acting oral opiate used for heroin detoxification or long-term maintenance.	
Naloxone + buprenorphine	Antagonist + partial agonist. Naloxone is not orally bioavailable, so withdrawal symptoms occur only if injected (lower abuse potential).	
Naltrexone	Long-acting opioid antagonist used for relapse prevention once detoxified.	

Alcoholism	Physiologic tolerance and dependence with symptoms of withdrawal (tremor, tachycardia, hypertension, malaise, nausea, DTs) when intake is interrupted. Complications: alcoholic cirrhosis, hepatitis, pancreatitis, peripheral neuropathy, testicular atrophy. Treatment: disulfiram (to condition the patient to abstain from alcohol use), acamprosate, naltrexone, supportive care. Support groups such as Alcoholics Anonymous are helpful in sustaining abstinence and supporting patient and family.
Wernicke-Korsakoff syndrome	Caused by vitamin B_1 deficiency. Triad of confusion, ophthalmoplegia, ataxia (Wernicke encephalopathy). May progress to irreversible memory loss, confabulation, personality change (Korsakoff psychosis). Associated with periventricular hemorrhage/necrosis of mammillary bodies. Treatment: IV vitamin B_1.
Mallory-Weiss syndrome	Partial thickness tear at gastroesophageal junction caused by excessive/forceful vomiting. Often presents with hematemesis and misdiagnosed as ruptured esophageal varices.

Delirium tremens (DTs)	Life-threatening alcohol withdrawal syndrome that peaks 2–4 days after last drink. Characterized by autonomic hyperactivity (e.g., tachycardia, tremors, anxiety, seizures). Classically occurs in hospital setting (e.g., 2–4 days postsurgery) in alcoholics not able to drink as inpatients. Treatment: benzodiazepines. Alcoholic hallucinosis is a distinct condition characterized by visual hallucinations 12–48 hours after last drink. Treatment: long-acting benzodiazepines (e.g., chlordiazepoxide, lorazepam, diazepam).

▶ PSYCHIATRY—PHARMACOLOGY

Medications for selected psychiatric conditions

PSYCHIATRIC CONDITION	PREFERRED DRUGS
ADHD	Stimulants (e.g., methylphenidate)
Alcohol withdrawal	Long-acting benzodiazepines (e.g., chlordiazepoxide, lorazepam, diazepam)
Bipolar disorder	Lithium, valproic acid, atypical antipsychotics
Bulimia	SSRIs
Depression	SSRIs
Generalized anxiety disorder	SSRIs, SNRIs
Obsessive-compulsive disorder	SSRIs, clomipramine (TCA)
Panic disorder	SSRIs, venlafaxine, benzodiazepines
PTSD	SSRIs, venlafaxine
Schizophrenia	Atypical antipsychotics
Social phobias	SSRIs, β-blockers
Tourette syndrome	Antipsychotics (e.g., fluphenazine, pimozide), tetrabenazine, clonidine

CNS stimulants	Methylphenidate, dextroamphetamine, methamphetamine.
MECHANISM	↑ catecholamines in the synaptic cleft, especially norepinephrine and dopamine.
CLINICAL USE	ADHD, narcolepsy, appetite control.

Antipsychotics (neuroleptics)	Haloperidol, trifluoperazine, fluphenazine, thioridazine, chlorpromazine (haloperidol + "-azines").	
MECHANISM	All typical antipsychotics block dopamine D_2 receptors (↑ [cAMP]).	**High** potency: **Tr**ifluoperazine, **Fl**uphenazine, **H**aloperidol (**Try to Fly High**)—neurologic side effects (e.g., Huntington disease, delirium, EPS symptoms).
CLINICAL USE	Schizophrenia (primarily positive symptoms), psychosis, acute mania, Tourette syndrome.	
TOXICITY	Highly lipid soluble and stored in body fat; thus, very slow to be removed from body. Extrapyramidal system side effects (e.g., dyskinesias). Treatment: benztropine or diphenhydramine. Endocrine side effects (e.g., dopamine receptor antagonism → hyperprolactinemia → galactorrhea). Side effects arising from blocking muscarinic (dry mouth, constipation), α_1 (hypotension), and histamine (sedation) receptors. Can cause QT prolongation.	**Low** potency: **Ch**lorpromazine, **Th**ioridazine (**Cheating Thieves are low**)—non-neurologic side effects (anticholinergic, antihistamine, and α_1-blockade effects). Chlorpromazine—**C**orneal deposits; Thioridazine—re**T**inal deposits; haloperidol— NMS, tardive dyskinesia. Evolution of EPS side effects: <ul><li>4 hr acute dystonia (muscle spasm, stiffness, oculogyric crisis)</li><li>4 day akathisia (restlessness)</li><li>4 wk bradykinesia (parkinsonism)</li><li>4 mo tardive dyskinesia</li></ul> For NMS, think **FEVER**: **F**ever **E**ncephalopathy **V**itals unstable **E**nzymes ↑ **R**igidity of muscles
OTHER TOXICITIES	**Neuroleptic malignant syndrome (NMS)**— rigidity, myoglobinuria, autonomic instability, hyperpyrexia. Treatment: dantrolene, D_2 agonists (e.g., bromocriptine). **Tardive dyskinesia**—stereotypic oral-facial movements as a result of long-term antipsychotic use.	

Atypical antipsychotics	Olanzapine, **cl**ozapine, **qu**etiapine, **risper**idone, aripiprazole, ziprasidone.	It's **atypical** for **old cl**osets to **quietly risper** from **A** to **Z**.
MECHANISM	Not completely understood. Varied effects on $5\text{-}HT_2$, dopamine, and $\alpha\text{-}$ and H_1-receptors.	
CLINICAL USE	Schizophrenia—both positive and negative symptoms. Also used for bipolar disorder, OCD, anxiety disorder, depression, mania, Tourette syndrome.	
TOXICITY	Fewer extrapyramidal and anticholinergic side effects than traditional antipsychotics. Olanzapine/clozapine may cause significant weight gain. Clozapine may cause agranulocytosis (requires weekly WBC monitoring) and seizure. Risperidone may increase prolactin (causing lactation and gynecomastia) → ↓ GnRH, LH, and FSH (causing irregular menstruation and fertility issues). All may prolong QT interval.	Must watch **cloz**apine **cloz**ely!

Lithium

MECHANISM	Not established; possibly related to inhibition of phosphoinositol cascade.	**LMNOP**—Lithium side effects:
CLINICAL USE	Mood stabilizer for bipolar disorder; blocks relapse and acute manic events. Also SIADH.	**M**ovement (tremor) **N**ephrogenic diabetes insipidus Hyp**O**thyroidism **P**regnancy problems
TOXICITY	Tremor, hypothyroidism, polyuria (causes nephrogenic diabetes insipidus), teratogenesis. Causes Ebstein anomaly in newborn if taken by pregnant mother. Narrow therapeutic window requires close monitoring of serum levels. Almost exclusively excreted by kidneys; most is reabsorbed at PCT with Na^+. Thiazide use is implicated in lithium toxicity in bipolar patients.	

Buspirone

MECHANISM	Stimulates $5\text{-}HT_{1A}$ receptors.	I'm always anxious if the **bus** will be **on** time, so I take **buspirone**.
CLINICAL USE	Generalized anxiety disorder. Does not cause sedation, addiction, or tolerance. Takes 1–2 weeks to take effect. Does not interact with alcohol (vs. barbiturates, benzodiazepines).	

Antidepressants

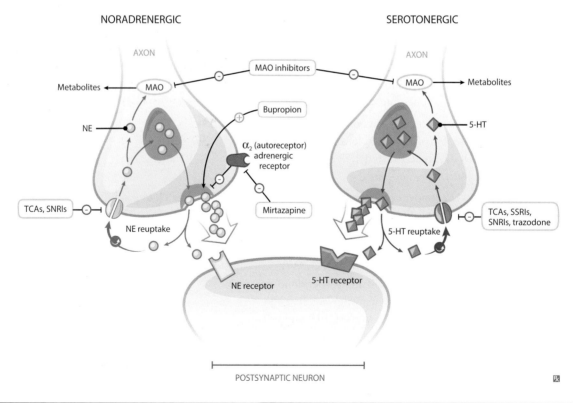

SSRIs	Fluoxetine, paroxetine, sertraline, citalopram.	Flashbacks paralyze senior citizens.
MECHANISM	5-HT–specific reuptake inhibitors.	It normally takes 4–8 weeks for antidepressants to have an effect.
CLINICAL USE	Depression, generalized anxiety disorder, panic disorder, OCD, bulimia, social phobias, PTSD.	
TOXICITY	Fewer than TCAs. GI distress, SIADH, sexual dysfunction (anorgasmia, ↓ libido). Serotonin syndrome with any drug that ↑ 5-HT (e.g., MAO inhibitors, SNRIs, TCAs)—hyperthermia, confusion, myoclonus, cardiovascular instability, flushing, diarrhea, seizures. Treatment: cyproheptadine (5-HT$_2$ receptor antagonist).	

SNRIs	Venlafaxine, duloxetine.
MECHANISM	Inhibit 5-HT and norepinephrine reuptake.
CLINICAL USE	Depression. Venlafaxine is also used in generalized anxiety disorder, panic disorder, PTSD. Duloxetine is also indicated for diabetic peripheral neuropathy.
TOXICITY	↑ BP most common; also stimulant effects, sedation, nausea.

Tricyclic antidepressants	Amitriptyline, nortriptyline, imipramine, desipramine, clomipramine, doxepin, amoxapine.
MECHANISM	Block reuptake of norepinephrine and 5-HT.
CLINICAL USE	Major depression, OCD (clomipramine), peripheral neuropathy, chronic pain, migraine prophylaxis.
TOXICITY	Sedation, α_1-blocking effects including postural hypotension, and atropine-like (anticholinergic) side effects (tachycardia, urinary retention, dry mouth). 3° TCAs (amitriptyline) have more anticholinergic effects than 2° TCAs (nortriptyline). Can prolong QT interval. Tri-C's: Convulsions, Coma, Cardiotoxicity (arrhythmias); also respiratory depression, hyperpyrexia. Confusion and hallucinations in elderly due to anticholinergic side effects (use nortriptyline). Treatment: NaHCO$_3$ to prevent arrhythmia.

Monoamine oxidase (MAO) inhibitors	Tranylcypromine, Phenelzine, Isocarboxazid, Selegiline (selective MAO-B inhibitor). (MAO Takes Pride In Shanghai).
MECHANISM	Nonselective MAO inhibition ↑ levels of amine neurotransmitters (norepinephrine, 5-HT, dopamine).
CLINICAL USE	Atypical depression, anxiety.
TOXICITY	Hypertensive crisis (most notably with ingestion of tyramine, which is found in many foods such as wine and cheese); CNS stimulation. Contraindicated with SSRIs, TCAs, St. John's wort, meperidine, dextromethorphan (to prevent serotonin syndrome).

Atypical antidepressants

Bupropion	Also used for smoking cessation. ↑ norepinephrine and dopamine via unknown mechanism. Toxicity: stimulant effects (tachycardia, insomnia), headache, seizures in anorexic/bulimic patients. No sexual side effects.
Mirtazapine	α_2-antagonist (↑ release of norepinephrine and 5-HT) and potent 5-HT$_2$ and 5-HT$_3$ receptor antagonist. Toxicity: sedation (which may be desirable in depressed patients with insomnia), ↑ appetite, weight gain (which may be desirable in elderly or anorexic patients), dry mouth.
Trazodone	Primarily blocks 5-HT$_2$ and α_1-adrenergic receptors. Used primarily for insomnia, as high doses are needed for antidepressant effects. Toxicity: sedation, nausea, priapism, postural hypotension. Called trazo**bone** due to male-specific side effects.

Renal

> "But I know all about love already. I know precious little still about kidneys."
>
> —Aldous Huxley, *Antic Hay*

> "This too shall pass. Just like a kidney stone."
>
> —Hunter Madsen

> "I drink too much. The last time I gave a urine sample it had an olive in it."
>
> —Rodney Dangerfield

▶ RENAL—EMBRYOLOGY

Kidney embryology	Pronephros—week 4; then degenerates.
	Mesonephros—functions as interim kidney for 1st trimester; later contributes to male genital system.
	Metanephros—permanent; first appears in 5th week of gestation; nephrogenesis continues through 32–36 weeks of gestation.
	  • Ureteric bud—derived from caudal end of mesonephric duct; gives rise to ureter, pelvises, calyces, collecting ducts; fully canalized by 10th week
	  • Metanephric mesenchyme—ureteric bud interacts with this tissue; interaction induces differentiation and formation of glomerulus through to distal convoluted tubule (DCT)
	  • Aberrant interaction between these 2 tissues may result in several congenital malformations of the kidney
	Ureteropelvic junction—last to canalize → most common site of obstruction (hydronephrosis) in fetus.

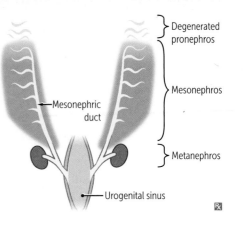

Degenerated pronephros

Mesonephric duct

Mesonephros

Metanephros

Urogenital sinus

Potter sequence (syndrome)
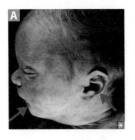
	Oligohydramnios → compression of developing fetus → limb deformities, facial anomalies (e.g., low-set ears and retrognathia [arrows in A]), compression of chest and lack of amniotic fluid aspiration into fetal lungs → pulmonary hypoplasia (cause of death).
	Causes include ARPKD, obstructive uropathy (e.g., posterior urethral valves), bilateral renal agenesis.
		Babies who can't "Pee" in utero develop Potter sequence.
		POTTER sequence associated with:
		  Pulmonary hypoplasia
		  Oligohydramnios (trigger)
		  Twisted face
		  Twisted skin
		  Extremity defects
		  Renal failure (in utero)

Horseshoe kidney

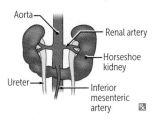

Aorta
Renal artery
Horseshoe kidney
Ureter
Inferior mesenteric artery

Inferior poles of both kidneys fuse 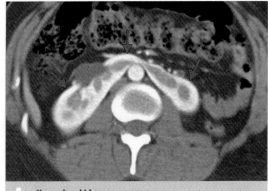 A. As they ascend from pelvis during fetal development, horseshoe kidneys get trapped under inferior mesenteric artery and remain low in the abdomen. Kidneys function normally. Associated with ureteropelvic junction obstruction, hydronephrosis, renal stones, infection, chromosomal aneuploidy syndromes (e.g., Edwards, Down, Patau, Turner), and rarely renal cancer.

A **Horseshoe kidney.** Axial CT of abdomen with contrast shows enhancing midline fused kidney (arrows). ℞

Multicystic dysplastic kidney

Due to abnormal interaction between ureteric bud and metanephric mesenchyme. Leads to a nonfunctional kidney consisting of cysts and connective tissue. If unilateral (most common), generally asymptomatic with compensatory hypertrophy of contralateral kidney. Often diagnosed prenatally via ultrasound.

Duplex collecting system

Bifurcation of ureteric bud before it enters metanephric blastema creates Y-shaped bifid ureter. Can alternatively occur when two ureteric buds reach and interact with metanephric blastema. Strongly associated with vesicoureteral reflux and/or ureteral obstruction, ↑ risk for UTIs.

Kidney anatomy and glomerular structure

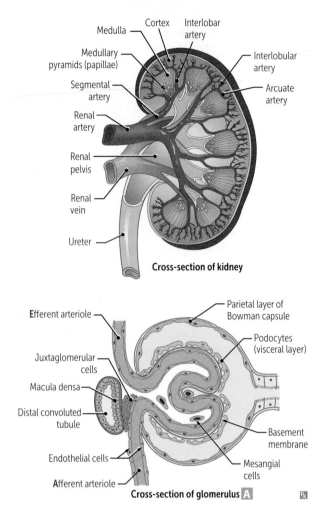

Medulla
Cortex
Interlobar artery
Medullary pyramids (papillae)
Interlobular artery
Segmental artery
Arcuate artery
Renal artery
Renal pelvis
Renal vein
Ureter

Cross-section of kidney

Left kidney is taken during donor transplantation because it has a longer renal vein.

Afferent = Arriving.

Efferent = Exiting.

Efferent arteriole
Parietal layer of Bowman capsule
Podocytes (visceral layer)
Juxtaglomerular cells
Macula densa
Distal convoluted tubule
Endothelial cells
Basement membrane
Mesangial cells
Afferent arteriole

Cross-section of glomerulus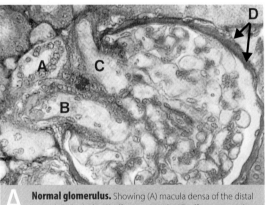

A   Normal glomerulus. Showing (A) macula densa of the distal convoluted tubule, (B) afferent arteriole, (C) efferent arteriole, and (D) Bowman capsule.

Ureters: course

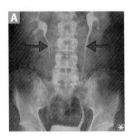

Ureters 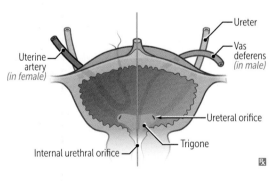 pass **under** uterine artery and **under** ductus deferens (retroperitoneal).

"Water (ureters) **under** the bridge (uterine artery, vas deferens)."

Gynecologic procedures involving ligation of uterine vessels traveling in cardinal ligament may damage ureter → ureteral obstruction or leak.

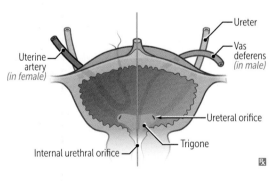

Uterine artery (in female)
Ureter
Vas deferens (in male)
Ureteral orifice
Trigone
Internal urethral orifice

▶ RENAL—PHYSIOLOGY

Fluid compartments

Body mass: ~70kg

Total body water (TBW) 60% of body mass = ~42 L = 42 kg

Non water mass (NWM) 40% of body mass = ~28 kg

Extracellular fluid (ECF) ~ 14 kg (20% of 70 kg)

1/3

Interstitial fluid = 75% ECF ~ 10.5 L = 10.5 kg

Plasma = 25% ECF ≈ 3.5 L = 3.5 kg

RBC volume = ~2.8 L

Intracellular fluid (ICF) ~ 28 kg (40% of 70 kg)

2/3

Blood volume ~6 L

Normal HCT = 45%

HCT (%) ~ 3×[Hb] in g/dL

HIKIN': HIgh K INtracellularly.
60–40–20 rule (% of body weight for average person):
- 60% total body water
- 40% ICF
- 20% ECF

Plasma volume measured by radiolabeled albumin.

Extracellular volume measured by inulin.

Osmolality = 285–295 mOsm/kg H_2O.

Glomerular filtration barrier	Responsible for filtration of plasma according to size and net charge. Composed of: - Fenestrated capillary endothelium (size barrier) - Fused basement membrane with heparan sulfate (negative charge barrier) - Epithelial layer consisting of podocyte foot processes	Charge barrier is lost in nephrotic syndrome → albuminuria, hypoproteinemia, generalized edema, hyperlipidemia.
Renal clearance	$C_x = U_x V/P_x$ = volume of plasma from which the substance is completely cleared per unit time. $C_x <$ GFR: net tubular reabsorption of X. $C_x >$ GFR: net tubular secretion of X. $C_x =$ GFR: no net secretion or reabsorption.	Be familiar with calculations. C_x = clearance of X (mL/min). U_x = urine concentration of X (e.g., mg/mL). P_x = plasma concentration of X (e.g., mg/mL). V = urine flow rate (mL/min).
Glomerular filtration rate	Inulin clearance can be used to calculate GFR because it is freely filtered and is neither reabsorbed nor secreted. GFR = $U_{inulin} \times V/P_{inulin} = C_{inulin}$ $= K_f [(P_{GC} - P_{BS}) - (\pi_{GC} - \pi_{BS})]$ (GC = glomerular capillary; BS = Bowman space.) π_{BS} normally equals zero.	Normal GFR ≈ 100 mL/min. Creatinine clearance is an approximate measure of GFR. Slightly overestimates GFR because creatinine is moderately secreted by renal tubules. Incremental reductions in GFR define the stages of chronic kidney disease.

Effective renal plasma flow

Effective renal plasma flow (eRPF) can be estimated using *para*-aminohippuric acid (PAH) clearance because it is both filtered and secreted in the proximal collecting tubule (PCT), resulting in near 100% excretion of all PAH entering kidney.

$eRPF = U_{PAH} \times V/P_{PAH} = C_{PAH}$.

$RBF = RPF/(1 - Hct)$.

eRPF underestimates true renal plasma flow (RPF) by ~ 10%.

Filtration

Filtration fraction (FF) = GFR/RPF.

Normal FF = 20%.

Filtered load (mg/min) = GFR (mL/min) × plasma concentration (mg/mL).

GFR can be estimated with creatinine clearance.

RPF is best estimated with PAH clearance.

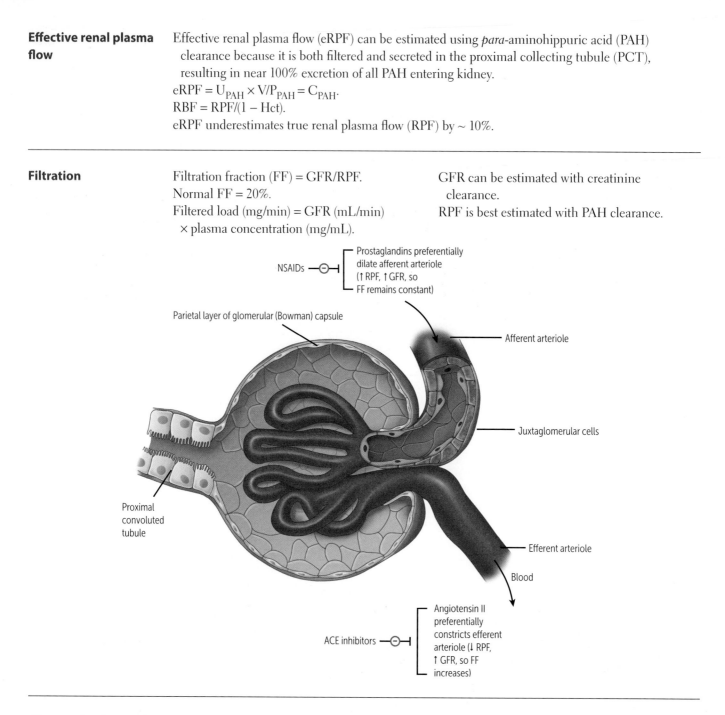

NSAIDs

Prostaglandins preferentially dilate afferent arteriole (↑ RPF, ↑ GFR, so FF remains constant)

Parietal layer of glomerular (Bowman) capsule

Afferent arteriole

Juxtaglomerular cells

Proximal convoluted tubule

Efferent arteriole

Blood

ACE inhibitors

Angiotensin II preferentially constricts efferent arteriole (↓ RPF, ↑ GFR, so FF increases)

Changes in glomerular dynamics

Effect	GFR	RPF	FF (GFR/RPF)
Afferent arteriole constriction	↓	↓	—
Efferent arteriole constriction	↑	↓	↑
↑ plasma protein concentration	↓	—	↓
↓ plasma protein concentration	↑	—	↑
Constriction of ureter	↓	—	↓

Calculation of reabsorption and secretion rate	Filtered load = $GFR \times P_x$. Excretion rate = $V \times U_x$. Reabsorption = filtered – excreted. Secretion = excreted – filtered.	
Glucose clearance	Glucose at a normal plasma level is completely reabsorbed in PCT by Na^+/glucose cotransport. At plasma glucose of ~ 200 mg/dL, glucosuria begins (threshold). At ~ 375 mg/dL, all transporters are fully saturated (T_m).	Glucosuria is an important clinical clue to diabetes mellitus. Normal pregnancy may decrease ability of PCT to reabsorb glucose and amino acids → glucosuria and aminoaciduria.
Amino acid clearance	Na^+-dependent transporters in PCT reabsorb amino acids. **Hartnup disease**—autosomal recessive. Deficiency of neutral amino acid (e.g., tryptophan) transporters in proximal renal tubular cells and on enterocytes → neutral aminoaciduria and ↓ absorption from the gut → ↓ tryptophan for conversion to niacin → pellagra-like symptoms. Treat with high-protein diet and nicotinic acid.	

Nephron physiology

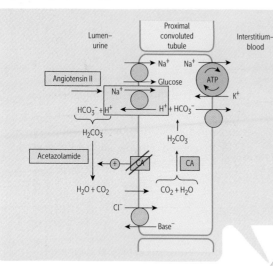

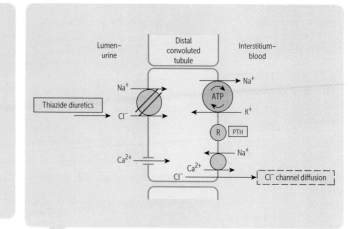

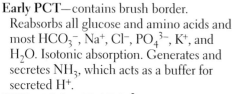

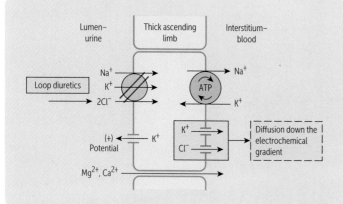

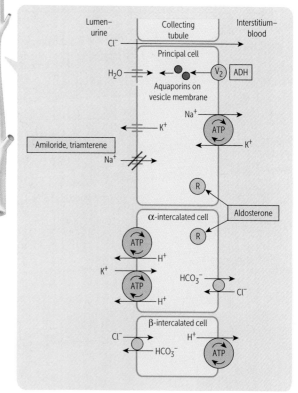

Early PCT—contains brush border. Reabsorbs all glucose and amino acids and most HCO_3^-, Na^+, Cl^-, PO_4^{3-}, K^+, and H_2O. Isotonic absorption. Generates and secretes NH_3, which acts as a buffer for secreted H^+.
PTH—inhibits Na^+/PO_4^{3-} cotransport → PO_4^{3-} excretion.
AT II—stimulates Na^+/H^+ exchange → ↑ Na^+, H_2O, and HCO_3^- reabsorption (permitting contraction alkalosis).
65–80% Na^+ reabsorbed.

Thin descending loop of Henle—passively reabsorbs H_2O via medullary hypertonicity (impermeable to Na^+). Concentrating segment. Makes urine hypertonic.

Thick ascending loop of Henle—reabsorbs Na^+, K^+, and Cl^-. Indirectly induces paracellular reabsorption of Mg^{2+} and Ca^{2+} through (+) lumen potential generated by K^+ backleak. Impermeable to H_2O. Makes urine less concentrated as it ascends.
10–20% Na^+ reabsorbed.

Early DCT—reabsorbs Na^+, Cl^-. Makes urine most dilute (hypotonic).
PTH—↑ Ca^{2+}/Na^+ exchange → Ca^{2+} reabsorption.
5–10% Na^+ reabsorbed.

Collecting tubule—reabsorbs Na^+ in exchange for secreting K^+ and H^+ (regulated by aldosterone).
Aldosterone—acts on mineralocorticoid receptor → mRNA → protein synthesis. In principal cells: ↑ apical K^+ conductance, ↑ Na^+/K^+ pump, ↑ ENaC channels → lumen negativity → K^+ loss. In α-intercalated cells: ↑ H^+ ATPase activity → ↑ HCO_3^-/Cl^- exchanger activity.
ADH—acts at V_2 receptor → insertion of aquaporin H_2O channels on apical side.
3–5% Na^+ reabsorbed.

Renal tubular defects	The kidneys put out **FAB**ulous **G**littering **L**iquid**S**:
	FAnconi syndrome is the 1st defect (PCT)
	Bartter syndrome is next (thick ascending loop of Henle)
	Gitelman syndrome is after Bartter (DCT)
	Liddle syndrome is last (collecting tubule)
	Syndrome of apparent mineralocorticoid excess (collecting tubule)

Fanconi syndrome	Generalized reabsorptive defect in PCT.
	Associated with ↑ excretion of nearly all amino acids, glucose, HCO_3^-, and PO_4^{3-}. May result in metabolic acidosis (proximal renal tubular acidosis).
	Causes include hereditary defects (e.g., Wilson disease, tyrosinemia, glycogen storage disease), ischemia, multiple myeloma, nephrotoxins/drugs (e.g., expired tetracyclines, tenofovir), lead poisoning.

Bartter syndrome	Reabsorptive defect in thick ascending loop of Henle. Autosomal recessive. Affects $Na^+/K^+/2Cl^-$ cotransporter.
	Results in hypokalemia and metabolic alkalosis with hypercalciuria.

Gitelman syndrome	Reabsorptive defect of NaCl in DCT.
	Autosomal recessive. Less severe than Bartter syndrome. Leads to hypokalemia, hypomagnesemia, metabolic alkalosis, hypocalciuria.

Liddle syndrome	Gain of function mutation → ↑ Na^+ reabsorption in collecting tubules (↑ activity of epithelial Na^+ channel).
	Autosomal dominant. Results in hypertension, hypokalemia, metabolic alkalosis, ↓ aldosterone. Treatment: Amiloride.

Syndrome of apparent mineralocorticoid excess	Hereditary deficiency of 11β-hydroxysteroid dehydrogenase, which normally converts cortisol into cortisone in mineralocorticoid receptor–containing cells before cortisol can act on the mineralocorticoid receptors. Excess cortisol in these cells from enzyme deficiency → ↑ mineralocorticoid receptor activity → hypertension, hypokalemia, metabolic alkalosis. Low serum aldosterone levels. Can acquire disorder from glycyrrhetic acid (present in licorice), which blocks activity of 11β-hydroxysteroid dehydrogenase.

Relative concentrations along proximal convoluted tubules	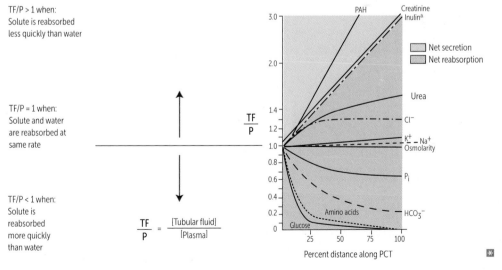

[a]Neither secreted nor reabsorbed; concentration increases as water is reabsorbed.

Tubular inulin ↑ in concentration (but not amount) along the PCT as a result of water reabsorption. Cl^- reabsorption occurs at a slower rate than Na^+ in early PCT and then matches the rate of Na^+ reabsorption more distally. Thus, its relative concentration ↑ before it plateaus.

Renin-angiotensin-aldosterone system

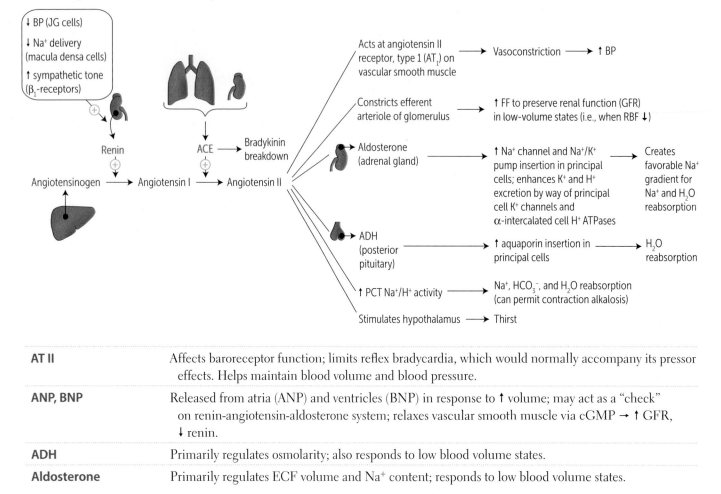

AT II	Affects baroreceptor function; limits reflex bradycardia, which would normally accompany its pressor effects. Helps maintain blood volume and blood pressure.
ANP, BNP	Released from atria (ANP) and ventricles (BNP) in response to ↑ volume; may act as a "check" on renin-angiotensin-aldosterone system; relaxes vascular smooth muscle via cGMP → ↑ GFR, ↓ renin.
ADH	Primarily regulates osmolarity; also responds to low blood volume states.
Aldosterone	Primarily regulates ECF volume and Na⁺ content; responds to low blood volume states.

Juxtaglomerular apparatus	Consists of mesangial cells, JG cells (modified smooth muscle of afferent arteriole) and the macula densa (NaCl sensor, part of DCT). JG cells secrete renin in response to ↓ renal blood pressure and ↑ sympathetic tone (β₁). Macula densa cells sense ↓ NaCl delivery to DCT → adenosine release → vasoconstriction.	JGA maintains GFR via renin-angiotensin-aldosterone system. β-blockers can decrease BP by inhibiting β₁-receptors of the JGA → ↓ renin release.

Kidney endocrine functions

Erythropoietin	Released by interstitial cells in peritubular capillary bed in response to hypoxia.	
1,25-(OH)₂ D₃	PCT cells convert 25-OH vitamin D to 1,25-(OH)₂ vitamin D (active form).	$25\text{-OH D}_3 \xrightarrow[\text{1α-hydroxylase}]{} 1,25\text{-(OH)}_2\,D_3$ ↑ ⊕ | PTH
Renin	Secreted by JG cells in response to ↓ renal arterial pressure and ↑ renal sympathetic discharge (β₁ effect).	
Prostaglandins	Paracrine secretion vasodilates the afferent arterioles to ↑ RBF.	NSAIDs block renal-protective prostaglandin synthesis → constriction of afferent arteriole and ↓ GFR; this may result in acute renal failure.

Hormones acting on kidney

Angiotensin II (AT II)

Synthesized in response to ↓ BP. Causes efferent arteriole constriction → ↑ GFR and ↑ FF but with compensatory Na^+ reabsorption in proximal and distal nephron. Net effect: preservation of renal function (↑ FF) in low-volume state with simultaneous Na^+ reabsorption (both proximal and distal) to maintain circulating volume.

Atrial natriuretic peptide (ANP)

Secreted in response to ↑ atrial pressure. Causes ↑ GFR and ↑ Na^+ filtration **with no compensatory Na^+ reabsorption** in distal nephron. Net effect: Na^+ loss and volume loss.

Aldosterone

Secreted in response to ↓ blood volume (via AT II) and ↑ plasma $[K^+]$; causes ↑ Na^+ reabsorption, ↑ K^+ secretion, ↑ H^+ secretion.

Parathyroid hormone (PTH)

Secreted in response to ↓ plasma $[Ca^{2+}]$, ↑ plasma $[PO_4^{3-}]$, or ↓ plasma $1,25-(OH)_2 D_3$. Causes ↑ $[Ca^{2+}]$ reabsorption (DCT), ↓ $[PO_4^{3-}]$ reabsorption (PCT), and ↑ $1,25-(OH)_2 D_3$ production (↑ Ca^{2+} and PO_4^{3-} absorption from gut via vitamin D).

ADH (vasopressin)

Secreted in response to ↑ plasma osmolarity and ↓ blood volume. Binds to receptors on principal cells, causing ↑ number of aquaporins and ↑ H_2O reabsorption.

Potassium shifts

SHIFTS K^+ OUT OF CELL (CAUSING HYPERKALEMIA)	SHIFTS K^+ INTO CELL (CAUSING HYPOKALEMIA)
Digitalis (blocks Na^+/K^+ ATPase)	
HyperOsmolarity	Hypo-osmolarity
Lysis of cells (e.g., crush injury, rhabdomyolysis, cancer)	
Acidosis	Alkalosis
β-blocker	β-adrenergic agonist (↑ Na^+/K^+ ATPase)
High blood Sugar (insulin deficiency)	Insulin (↑ Na^+/K^+ ATPase)
Patient with hyperkalemia? **DO LAβS.**	Insulin shifts K^+ into cells

Electrolyte disturbances

ELECTROLYTE	LOW SERUM CONCENTRATION	HIGH SERUM CONCENTRATION
Na^+	Nausea and malaise, stupor, coma, seizures	Irritability, stupor, coma
K^+	U waves on ECG, flattened T waves, arrhythmias, muscle spasm	Wide QRS and peaked T waves on ECG, arrhythmias, muscle weakness
Ca^{2+}	Tetany, seizures, QT prolongation	**Stones** (renal), **bones** (pain), **groans** (abdominal pain), **thrones** (↑ urinary frequency), **psychiatric overtones** (anxiety, altered mental status), but not necessarily calciuria
Mg^{2+}	Tetany, torsades de pointes, hypokalemia	↓ DTRs, lethargy, bradycardia, hypotension, cardiac arrest, hypocalcemia
PO_4^{3-}	Bone loss, osteomalacia (adults), rickets (children)	Renal stones, metastatic calcifications, hypocalcemia

Acid-base physiology

	pH	P_{CO_2}	$[HCO_3^-]$	COMPENSATORY RESPONSE
Metabolic acidosis	↓	↓	↓	Hyperventilation (immediate)
Metabolic alkalosis	↑	↑	↑	Hypoventilation (immediate)
Respiratory acidosis	↓	↑	↑	↑ renal $[HCO_3^-]$ reabsorption (delayed)
Respiratory alkalosis	↑	↓	↓	↓ renal $[HCO_3^-]$ reabsorption (delayed)

Key: ↑ ↓ = 1° disturbance; ↓ ↑ = compensatory response.

Henderson-Hasselbalch equation: $pH = 6.1 + \log \dfrac{[HCO_3^-]}{0.03\ P_{CO_2}}$

Predicted respiratory compensation for a simple metabolic acidosis can be calculated using the Winters formula. If measured P_{CO_2} differs significantly from predicted P_{CO_2}, then a mixed acid-base disorder is likely present:

$$P_{CO_2} = 1.5\ [HCO_3^-] + 8 \pm 2$$

Acidosis/alkalosis

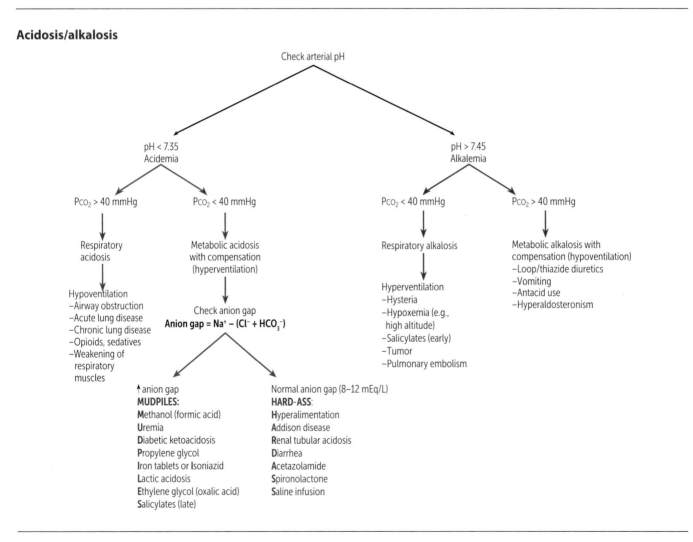

Renal tubular acidosis	A disorder of the renal tubules that leads to normal anion gap (hyperchloremic) metabolic acidosis.
RTA TYPE	**NOTES**
Distal (type 1), urine pH > 5.5	Defect in ability of α intercalated cells to secrete H^+ → no new HCO_3^- is generated → metabolic acidosis. Associated with **hypokalemia**, ↑ risk for calcium phosphate kidney stones (due to ↑ urine pH and ↑ bone turnover). Causes: amphotericin B toxicity, analgesic nephropathy, congenital anomalies (obstruction) of urinary tract.
Proximal (type 2), urine pH < 5.5	Defect in PCT HCO_3^- reabsorption → ↑ excretion of HCO_3^- in urine and subsequent metabolic acidosis. Urine is acidified by α-intercalated cells in collecting tubule. Associated with **hypokalemia**, ↑ risk for hypophosphatemic rickets. Causes: Fanconi syndrome and carbonic anhydrase inhibitors.
Hyperkalemic (type 4), urine pH < 5.5	Hypoaldosteronism → **hyperkalemia** → ↓ NH_3 synthesis in PCT → ↓ NH_4^+ excretion. Causes: ↓ aldosterone production (e.g., diabetic hyporeninism, ACE inhibitors, ARBs, NSAIDs, heparin, cyclosporine, adrenal insufficiency) or aldosterone resistance (e.g., K^+-sparing diuretics, nephropathy due to obstruction, TMP/SMX).

▶ RENAL—PATHOLOGY

Casts in urine	Presence of casts indicates that hematuria/pyuria is of glomerular or renal tubular origin. Bladder cancer, kidney stones → hematuria, no casts. Acute cystitis → pyuria, no casts.
RBC casts	Glomerulonephritis, malignant hypertension.
WBC casts	Tubulointerstitial inflammation, acute pyelonephritis, transplant rejection.
Fatty casts ("oval fat bodies")	Nephrotic syndrome.
Granular ("muddy brown") casts	Acute tubular necrosis.
Waxy casts	End-stage renal disease/chronic renal failure.
Hyaline casts	Nonspecific, can be a normal finding, often seen in concentrated urine samples.

Nomenclature of glomerular disorders

TYPE	CHARACTERISTICS	EXAMPLE
Focal	< 50% of glomeruli are involved	Focal segmental glomerulosclerosis
Diffuse	> 50% of glomeruli are involved	Diffuse proliferative glomerulonephritis
Proliferative	Hypercellular glomeruli	Membranoproliferative glomerulonephritis
Membranous	Thickening of glomerular basement membrane (GBM)	Membranous nephropathy
1° glomerular disease	A 1° disease of the kidney specifically impacting the glomeruli	Minimal change disease
2° glomerular disease	A systemic disease or disease of another organ system that also impacts the glomeruli	SLE, diabetic nephropathy

Glomerular diseases

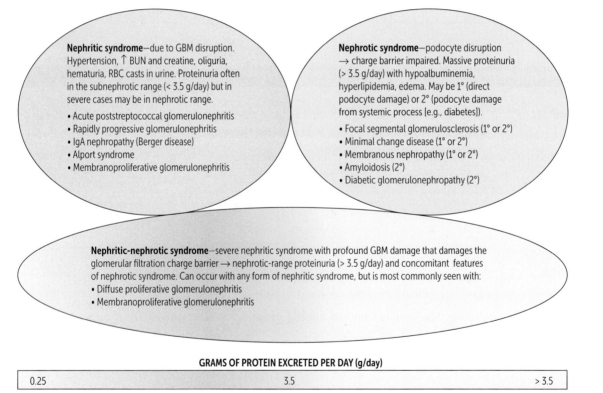

Nephritic syndrome—due to GBM disruption. Hypertension, ↑ BUN and creatine, oliguria, hematuria, RBC casts in urine. Proteinuria often in the subnephrotic range (< 3.5 g/day) but in severe cases may be in nephrotic range.
- Acute poststreptococcal glomerulonephritis
- Rapidly progressive glomerulonephritis
- IgA nephropathy (Berger disease)
- Alport syndrome
- Membranoproliferative glomerulonephritis

Nephrotic syndrome—podocyte disruption → charge barrier impaired. Massive proteinuria (> 3.5 g/day) with hypoalbuminemia, hyperlipidemia, edema. May be 1° (direct podocyte damage) or 2° (podocyte damage from systemic process [e.g., diabetes]).
- Focal segmental glomerulosclerosis (1° or 2°)
- Minimal change disease (1° or 2°)
- Membranous nephropathy (1° or 2°)
- Amyloidosis (2°)
- Diabetic glomerulonephropathy (2°)

Nephritic-nephrotic syndrome—severe nephritic syndrome with profound GBM damage that damages the glomerular filtration charge barrier → nephrotic-range proteinuria (> 3.5 g/day) and concomitant features of nephrotic syndrome. Can occur with any form of nephritic syndrome, but is most commonly seen with:
- Diffuse proliferative glomerulonephritis
- Membranoproliferative glomerulonephritis

GRAMS OF PROTEIN EXCRETED PER DAY (g/day)

| 0.25 | 3.5 | > 3.5 |

Nephritic syndrome	NephrItic syndrome = Inflammatory process. When it involves glomeruli, it leads to hematuria and RBC casts in urine. Associated with azotemia, oliguria, hypertension (due to salt retention), proteinuria.	
Acute poststreptococcal glomerulonephritis	LM—glomeruli enlarged and hypercellular **A**. IF—("starry sky") granular appearance ("lumpy-bumpy") **B** due to IgG, IgM, and C3 deposition along GBM and mesangium. EM—subepithelial immune complex (IC) humps.	Most frequently seen in children. Occurs ~ 2 weeks after group A streptococcal infection of pharynx or skin. Resolves spontaneously. Type III hypersensitivity reaction. Presents with peripheral and periorbital edema, cola-colored urine, hypertension. ↑ anti-DNase B titers, ↓ complement levels.

Nephritic syndrome *(continued)*

Rapidly progressive (crescentic) glomerulonephritis (RPGN)	LM and IF—crescent moon shape 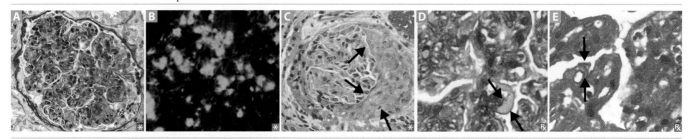. Crescents consist of fibrin and plasma proteins (e.g., C3b) with glomerular parietal cells, monocytes, macrophages. Several disease processes may result in this pattern, in particular: ■ Goodpasture syndrome—type II hypersensitivity; antibodies to GBM and alveolar basement membrane → linear IF ■ Granulomatosis with polyangiitis (Wegener) ■ Microscopic polyangiitis	Poor prognosis. Rapidly deteriorating renal function (days to weeks). Hematuria/hemoptysis. Treatment: emergent plasmapheresis. PR3-ANCA/c-ANCA. MPO-ANCA/p-ANCA.
Diffuse proliferative glomerulonephritis (DPGN)	Due to SLE or membranoproliferative glomerulonephritis. LM—"**wire loop**ing" of capillaries. EM—subendothelial and sometimes intramembranous IgG-based ICs often with C3 deposition. IF—granular.	Most common cause of death in SLE (think "**wire lupus**"). DPGN and MPGN often present as nephrotic syndrome and nephritic syndrome concurrently.
IgA nephropathy (Berger disease)	LM—mesangial proliferation. EM—mesangial IC deposits. IF—IgA-based IC deposits in mesangium. Renal pathology of Henoch-Schönlein purpura.	Often presents with renal insufficiency or acute gastroenteritis. Episodic hematuria with RBC casts. Not to be confused with Buerger disease (thromboangiitis obliterans).
Alport syndrome	Mutation in type IV collagen → thinning and splitting of glomerular basement membrane. Most commonly X-linked.	Eye problems (e.g., retinopathy, lens dislocation), glomerulonephritis, sensorineural deafness; "can't see, can't pee, can't hear a buzzing bee." "Basket-weave" appearance on EM.
Membrano-proliferative glomerulonephritis (MPGN)	Type I—subendothelial immune complex (IC) deposits with granular IF; "tram-track" appearance on PAS stain and H&E stain due to GBM splitting caused by mesangial ingrowth. Type II—intramembranous IC deposits; "dense deposits."	MPGN is a nephritic syndrome that often copresents with nephrotic syndrome. Type 1 may be 2° to hepatitis B or C infection. May also be idiopathic. Type II is associated with C3 nephritic factor (stabilizes C3 convertase → ↓ serum C3 levels).

LM = light microscopy; EM = electron microscopy; IF = immunofluorescence.

Nephrotic syndrome	NephrOtic syndrome—massive prOteinuria (> 3.5 g/day) with hypoalbuminemia, resulting edema, hyperlipidemia. Frothy urine with fatty casts. Due to podocyte damage disrupting glomerular filtration charge barrier. May be 1° (direct sclerosis of podocytes) or 2° (systemic process [e.g., diabetes] secondarily damages podocytes). Severe nephritic syndrome may present with nephrotic syndrome features (nephritic-nephrotic syndrome) if damage to GBM is severe enough to damage charge barrier. Associated with hypercoagulable state (e.g., thromboembolism) due to antithrombin (AT) III loss in urine and ↑ risk of infection (due to loss of immunoglobulins in urine and soft tissue compromise by edema).

Focal segmental glomerulosclerosis	LM—segmental sclerosis and hyalinosis **A**. IF—nonspecific for focal deposits of IgM, C3, Cl. EM—effacement of foot process similar to minimal change disease. Most common cause of nephrotic syndrome in African Americans and Hispanics. Can be 1° (idiopathic) or 2° to other conditions (e.g., HIV infection, sickle cell disease, heroin abuse, massive obesity, interferon treatment, chronic kidney disease due to congenital malformations). 1° disease has inconsistent response to steroids. May progress to chronic renal disease.	 **Focal segmental glomerulosclerosis.**
Minimal change disease (lipoid nephrosis)	LM—normal glomeruli (lipid may be seen in PCT cells). IF ⊖. EM—effacement (fusion) of foot processes **B**. Most common cause of nephrotic syndrome in children. Often 1° (idiopathic) and may be triggered by recent infection, immunization, immune stimulus. Rarely, may be 2° to lymphoma (e.g., cytokine-mediated damage). 1° disease has excellent response to corticosteroids.	 **Minimal change disease (lipoid nephrosis).** Note effacement of foot processes on EM (arrow).
Membranous nephropathy	LM—diffuse capillary and GBM thickening **C**. IF—granular as a result of immune complex deposition. Nephrotic presentation of SLE. EM—"spike and dome" appearance with subepithelial deposits. Most common cause of 1° nephrotic syndrome in Caucasian adults. Can be 1° (idiopathic) or 2° to other conditions (e.g., antibodies to phospholipase A_2 receptor, drugs [e.g., NSAIDs, penicillamine], infections [e.g., HBV, HCV], SLE, solid tumors). 1° disease has poor response to steroids. May progress to chronic renal disease.	 **Membranous nephropathy.**

Nephrotic syndrome (continued)

Amyloidosis	LM—Congo red stain shows apple-green birefringence under polarized light. Kidney is the most commonly involved organ (systemic amyloidosis). Associated with chronic conditions (e.g., multiple myeloma, TB, rheumatoid arthritis).
Diabetic glomerulo-nephropathy	LM—mesangial expansion, GBM thickening, eosinophilic nodular glomerulosclerosis (Kimmelstiel-Wilson lesions) **D**. Nonenzymatic glycosylation of GBM → ↑ permeability, thickening. Nonenzymatic glycosylation of efferent arterioles → ↑ GFR → mesangial expansion.

D **Diabetic glomerulosclerosis.** Arrows point to one of several Kimmelstiel-Wilson lesions. Note the light pink diffuse mesangial expansion. ✶

Kidney stones   Can lead to severe complications, such as hydronephrosis, pyelonephritis. Presents with unilateral flank tenderness, colicky pain radiating to groin, hematuria. Treat and prevent by encouraging fluid intake.

CONTENT	PRECIPITATES AT	X-RAY FINDINGS	URINE CRYSTAL	NOTES
Calcium (80%)	↑ pH (calcium phosphate) ↓ pH (calcium oxalate)	Radiopaque	Envelope- or dumbbell-shaped calcium oxalate	Oxalate crystals can result from ethylene glycol (antifreeze) ingestion, vitamin C abuse, hypocitraturia, malabsorption (e.g., Crohn disease). Most common kidney stone presentation: calcium oxalate stone in patient with hypercalciuria and normocalcemia. Treatment: hydration, thiazides, citrate.
Ammonium magnesium phosphate (15%)	↑ pH	Radiopaque	Coffin lid	Also known as struvite. Caused by infection with urease ⊕ bugs (e.g., *Proteus mirabilis*, *Staphylococcus saprophyticus*, *Klebsiella*) that hydrolyze urea to ammonia → urine alkalinization. Commonly form staghorn calculi . Treatment: eradication of underlying infection, surgical removal of stone.
Uric acid (5%)	↓ pH	RadiolUcent	Rhomboid or rosettes	Risk factors: ↓ urine volume, arid climates, acidic pH. Visible on CT and ultrasound, but not x-ray. Strong association with hyperuricemia (e.g., gout). Often seen in diseases with ↑ cell turnover, such as leukemia. Treatment: alkalinization of urine, allopurinol.
Cystine (1%)	↓ pH	Radiolucent	Hexagonal	Hereditary (autosomal recessive) condition in which cystine-reabsorbing PCT transporter loses function, causing cystinuria. Cystine is poorly soluble, thus stones form in urine. Mostly seen in children. Can form staghorn calculi. Sodium cyanide nitroprusside test ⊕. "**SIX**tine" stones have **SIX** sides. Treatment: alkalinization of urine.

Hydronephrosis

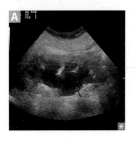

Distention/dilation of renal pelvis and calyces 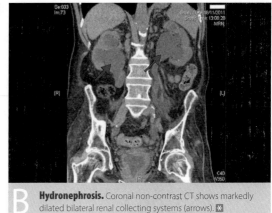 **B**. Usually caused by urinary tract obstruction (e.g., renal stones, BPH, cervical cancer, injury to ureter); other causes include retroperitoneal fibrosis, vesicoureteral reflux. Dilation occurs proximal to site of pathology. Serum creatinine becomes elevated only if obstruction is bilateral or if patient has only one kidney. Leads to compression and possible atrophy of renal cortex and medulla.

B **Hydronephrosis.** Coronal non-contrast CT shows markedly dilated bilateral renal collecting systems (arrows). ✺

Renal cell carcinoma

Originates from PCT cells → polygonal clear cells **A** filled with accumulated lipids and carbohydrates. Most common in men 50–70 years old. ↑ incidence with smoking and obesity. Manifests clinically with hematuria, palpable mass, 2° polycythemia, flank pain, fever, weight loss. Invades renal vein then IVC and spreads hematogenously; metastasizes to lung and bone.

Treatment: resection if localized disease. Immunotherapy or targeted therapy for advanced/metastatic disease. Resistant to chemotherapy and radiation therapy.

Most common 1° renal malignancy **B C**. Associated with gene deletion on chromosome 3 (sporadic or inherited as von Hippel-Lindau syndrome). RCC = 3 letters = chromosome 3. Associated with paraneoplastic syndromes (e.g., ectopic EPO, ACTH, PTHrP).
"Silent" cancer because commonly presents as a metastatic neoplasm.

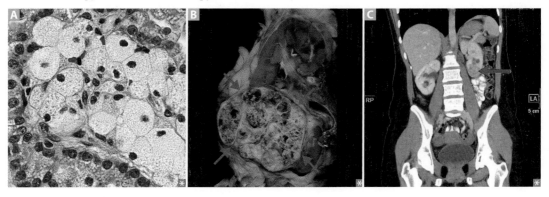

Renal oncocytoma

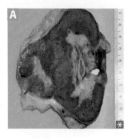

Benign epithelial cell tumor (arrows in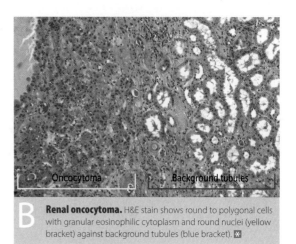
point to well-circumscribed mass with central
scar). Large eosinophilic cells with abundant
mitochondria without perinuclear clearing B
(vs. chromophobe renal cell carcinoma).
Presents with painless hematuria, flank pain,
abdominal mass.

Often resected to exclude malignancy (e.g.,
renal cell carcinoma).

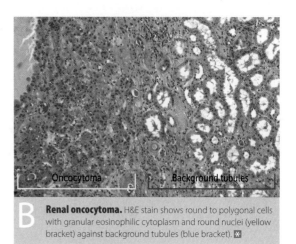

Oncocytoma   Background tubules

Renal oncocytoma. H&E stain shows round to polygonal cells
with granular eosinophilic cytoplasm and round nuclei (yellow
bracket) against background tubules (blue bracket). ✲

**Wilms tumor
(nephroblastoma)**

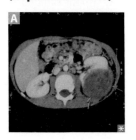

Most common renal malignancy of early childhood (ages 2–4). Contains embryonic glomerular
structures. Presents with large, palpable, unilateral flank mass A and/or hematuria.

"Loss of function" mutations of tumor suppressor genes *WT1* or *WT2* on chromosome 11.

May be part of Beckwith-Wiedemann syndrome (Wilms tumor, macroglossia, organomegaly,
hemihypertrophy) or **WAGR** complex: **W**ilms tumor, **A**niridia, **G**enitourinary malformation,
mental **R**etardation (intellectual disability).

Transitional cell carcinoma

Most common tumor of urinary tract system (can occur in renal calyces, renal pelvis, ureters, and bladder) A B. Painless hematuria (no casts) suggests bladder cancer.

Associated with problems in your Pee SAC: Phenacetin, Smoking, Aniline dyes, and Cyclophosphamide.

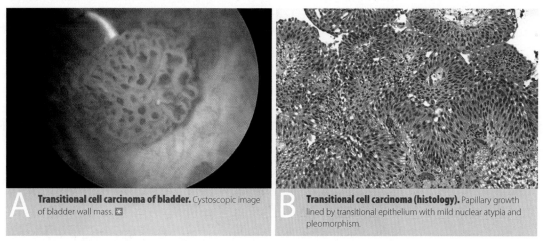

A **Transitional cell carcinoma of bladder.** Cystoscopic image of bladder wall mass. ✱

B **Transitional cell carcinoma (histology).** Papillary growth lined by transitional epithelium with mild nuclear atypia and pleomorphism.

Squamous cell carcinoma of the bladder

Chronic irritation of urinary bladder → squamous metaplasia → dysplasia and squamous cell carcinoma.

Risk factors include *Schistosoma haematobium* infection (Middle East), chronic cystitis, smoking, chronic nephrolithiasis. Presents with painless hematuria.

Urinary tract infection (acute bacterial cystitis)

Inflammation of urinary bladder. Presents as suprapubic pain, dysuria, urinary frequency, urgency. Systemic signs (e.g., high fever, chills) are usually absent.

Risk factors include female gender (short urethra), sexual intercourse ("honeymoon cystitis"), indwelling catheter, diabetes mellitus, impaired bladder emptying.

Causes:

- *E. coli* (most common).
- *Staphylococcus saprophyticus*—seen in sexually active young women (*E. coli* is still more common in this group).
- *Klebsiella*.
- *Proteus mirabilis*—urine has ammonia scent.

Lab findings: ⊕ leukocyte esterase. ⊕ nitrites for gram-negative organisms (especially *E. coli*). Sterile pyuria and ⊖ urine cultures suggest urethritis by *Neisseria gonorrhoeae* or *Chlamydia trachomatis*.

Pyelonephritis

Acute	Neutrophils infiltrate renal interstitium A. Affects cortex with relative sparing of glomeruli/vessels. Presents with fevers, flank pain (costovertebral angle tenderness).
	Causes include ascending UTI (*E. coli* is most common), hematogenous spread to kidney. Presents with WBCs in urine +/– WBC casts. CT shows striated parenchymal enhancement (arrow in B).
	Risk factors include indwelling urinary catheter, urinary tract obstruction, vesicoureteral reflux, diabetes mellitus, pregnancy.
	Complications include chronic pyelonephritis, renal papillary necrosis, perinephric abscess, urosepsis.
	Treatment: antibiotics.
Chronic	The result of recurrent episodes of acute pyelonephritis. Typically requires predisposition to infection such as vesicoureteral reflux or chronically obstructing kidney stones.
	Coarse, asymmetric corticomedullary scarring, blunted calyx. Tubules can contain eosinophilic casts resembling thyroid tissue C (thyroidization of kidney).

Drug-induced interstitial nephritis (tubulointerstitial nephritis)	Acute interstitial renal inflammation. Pyuria (classically eosinophils) and azotemia occurring after administration of drugs that act as haptens, inducing hypersensitivity. Nephritis typically occurs 1–2 weeks after certain drugs (e.g., diuretics, penicillin derivatives, proton pump inhibitors, sulfonamides, rifampin), but can occur months after starting NSAIDs.	Associated with fever, rash, hematuria, and costovertebral angle tenderness, but can be asymptomatic.
Diffuse cortical necrosis	Acute generalized cortical infarction of both kidneys. Likely due to a combination of vasospasm and DIC.	Associated with obstetric catastrophes (e.g., abruptio placentae), septic shock.

Acute tubular necrosis

Most common cause of acute kidney injury in hospitalized patients. Spontaneously resolves in many cases. Can be fatal, especially during initial oliguric phase. ↑ FENa.

Key finding: granular ("muddy brown") casts 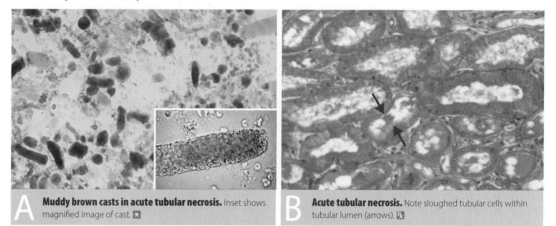.

3 stages:

1. Inciting event
2. Maintenance phase—oliguric; lasts 1–3 weeks; risk of hyperkalemia, metabolic acidosis, uremia
3. Recovery phase—polyuric; BUN and serum creatinine fall; risk of hypokalemia

Can be caused by ischemic or nephrotoxic injury:

- Ischemic—2° to ↓ renal blood flow (e.g., hypotension, shock, sepsis, hemorrhage, HF). Results in death of tubular cells that may slough into tubular lumen B (PCT and thick ascending limb are highly susceptible to injury).
- Nephrotoxic—2° to injury resulting from toxic substances (e.g., aminoglycosides, radiocontrast agents, lead, cisplatin), crush injury (myoglobinuria), hemoglobinuria. PCT is particularly susceptible to injury.

A **Muddy brown casts in acute tubular necrosis.** Inset shows magnified image of cast. ✱

B **Acute tubular necrosis.** Note sloughed tubular cells within tubular lumen (arrows). ℞

Renal papillary necrosis

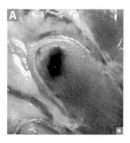

Sloughing of necrotic renal papillae A → gross hematuria and proteinuria. May be triggered by recent infection or immune stimulus. Associated with sickle cell disease or trait, acute pyelonephritis, NSAIDs, diabetes mellitus.

SAAD papa with papillary necrosis:
Sickle cell disease or trait
Acute pyelonephritis
Analgesics (NSAIDs)
Diabetes mellitus

Acute kidney injury (acute renal failure)	Acute kidney injury is defined as an abrupt decline in renal function as measured by ↑ creatinine and ↑ BUN.
Prerenal azotemia	Due to ↓ RBF (e.g., hypotension) → ↓ GFR. Na^+/H_2O and BUN retained by kidney in an attempt to conserve volume → ↑ BUN/creatinine ratio (BUN is reabsorbed, creatinine is not) and ↓ FENa.
Intrinsic renal failure	Generally due to acute tubular necrosis or ischemia/toxins; less commonly due to acute glomerulonephritis (e.g., RPGN, hemolytic uremic syndrome). In ATN, patchy necrosis → debris obstructing tubule and fluid backflow across necrotic tubule → ↓ GFR. Urine has epithelial/granular casts. BUN reabsorption is impaired → ↓ BUN/creatinine ratio.
Postrenal azotemia	Due to outflow obstruction (stones, BPH, neoplasia, congenital anomalies). Develops only with bilateral obstruction.

Variable	Prerenal	Intrinsic Renal	Postrenal
Urine osmolality (mOsm/kg)	> 500	< 350	< 350
Urine Na^+ (mEq/L)	< 20	> 40	> 40
FENa	< 1%	> 2%	> 1% (mild) > 2% (severe)
Serum BUN/Cr	> 20	< 15	Varies

Consequences of renal failure	Inability to make urine and excrete nitrogenous wastes. Consequences (**MAD HUNGER**): <ul><li>**M**etabolic Acidosis</li><li>**D**yslipidemia (especially ↑ triglycerides)</li><li>**H**yperkalemia</li><li>**U**remia—clinical syndrome marked by ↑ BUN:<ul><li>Nausea and anorexia</li><li>Pericarditis</li><li>Asterixis</li><li>Encephalopathy</li><li>Platelet dysfunction</li></ul></li><li>**N**a$^+$/H$_2$O retention (HF, pulmonary edema, hypertension)</li><li>**G**rowth retardation and developmental delay</li><li>**E**rythropoietin failure (anemia)</li><li>**R**enal osteodystrophy</li></ul>	2 forms of renal failure: acute (e.g., ATN) and chronic (e.g., hypertension, diabetes mellitus, congenital anomalies).

Renal osteodystrophy	Failure of vitamin D hydroxylation, hypocalcemia, and hyperphosphatemia → 2° hyperparathyroidism. Hyperphosphatemia also independently ↓ serum Ca^{2+} by causing tissue calcifications, whereas ↓ 1,25-$(OH)_2$ D_3 → ↓ intestinal Ca^{2+} absorption. Causes subperiosteal thinning of bones.

Renal cyst disorders

ADPKD	Formerly adult polycystic kidney disease. Numerous cysts causing bilateral enlarged kidneys ultimately destroy kidney parenchyma. Presents with flank pain, hematuria, hypertension, urinary infection, progressive renal failure. Autosomal Dominant; mutation in *PKD1* (85% of cases, chromosome 16) or *PKD2* (15% of cases, chromosome 4). Death from complications of chronic kidney disease or hypertension (caused by ↑ renin production). Associated with berry aneurysms, mitral valve prolapse, benign hepatic cysts.
ARPKD	Formerly infantile polycystic kidney disease ◼. Presents in infancy. Autosomal Recessive. Associated with congenital hepatic fibrosis. Significant oliguric renal failure in utero can lead to Potter sequence. Concerns beyond neonatal period include systemic hypertension, progressive renal insufficiency, and portal hypertension from congenital hepatic fibrosis.
Medullary cystic disease	Inherited disease causing tubulointerstitial fibrosis and progressive renal insufficiency with inability to concentrate urine. Medullary cysts usually not visualized; shrunken kidneys on ultrasound. Poor prognosis.
Simple vs. complex renal cysts	Simple cysts are filled with ultrafiltrate (anechoic on ultrasound ◼). Very common and account for majority of all renal masses. Found incidentally and typically asymptomatic. Complex cysts, including those that are septated, enhanced, or have solid components on imaging require follow-up or removal due to risk of renal cell carcinoma.

Diuretics: site of action

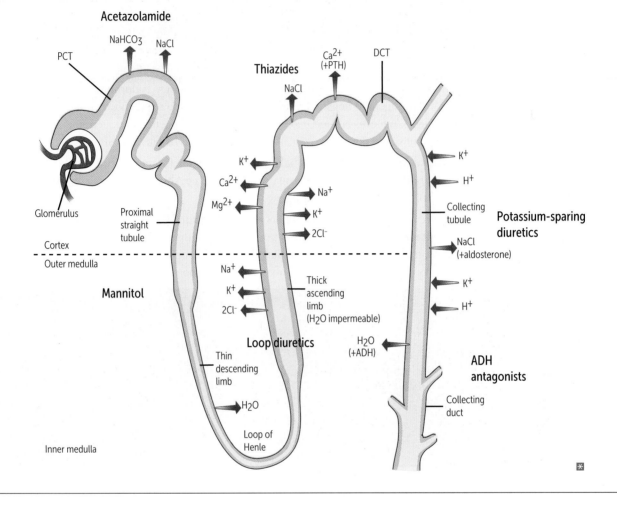

Mannitol

MECHANISM	Osmotic diuretic. ↑ tubular fluid osmolarity → ↑ urine flow, ↓ intracranial/intraocular pressure.
CLINICAL USE	Drug overdose, elevated intracranial/intraocular pressure.
TOXICITY	Pulmonary edema, dehydration. Contraindicated in anuria, HF.

Acetazolamide

MECHANISM	Carbonic anhydrase inhibitor. Causes self-limited $NaHCO_3$ diuresis and ↓ total body HCO_3^- stores.
CLINICAL USE	Glaucoma, urinary alkalinization, metabolic alkalosis, altitude sickness, pseudotumor cerebri.
TOXICITY	Hyperchloremic metabolic acidosis, paresthesias, NH_3 toxicity, sulfa allergy.

"ACID"azolamide causes ACIDosis.

Loop diuretics

Furosemide, bumetanide, torsemide

MECHANISM	Sulfonamide loop diuretics. Inhibit cotransport system ($Na^+/K^+/2Cl^-$) of thick ascending limb of loop of Henle. Abolish hypertonicity of medulla, preventing concentration of urine. Stimulate PGE release (vasodilatory effect on afferent arteriole); inhibited by NSAIDs. ↑ Ca^{2+} excretion. Loops Lose Ca^{2+}.
CLINICAL USE	Edematous states (HF, cirrhosis, nephrotic syndrome, pulmonary edema), hypertension, hypercalcemia.
TOXICITY	Ototoxicity, Hypokalemia, Dehydration, Allergy (sulfa), Nephritis (interstitial), Gout.

OH DANG!

Ethacrynic acid

MECHANISM	Phenoxyacetic acid derivative (not a sulfonamide). Essentially same action as furosemide.
CLINICAL USE	Diuresis in patients allergic to sulfa drugs.
TOXICITY	Similar to furosemide; can cause hyperuricemia; never use to treat gout.

Thiazide diuretics	Chlorthalidone, hydrochlorothiazide.	
MECHANISM	Inhibit NaCl reabsorption in early DCT → ↓ diluting capacity of nephron. ↓ Ca^{2+} excretion.	
CLINICAL USE	Hypertension, HF, idiopathic hypercalciuria, nephrogenic diabetes insipidus, osteoporosis.	
TOXICITY	Hypokalemic metabolic alkalosis, hyponatremia, hyperGlycemia, hyperLipidemia, hyperUricemia, hyperCalcemia. Sulfa allergy.	HyperGLUC.

K⁺-sparing diuretics	Spironolactone and eplerenone; Triamterene, and Amiloride.	The K^+ STAys.
MECHANISM	Spironolactone and eplerenone are competitive aldosterone receptor antagonists in cortical collecting tubule. Triamterene and amiloride act at the same part of the tubule by blocking Na^+ channels in the cortical collecting tubule.	
CLINICAL USE	Hyperaldosteronism, K^+ depletion, HF.	
TOXICITY	Hyperkalemia (can lead to arrhythmias), endocrine effects with spironolactone (e.g., gynecomastia, antiandrogen effects).	

Diuretics: electrolyte changes

Urine NaCl	↑ with all diuretics except acetazolamide. Serum NaCl may decrease as a result.
Urine K⁺	↑ with loop and thiazide diuretics. Serum K^+ may decrease as a result.
Blood pH	↓ (**acidemia**): carbonic anhydrase inhibitors: ↓ HCO_3^- reabsorption. K^+ sparing: aldosterone blockade prevents K^+ secretion and H^+ secretion. Additionally, hyperkalemia leads to K^+ entering all cells (via H^+/K^+ exchanger) in exchange for H^+ exiting cells. ↑ (**alkalemia**): loop diuretics and thiazides cause alkalemia through several mechanisms: ▪ Volume contraction → ↑ AT II → ↑ Na^+/H^+ exchange in PCT → ↑ HCO_3^- reabsorption ("contraction alkalosis") ▪ K^+ loss leads to K^+ exiting all cells (via H^+/K^+ exchanger) in exchange for H^+ entering cells ▪ In low K^+ state, H^+ (rather than K^+) is exchanged for Na^+ in cortical collecting tubule → alkalosis and "paradoxical aciduria"
Urine Ca²⁺	↑ with loop diuretics: ↓ paracellular Ca^{2+} reabsorption → hypocalcemia. ↓ with thiazides: Enhanced Ca^{2+} reabsorption in DCT.

ACE inhibitors	Captopril, enalapril, lisinopril, ramipril.	
MECHANISM	Inhibit ACE → ↓ AT II → ↓ GFR by preventing constriction of efferent arterioles. Levels of renin ↑ as a result of loss of feedback inhibition. Inhibition of ACE also prevents inactivation of bradykinin, a potent vasodilator.	
CLINICAL USE	Hypertension, HF, proteinuria, diabetic nephropathy. Prevent unfavorable heart remodeling as a result of chronic hypertension.	In diabetic nephropathy, ↓ intraglomerular pressure, slowing GBM thickening.
TOXICITY	Cough, Angioedema (contraindicated in C1 esterase inhibitor deficiency), Teratogen (fetal renal malformations), ↑ Creatinine (↓ GFR), Hyperkalemia, and Hypotension. Avoid in bilateral renal artery stenosis, because ACE inhibitors will further ↓ GFR → renal failure.	Captopril's **CATCHH**.

Angiotensin II receptor blockers	Losartan, candesartan, valsartan.
MECHANISM	Selectively block binding of angiotensin II to AT_1 receptor. Effects similar to ACE inhibitors, but ARBs do not increase bradykinin.
CLINICAL USE	Hypertension, HF, proteinuria, or diabetic nephropathy with intolerance to ACE inhibitors (e.g., cough, angioedema).
TOXICITY	Hyperkalemia, ↓ renal function, hypotension; teratogen.

Aliskiren	
MECHANISM	Direct renin inhibitor, blocks conversion of angiotensinogen to angiotensin I.
CLINICAL USE	Hypertension.
TOXICITY	Hyperkalemia, ↓ renal function, hypotension. Contraindicated in diabetics taking ACE inhibitors or ARBs.

▶ NOTES

Reproductive

"Artificial insemination is when the farmer does it to the cow instead of the bull."

—Student essay

"Whoever called it necking was a poor judge of anatomy."

—Groucho Marx

"See, the problem is that God gives men a brain and a penis, and only enough blood to run one at a time."

—Robin Williams

▶ REPRODUCTIVE—EMBRYOLOGY

Important genes of embryogenesis

Sonic hedgehog gene	Produced at base of limbs in zone of polarizing activity. Involved in patterning along anterior-posterior axis. Involved in CNS development; mutation can cause holoprosencephaly.
Wnt-7 gene	Produced at apical ectodermal ridge (thickened ectoderm at distal end of each developing limb). Necessary for proper organization along dorsal-ventral axis.
FGF gene	Produced at apical ectodermal ridge. Stimulates mitosis of underlying mesoderm, providing for lengthening of limbs.
Homeobox (Hox) genes	Involved in segmental organization of embryo in a craniocaudal direction. Code for transcription factors. Hox mutations → appendages in wrong locations.

Early fetal development

Day 0	Fertilization by sperm, forming zygote, initiating embryogenesis.	
Within week 1	hCG secretion begins around the time of implantation of blastocyst ("it 'sticks' at day 6").	
Within week 2	Bilaminar disc (epiblast, hypoblast). 2 weeks = 2 layers.	
Within week 3	Trilaminar disc. 3 weeks = 3 layers. Gastrulation. Primitive streak, notochord, mesoderm and its organization, and neural plate begin to form.	
Weeks 3–8 (embryonic period)	Neural tube formed by neuroectoderm and closes by week 4. Organogenesis. Extremely susceptible to teratogens.	
Week 4	Heart begins to beat. Upper and lower limb buds begin to form. 4 weeks = 4 limbs.	
Week 6	Fetal cardiac activity visible by transvaginal ultrasound.	
Week 10	Genitalia have male/female characteristics.	

Gastrulation	Process that forms the trilaminar embryonic disc. Establishes the ectoderm, mesoderm, and endoderm germ layers. Starts with the epiblast invaginating to form the primitive streak.

Embryologic derivatives

Ectoderm		External/outer layer
Surface ectoderm	Epidermis; adenohypophysis (from Rathke pouch); lens of eye; epithelial linings of oral cavity, sensory organs of ear, and olfactory epithelium; epidermis; anal canal below the pectinate line; parotid, sweat, and mammary glands.	Craniopharyngioma—benign Rathke pouch tumor with cholesterol crystals, calcifications.
Neuroectoderm	Brain (neurohypophysis, CNS neurons, oligodendrocytes, astrocytes, ependymal cells, pineal gland), retina and optic nerve, spinal cord.	Neuroectoderm—think CNS.
Neural crest	PNS (dorsal root ganglia, cranial nerves, celiac ganglion, Schwann cells, ANS), melanocytes, chromaffin cells of adrenal medulla, parafollicular (C) cells of thyroid, pia and arachnoid, bones of the skull, odontoblasts, aorticopulmonary septum.	Neural crest—think PNS and non-neural structures nearby.
Mesoderm	Muscle, bone, connective tissue, serous linings of body cavities (e.g., peritoneum), spleen (derived from foregut mesentery), cardiovascular structures, lymphatics, blood, wall of gut tube, vagina, kidneys, adrenal cortex, dermis, testes, ovaries. Notochord induces ectoderm to form neuroectoderm (neural plate). Its only postnatal derivative is the nucleus pulposus of the intervertebral disc.	Middle/"meat" layer. Mesodermal defects = **VACTERL**: **V**ertebral defects **A**nal atresia **C**ardiac defects **T**racheo-**E**sophageal fistula **R**enal defects **L**imb defects (bone and muscle)
Endoderm	Gut tube epithelium (including anal canal above the pectinate line), most of urethra (derived from urogenital sinus), luminal epithelial derivatives (e.g., lungs, liver, gallbladder, pancreas, eustachian tube, thymus, parathyroid, thyroid follicular cells).	Enternal layer.

Types of errors in organ morphogenesis

Agenesis	Absent organ due to absent primordial tissue.
Aplasia	Absent organ despite presence of primordial tissue.
Hypoplasia	Incomplete organ development; primordial tissue present.
Deformation	Extrinsic disruption; occurs after embryonic period.
Disruption	2° breakdown of previously normal tissue or structure (e.g., amniotic band syndrome).
Malformation	Intrinsic disruption; occurs during embryonic period (weeks 3–8).
Sequence	Abnormalities result from a single 1° embryologic event (e.g., oligohydramnios → Potter sequence).

Teratogens	Most susceptible in 3rd–8th weeks (embryonic period—organogenesis) of pregnancy. Before week 3, "all-or-none" effects. After week 8, growth and function affected.

TERATOGEN	EFFECTS ON FETUS	NOTES
Medications		
ACE inhibitors	Renal damage	
Alkylating agents	Absence of digits, multiple anomalies	
Aminoglycosides	CN VIII toxicity	**A mean guy** hit the baby in the ear.
Carbamazepine	Facial dysmorphism, developmental delay, neural tube defects, phalanx/fingernail hypoplasia	
Diethylstilbestrol (DES)	Vaginal clear cell adenocarcinoma, congenital Müllerian anomalies	
Folate antagonists	Neural tube defects	
Isotretinoin	Multiple severe birth defects	Contraception mandatory
Lithium	Ebstein anomaly (atrialized right ventricle)	
Methimazole	Aplasia cutis congenita	
Phenytoin	Fetal hydantoin syndrome—cleft palate, cardiac defects, phalanx/fingernail hypoplasia	
Tetracyclines	Discolored teeth	"**Teeth**racyclines."
Thalidomide	Limb defects (phocomelia, micromelia—"flipper" limbs)	**Limb** defects with "tha-**limb**-domide."
Valproate	Inhibition of maternal folate absorption → neural tube defects	Valproate inhibits folate absorption.
Warfarin	Bone deformities, fetal hemorrhage, abortion, ophthalmologic abnormalities	Do not wage **warfar**e on the baby; keep it **hep**py with **hep**arin (does not cross placenta).
Substance abuse		
Alcohol	Common cause of birth defects and intellectual disability; fetal alcohol syndrome	
Cocaine	Abnormal fetal growth and fetal addiction; placental abruption	
Smoking (nicotine, CO)	Low birth weight (leading cause in developed countries), preterm labor, placental problems, IUGR, ADHD	Nicotine → vasoconstriction. CO → impaired O_2 delivery.
Other		
Iodine (lack or excess)	Congenital goiter or hypothyroidism (cretinism)	
Maternal diabetes	Caudal regression syndrome (anal atresia to sirenomelia), congenital heart defects, neural tube defects	
Vitamin A (excess)	Extremely high risk for spontaneous abortions and birth defects (cleft palate, cardiac)	
X-rays	Microcephaly, intellectual disability	Minimized by lead shielding.

Fetal alcohol syndrome	Leading cause of intellectual disability in the U.S. Newborns of alcohol-consuming mothers have ↑ incidence of congenital abnormalities, including pre- and postnatal developmental retardation, microcephaly, facial abnormalities (e.g., smooth philtrum, hypertelorism), limb dislocation, heart defects. Heart-lung fistulas and holoprosencephaly in most severe form. Mechanism is failure of cell migration.
Twinning	Dizygotic twins arise from 2 eggs that are separately fertilized by 2 different sperm (always 2 zygotes) and will have 2 separate amniotic sacs and 2 separate placentas (chorions). Monozygotic twins arise from 1 fertilized egg (1 egg + 1 sperm) that splits into 2 zygotes in early pregnancy. The degree of separation between monozygotic twins depends on when the fertilized egg splits into 2 zygotes. The timing of this separation determines the number of chorions and the number of amnions.

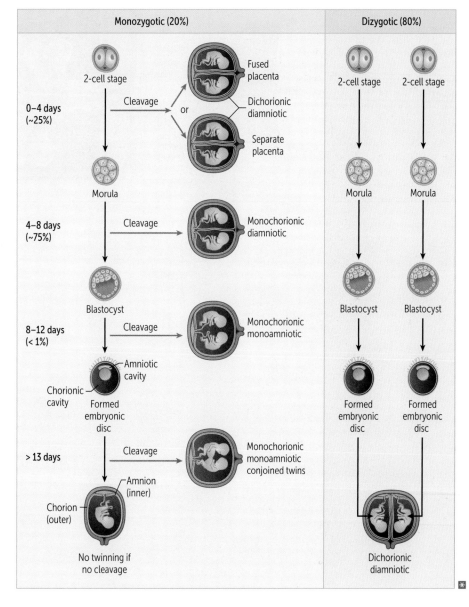

Placenta	1° site of nutrient and gas exchange between mother and fetus.	
Fetal component		
Cytotrophoblast	Inner layer of chorionic villi.	Cytotrophoblast makes Cells.
Syncytiotrophoblast	Outer layer of chorionic villi; secretes hCG (structurally similar to LH; stimulates corpus luteum to secrete progesterone during first trimester).	Lacks MHC-I expression → ↓ chance of attack by maternal immune system.
Maternal component		
Decidua basalis	Derived from endometrium. Maternal blood in lacunae.	

| **Umbilical cord** | Umbilical arteries (2)—return deoxygenated blood from fetal internal iliac arteries to placenta 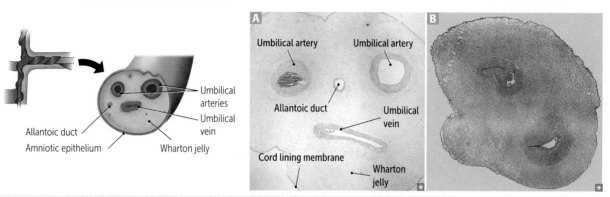. Umbilical vein (1)—supplies oxygenated blood from placenta to fetus; drains into IVC via liver or via ductus venosus. | Single umbilical artery (2-vessel cord B) is associated with congenital and chromosomal anomalies. Umbilical arteries and vein are derived from allantois. |

Labels on diagram: Allantoic duct, Amniotic epithelium, Wharton jelly, Umbilical arteries, Umbilical vein

Labels on image A: Umbilical artery, Umbilical artery, Allantoic duct, Umbilical vein, Cord lining membrane, Wharton jelly

Urachus	In the 3rd week the yolk sac forms the allantois, which extends into urogenital sinus. Allantois becomes the urachus, a duct between fetal bladder and yolk sac.
Patent urachus	Total failure of urachus to obliterate → urine discharge from umbilicus.
Urachal cyst	Partial failure of urachus to obliterate; fluid-filled cavity lined with uroepithelium, between umbilicus and bladder. Can lead to infection, adenocarcinoma.
Vesicourachal diverticulum	Slight failure of urachus to obliterate → outpouching of bladder.

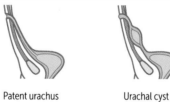 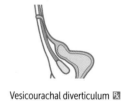

Patent urachus   Urachal cyst   Vesicourachal diverticulum

Vitelline duct	7th week—obliteration of vitelline duct (omphalo-mesenteric duct), which connects yolk sac to midgut lumen.
Vitelline fistula	Vitelline duct fails to close → meconium discharge from umbilicus.
Meckel diverticulum	Partial closure of vitelline duct, with patent portion attached to ileum (true diverticulum). May have heterotopic gastric and/or pancreatic tissue → melena, hematochezia, abdominal pain.

 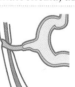

Normal   Vitelline fistula   Meckel diverticulum

Aortic arch derivatives	Develop into arterial system.	
1st	Part of **maxillary** artery (branch of external carotid).	1st arch is **maximal**.
2nd	Stapedial artery and hyoid artery.	Second = Stapedial.
3rd	Common Carotid artery and proximal part of internal Carotid artery.	C is 3rd letter of alphabet.
4th	On left, aortic arch; on right, proximal part of right subclavian artery.	4th arch (4 limbs) = systemic.
6th	Proximal part of pulmonary arteries and (on left only) ductus arteriosus.	6th arch = pulmonary and the pulmonary-to-systemic shunt (ductus arteriosus).

Right recurrent laryngeal nerve loops around here

Left recurrent laryngeal nerve gets caught here by the ductus arteriosus; ductus arteriosus turns into the ligamentum arteriosum shortly after birth

6 months postnatal

Branchial apparatus	Also called pharyngeal apparatus. Composed of branchial clefts, arches, pouches. Branchial clefts—derived from ectoderm. Also called branchial grooves. Branchial arches—derived from mesoderm (muscles, arteries) and neural crest (bones, cartilage). Branchial pouches—derived from endoderm.	**CAP** covers outside to inside: Clefts = ectoderm Arches = mesoderm Pouches = endoderm

Primitive pharynx

Arch
Cleft
Pouch

1st
2nd
3rd
4th

Pharyngeal arches

Epicardial ridge

Primitive esophagus

Branchial cleft derivatives	1st cleft develops into external auditory meatus. 2nd through 4th clefts form temporary cervical sinuses, which are obliterated by proliferation of 2nd arch mesenchyme. Persistent cervical sinus → branchial cleft cyst within lateral neck.

Branchial arch derivatives

ARCH	CARTILAGE	MUSCLES	NERVES[a]	ABNORMALITIES/COMMENTS
1st arch	Meckel cartilage: Mandible, Malleus, incus, spheno-Mandibular ligament	Muscles of Mastication (temporalis, Masseter, lateral and Medial pterygoids), Mylohyoid, anterior belly of digastric, tensor tympani, tensor veli palatini	CN V_2 and V_3 chew	Treacher Collins syndrome—1st-arch neural crest fails to migrate → mandibular hypoplasia, facial abnormalities
2nd arch	Reichert cartilage: Stapes, Styloid process, lesser horn of hyoid, Stylohyoid ligament	Muscles of facial expression, Stapedius, Stylohyoid, platySma, posterior belly of digastric	CN VII (facial expression) smile	Congenital pharyngo-cutaneous fistula—persistence of cleft and pouch → fistula between tonsillar area and lateral neck
3rd arch	Cartilage: greater horn of hyoid	Stylopharyngeus (think of stylo**pharyngeus** innervated by glosso**pharyngeal** nerve)	CN IX (stylo-pharyngeus) **swallow stylishly**	
4th–6th arches	Cartilages: thyroid, cricoid, arytenoids, corniculate, cuneiform	4th arch: most pharyngeal constrictors; cricothyroid, levator veli palatini 6th arch: all intrinsic muscles of larynx except cricothyroid	4th arch: CN X (superior laryngeal branch) **simply swallow** 6th arch: CN X (recurrent laryngeal branch) **speak**	Arches 3 and 4 form posterior ⅓ of tongue; arch 5 makes no major developmental contributions

[a]These are the only CNs with both motor and sensory components (except V_2, which is sensory only).

When at the restaurant of the golden **arches**, children tend to first **chew** (1), then **smile** (2), then **swallow styl**ishly (3) or **simply swallow** (4), and then **speak** (6).

Branchial pouch derivatives

POUCH	DERIVATIVES	NOTES	MNEMONIC
1st pouch	Develops into middle ear cavity, eustachian tube, mastoid air cells.	1st pouch contributes to endoderm-lined structures of ear.	**Ear, tonsils, bottom-to-top:** 1 (**ear**), 2 (**tonsils**), 3 dorsal (**bottom** for inferior parathyroids), 3 ventral (**to** = **thymus**), 4 (**top** = superior parathyroids).
2nd pouch	Develops into epithelial lining of palatine tonsil.		
3rd pouch	Dorsal wings—develop into **inferior** parathyroids. Ventral wings—develop into thymus.	3rd pouch contributes to 3 structures (thymus, left and right inferior parathyroids). 3rd-pouch structures end up **below** 4th-pouch structures.	
4th pouch	Dorsal wings—develop into **superior** parathyroids.		
DiGeorge syndrome	Aberrant development of 3rd and 4th pouches → T-cell deficiency (thymic aplasia) and hypocalcemia (failure of parathyroid development). Associated with cardiac defects (conotruncal anomalies).		
MEN 2A	Mutation of germline *RET* (neural crest cells): ▪ Adrenal medulla (pheochromocytoma). ▪ Parathyroid (tumor): 3rd/4th pharyngeal pouch. ▪ Parafollicular cells (medullary thyroid cancer): derived from neural crest cells; associated with 4th/5th pharyngeal pouches.		

Cleft lip and cleft palate

Cleft lip—failure of fusion of the maxillary and medial nasal processes (formation of 1° palate).

Cleft palate—failure of fusion of the two lateral palatine processes or failure of fusion of lateral palatine processes with the nasal septum and/or median palatine process (formation of 2° palate).

Cleft lip and cleft palate have two distinct etiologies, but often occur together.

Cleft lip

Roof of mouth — Nasal cavity
Palatine shelves (2° palate)
Uvula
Cleft palate (partial)

Genital embryology

Female	Default development. Mesonephric duct degenerates and paramesonephric duct develops.	
Male	SRY gene on Y chromosome—produces testis-determining factor → testes development. Sertoli cells secrete Müllerian inhibitory factor (MIF) that suppresses development of paramesonephric ducts. Leydig cells secrete androgens that stimulate development of mesonephric ducts.	
Paramesonephric (Müllerian) duct	Develops into female internal structures—fallopian tubes, uterus, upper portion of vagina (lower portion from urogenital sinus). **Müllerian agenesis**—may present as 1° amenorrhea (due to a lack of uterine development) in females with fully developed 2° sexual characteristics (functional ovaries).	
Mesonephric (Wolffian) duct	Develops into male internal structures (except prostate)—Seminal vesicles, Epididymis, Ejaculatory duct, Ductus deferens (**SEED**). In females, remnant of mesonephric duct → Gartner duct.	

Diagram labels (right side): Gubernaculum, Indifferent gonad, Mesonephros, Paramesonephric duct, Mesonephric duct, Urogenital sinus

---

SRY gene

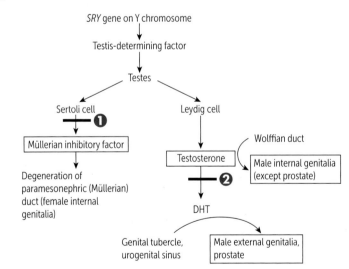

SRY gene on Y chromosome
↓
Testis-determining factor
↓
Testes
↙   ↘
Sertoli cell ❶   Leydig cell
↓   ↓   Wolffian duct
Müllerian inhibitory factor   Testosterone ──→ Male internal genitalia (except prostate)
↓   ↓ ❷
Degeneration of paramesonephric (Müllerian) duct (female internal genitalia)   DHT
                           ↓
Genital tubercle, urogenital sinus   Male external genitalia, prostate

❶ No Sertoli cells or lack of Müllerian inhibitory factor → develop both male and female internal genitalia and male external genitalia

❷ 5α-reductase deficiency—inability to convert testosterone into DHT → male internal genitalia, ambiguous external genitalia until puberty (when ↑ testosterone levels cause masculinization)

Uterine (Müllerian duct) anomalies

Septate uterus	Common anomaly vs. normal **A** uterus. Incomplete resorption of septum **B**. ↓ fertility. Treat with septoplasty.
Bicornuate uterus	Incomplete fusion of Müllerian ducts **C**. ↑ risk of complicated pregnancy.
Uterus didelphys	Complete failure of fusion → double uterus, vagina, and cervix **D**. Pregnancy possible.

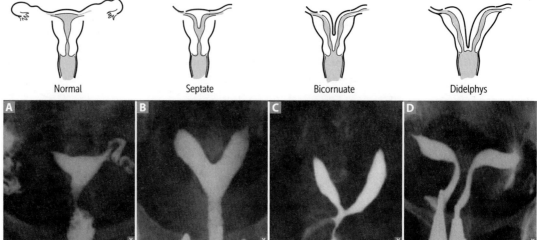

Normal   Septate   Bicornuate   Didelphys

Male/female genital homologs

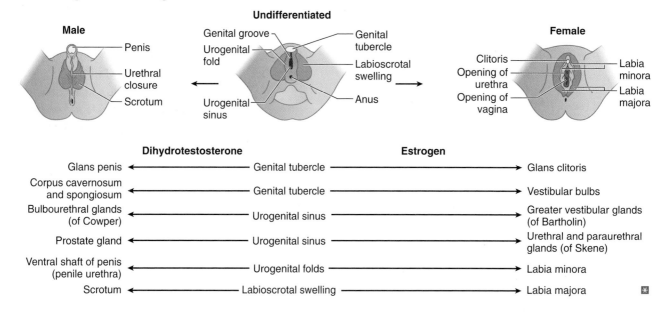

Congenital penile abnormalities

Hypospadias	Abnormal opening of penile urethra on ventral surface of penis due to failure of urethral folds to fuse.	Hypospadias is more common than epispadias. Associated with inguinal hernia and cryptorchidism. **Hypo** is below.
Epispadias	Abnormal opening of penile urethra on dorsal surface of penis due to faulty positioning of genital tubercle.	Exstrophy of the bladder is associated with Epispadias. When you have Epispadias, you hit your Eye when you pEE.

Descent of testes and ovaries

	MALE REMNANT	FEMALE REMNANT
Gubernaculum (band of fibrous tissue)	Anchors testes within scrotum.	Ovarian ligament + round ligament of uterus.
Processus vaginalis (evagination of peritoneum)	Forms tunica vaginalis.	Obliterated.

▶ REPRODUCTIVE—ANATOMY

Gonadal drainage

Venous drainage	Left ovary/testis → left gonadal vein → left renal vein → IVC. Right ovary/testis → right gonadal vein → IVC.	"Left gonadal vein takes the Longest way." Because the left spermatic vein enters the left renal vein at a 90° angle, flow is less laminar on left than on right → left venous pressure > right venous pressure → varicocele more common on the left.
Lymphatic drainage	Ovaries/testes → para-aortic lymph nodes. Distal vagina/vulva/scrotum → superficial inguinal nodes. Proximal vagina/uterus → obturator, external iliac and hypogastric nodes.	

Female reproductive anatomy

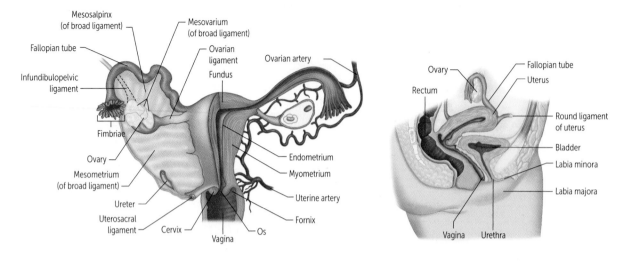

Posterior view   Sagittal view

LIGAMENT	CONNECTS	STRUCTURES CONTAINED	NOTES
Infundibulopelvic ligament (suspensory ligament of the ovary)	Ovaries to lateral pelvic wall	Ovarian vessels	Ligate vessels during oophorectomy to avoid bleeding. Ureter courses retroperitoneally, close to gonadal vessels → at risk of injury during ligation of ovarian vessels.
Cardinal ligament (not labeled)	Cervix to side wall of pelvis	Uterine vessels	Ureter at risk of injury during ligation of uterine vessels in hysterectomy.
Round ligament of the uterus	Uterine fundus to labia majora		Derivative of gubernaculum. Travels through **round** inguinal canal; above the artery of Sampson.
Broad ligament	Uterus, fallopian tubes, and ovaries to pelvic side wall	Ovaries, fallopian tubes, round ligaments of uterus	Mesosalpinx, mesometrium, and mesovarium comprise the broad ligament.
Ovarian ligament	Medial pole of ovary to lateral uterus	—	Derivative of gubernaculum. Ovarian Ligament Latches to Lateral uterus.

Female reproductive epithelial histology

TISSUE	HISTOLOGY/NOTES
Vagina	Stratified squamous epithelium, nonkeratinized
Ectocervix	Stratified squamous epithelium, nonkeratinized
Transformation zone	Squamocolumnar junction A (most common area for cervical cancer)
Endocervix	Simple columnar epithelium
Uterus	Simple columnar epithelium with long tubular glands in follicular phase; coiled glands in luteal phase
Fallopian tube	Simple columnar epithelium, ciliated
Ovary, outer surface	Simple cuboidal epithelium (germinal epithelium covering surface of ovary)

Female sexual response cycle	Most commonly described as phase of excitement (uterus elevates, vaginal lubrication), plateau (expansion of inner vagina), orgasm (contraction of uterus), resolution; mediated by autonomic nervous system. Also causes tachycardia and skin flushing.

Male reproductive anatomy

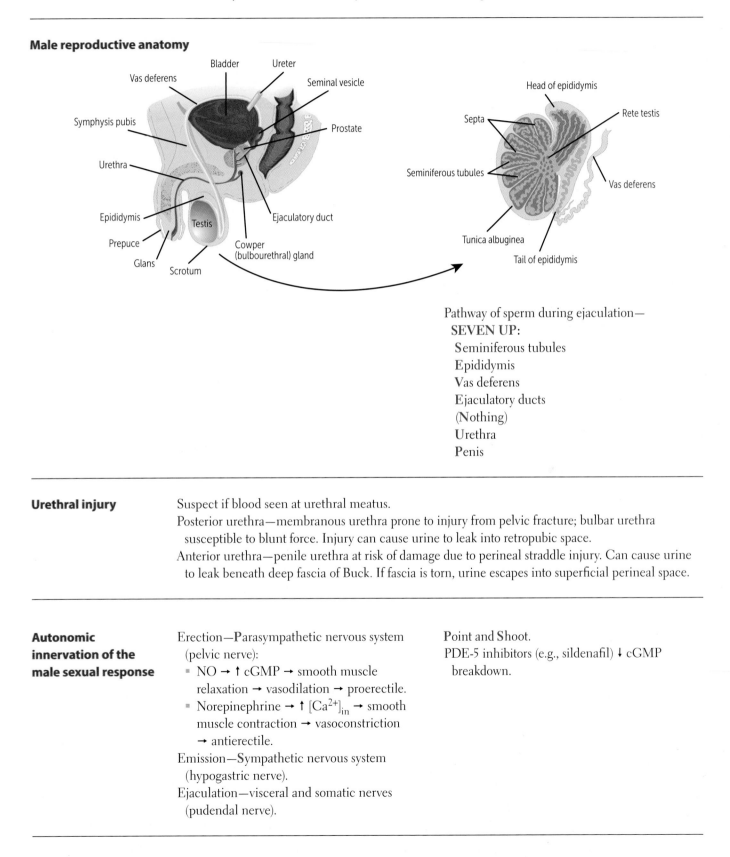

Pathway of sperm during ejaculation—
  SEVEN UP:
  Seminiferous tubules
  Epididymis
  Vas deferens
  Ejaculatory ducts
  (Nothing)
  Urethra
  Penis

Urethral injury	Suspect if blood seen at urethral meatus. Posterior urethra—membranous urethra prone to injury from pelvic fracture; bulbar urethra susceptible to blunt force. Injury can cause urine to leak into retropubic space. Anterior urethra—penile urethra at risk of damage due to perineal straddle injury. Can cause urine to leak beneath deep fascia of Buck. If fascia is torn, urine escapes into superficial perineal space.

Autonomic innervation of the male sexual response	Erection—Parasympathetic nervous system (pelvic nerve): ▪ NO → ↑ cGMP → smooth muscle relaxation → vasodilation → proerectile. ▪ Norepinephrine → ↑ $[Ca^{2+}]_{in}$ → smooth muscle contraction → vasoconstriction → antierectile. Emission—Sympathetic nervous system (hypogastric nerve). Ejaculation—visceral and somatic nerves (pudendal nerve).	Point and Shoot. PDE-5 inhibitors (e.g., sildenafil) ↓ cGMP breakdown.

Seminiferous tubules

CELL	FUNCTION	LOCATION/NOTES
Spermatogonia (germ cells)	Maintain germ pool and produce 1° spermatocytes.	Line seminiferous tubules
Sertoli cells (non–germ cells)	Secrete inhibin → inhibit FSH. Secrete androgen-binding protein → maintain local levels of testosterone. Tight junctions between adjacent Sertoli cells form blood-testis barrier → isolate gametes from autoimmune attack. Support and nourish developing spermatozoa. Regulate spermatogenesis. Produce MIF.	Line seminiferous tubules Convert testosterone and androstenedione to estrogens via aromatase Sertoli cells Support Sperm Synthesis Homolog of female granulosa cells
	Temperature sensitive; ↓ sperm production and ↓ inhibin with ↑ temperature.	↑ temperature seen in varicocele, cryptorchidism
Leydig cells (endocrine cells)	Secrete testosterone in the presence of LH; testosterone production unaffected by temperature.	Interstitium Homolog of female theca interna cells

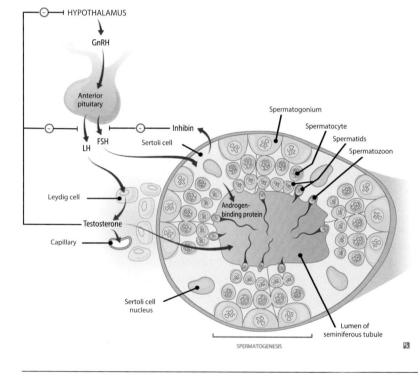

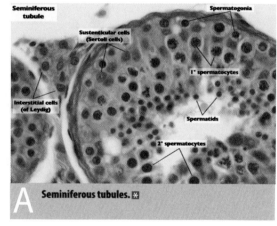

A Seminiferous tubules.

Estrogen

SOURCE	Ovary (17β-estradiol), placenta (estriol), adipose tissue (estrone via aromatization).	Potency: estradiol > estrone > estriol
FUNCTION	Development of genitalia and breast, female fat distribution. Growth of follicle, endometrial proliferation, ↑ myometrial excitability. Upregulation of estrogen, LH, and progesterone receptors; feedback inhibition of FSH and LH, then LH surge; stimulation of prolactin secretion. ↑ transport proteins, SHBG; ↑ HDL; ↓ LDL.	Pregnancy: • 50-fold ↑ in estradiol and estrone • 1000-fold ↑ in estriol (indicator of fetal well-being) Estrogen receptors expressed in cytoplasm; translocate to nucleus when bound by estrogen

Progesterone

SOURCE	Corpus luteum, placenta, adrenal cortex, testes.	Fall in progesterone after delivery disinhibits prolactin → lactation. ↑ progesterone is indicative of ovulation. Progesterone is **pro-gest**ation. Prolactin is **pro-lact**ation.
FUNCTION	Stimulation of endometrial glandular secretions and spiral artery development. Maintenance of pregnancy. ↓ myometrial excitability. Production of thick cervical mucus, which inhibits sperm entry into uterus. ↑ body temperature. Inhibition of gonadotropins (LH, FSH). Uterine smooth muscle relaxation (preventing contractions). ↓ estrogen receptor expression. Prevents endometrial hyperplasia.	

Tanner stages of sexual development

Tanner stage is assigned independently to genitalia, pubic hair, and breast (e.g., a person can have Tanner stage 2 genitalia, Tanner stage 3 pubic hair).

   I. Childhood (prepubertal)

   II. Pubic hair appears (pubarche); breast buds form (thelarche)

   III. Pubic hair darkens and becomes curly; penis size/length ↑; breasts enlarge

   IV. Penis width ↑, darker scrotal skin, development of glans; raised areolae

   V. Adult; areolae are no longer raised

Menstrual cycle

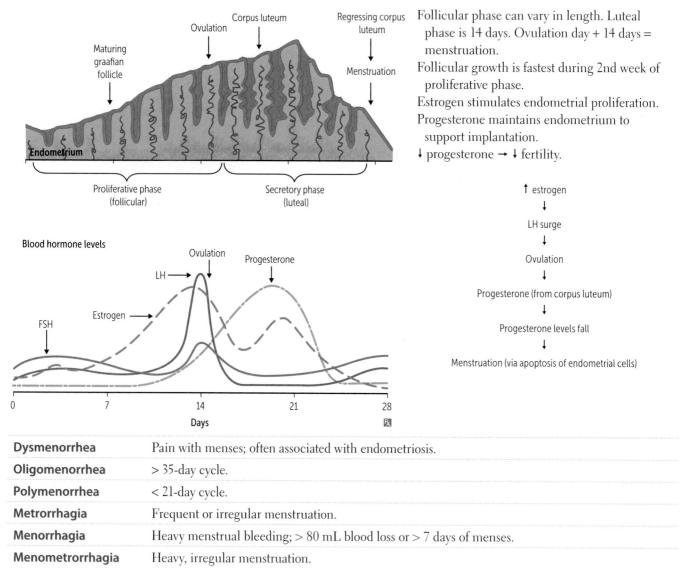

Follicular phase can vary in length. Luteal phase is 14 days. Ovulation day + 14 days = menstruation.

Follicular growth is fastest during 2nd week of proliferative phase.

Estrogen stimulates endometrial proliferation.

Progesterone maintains endometrium to support implantation.

↓ progesterone → ↓ fertility.

↑ estrogen
↓
LH surge
↓
Ovulation
↓
Progesterone (from corpus luteum)
↓
Progesterone levels fall
↓
Menstruation (via apoptosis of endometrial cells)

Dysmenorrhea	Pain with menses; often associated with endometriosis.
Oligomenorrhea	> 35-day cycle.
Polymenorrhea	< 21-day cycle.
Metrorrhagia	Frequent or irregular menstruation.
Menorrhagia	Heavy menstrual bleeding; > 80 mL blood loss or > 7 days of menses.
Menometrorrhagia	Heavy, irregular menstruation.

Oogenesis

1° oocytes begin meiosis I during fetal life and complete meiosis I just prior to ovulation.

Meiosis I is arrested in prOphase I for years until Ovulation (1° oocytes).

Meiosis II is arrested in **meta**phase II until fertilization (2° oocytes).

An egg **met** a sperm.

If fertilization does not occur within 1 day, the 2° oocyte degenerates.

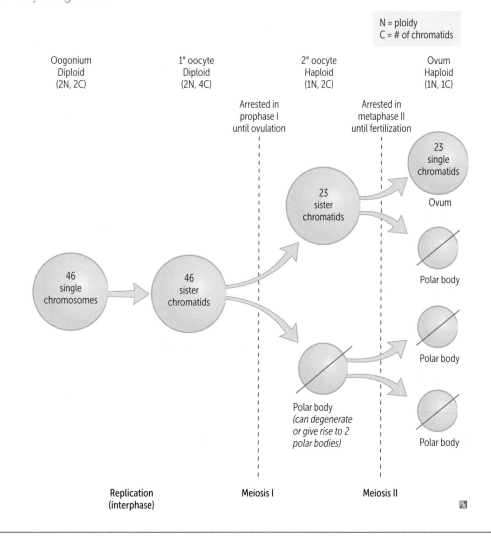

| **Ovulation** | ↑ estrogen, ↑ GnRH receptors on anterior pituitary. Estrogen surge then stimulates LH release → ovulation (rupture of follicle). ↑ temperature (progesterone induced). | Mittelschmerz—transient mid-cycle ovulatory pain; classically associated with peritoneal irritation (e.g., follicular swelling/rupture, fallopian tube contraction). Can mimic appendicitis. |

Pregnancy

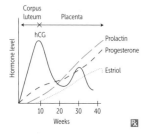

Fertilization most commonly occurs in upper end of fallopian tube (the ampulla). Occurs within 1 day of ovulation.

Implantation within the wall of the uterus occurs 6 days after fertilization. Syncytiotrophoblasts secrete hCG, which is detectable in blood 1 week after conception and on home test in urine 2 weeks after conception.

Lactation

After labor, the ↓ in progesterone and estrogen disinhibits lactation. Suckling is required to maintain milk production, since ↑ nerve stimulation → ↑ oxytocin and prolactin.

Prolactin—induces and maintains lactation and ↓ reproductive function.

Oxytocin—assists in milk letdown; also promotes uterine contractions.

Breast milk is the ideal nutrition for infants < 6 months old. Contains maternal immunoglobulins (conferring passive immunity; mostly IgA), macrophages, lymphocytes. Breast milk reduces infant infections and is associated with ↓ risk for child to develop asthma, allergies, diabetes mellitus, and obesity. Exclusively breastfed infants require vitamin D supplementation.

Breastfeeding ↓ maternal risk of breast and ovarian cancer and facilitates mother-child bonding.

---

hCG

SOURCE	Syncytiotrophoblast of placenta.
FUNCTION	Maintains corpus luteum (and thus progesterone) for first 8–10 weeks of pregnancy by acting like LH (otherwise no luteal cell stimulation → abortion). After 8–10 weeks, placenta synthesizes its own estriol and progesterone and corpus luteum degenerates. Used to detect pregnancy because it appears early in urine (see above). Has identical α subunit as LH, FSH, TSH. β subunit is unique (pregnancy tests detect β subunit). hCG is ↑ in multiple gestations, hydatidiform moles, choriocarcinomas, and Down syndrome; hCG is ↓ in ectopic/failing pregnancy, Edward syndrome, and Patau syndrome.

| **Menopause** | ↓ estrogen production due to age-linked decline in number of ovarian follicles. Average age at onset is 51 years (earlier in smokers).

Usually preceded by 4–5 years of abnormal menstrual cycles. Source of estrogen (estrone) after menopause becomes peripheral conversion of androgens, ↑ androgens → hirsutism.

↑↑ FSH is specific for menopause (loss of negative feedback on FSH due to ↓ estrogen). | Hormonal changes: ↓ estrogen, ↑↑ FSH, ↑ LH (no surge), ↑ GnRH.

Menopause causes **HAVOCS**: Hot flashes, Atrophy of the Vagina, Osteoporosis, Coronary artery disease, Sleep disturbances.

Menopause before age 40 can indicate premature ovarian failure. |

Spermatogenesis	Spermatogenesis begins at puberty with spermatogonia. Full development takes 2 months. Occurs in seminiferous tubules. Produces spermatids that undergo spermiogenesis (loss of cytoplasmic contents, gain of acrosomal cap) to form mature spermatozoon.	"Gonium" is going to be a sperm; "Zoon" is "Zooming" to egg.

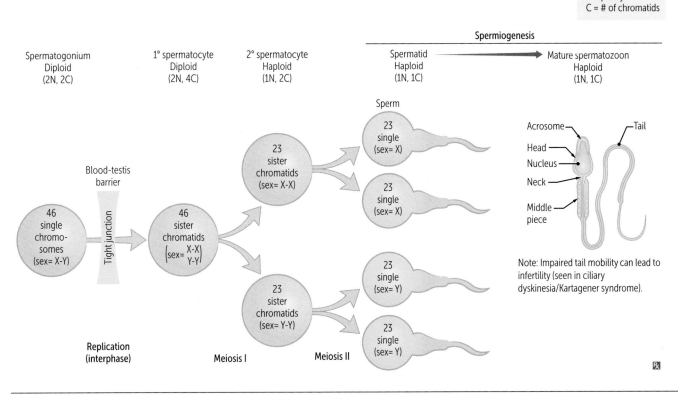

Androgens	Testosterone, dihydrotestosterone (DHT), androstenedione.	
SOURCE	DHT and testosterone (testis), AnDrostenedione (ADrenal)	Potency: DHT > testosterone > androstenedione.
FUNCTION	Testosterone: ▪ Differentiation of epididymis, vas deferens, seminal vesicles (genitalia, except prostate). ▪ Growth spurt: penis, seminal vesicles, sperm, muscle, RBCs. ▪ Deepening of voice. ▪ Closing of epiphyseal plates (via estrogen converted from testosterone). ▪ Libido. DHT: ▪ Early—differentiation of penis, scrotum, prostate. ▪ Late—prostate growth, balding, sebaceous gland activity.	Testosterone is converted to DHT by 5α-reductase, which is inhibited by finasteride. In the male, androgens are converted to estrogen by cytochrome P-450 aromatase (primarily in adipose tissue and testis). Aromatase is the key enzyme in conversion of androgens to estrogen. Exogenous testosterone → inhibition of hypothalamic–pituitary–gonadal axis → ↓ intratesticular testosterone → ↓ testicular size → azoospermia.

▸ REPRODUCTIVE—PATHOLOGY

Sex chromosome disorders of sexual development

Klinefelter syndrome [male] (47,XXY), 1:850 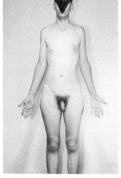	Testicular atrophy, eunuchoid body shape, tall, long extremities, gynecomastia, female hair distribution **A**. May present with developmental delay. Presence of inactivated X chromosome (Barr body). Common cause of hypogonadism seen in infertility work-up.	Dysgenesis of seminiferous tubules → ↓ inhibin → ↑ FSH. Abnormal Leydig cell function → ↓ testosterone → ↑ LH → ↑ estrogen.
Turner syndrome [female] (45,XO) **B**	Short stature (if untreated), ovarian dysgenesis (streak ovary), shield chest, bicuspid aortic valve, preductal coarctation (femoral < brachial pulse), lymphatic defects (result in webbed neck or cystic hygroma; lymphedema in feet, hands), horseshoe kidney **B**. Most common cause of 1° amenorrhea. No Barr body.	"Hugs and kisses" (XO) from Tina **Turner**. Menopause before menarche. ↓ estrogen leads to ↑ LH, FSH. Can result from mitotic or meiotic error. Can be complete monosomy (45,XO) or mosaicism (e.g., 45,XO/46,XX). Pregnancy is possible in some cases (oocyte donation, exogenous estradiol-17β and progesterone).
Double Y males [male] (XYY), 1:1000	Phenotypically normal (usually undiagnosed), very tall. Random nondisjunction event (paternal meiosis II); noninherited; normal fertility. May be associated with severe acne, learning disability, autism spectrum disorders.	
True hermaphroditism (46,XX or 47,XXY)	Also called ovotesticular disorder of sex development. Both ovarian and testicular tissue present (ovotestis); ambiguous genitalia.	

Diagnosing disorders of sex hormones	Testosterone	LH	Diagnosis
	↑	↑	Defective androgen receptor
	↑	↓	Testosterone-secreting tumor, exogenous steroids
	↓	↑	1° hypogonadism
	↓	↓	Hypogonadotropic hypogonadism

Other disorders of sex development	Disagreement between the phenotypic (external genitalia) and gonadal (testes vs. ovaries) sex. Include terms pseudohermaphrodite, hermaphrodite, and intersex.
Female pseudo-hermaphrodite (XX)	Ovaries present, but external genitalia are virilized or ambiguous. Due to excessive and inappropriate exposure to androgenic steroids during early gestation (e.g., congenital adrenal hyperplasia or exogenous administration of androgens during pregnancy).
Male pseudo-hermaphrodite (XY)	Testes present, but external genitalia are female or ambiguous. Most common form is androgen insensitivity syndrome (testicular feminization).

Aromatase deficiency	Inability to synthesize estrogens from androgens. Masculinization of female (46,XX) infants (ambiguous genitalia), ↑ serum testosterone and androstenedione. Can present with maternal virilization during pregnancy (fetal androgens cross the placenta).

Androgen insensitivity syndrome (46,XY)	Defect in androgen receptor resulting in normal-appearing female; female external genitalia with scant sexual hair, rudimentary vagina; uterus and fallopian absent. Patients develop testes (often found in labia majora; surgically removed to prevent malignancy). ↑ testosterone, estrogen, LH (vs. sex chromosome disorders).

5α-reductase deficiency	Autosomal recessive; sex limited to genetic males (46,XY). Inability to convert testosterone to DHT. Ambiguous genitalia until puberty, when ↑ testosterone causes masculinization/↑ growth of external genitalia. Testosterone/estrogen levels are normal; LH is normal or ↑. Internal genitalia are normal.

Kallmann syndrome	Failure to complete puberty; a form of hypogonadotropic hypogonadism. Defective migration of GnRH cells and formation of olfactory bulb; ↓ synthesis of GnRH in the hypothalamus; anosmia; ↓ GnRH, FSH, LH, testosterone. Infertility (low sperm count in males; amenorrhea in females).

Hydatidiform mole

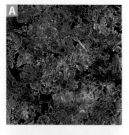

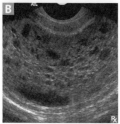

Cystic swelling of chorionic villi and proliferation of chorionic epithelium (only trophoblast).
Associated with theca-lutein cysts, hyperemesis gravidarum, hyperthyroidism.
Treatment: dilation and curettage and methotrexate. Monitor β-hCG.

	Complete mole	Partial mole
KARYOTYPE	46,XX; 46,XY	69,XXX; 69,XXY; 69,XYY
hCG	↑↑↑↑	↑
UTERINE SIZE	↑	—
CONVERT TO CHORIOCARCINOMA	2%	Rare
FETAL PARTS	No	Yes (partial = fetal parts)
COMPONENTS	Most commonly enucleated egg + single sperm (subsequently duplicates paternal DNA)	2 sperm + 1 egg
RISK OF COMPLICATIONS	15–20% malignant trophoblastic disease	Low risk of malignancy (< 5%)
SYMPTOMS	First-trimester bleeding, enlarged uterus, hyperemesis, pre-eclampsia, hyperthyroidism	Vaginal bleeding, abdominal pain
IMAGING	"Honeycombed" uterus or "clusters of grapes" , "snowstorm" on ultrasound	Fetal parts

Hypertension in pregnancy

Gestational hypertension (pregnancy-induced hypertension)	BP > 140/90 mmHg after 20th week of gestation. No pre-existing hypertension. No proteinuria or end-organ damage.	Treatment: antihypertensives (α-methyldopa, labetalol, hydralazine, nifedipine), deliver at 37–39 weeks.
Preeclampsia	New-onset hypertension with either proteinuria or end-organ dysfunction after 20th week of gestation (< 20 weeks suggests molar pregnancy). May proceed to eclampsia (+ seizures) and/or HELLP syndrome. Caused by abnormal placental spiral arteries → endothelial dysfunction, vasoconstriction, ischemia. Incidence ↑ in patients with pre-existing hypertension, diabetes, chronic renal disease, autoimmune disorders. Complications: placental abruption, coagulopathy, renal failure, uteroplacental insufficiency, eclampsia.	Treatment: antihypertensives, IV magnesium sulfate (to prevent seizure); definitive is delivery of fetus.
Eclampsia	Preeclampsia + maternal seizures. Maternal death due to stroke, intracranial hemorrhage, or ARDS.	Treatment: IV magnesium sulfate, antihypertensives, immediate delivery.
HELLP syndrome	Hemolysis, Elevated Liver enzymes, Low Platelets. A manifestation of severe preeclampsia. Blood smear shows schistocytes. Can lead to hepatic subcapsular hematomas → rupture → severe hypotension.	Treatment: immediate delivery.

Pregnancy complications

Placental abruption (abruptio placentae)	Premature separation (partial or complete) of placenta from uterine wall before delivery of infant. Risk factors: trauma (e.g., motor vehicle accident), smoking, hypertension, preeclampsia, cocaine abuse. Presentation: **abrupt**, painful bleeding (concealed or apparent) in third trimester; possible DIC, maternal shock, fetal distress. Life threatening for mother and fetus.	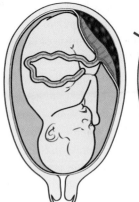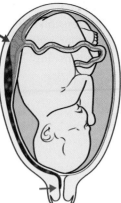 Complete abruption with concealed hemorrhage Partial abruption **with** apparent hemorrhage
Placenta accreta/ increta/percreta	Defective decidual layer → abnormal attachment and separation after delivery. Risk factors: prior C-section, inflammation, placenta previa. Three types distinguishable by the depth of penetration: Placenta accreta—placenta **attaches** to myometrium without penetrating it; most common type. Placenta increta—placenta penetrates **into** myometrium. Placenta percreta—placenta penetrates ("**perforates**") through myometrium and into uterine serosa (invades entire uterine wall); can result in placental attachment to rectum or bladder. Presentation: often detected on ultrasound prior to delivery. No separation of placenta after delivery → postpartum bleeding (can cause Sheehan syndrome).	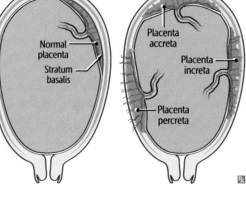
Placenta previa	Attachment of placenta to lower uterine segment over (or < 2 cm from) internal cervical os. Risk factors: multiparity, prior C-section. Associated with painless third-trimester bleeding.	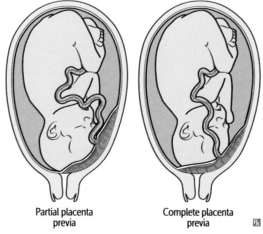 Partial placenta previa Complete placenta previa

Pregnancy complications *(continued)*

Vasa previa	Fetal vessels run over, or in close proximity to, cervical os. May result in vessel rupture, exsanguination, fetal death. Presents with triad of membrane rupture, painless vaginal bleeding, fetal bradycardia (< 110 beats/min). Emergency C-section usually indicated. Frequently associated with velamentous umbilical cord insertion (cord inserts in chorioamniotic membrane rather than placenta → fetal vessels travel to placenta unprotected by Wharton jelly).
Retained placental tissue	May cause postpartum hemorrhage, ↑ risk of infection.

Labels: Umbilical cord; Placenta (succenturiate lobe); Velamentous attachment; Vasa previa; Placenta

Ectopic pregnancy

Most often in ampulla of fallopian tube (**A** shows 10-mm embryo in oviduct at 7 weeks of gestation). Suspect with history of amenorrhea, lower-than-expected rise in hCG based on dates, and sudden lower abdominal pain; confirm with ultrasound. Often clinically mistaken for appendicitis.

Pain with or without bleeding.
Risk factors:
- History of infertility
- Salpingitis (PID)
- Ruptured appendix
- Prior tubal surgery

Amniotic fluid abnormalities

Polyhydramnios	Too much (> 1.5–2 L) amniotic fluid; associated with fetal malformations (e.g., esophageal/duodenal atresia, anencephaly; both result in inability to swallow amniotic fluid), maternal diabetes, fetal anemia, multiple gestations.
Oligohydramnios	Too little (< 0.5 L) amniotic fluid; associated with placental insufficiency, bilateral renal agenesis, posterior urethral valves (in males) and resultant inability to excrete urine. Any profound oligohydramnios can cause Potter sequence.

Gynecologic tumor epidemiology	Incidence (U.S.)—endometrial > ovarian > cervical; cervical cancer is more common worldwide due to lack of screening or HPV vaccination. Worst prognosis—ovarian > cervical > endometrial.

Vaginal tumors

Squamous cell carcinoma (SCC)	Usually 2° to cervical SCC; 1° vaginal carcinoma rare.
Clear cell adenocarcinoma	Affects women who had exposure to DES in utero.
Sarcoma botryoides (rhabdomyosarcoma variant)	Affects girls < 4 years old; spindle-shaped cells; desmin ⊕. Presents with clear, grape-like, polypoid mass emerging from vagina.

Cervical pathology

Dysplasia and carcinoma in situ	Disordered epithelial growth; begins at basal layer of squamocolumnar junction (transition zone) and extends outward. Classified as CIN 1, CIN 2, or CIN 3 (severe dysplasia or carcinoma in situ), depending on extent of dysplasia. Associated with HPV 16 and HPV 18, which produce both the E6 gene product (inhibits $p53$ suppressor gene) and E7 gene product (inhibits RB suppressor gene). May progress slowly to invasive carcinoma if left untreated. Typically asymptomatic (detected with Pap smear) or presents as abnormal vaginal bleeding (often postcoital). Risk factors: multiple sexual partners (#1), smoking, starting sexual intercourse at young age, HIV infection.

A **Koilocytes in cervical condyloma.** Note the wrinkled, "raisinoid" nuclei, some of which have clearing or a perinuclear halo (arrow). ℞

Invasive carcinoma	Often squamous cell carcinoma. Pap smear can catch cervical dysplasia (koilocytes **A**) before it progresses to invasive carcinoma. Diagnose via colposcopy and biopsy. Lateral invasion can block ureters → renal failure.

Premature ovarian failure	Premature atresia of ovarian follicles in women of reproductive age. Patients present with signs of menopause after puberty but before age 40.	↓ estrogen, ↑ LH, ↑ FSH.

Most common causes of anovulation	Pregnancy, polycystic ovarian syndrome, obesity, HPO axis abnormalities, premature ovarian failure, hyperprolactinemia, thyroid disorders, eating disorders, competitive athletics, Cushing syndrome, adrenal insufficiency.

Polycystic ovarian syndrome (Stein-Leventhal syndrome)	Hyperinsulinemia and/or insulin resistance hypothesized to alter hypothalamic hormonal feedback response → ↑ LH:FSH, ↑ androgens from theca interna cells, ↓ rate of follicular maturation → unruptured follicles (cysts) + anovulation. Common cause of subfertility in women. Enlarged, bilateral cystic ovaries A; presents with amenorrhea/oligomenorrhea, hirsutism, acne, subfertility. Associated with obesity. ↑ risk of endometrial cancer 2° to unopposed estrogen from repeated anovulatory cycles. Treatment: weight reduction, OCPs, clomiphene citrate, ketoconazole, spironolactone.

Ovarian cysts

Follicular cyst	Distention of unruptured graafian follicle. May be associated with hyperestrogenism, endometrial hyperplasia. Most common ovarian mass in young women.
Theca-lutein cyst	Often bilateral/multiple. Due to gonadotropin stimulation. Associated with choriocarcinoma and hydatidiform moles.

Ovarian neoplasms	Most common adnexal mass in women > 55 years old. Can be benign or malignant. Arise from surface epithelium, germ cells, or sex cord stromal tissue. Majority of malignant tumors are epithelial (serous cystadenocarcinoma most common). Risk ↑ with advanced age, infertility, endometriosis, PCOS, genetic predisposition (*BRCA-1* or *BRCA-2* mutation, hereditary nonpolyposis colorectal cancer [HNPCC], strong family history). Risk ↓ with previous pregnancy, history of breastfeeding, OCPs, tubal ligation. Presents with adnexal mass, abdominal distension, bowel obstruction, pleural effusion. Diagnose surgically. Monitor progression by measuring CA 125 levels (not good for screening).

Benign ovarian neoplasms

Serous cystadenoma	Most common ovarian neoplasm. Lined with fallopian tube–like epithelium. Often bilateral.
Mucinous cystadenoma	Multiloculated, large. Lined by mucus-secreting epithelium A.
Endometrioma	Endometriosis (ectopic endometrial tissue) within ovary with cyst formation. Presents with pelvic pain, dysmenorrhea, dyspareunia; symptoms may vary with menstrual cycle. "Chocolate cyst"—endometrioma filled with dark, reddish-brown blood. Complex mass on ultrasound.
Mature cystic teratoma (dermoid cyst)	Germ cell tumor, most common ovarian tumor in women 20–30 years old. Cystic mass containing elements from all 3 germ layers (e.g., teeth, hair, sebum) B. Can present with pain 2° to ovarian enlargement or torsion. Can also contain functional thyroid tissue and present as hyperthyroidism (struma ovarii) C.
Brenner tumor	Looks like bladder. Solid tumor that is pale yellow-tan and appears encapsulated. "Coffee bean" nuclei on H&E stain.
Fibromas	Bundles of spindle-shaped fibroblasts. Meigs syndrome—triad of ovarian fibroma, ascites, hydrothorax. "Pulling" sensation in groin.
Thecoma	Like granulosa cell tumors, may produce estrogen. Usually presents as abnormal uterine bleeding in a postmenopausal woman.

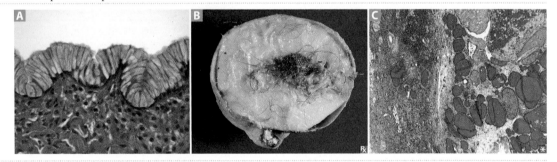

Ovarian neoplasms *(continued)*

Malignant ovarian neoplasms	
Immature teratoma	Aggressive, contains fetal tissue, neuroectoderm. Immature teratoma is most typically represented by immature/embryonic-like neural tissue. Mature teratoma are more likely to contain thyroid tissue.
Granulosa cell tumor	Most common malignant stromal tumor. Predominantly women in their 50s. Often produces estrogen and/or progesterone and presents with abnormal uterine bleeding, sexual precocity (in pre-adolescents), breast tenderness. Histology shows Call-Exner bodies (granulosa cells arranged haphazardly around collections of eosinophilic fluid, resembling primordial follicles).
Serous cystadenocarcinoma	Most common ovarian neoplasm, frequently bilateral. Psammoma bodies.
Mucinous cystadenocarcinoma	Pseudomyxoma peritonei—intraperitoneal accumulation of mucinous material from ovarian or appendiceal tumor.
Dysgerminoma	Most common in adolescents. Equivalent to male seminoma but rarer. 1% of all ovarian tumors; 30% of germ cell tumors. Sheets of uniform "fried egg" cells **D**. hCG, LDH = tumor markers.
Choriocarcinoma	Rare; can develop during or after pregnancy in mother or baby. Malignancy of trophoblastic tissue **E** (cytotrophoblasts, syncytiotrophoblasts); **no** chorionic villi present. ↑ frequency of bilateral/multiple theca-lutein cysts. Presents with abnormal ↑ β-hCG, shortness of breath, hemoptysis. Hematogenous spread to lungs. Very responsive to chemotherapy.
Yolk sac (endodermal sinus) tumor	Aggressive, in ovaries or testes (boys) and sacrococcygeal area in young children. Most common tumor in male infants. Yellow, friable (hemorrhagic), solid mass. 50% have Schiller-Duval bodies (resemble glomeruli) **F**. AFP = tumor marker.
Krukenberg tumor	GI malignancy that metastasizes to ovaries → mucin-secreting signet cell adenocarcinoma.

Endometrial conditions

Polyp	Well-circumscribed collection of endometrial tissue within uterine wall. May contain smooth muscle cells. Can extend into endometrial cavity in the form of a polyp.
Leiomyoma (fibroid)	Most common tumor in females. Often presents with multiple discrete tumors A. ↑ incidence in blacks. Benign smooth muscle tumor; malignant transformation is rare. Estrogen sensitive—tumor size ↑ with pregnancy and ↓ with menopause. Peak occurrence at 20–40 years old. May be asymptomatic, cause abnormal uterine bleeding, or result in miscarriage. Severe bleeding may lead to iron deficiency anemia. Usually does not progress to leiomyosarcoma. Whorled pattern of smooth muscle bundles with well-demarcated borders B.
Adenomyosis	Extension of endometrial tissue (glandular) into uterine myometrium. Caused by hyperplasia of basal layer of endometrium. Presents with dysmenorrhea, menorrhagia, uniformly enlarged, soft, globular uterus. Treatment: GnRH agonists, hysterectomy.
Endometriosis	Non-neoplastic endometrial glands/stroma outside endometrial cavity C. Can be found anywhere; most common sites are ovary (frequently bilateral), pelvis, peritoneum. In ovary, appears as endometrioma (blood-filled "chocolate cyst"). May be due to retrograde flow, metaplastic transformation of multipotent cells, transportation of endometrial tissue via lymphatic system. Characterized by cyclic pelvic pain, bleeding, dysmenorrhea, dyspareunia, dyschezia (pain with defecation), infertility; normal-sized uterus. Treatment: NSAIDs, OCPs, progestins, GnRH agonists, danazol, laparoscopic removal.
Endometritis	Inflammation of endometrium D associated with retained products of conception following delivery, miscarriage, abortion, or with foreign body (e.g., IUD). Retained material in uterus promotes infection by bacterial flora from vagina or intestinal tract. Treatment: gentamicin + clindamycin with or without ampicillin.
Endometrial hyperplasia	Abnormal endometrial gland proliferation E usually caused by excess estrogen stimulation. ↑ risk for endometrial carcinoma. Presents as postmenopausal vaginal bleeding. Risk factors include anovulatory cycles, hormone replacement therapy, polycystic ovarian syndrome, granulosa cell tumor.
Endometrial carcinoma	Most common gynecologic malignancy F. Peak occurrence at 55–65 years old. Presents with vaginal bleeding. Typically preceded by endometrial hyperplasia. Risk factors include prolonged use of estrogen without progestins, obesity, diabetes, hypertension, nulliparity, late menopause, Lynch syndrome.

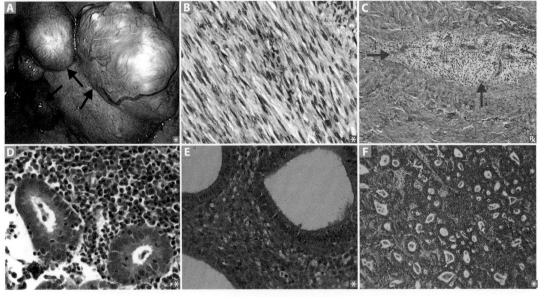

Breast pathology

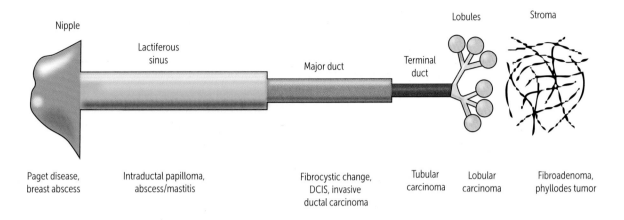

Paget disease, breast abscess	Intraductal papilloma, abscess/mastitis	Fibrocystic change, DCIS, invasive ductal carcinoma	Tubular carcinoma	Lobular carcinoma	Fibroadenoma, phyllodes tumor

Benign breast tumors

TYPE	CHARACTERISTICS	EPIDEMIOLOGY	NOTES
Fibroadenoma	Small, mobile, firm mass with sharp edges.	Most common tumor in those < 35 years old.	↑ size and tenderness with ↑ estrogen (e.g., pregnancy, prior to menstruation). Not a precursor to breast cancer.
Intraductal papilloma	Small tumor that grows in lactiferous ducts. Typically beneath areola.		Serous or bloody nipple discharge. Slight (1.5–2×) ↑ in risk for carcinoma.
Phyllodes tumor	Large, bulky mass of connective tissue and cysts. "Leaf-like" projections.	Most common in 5th decade.	Some may become malignant.

Common breast conditions

Proliferative breast disease	Most common cause of "breast lumps" from age 25 to menopause. Presents with premenstrual breast pain and multiple lesions, often bilateral. Fluctuation in size of mass. Usually does not indicate increased risk of carcinoma. Histologic types: ▪ Fibrosis—hyperplasia of breast stroma. ▪ Cystic—fluid filled, blue dome. Ductal dilation. ▪ Sclerosing adenosis—↑ acini and intralobular fibrosis. Associated with calcifications. Often confused with cancer. ↑ risk (1.5–2×) of developing cancer. ▪ Epithelial hyperplasia—↑ in number of epithelial cell layers in terminal duct lobule. ↑ risk of carcinoma with atypical cells. Occurs in women > 30 years old.
Lactational mastitis	During breastfeeding, ↑ risk of bacterial infection through cracks in the nipple; *S. aureus* is most common pathogen. Treat with dicloxacillin and continued breastfeeding.
Fat necrosis	Benign, usually painless lump; forms as a result of injury to breast tissue. Abnormal calcification on mammography; biopsy shows necrotic fat, giant cells. Up to 50% of patients may not report trauma.
Gynecomastia	Breast enlargement in males. Results from hyperestrogenism (cirrhosis, testicular tumor, puberty, old age), Klinefelter syndrome, drugs (Spironolactone, Digoxin, Cimetidine, Alcohol, Ketoconazole). "Some Drugs Create Awesome Knockers." Physiologic (not pathologic) at birth, puberty, old age.

Malignant breast tumors	Commonly postmenopausal. Usually arise from terminal duct lobular unit. Overexpression of estrogen/progesterone receptors or *c-erbB2* (HER-2, an EGF receptor) is common; triple negative (ER ⊖, PR ⊖, and Her2/Neu ⊖) more aggressive; type affects therapy and prognosis. Axillary lymph node involvement indicating metastasis is the single most important prognostic factor. Most often located in upper-outer quadrant of breast.	Risk factors: ↑ estrogen exposure, ↑ total number of menstrual cycles, older age at 1st live birth, obesity (↑ estrogen exposure as adipose tissue converts androstenedione to estrone), *BRCA1* and *BRCA2* gene mutations, African American ethnicity (↑ risk for triple ⊖ breast cancer).

TYPE	CHARACTERISTICS	NOTES
Noninvasive		
Ductal carcinoma in situ (DCIS)	Fills ductal lumen (black arrow in **A** indicates neoplastic cells in duct; blue arrow shows engorged blood vessel). Arises from ductal atypia. Often seen early as microcalcifications on mammography.	Early malignancy without basement membrane penetration.
Comedocarcinoma	Ductal, central necrosis (arrow in **B**). Subtype of DCIS.	
Paget disease	Results from underlying DCIS or invasive breast cancer. Eczematous patches on nipple **C**. Paget cells = large cells in epidermis with clear halo.	Extramammary Paget disease seen on vulva does not suggest underlying malignancy.

Malignant breast tumors *(continued)*

Invasive		
Invasive ductal	Firm, fibrous, "rock-hard" mass with sharp margins and small, glandular, duct-like cells **D**. Grossly, see classic "stellate" infiltration.	Worst and most invasive. Most common (~75% of all breast cancers).
Invasive lobular	Orderly row of cells ("Indian file" **E**), due to ↓ E-cadherin expression.	Often bilateral with multiple lesions in the same location.
Medullary	Fleshy, cellular, lymphocytic infiltrate.	Good prognosis.
Inflammatory	Dermal lymphatic invasion by breast carcinoma. Peau d'orange (breast skin resembles orange peel **F**); neoplastic cells block lymphatic drainage.	50% survival at 5 years. Often mistaken for mastitis or Paget disease.

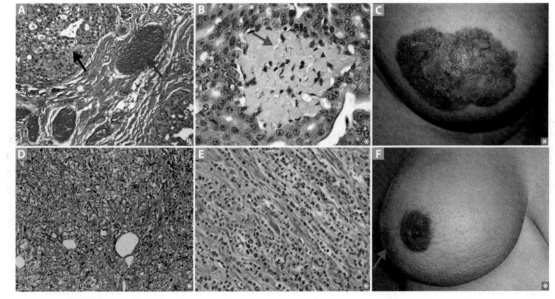

Penile pathology

Peyronie disease	Abnormal curvature of penis due to fibrous plaque within tunica albuginea. Associated with erectile dysfunction. Can cause pain, anxiety. Consider surgical repair once curvature stabilizes. Distinct from penile fracture (rupture of corpora cavernosa due to forced bending).
Priapism	Painful sustained erection lasting > 4 hours. Associated with trauma, sickle cell disease (sickled RBCs get trapped in vascular channels), medications (e.g., sildenafil, trazodone). Treat immediately with corporal aspiration, intracavernosal phenylephrine, or surgical decompression to prevent ischemia.
Squamous cell carcinoma	More common in Asia, Africa, South America. Precursor in situ lesions: Bowen disease (in penile shaft, presents as leukoplakia), erythroplasia of Queyrat (cancer of glans, presents as erythroplakia), Bowenoid papulosis (carcinoma in situ of unclear malignant potential, presenting as reddish papules). Associated with HPV, lack of circumcision.

Cryptorchidism	Undescended testis (one or both); impaired spermatogenesis (since sperm develop best at temperatures < 37°C); can have normal testosterone levels (Leydig cells are unaffected by temperature); associated with ↑ risk of germ cell tumors. Prematurity ↑ risk of cryptorchidism. ↓ inhibin, ↑ FSH, ↑ LH; testosterone ↓ in bilateral cryptorchidism, normal in unilateral.

Varicocele	Dilated veins in pampiniform plexus due to ↑ venous pressure; most common cause of scrotal enlargement in adult males; most often on left side because of ↑ resistance to flow from left gonadal vein drainage into left renal vein; can cause infertility because of ↑ temperature; "bag of worms" on palpation; diagnose by ultrasound with Doppler **A**; does not transilluminate. Treatment: varicocelectomy, embolization by interventional radiologist.	

Varicocele. Dilated pampiniform veins ("bag of worms" appearance). These voids fill in with color on flow ultrasound. ℞

Extragonadal germ cell tumors	Arise in midline locations. In adults, most commonly in retroperitoneum, mediastinum, pineal, and suprasellar regions. In infants and young children, sacrococcygeal teratomas are most common.

Scrotal masses	Benign scrotal lesions present as testicular masses that can be transilluminated (vs. solid testicular tumors).	
Congenital hydrocele	Common cause of scrotal swelling in infants, due to incomplete obliteration of processus vaginalis.	Transilluminating swelling.
Acquired hydrocele	Benign scrotal fluid collection usually 2° to infection, trauma, tumor. If bloody → hematocele.	
Spermatocele	Cyst due to dilated epididymal duct or rete testis.	Paratesticular fluctuant nodule.

Testicular germ cell tumors	~95% of all testicular tumors. Most often occur in young men. Risk factors: cryptorchidism, Klinefelter syndrome. Can present as a mixed germ cell tumor. Differential diagnosis for testicular mass that does not transilluminate: cancer.
Seminoma	Malignant; painless, homogenous testicular enlargement; most common testicular tumor, most common in 3rd decade, never in infancy. Large cells in lobules with watery cytoplasm and "fried egg" appearance. ↑ placental ALP. Radiosensitive. Late metastasis, excellent prognosis.
Yolk sac (endodermal sinus) tumor	Yellow, mucinous. Aggressive malignancy of testes, analogous to ovarian yolk sac tumor. Schiller-Duval bodies resemble primitive glomeruli. ↑ AFP is highly characteristic. Most common testicular tumor in boys < 3 years old.
Choriocarcinoma	Malignant, ↑ hCG. Disordered syncytiotrophoblastic and cytotrophoblastic elements. Hematogenous metastases to lungs and brain (may present with "hemorrhagic stroke" due to bleeding into metastasis. May produce gynecomastia, symptoms of hyperthyroidism (hCG is structurally similar to LH, FSH, TSH).
Teratoma	Unlike in females, mature teratoma in adult males may be malignant. Benign in children. ↑ hCG and/or AFP in 50% of cases.
Embryonal carcinoma	Malignant, hemorrhagic mass with necrosis; painful; worse prognosis than seminoma. Often glandular/papillary morphology. "Pure" embryonal carcinoma is rare; most commonly mixed with other tumor types. May be associated with increased hCG and normal AFP levels when pure (↑ AFP when mixed).

Testicular non–germ cell tumors	5% of all testicular tumors. Mostly benign.
Leydig cell	Contains Reinke crystals (eosinophilic cytoplasmic inclusions); usually produce androgens → gynecomastia in men, precocious puberty in boys. Golden brown color.
Sertoli cell	Androblastoma from sex cord stroma.
Testicular lymphoma	Most common testicular cancer in older men. Not a 1° cancer; arises from metastatic lymphoma to testes. Aggressive.

Benign prostatic hyperplasia

Common in men > 50 years old. Characterized by smooth, elastic, firm nodular enlargement (hyperplasia not hypertrophy) of periurethral (lateral and middle) lobes, which compress the urethra into a vertical slit. Not premalignant. Often presents with ↑ frequency of urination, nocturia, difficulty starting and stopping urine stream, dysuria. May lead to distention and hypertrophy of bladder, hydronephrosis, UTIs. ↑ free prostate-specific antigen (PSA).
Treatment: α_1-antagonists (terazosin, tamsulosin), which cause relaxation of smooth muscle; 5α-reductase inhibitors (e.g., finasteride); PDE-5 inhibitors.

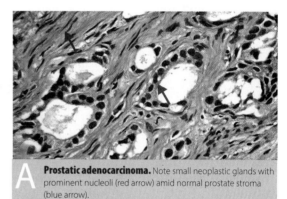

Prostatitis

Dysuria, frequency, urgency, low back pain. Acute: bacterial (e.g., *E. coli*); chronic: bacterial or abacterial (most common).

Prostatic adenocarcinoma

Common in men > 50 years old. Arises most often from posterior lobe (peripheral zone) of prostate gland **A** and is most frequently diagnosed by ↑ PSA and subsequent needle core biopsies. Prostatic acid phosphatase (PAP) and PSA are useful tumor markers (↑ total PSA, with ↓ fraction of free PSA). Osteoblastic metastases in bone may develop in late stages, as indicated by lower back pain and ↑ serum ALP and PSA.

Prostatic adenocarcinoma. Note small neoplastic glands with prominent nucleoli (red arrow) amid normal prostate stroma (blue arrow).

▶ REPRODUCTIVE—PHARMACOLOGY

Control of reproductive hormones

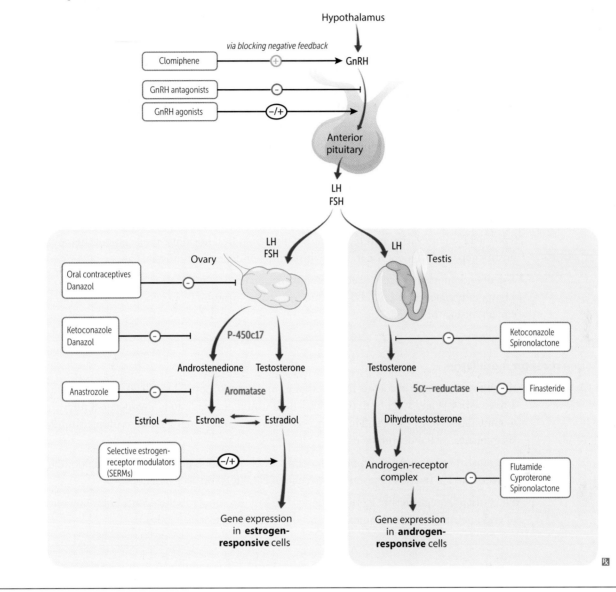

Leuprolide

MECHANISM	GnRH analog with agonist properties when used in pulsatile fashion; antagonist properties when used in continuous fashion (downregulates GnRH receptor in pituitary → ↓ FSH/LH).
CLINICAL USE	Infertility (pulsatile), prostate cancer (continuous use following androgen receptor blockade with flutamide), uterine fibroids (continuous), precocious puberty (continuous).
TOXICITY	Antiandrogen, nausea, vomiting.

Leuprolide can be used in **lieu** of GnRH.

Estrogens (ethinyl estradiol, DES, mestranol)

MECHANISM	Bind estrogen receptors.
CLINICAL USE	Hypogonadism or ovarian failure, menstrual abnormalities, hormone replacement therapy in postmenopausal women; use in men with androgen-dependent prostate cancer.
TOXICITY	↑ risk of endometrial cancer, bleeding in postmenopausal women, clear cell adenocarcinoma of vagina in females exposed to DES in utero, ↑ risk of thrombi. Contraindications—ER ⊕ breast cancer, history of DVTs.

Selective estrogen receptor modulators

Clomiphene	Antagonist at estrogen receptors in hypothalamus. Prevents normal feedback inhibition and ↑ release of LH and FSH from pituitary, which stimulates ovulation. Used to treat infertility due to anovulation (e.g., PCOS). May cause hot flashes, ovarian enlargement, multiple simultaneous pregnancies, visual disturbances.
Tamoxifen	Antagonist at breast; agonist at bone, uterus; ↑ risk of thromboembolic events and endometrial cancer. Used to treat and prevent recurrence of ER/PR ⊕ breast cancer.
Raloxifene	Antagonist at breast, uterus; agonist at bone; ↑ risk of thromboembolic events but no increased risk of endometrial cancer (vs. tamoxifen); used primarily to treat osteoporosis.

Hormone replacement therapy	Used for relief or prevention of menopausal symptoms (e.g., hot flashes, vaginal atrophy), osteoporosis (↑ estrogen, ↓ osteoclast activity). Unopposed estrogen replacement therapy ↑ risk of endometrial cancer, so progesterone is added. Possible increased cardiovascular risk.

Anastrozole/ exemestane	Aromatase inhibitors used in postmenopausal women with ER ⊕ breast cancer.

Progestins

MECHANISM	Bind progesterone receptors, ↓ growth and ↑ vascularization of endometrium.
CLINICAL USE	Used in oral contraceptives and to treat endometrial cancer, abnormal uterine bleeding.

Mifepristone (RU-486)

MECHANISM	Competitive inhibitor of progestins at progesterone receptors.
CLINICAL USE	Termination of pregnancy. Administered with misoprostol (PGE_1).
TOXICITY	Heavy bleeding, GI effects (nausea, vomiting, anorexia), abdominal pain.

Oral contraception (synthetic progestins, estrogen)

Estrogen and progestins inhibit LH/FSH and thus prevent estrogen surge. No estrogen surge → no LH surge → no ovulation.

Progestins cause thickening of cervical mucus, thereby limiting access of sperm to uterus. Progestins also inhibit endometrial proliferation → endometrium is less suitable to the implantation of an embryo.

Contraindications: smokers > 35 years old (↑ risk of cardiovascular events), patients with history of thromboembolism and stroke or history of estrogen-dependent tumor.

Terbutaline, ritodrine

β_2-agonists that relax the uterus; used to ↓ contraction frequency in women during labor.

Danazol

MECHANISM	Synthetic androgen that acts as partial agonist at androgen receptors.
CLINICAL USE	Endometriosis, hereditary angioedema.
TOXICITY	Weight gain, edema, acne, hirsutism, masculinization, ↓ HDL levels, hepatotoxicity.

Testosterone, methyltestosterone

MECHANISM	Agonists at androgen receptors.
CLINICAL USE	Treats hypogonadism and promotes development of 2° sex characteristics; stimulation of anabolism to promote recovery after burn or injury.
TOXICITY	Causes masculinization in females; ↓ intratesticular testosterone in males by inhibiting release of LH (via negative feedback) → gonadal atrophy. Premature closure of epiphyseal plates. ↑ LDL, ↓ HDL.

Antiandrogens

Testosterone $\xrightarrow{5\alpha\text{-reductase}}$ DHT (more potent).

Finasteride	A 5α-reductase inhibitor (↓ conversion of testosterone to DHT). Useful in BPH and male-pattern baldness.
Flutamide	A nonsteroidal competitive inhibitor at androgen receptors. Used for prostate carcinoma.
Ketoconazole	Inhibits steroid synthesis (inhibits 17,20-desmolase).
Spironolactone	Inhibits steroid binding, 17α-hydroxylase, and 17,20-desmolase.

Ketoconazole and spironolactone are used to treat polycystic ovarian syndrome to reduce androgenic symptoms. Both have side effects of gynecomastia and amenorrhea.

Tamsulosin α_1-antagonist used to treat BPH by inhibiting smooth muscle contraction. Selective for $\alpha_{1A,D}$ receptors (found on prostate) vs. vascular α_{1B} receptors.

Sildenafil, vardenafil, tadalafil

MECHANISM	Inhibit PDE-5 → ↑ cGMP, smooth muscle relaxation in corpus cavernosum, ↑ blood flow, penile erection.	Sildenafil, vardenafil, and tadalafil **fill** the penis.
CLINICAL USE	Erectile dysfunction.	
TOXICITY	Headache, flushing, dyspepsia, cyanopsia (blue-tinted vision). Risk of life-threatening hypotension in patients taking nitrates.	"Hot and sweaty," but then Headache, Heartburn, Hypotension.

Minoxidil

MECHANISM	Direct arteriolar vasodilator.
CLINICAL USE	Androgenetic alopecia; severe refractory hypertension.

Respiratory

"There's so much pollution in the air now that if it weren't for our lungs, there'd be no place to put it all."

—Robert Orben

"Mars is essentially in the same orbit. Somewhat the same distance from the Sun, which is very important. We have seen pictures where there are canals, we believe, and water. If there is water, that means there is oxygen. If there is oxygen, that means we can breathe."

—Former Vice President Dan Quayle

"None of us is different either as barbarian or as Greek; for we all breathe into the air with mouth and nostrils."

—Antiphon

"Life is not the amount of breaths you take; it's the moments that take your breath away."

—Hitch

Respiratory tree

Conducting zone	Large airways consist of nose, pharynx, larynx, trachea, and bronchi. Small airways consist of bronchioles that further divide into terminal bronchioles (large numbers in parallel → least airway resistance). Warms, humidifies, and filters air but does not participate in gas exchange → "anatomic dead space." Cartilage and goblet cells extend to end of bronchi. Pseudostratified ciliated columnar cells (clear mucus from lungs) extend to beginning of terminal bronchioles, then transition to cuboidal cells. Airway smooth muscle cells extend to end of terminal bronchioles (sparse beyond this point).
Respiratory zone	Lung parenchyma; consists of respiratory bronchioles, alveolar ducts, and alveoli. Participates in gas exchange. Mostly cuboidal cells in respiratory bronchioles, then simple squamous cells up to alveoli. Cilia terminate in respiratory bronchioles. Alveolar macrophages clear debris and participate in immune response.

Pneumocytes

Type I cells	97% of alveolar surfaces. Line the alveoli. Squamous; thin for optimal gas diffusion.
Type II cells	Secrete pulmonary surfactant → ↓ alveolar surface tension and prevents alveolar collapse (atelectasis). Cuboidal and clustered **A**. Also serve as precursors to type I cells and other type II cells. Type II cells proliferate during lung damage.
Club (Clara) cells	Nonciliated; low-columnar/cuboidal with secretory granules. Secrete component of surfactant; degrade toxins; act as reserve cells.

$$\text{Collapsing pressure } (P) = \frac{2 \text{ (surface tension)}}{\text{radius}}$$

Alveoli have ↑ tendency to collapse on expiration as radius ↓ (law of Laplace).

Pulmonary surfactant is a complex mix of lecithins, the most important of which is dipalmitoylphosphatidylcholine.

Surfactant synthesis begins around week 26 of gestation, but mature levels are not achieved until around week 35.

Lecithin-to-sphingomyelin ratio > 2.0 in amniotic fluid indicates fetal lung maturity.

Lung relations

Right lung has 3 lobes; Left has Less Lobes (2) and **L**ingula (homolog of right middle lobe). Right lung is more common site for inhaled foreign body because the right main stem bronchus is wider and more vertical than the left.

If you aspirate a peanut:
- While upright—enters lower portion of right inferior lobe.
- While supine—enters superior portion of right inferior lobe.

Instead of a middle lobe, the left lung has a space occupied by the heart.

The relation of the pulmonary artery to the bronchus at each lung hilum is described by **RALS**—**R**ight **A**nterior; **L**eft **S**uperior.

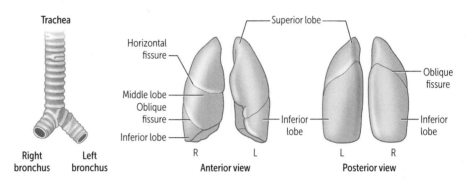

Trachea · Right bronchus · Left bronchus · Horizontal fissure · Superior lobe · Middle lobe · Oblique fissure · Inferior lobe · Inferior lobe · Oblique fissure · Inferior lobe · R · L Anterior view · L · R Posterior view

Diaphragm structures

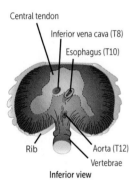

Central tendon · Inferior vena cava (T8) · Esophagus (T10) · Rib · Aorta (T12) · Vertebrae · Inferior view

Structures perforating diaphragm:
- At T8: IVC
- At T10: esophagus, vagus (CN 10; 2 trunks)
- At T12: aorta (red), thoracic duct (white), azygos vein (blue) ("At **T-1-2** it's the **red**, **white**, and **blue**")

Diaphragm is innervated by C3, 4, and 5 (phrenic nerve). Pain from diaphragm irritation (e.g., air or blood in peritoneal cavity) can be referred to shoulder (C5) and trapezius ridge (C3, 4).

Number of letters = T level:
T8: vena cava
T10: "oesophagus"
T12: aortic hiatus

I (IVC) **ate** (8) **ten** (10) **eggs** (esophagus) **at** (aorta) **twelve** (12).

C3, 4, 5 keeps the diaphragm **alive**.
Other bifurcations:
- The common carotid bi**four**cates at C4.
- The trachea bi**four**cates at T4.
- The abdominal aorta bi**four**cates at L4.

▶ RESPIRATORY—PHYSIOLOGY

Lung volumes

Inspiratory reserve volume (IRV)	Air that can still be breathed in after normal inspiration	Lung volumes (**LITER**):
Tidal volume (TV)	Air that moves into lung with each quiet inspiration, typically 500 mL	
Expiratory reserve volume (ERV)	Air that can still be breathed out after normal expiration	
Residual volume (RV)	Air in lung after maximal expiration; cannot be measured on spirometry	
Inspiratory capacity (IC)	IRV + TV	
Functional residual capacity (FRC)	RV + ERV Volume of gas in lungs after normal expiration	
Vital capacity (VC)	TV + IRV + ERV Maximum volume of gas that can be expired after a maximal inspiration	A capacity is a sum of ≥ 2 physiologic volumes.
Total lung capacity (TLC)	IRV + TV + ERV + RV Volume of gas present in lungs after a maximal inspiration	

Determination of physiologic dead space	$V_D = V_T \times \dfrac{P_{aCO_2} - P_{ECO_2}}{P_{aCO_2}}$ V_D = physiologic dead space = anatomic dead space of conducting airways plus alveolar dead space; apex of healthy lung is largest contributor of alveolar dead space. Volume of inspired air that does not take part in gas exchange. V_T = tidal volume. P_{aCO_2} = arterial P_{CO_2}. P_{ECO_2} = expired air P_{CO_2}.	Taco, Paco, Peco, Paco (refers to order of variables in equation)

Ventilation

Minute ventilation (V_E)	Total volume of gas entering lungs per minute $V_E = V_T \times$ respiratory rate (RR)
Alveolar ventilation (V_A)	Volume of gas per unit time that reaches alveoli $V_A = (V_T - V_D) \times$ RR

Lung and chest wall

Elastic recoil—tendency for lungs to collapse inward and chest wall to spring outward.

At FRC, inward pull of lung is balanced by outward pull of chest wall, and system pressure is atmospheric.

Elastic properties of both chest wall and lungs determine their combined volume.

At FRC, airway and alveolar pressures are 0, and intrapleural pressure is negative (prevents pneumothorax). PVR is at minimum.

Compliance—change in lung volume for a given change in pressure; ↓ in pulmonary fibrosis, pneumonia, pulmonary edema; ↑ in emphysema, normal aging.

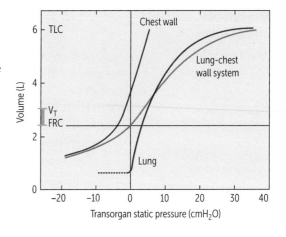

Hemoglobin

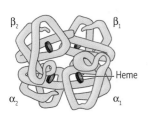

Hemoglobin (Hb) is composed of 4 polypeptide subunits (2 α and 2 β) and exists in 2 forms:
- T (taut; deoxygenated) form has low affinity for O_2.
- R (relaxed; oxygenated) form has high affinity for O_2 (300×). Hb exhibits positive cooperativity and negative allostery.

↑ Cl^-, H^+, CO_2, 2,3-BPG, and temperature favor taut form over relaxed form (shifts dissociation curve right → ↑ O_2 unloading).

Fetal Hb (2 α and 2 γ subunits) has lower affinity for 2,3-BPG than adult Hb and thus has higher affinity for O_2.

Taut in **T**issues.

Relaxed in **R**espiratory tract.

Hemoglobin acts as buffer for H^+ ions.

Hemoglobin modifications	Lead to tissue hypoxia from ↓ O_2 saturation and ↓ O_2 content.	
Methemoglobin	Oxidized form of Hb (ferric, Fe^{3+}) that does not bind O_2 as readily, but has ↑ affinity for cyanide. Iron in Hb is normally in a reduced state (ferrous, Fe^{2+}). Methemoglobinemia may present with cyanosis and chocolate-colored blood. Induced methemoglobinemia (using nitrites, followed by thiosulfate) may be used to treat cyanide poisoning.	Methemoglobinemia can be treated with **methylene blue.** Nitrites and benzocaine cause poisoning by oxidizing Fe^{2+} to Fe^{3+}. Just the **2 of us:** ferrous is Fe^{2+}.
Carboxyhemoglobin	Form of Hb bound to CO in place of O_2. Causes ↓ oxygen-binding capacity with left shift in oxygen-hemoglobin dissociation curve. ↓ O_2 unloading in tissues. CO binds competitively to Hb and with 200× greater affinity than O_2. Treat with 100% O_2 and hyperbaric O_2.	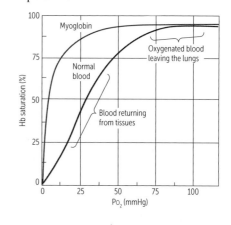

Oxygen-hemoglobin dissociation curve

Sigmoidal shape due to positive cooperativity (i.e., tetrameric Hb molecule can bind 4 O_2 molecules and has higher affinity for each subsequent O_2 molecule bound). Myoglobin is monomeric and thus does not show positive cooperativity; curve lacks sigmoidal appearance.

When curve shifts to the right, ↓ affinity of Hb for O_2 (facilitates unloading of O_2 to tissue).

An ↑ in all factors (including H^+) causes a shift of the curve to the right.

A ↓ in all factors (including H^+) causes a shift of the curve to the left.

Fetal Hb has higher affinity for O_2 than adult Hb, so its dissociation curve is shifted left.

Right shift—**ACE BAT**s **right** handed:
Acid
CO_2
Exercise
2,3-BPG
Altitude
Temperature

Oxygen content of blood

O_2 content = (O_2 binding capacity × % saturation) + dissolved O_2.

Normally 1 g Hb can bind 1.34 mL O_2; normal Hb amount in blood is 15 g/dL. Cyanosis results when deoxygenated Hb > 5 g/dL.

O_2 binding capacity ≈ 20.1 mL O_2/dL.

With ↓ Hb there is ↓ O_2 content of arterial blood, but no change in O_2 saturation and arterial P_{O_2}.

O_2 delivery to tissues = cardiac output × O_2 content of blood.

	Hb concentration	% O_2 sat of Hb	Dissolved O_2 (Pa_{O_2})	Total O_2 content
CO poisoning	Normal	↓ (CO competes with O_2)	Normal	↓
Anemia	↓	Normal	Normal	↓
Polycythemia	↑	Normal	Normal	↑

Pulmonary circulation

Normally a low-resistance, high-compliance system. P_{O_2} and P_{CO_2} exert opposite effects on pulmonary and systemic circulation. A ↓ in PA_{O_2} causes a hypoxic vasoconstriction that shifts blood away from poorly ventilated regions of lung to well-ventilated regions of lung.

Perfusion limited—O_2 (normal health), CO_2, N_2O. Gas equilibrates early along the length of the capillary. Diffusion can be ↑ only if blood flow ↑.

Diffusion limited—O_2 (emphysema, fibrosis), CO. Gas does not equilibrate by the time blood reaches the end of the capillary.

A consequence of pulmonary hypertension is cor pulmonale and subsequent right ventricular failure (jugular venous distention, edema, hepatomegaly).

Diffusion: $V_{gas} = A/T × D_k(P_1 - P_2)$ where A = area, T = alveolar wall thickness, and $D_k(P_1 - P_2)$ ≈ difference in partial pressures:
- A ↓ in emphysema.
- T ↑ in pulmonary fibrosis.

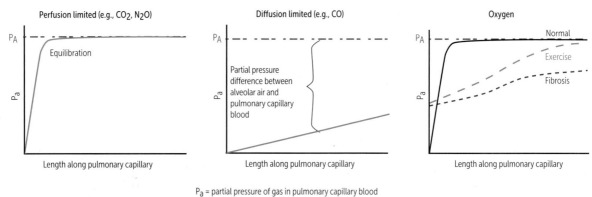

P_a = partial pressure of gas in pulmonary capillary blood
P_A = partial pressure of gas in alveolar air

Pulmonary vascular resistance

$$PVR = \frac{P_{pulm\ artery} - P_{L\ atrium}}{cardiac\ output}$$

Remember: $\Delta P = Q \times R$, so $R = \Delta P / Q$

$R = 8\eta l / \pi r^4$

$P_{pulm\ artery}$ = pressure in pulmonary artery
$P_{L\ atrium}$ = pulmonary wedge pressure

η = viscosity of blood; l = vessel length;
r = vessel radius

Alveolar gas equation

$$PAo_2 = PIo_2 - \frac{Paco_2}{R}$$

$$\approx 150\ mmHg^a - \frac{Paco_2}{0.8}$$

[a]At sea level breathing room air.

PAo_2 = alveolar Po_2 (mmHg).
PIo_2 = Po_2 in inspired air (mmHg).
$Paco_2$ = arterial Pco_2 (mmHg).
R = respiratory quotient = CO_2 produced/O_2 consumed.
A-a gradient = $PAo_2 - Pao_2$ = 10–15 mmHg.
↑ A-a gradient may occur in hypoxemia; causes include shunting, V/Q mismatch, fibrosis (impairs diffusion).

Oxygen deprivation

Hypoxemia (↓ Pao₂)	Hypoxia (↓ O₂ delivery to tissue)	Ischemia (loss of blood flow)
Normal A-a gradient	↓ cardiac output	Impeded arterial flow
▪ High altitude	Hypoxemia	↓ venous drainage
▪ Hypoventilation (e.g., opioid use)	Anemia	
↑ A-a gradient	CO poisoning	
▪ V/Q mismatch		
▪ Diffusion limitation		
▪ Right-to-left shunt		

V/Q mismatch

Ideally, ventilation is matched to perfusion (i.e., V/Q = 1) for adequate gas exchange.

Lung zones:
- V/Q at apex of lung = 3 (wasted ventilation)
- V/Q at base of lung = 0.6 (wasted perfusion)

Both ventilation and perfusion are greater at the base of the lung than at the apex of the lung.

With exercise (↑ cardiac output), there is vasodilation of apical capillaries → V/Q ratio approaches 1.

Certain organisms that thrive in high O_2 (e.g., TB) flourish in the apex.

V/Q = 0 = "airway" obstruction (shunt). In shunt, 100% O_2 does not improve Pao_2.

V/Q = ∞ = blood flow obstruction (physiologic dead space). Assuming < 100% dead space, 100% O_2 improves Pao_2.

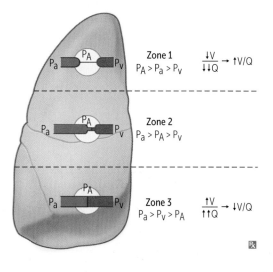

CO$_2$ transport	CO$_2$ is transported from tissues to lungs in 3 forms:	In lungs, oxygenation of Hb promotes dissociation of H$^+$ from Hb. This shifts equilibrium toward CO$_2$ formation; therefore, CO$_2$ is released from RBCs (Haldane effect).

CO$_2$ is transported from tissues to lungs in 3 forms:
- HCO$_3^-$ (90%).
- Carbaminohemoglobin or HbCO$_2$ (5%). CO$_2$ bound to Hb at N-terminus of globin (not heme). CO$_2$ binding favors taut form (O$_2$ unloaded).
- Dissolved CO$_2$ (5%).

In lungs, oxygenation of Hb promotes dissociation of H$^+$ from Hb. This shifts equilibrium toward CO$_2$ formation; therefore, CO$_2$ is released from RBCs (Haldane effect).

In peripheral tissue, ↑ H$^+$ from tissue metabolism shifts curve to right, unloading O$_2$ (Bohr effect).

Majority of blood CO$_2$ is carried as HCO$_3^-$ in the plasma.

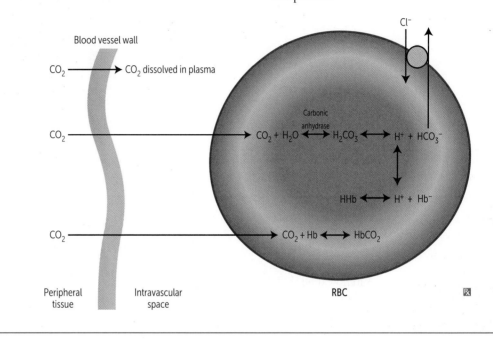

Response to high altitude

↓ atmospheric oxygen (PO$_2$) → ↓ Pao$_2$ → ↑ ventilation → ↓ Paco$_2$.

Chronic ↑ in ventilation.

↑ erythropoietin → ↑ hematocrit and Hb (chronic hypoxia).

↑ 2,3-BPG (binds to Hb so that Hb releases more O$_2$).

Cellular changes (↑ mitochondria).

↑ renal excretion of HCO$_3^-$ to compensate for respiratory alkalosis (can augment with acetazolamide).

Chronic hypoxic pulmonary vasoconstriction results in RVH.

Response to exercise

↑ CO$_2$ production.

↑ O$_2$ consumption.

↑ ventilation rate to meet O$_2$ demand.

V/Q ratio from apex to base becomes more uniform.

↑ pulmonary blood flow due to ↑ cardiac output.

↓ pH during strenuous exercise (2° to lactic acidosis).

No change in Pao$_2$ and Paco$_2$, but ↑ in venous CO$_2$ content and ↓ in venous O$_2$ content.

▶ RESPIRATORY—PATHOLOGY

Rhinosinusitis

Obstruction of sinus drainage into nasal cavity → inflammation and pain over affected area (typically maxillary sinuses in adults 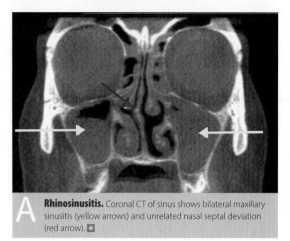). Most common acute cause is viral URI; may cause superimposed bacterial infection, most commonly *S. pneumoniae, H. influenzae, M. catarrhalis.*

Rhinosinusitis. Coronal CT of sinus shows bilateral maxillary sinusitis (yellow arrows) and unrelated nasal septal deviation (red arrow). ✴

Epistaxis

Nose bleed. Most commonly occurs in anterior segment of nostril (Kiesselbach plexus). Life-threatening hemorrhages occur in posterior segment (sphenopalatine artery, a branch of maxillary artery).

Deep venous thrombosis

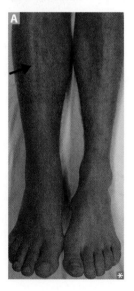

Blood clot within a deep vein → swelling, redness A, warmth, pain. Predisposed by Virchow triad (**SHE**):
- Stasis
- Hypercoagulability (e.g., defect in coagulation cascade proteins, such as factor V Leiden)
- Endothelial damage (exposed collagen triggers clotting cascade)

Approximately 95% of pulmonary emboli arise from proximal deep veins of lower extremity. Homan sign—dorsiflexion of foot → calf pain. Use unfractionated heparin or low-molecular-weight heparins (e.g., enoxaparin) for prophylaxis and acute management. Use oral anticoagulants (e.g., warfarin, rivaroxaban) for treatment (long-term prevention).

Pulmonary emboli

V/Q mismatch → hypoxemia → respiratory alkalosis. Sudden-onset dyspnea, chest pain, tachypnea, tachycardia. May present as sudden death **A**. Lines of Zahn are interdigitating areas of pink (platelets, fibrin) and red (RBCs) found only in thrombi formed before death; help distinguish pre- and postmortem thrombi **B**.

Types: Fat, Air, Thrombus, Bacteria, Amniotic fluid, Tumor.

Fat emboli—associated with long bone fractures and liposuction; classic triad of hypoxemia, neurologic abnormalities, petechial rash.

Amniotic fluid emboli—can lead to DIC, especially postpartum.

Air emboli—nitrogen bubbles precipitate in ascending divers; treat with hyperbaric O_2.

CT pulmonary angiography is imaging test of choice for PE (look for filling defects) **C**.

An embolus moves like a **FAT BAT**.

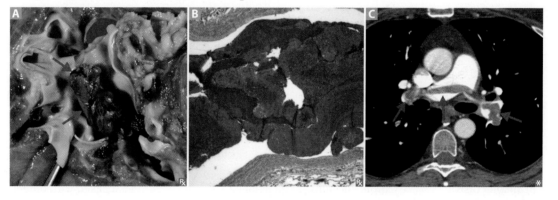

Obstructive lung diseases	Obstruction of air flow resulting in air trapping in lungs. Airways close prematurely at high lung volumes → ↑ RV and ↓ FVC. PFTs: ↓↓ FEV_1, ↓ FVC → ↓ FEV_1/FVC ratio (hallmark), V/Q mismatch. Chronic, hypoxic pulmonary vasoconstriction can lead to cor pulmonale.	

TYPE	PATHOLOGY	OTHER
Chronic bronchitis ("blue bloater")	Hyperplasia of mucus-secreting glands in bronchi → Reid index (thickness of gland layer/total thickness of bronchial wall) > 50%.	Productive cough for > 3 months per year (not necessarily consecutive) for > 2 years. Findings: wheezing, crackles, cyanosis (early-onset hypoxemia due to shunting), late-onset dyspnea, CO_2 retention (hypercapnia), 2° polycythemia.
Emphysema ("pink puffer")	Enlargement of air spaces, ↓ recoil, ↑ compliance, ↓ diffusing capacity for CO resulting from destruction of alveolar walls (arrow in A). Two types: ▪ Centriacinar—associated with smoking B C. ▪ Panacinar—associated with α_1-antitrypsin deficiency.	↑ elastase activity → loss of elastic fibers → ↑ lung compliance. Exhalation through pursed lips to ↑ airway pressure and prevent airway collapse during respiration. Barrel-shaped chest D.
Asthma	Bronchial hyperresponsiveness causes reversible bronchoconstriction. Smooth muscle hypertrophy, Curschmann spirals E (shed epithelium forms whorled mucus plugs), and Charcot-Leyden crystals (eosinophilic, hexagonal, double-pointed, needle-like crystals formed from breakdown of eosinophils in sputum).	Can be triggered by viral URIs, allergens, stress. Test with methacholine challenge. Findings: cough, wheezing, tachypnea, dyspnea, hypoxemia, ↓ inspiratory/expiratory ratio, pulsus paradoxus, mucus plugging F.
Bronchiectasis	Chronic necrotizing infection of bronchi → permanently dilated airways, purulent sputum, recurrent infections, hemoptysis.	Associated with bronchial obstruction, poor ciliary motility (e.g., smoking, Kartagener syndrome), cystic fibrosis G, allergic bronchopulmonary aspergillosis.

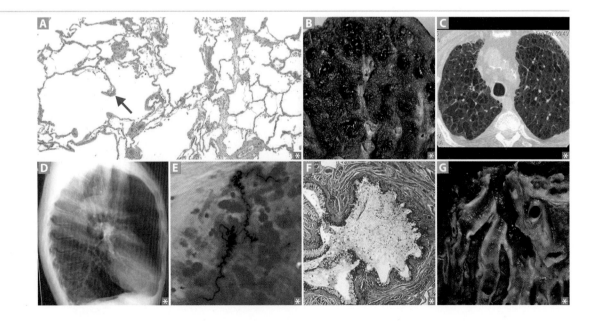

Restrictive lung disease

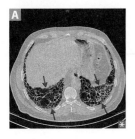

Restricted lung expansion causes ↓ lung volumes (↓ FVC and TLC). PFTs: FEV_1/FVC ratio ≥ 80%.

Types:

- Poor breathing mechanics (extrapulmonary, peripheral hypoventilation, normal A-a gradient):
  - Poor muscular effort—polio, myasthenia gravis
  - Poor structural apparatus—scoliosis, morbid obesity
- Interstitial lung diseases (pulmonary ↓ diffusing capacity, ↑ A-a gradient):
  - Acute respiratory distress syndrome (ARDS)
  - Neonatal respiratory distress syndrome (NRDS; hyaline membrane disease)
  - Pneumoconioses (e.g., anthracosis, silicosis, asbestosis)
  - Sarcoidosis: bilateral hilar lymphadenopathy, noncaseating granuloma; ↑ ACE and Ca^{2+}
  - Idiopathic pulmonary fibrosis **A** (repeated cycles of lung injury and wound healing with ↑ collagen deposition)
  - Goodpasture syndrome
  - Granulomatosis with polyangiitis (Wegener)
  - Langerhans cell histiocytosis (eosinophilic granuloma)
  - Hypersensitivity pneumonitis
  - Drug toxicity (bleomycin, busulfan, amiodarone, methotrexate)

Obstructive vs. restrictive lung disease

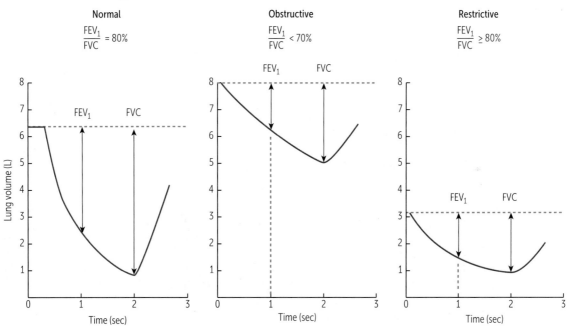

Normal
$$\frac{FEV_1}{FVC} = 80\%$$

Obstructive
$$\frac{FEV_1}{FVC} < 70\%$$

Restrictive
$$\frac{FEV_1}{FVC} \geq 80\%$$

Note: Obstructive lung volumes > normal (↑ TLC, ↑ FRC, ↑ RV); restrictive lung volumes < normal. In both obstructive and restrictive, FEV_1 and FVC are reduced. In obstructive, however, FEV_1 is more dramatically reduced compared to FVC, resulting in a ↓ FEV_1/FVC ratio.

Hypersensitivity pneumonitis	Mixed type III/IV hypersensitivity reaction to environmental antigen → dyspnea, cough, chest tightness, headache. Often seen in farmers and those exposed to birds.	

Pneumoconioses	Coal workers' pneumoconiosis, silicosis, and asbestosis → ↑ risk of cor pulmonale and Caplan syndrome (rheumatoid arthritis and pneumoconioses with intrapulmonary nodules).	
Asbestosis	Associated with shipbuilding, roofing, plumbing. "Ivory white," calcified, supradiaphragmatic and pleural plaques **A B** are pathognomonic of asbestosis. Associated with ↑ incidence of lung cancer (bronchogenic carcinoma > mesothelioma).	Affects lower lobes. Asbestos (ferruginous) bodies are golden-brown fusiform rods resembling dumbbells **C**, found in alveolar septum.
Berylliosis	Associated with exposure to beryllium in aerospace and manufacturing industries. Granulomatous on histology and therefore occasionally responsive to steroids.	Affects upper lobes.
Coal workers' pneumoconiosis	Prolonged coal dust exposure → macrophages laden with carbon → inflammation and fibrosis. Also known as black lung disease.	Affects upper lobes. Anthracosis—asymptomatic condition found in many urban dwellers exposed to sooty air.
Silicosis	Associated with foundries, sandblasting, mines. Macrophages respond to silica and release fibrogenic factors, leading to fibrosis. It is thought that silica may disrupt phagolysosomes and impair macrophages, increasing susceptibility to TB. Also ↑ risk of bronchogenic carcinoma.	Affects upper lobes. "Eggshell" calcification of hilar lymph nodes. **Asbestos** is from the **roof** (was common in insulation), but affects the **base** (lower lobes). **Silica and coal** are from the **base** (earth), but affect the **roof** (upper lobes).

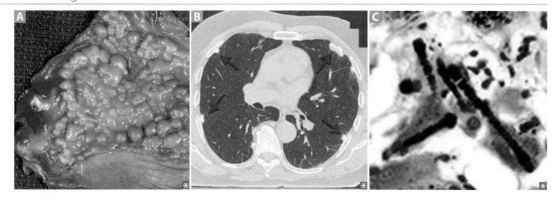

Neonatal respiratory distress syndrome

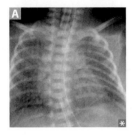

Surfactant deficiency → ↑ surface tension → alveolar collapse ("ground-glass" appearance of lung fields) **A**. A lecithin:sphingomyelin ratio < 1.5 in amniotic fluid is predictive of NRDS. Persistently low O_2 tension → risk of PDA. Therapeutic supplemental O_2 can result in **R**etinopathy of prematurity, **I**ntraventricular hemorrhage, **B**ronchopulmonary dysplasia (**RIB**).

Risk factors: prematurity, maternal diabetes (due to ↑ fetal insulin), C-section delivery (↓ release of fetal glucocorticoids).

Complications: metabolic acidosis, PDA, necrotizing enterocolitis.

Treatment: maternal steroids before birth; artificial surfactant for infant.

Acute respiratory distress syndrome

Clinical syndrome characterized by acute onset respiratory failure, bilateral lung opacities, ↓ PaO_2/FiO_2, no HF. May be caused by trauma, sepsis, shock, gastric aspiration, uremia, acute pancreatitis, amniotic fluid embolism. Diffuse alveolar damage → ↑ alveolar capillary permeability → protein-rich leakage into alveoli and noncardiogenic pulmonary edema (normal PCWP) **A**. Results in formation of intra-alveolar hyaline membranes **B**. Initial damage due to release of neutrophilic substances toxic to alveolar wall, activation of coagulation cascade, and oxygen-derived free radicals.

Management: mechanical ventilation with low tidal volumes, address underlying cause.

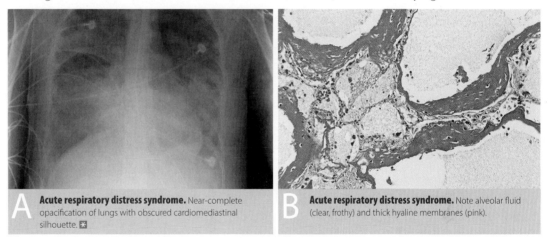

A **Acute respiratory distress syndrome.** Near-complete opacification of lungs with obscured cardiomediastinal silhouette. ✴

B **Acute respiratory distress syndrome.** Note alveolar fluid (clear, frothy) and thick hyaline membranes (pink).

Sleep apnea

Repeated cessation of breathing > 10 seconds during sleep → disrupted sleep → daytime somnolence. Normal PaO_2 during the day.

Nocturnal hypoxia → systemic/pulmonary hypertension, arrhythmias (atrial fibrillation/flutter), sudden death.

Obstructive sleep apnea—respiratory effort against airway obstruction. Associated with obesity, loud snoring. Caused by excess parapharyngeal tissue in adults, adenotonsillar hypertrophy in children. Treatment: weight loss, CPAP, surgery.

Central sleep apnea—no respiratory effort (due to **CNS** injury/toxicity).

Hypoxia → ↑ EPO release → ↑ erythropoiesis.

Obesity hypoventilation syndrome—obesity (BMI ≥ 30 kg/m²) → hypoventilation (↓ respiratory rate) → ↓ PaO_2 and ↑ $PaCO_2$ during sleep → ↑ $PaCO_2$ during waking hours (retention).

Pulmonary hypertension	Normal mean pulmonary artery pressure = 10–14 mmHg; pulmonary hypertension (PH) ≥ 25 mmHg at rest. Results in arteriosclerosis, medial hypertrophy, intimal fibrosis of pulmonary arteries. Course: severe respiratory distress → cyanosis and RVH → death from decompensated cor pulmonale. Five classification groups based on cause and treatment options.
Pulmonary arterial hypertension (PAH)	Idiopathic PAH; heritable—often due to an inactivating mutation in *BMPR2* gene (normally inhibits vascular smooth muscle proliferation); poor prognosis. Includes pulmonary venous occlusive disease and persistent PH of newborn. Other causes include drugs (e.g., amphetamines, cocaine), connective tissue disease, HIV infection, portal hypertension, congenital heart disease, schistosomiasis.
PH due to left heart disease	Causes includes systolic/diastolic dysfunction and valvular disease such as mitral stenosis.
PH due to lung diseases or hypoxia	Destruction of lung parenchyma (e.g., COPD), hypoxemic vasoconstriction (e.g., obstructive sleep apnea, living in high altitude).
Chronic thromboembolic PH	Recurrent microthrombi → ↓ cross-sectional area of pulmonary vascular bed.
Multifactorial PH	Causes include hematologic, systemic, and metabolic disorders.

Lung—physical findings

ABNORMALITY	BREATH SOUNDS	PERCUSSION	FREMITUS	TRACHEAL DEVIATION
Pleural effusion	↓	Dull	↓	— or away from side of lesion (if large)
Atelectasis (bronchial obstruction)	↓	Dull	↓	Toward side of lesion
Simple pneumothorax	↓	Hyperresonant	↓	—
Tension pneumothorax	↓	Hyperresonant	↓	Away from side of lesion
Consolidation (lobar pneumonia, pulmonary edema)	Bronchial breath sounds; late inspiratory crackles	Dull	↑	—

Pleural effusions	Excess accumulation of fluid between pleural layers **A** → restricted lung expansion during inspiration. Can be treated with thoracentesis to remove fluid **B**.
Transudate	↓ protein content. Due to ↑ hydrostatic pressure or ↓ oncotic pressure (e.g., HF, nephrotic syndrome, hepatic cirrhosis).
Exudate	↑ protein content, cloudy. Due to malignancy, pneumonia, collagen vascular disease, trauma (occurs in states of ↑ vascular permeability). Must be drained due to risk of infection.
Lymphatic	Also known as chylothorax. Due to thoracic duct injury from trauma or malignancy. Milky-appearing fluid; ↑ triglycerides.

A **Pleural effusion before treatment.** Note small right-sided pleural effusion on CXR (left) and CT (right). ✲

B **Pleural effusion after treatment.** Almost complete resolution after therapy seen on CXR (left) and CT (right). ✲

Pneumothorax	Accumulation of air in pleural space **A**. Unilateral chest pain and dyspnea, unilateral chest expansion, ↓ tactile fremitus, hyperresonance, diminished breath sounds, all on the affected side.
Primary spontaneous	Due to rupture of apical blebs or cysts. Occurs most frequently in tall, thin, young males.
Secondary spontaneous	Due to diseased lung (e.g., bullae in emphysema, infections), mechanical ventilation with use of high pressures → barotrauma.
Traumatic pneumothorax	Caused by blunt (e.g., rib fracture) or penetrating (e.g., gunshot) trauma.
Tension	Can be any of the above. Air enters pleural space but cannot exit. Increasing trapped air → tension pneumothorax. Trachea deviates away from affected lung **B**.

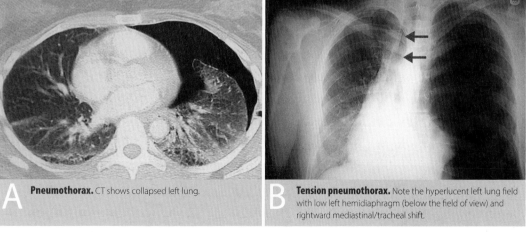

A **Pneumothorax.** CT shows collapsed left lung.

B **Tension pneumothorax.** Note the hyperlucent left lung field with low left hemidiaphragm (below the field of view) and rightward mediastinal/tracheal shift.

Pneumonia

TYPE	TYPICAL ORGANISMS	CHARACTERISTICS
Lobar	*S. pneumoniae* most frequently, also *Legionella*, *Klebsiella*	Intra-alveolar exudate → consolidation 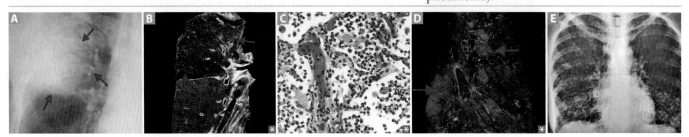; may involve entire lobe B or lung.
Bronchopneumonia	*S. pneumoniae*, *S. aureus*, *H. influenzae*, *Klebsiella*	Acute inflammatory infiltrates C from bronchioles into adjacent alveoli; patchy distribution involving ≥ 1 lobe D.
Interstitial (atypical) pneumonia	Viruses (influenza, CMV, RSV, adenoviruses), *Mycoplasma*, *Legionella*, *Chlamydia*	Diffuse patchy inflammation localized to interstitial areas at alveolar walls; diffuse distribution involving ≥ 1 lobe E. Generally follows a more indolent course ("walking" pneumonia).

Lung abscess

Localized collection of pus within parenchyma 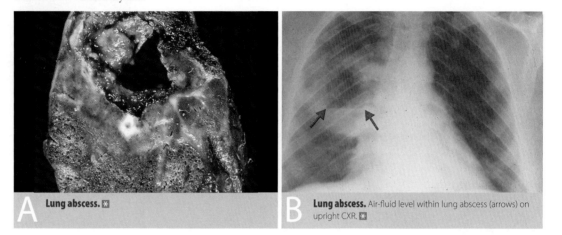. Caused by aspiration of oropharyngeal contents (especially in patients predisposed to loss of consciousness [e.g., alcoholics, epileptics]) or bronchial obstruction (e.g., cancer).

Treatment: clindamycin.

Air-fluid levels **B** often seen on CXR. Fluid levels common in cavities; presence suggests cavitation. Due to anaerobes (e.g., *Bacteroides, Fusobacterium, Peptostreptococcus*) or *S. aureus.*

A Lung abscess. ✴

B Lung abscess. Air-fluid level within lung abscess (arrows) on upright CXR. ✴

Mesothelioma

Malignancy of the pleura associated with asbestosis. May result in hemorrhagic pleural effusion (exudative), pleural thickening.

Psammoma bodies seen on histology. Smoking not a risk factor.

Pancoast tumor (superior sulcus tumor)

Carcinoma that occurs in apex of lung **A** may cause Pancoast syndrome by invading cervical sympathetic chain, causing Horner syndrome (ipsilateral ptosis, miosis, anhidrosis), SVC syndrome, sensorimotor deficits, hoarseness.

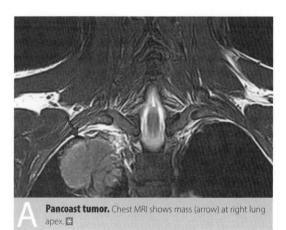

A Pancoast tumor. Chest MRI shows mass (arrow) at right lung apex. ✴

Superior vena cava syndrome

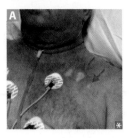

An obstruction of the SVC that impairs blood drainage from the head ("facial plethora"; note blanching after fingertip pressure in), neck (jugular venous distention), and upper extremities (edema). Commonly caused by malignancy (e.g., Pancoast tumor) and thrombosis from indwelling catheters 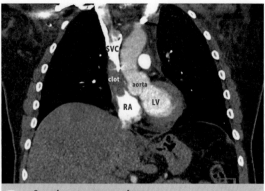. Medical emergency. Can raise intracranial pressure (if obstruction is severe) → headaches, dizziness, ↑ risk of aneurysm/rupture of intracranial arteries.

Superior vena cava syndrome. Coronal contrast-enhanced CT of chest shows low-density clot at junction of SVC and right atrium (RA). ✖

Lung cancer	Leading cause of cancer death.	SPHERE of complications:

Leading cause of cancer death.
Presentation: cough, hemoptysis, bronchial obstruction, wheezing, pneumonic "coin" lesion on CXR or noncalcified nodule on CT.
Sites of metastases from lung cancer: adrenals, brain, bone (pathologic fracture), liver (jaundice, hepatomegaly).
In the lung, metastases (usually multiple lesions) are more common than 1° neoplasms. Most often from breast, colon, prostate, and bladder cancer.

SPHERE of complications:
Superior vena cava syndrome
Pancoast tumor
Horner syndrome
Endocrine (paraneoplastic)
Recurrent laryngeal nerve compression (hoarseness)
Effusions (pleural or pericardial)
Risk factors include smoking, secondhand smoke, radon, asbestos, family history.
Squamous and Small cell carcinomas are Sentral (central).

TYPE	LOCATION	CHARACTERISTICS	HISTOLOGY
Small cell			
Small cell (oat cell) carcinoma	Central	Undifferentiated → very aggressive. May produce ACTH (Cushing syndrome), SIADH, or Antibodies against presynaptic Ca^{2+} channels (Lambert-Eaton myasthenic syndrome) or neurons (paraneoplastic myelitis/encephalitis). Amplification of *myc* oncogenes common. Inoperable; treat with chemotherapy.	Neoplasm of neuroendocrine Kulchitsky cells → small dark blue cells A. Chromogranin A ⊕.
Non–small cell			
Adenocarcinoma	Peripheral	Most common lung cancer in nonsmokers and overall (except for metastases). Activating mutations include *KRAS*, *EGFR*, and *ALK*. Associated with hypertrophic osteoarthropathy (clubbing). Bronchioloalveolar subtype (adenocarcinoma in situ): CXR often shows hazy infiltrates similar to pneumonia; excellent prognosis.	Glandular pattern on histology, often stains mucin ⊕ B. Bronchioloalveolar subtype: grows along alveolar septa → apparent "thickening" of alveolar walls.
Squamous cell carcinoma	Central	Hilar mass arising from bronchus C; Cavitation; Cigarettes; hyperCalcemia (produces PTHrP).	Keratin pearls D and intercellular bridges.
Large cell carcinoma	Peripheral	Highly anaplastic undifferentiated tumor; poor prognosis. Less responsive to chemotherapy; removed surgically.	Pleomorphic giant cells. Can secrete β-hCG.
Bronchial carcinoid tumor	—	Excellent prognosis; metastasis rare. Symptoms usually due to mass effect; occasionally carcinoid syndrome (5-HT secretion → flushing, diarrhea, wheezing).	Nests of neuroendocrine cells; chromogranin A ⊕.

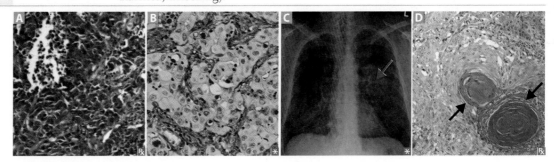

▶ RESPIRATORY—PHARMACOLOGY

H₁ blockers	Reversible inhibitors of H₁ histamine receptors.	
1st generation	Diphenhydramine, dimenhydrinate, chlorpheniramine.	Names contain "-en/-ine" or "-en/-ate."
CLINICAL USES	Allergy, motion sickness, sleep aid.	
TOXICITY	Sedation, antimuscarinic, anti-α-adrenergic.	
2nd generation	Loratadine, fexofenadine, desloratadine, cetirizine.	Names usually end in "-adine."
CLINICAL USES	Allergy.	
TOXICITY	Far less sedating than 1st generation because of ↓ entry into CNS.	

Expectorants	
Guaifenesin	Expectorant—thins respiratory secretions; does not suppress cough reflex.
***N*-acetylcysteine**	Mucolytic—can loosen mucous plugs in CF patients by disrupting disulfide bonds. Also used as an antidote for acetaminophen overdose.

Dextromethorphan	Antitussive (antagonizes NMDA glutamate receptors). Synthetic codeine analog. Has mild opioid effect when used in excess. Naloxone can be given for overdose. Mild abuse potential. May cause serotonin syndrome if combined with other serotonergic agents.

Pseudoephedrine, phenylephrine	
MECHANISM	α-adrenergic agonists, used as nasal decongestants.
CLINICAL USE	Reduce hyperemia, edema, nasal congestion; open obstructed eustachian tubes. Pseudoephedrine also illicitly used to make methamphetamine.
TOXICITY	Hypertension. Can also cause CNS stimulation/anxiety (pseudoephedrine).

Pulmonary hypertension drugs	
Endothelin receptor antagonists	Include bosentan. Competitively antagonize endothelin-1 receptors → ↓ pulmonary vascular resistance. Hepatotoxic (monitor LFTs).
PDE-5 inhibitors	Include sildenafil. Inhibit cGMP PDE5 and prolong vasodilatory effect of nitric oxide. Also used to treat erectile dysfunction.
Prostacyclin analogs	Include epoprostenol, iloprost. Prostacyclins (PGI_2) with direct vasodilatory effects on pulmonary and systemic arterial vascular beds. Inhibit platelet aggregation. Side effects: flushing, jaw pain.

Asthma drugs	Bronchoconstriction is mediated by (1) inflammatory processes and (2) parasympathetic tone; therapy is directed at these 2 pathways.
β$_2$-agonists	**Albuterol**—relaxes bronchial smooth muscle (β$_2$). Used during acute exacerbation.
	Salmeterol, formoterol—long-acting agents for prophylaxis. Adverse effects are tremor and arrhythmia.
Corticosteroids	**Fluticasone, budesonide**—inhibit the synthesis of virtually all cytokines. Inactivate NF-κB, the transcription factor that induces production of TNF-α and other inflammatory agents. 1st-line therapy for chronic asthma.
Muscarinic antagonists	**Ipratropium**—competitively blocks muscarinic receptors, preventing bronchoconstriction. Also used for COPD. Tiotropium is long acting.
Antileukotrienes	**Montelukast, zafirlukast**—block leukotriene receptors (CysLT1). Especially good for aspirin-induced asthma.
	Zileuton—5-lipoxygenase pathway inhibitor. Blocks conversion of arachidonic acid to leukotrienes. Hepatotoxic.
Omalizumab	Monoclonal anti-IgE antibody. Binds mostly unbound serum IgE and blocks binding to FcεRI. Used in allergic asthma resistant to inhaled steroids and long-acting β$_2$-agonists.
Methylxanthines	**Theophylline**—likely causes bronchodilation by inhibiting phosphodiesterase → ↑ cAMP levels due to ↓ cAMP hydrolysis. Usage is limited because of narrow therapeutic index (cardiotoxicity, neurotoxicity); metabolized by cytochrome P-450. Blocks actions of adenosine.

Methacholine	Muscarinic receptor (M$_3$) agonist. Used in bronchial challenge test to help diagnose asthma.

▶ NOTES

Rapid Review

"Study without thought is vain: thought without study is dangerous."
—Confucius

"It is better, of course, to know useless things than to know nothing."
—Lucius Annaeus Seneca

The following tables represent a collection of high-yield associations of diseases with their clinical findings, treatments, and pathophysiology. They serve as a quick review before the exam to tune your senses to commonly tested cases.

▶ CLASSIC PRESENTATIONS

CLINICAL PRESENTATION	DIAGNOSIS/DISEASE
Abdominal pain, ascites, hepatomegaly	Budd-Chiari syndrome (posthepatic venous thrombosis)
Abdominal pain, diarrhea, leukocytosis, recent antibiotic use	*Clostridium difficile* infection
Achilles tendon xanthoma	Familial hypercholesterolemia ($\downarrow$ LDL receptor signaling)
Adrenal hemorrhage, hypotension, DIC	Waterhouse-Friderichsen syndrome (meningococcemia)
Anaphylaxis following blood transfusion	IgA deficiency
Anterior "drawer sign" $\oplus$	Anterior cruciate ligament injury
Arachnodactyly, lens dislocation, aortic dissection, hyperflexible joints	Marfan syndrome (fibrillin defect)
Athlete with polycythemia	2° to erythropoietin injection
Back pain, fever, night sweats	Pott disease (vertebral TB)
Bilateral acoustic schwannomas	Neurofibromatosis type 2
Bilateral hilar adenopathy, uveitis	Sarcoidosis (noncaseating granulomas)
Black eschar on face of patient with diabetic ketoacidosis	*Mucor* or *Rhizopus* fungal infection
Blue sclera	Osteogenesis imperfecta (type I collagen defect)
Bluish line on gingiva	Burton line (lead poisoning)
Bone pain, bone enlargement, arthritis	Paget disease of bone ($\uparrow$ osteoblastic and osteoclastic activity)
Bounding pulses, diastolic heart murmur, head bobbing	Aortic regurgitation
"Butterfly" facial rash and Raynaud phenomenon in a young female	Systemic lupus erythematosus
Café-au-lait spots, Lisch nodules (iris hamartoma), cutaneous neurofibromas, pheochromocytomas, optic gliomas	Neurofibromatosis type I, pheochromocytoma, optic gliomas
Café-au-lait spots (unilateral), polyostotic fibrous dysplasia, precocious puberty, multiple endocrine abnormalities	McCune-Albright syndrome (mosaic G-protein signaling mutation)
Calf pseudohypertrophy	Muscular dystrophy (most commonly Duchenne, due to X-linked recessive frameshift mutation of dystrophin gene)
Cervical lymphadenopathy, desquamating rash, coronary aneurysms, red conjunctivac and tongue	Kawasaki disease (treat with IVIG and aspirin)
"Cherry-red spots" on macula	Tay-Sachs (ganglioside accumulation) or Niemann-Pick (sphingomyelin accumulation), central retinal artery occlusion
Chest pain on exertion	Angina (stable: with moderate exertion; unstable: with minimal exertion or at rest)
Chest pain, pericardial effusion/friction rub, persistent fever following MI	Dressler syndrome (autoimmune-mediated post-MI fibrinous pericarditis, 2–12 weeks after acute episode)
Chest pain with ST depressions on EKG	Unstable angina (troponins −) or NSTEMI (troponins +)
Child uses arms to stand up from squat	Gowers sign (Duchenne muscular dystrophy)
Child with fever later develops red rash on face that spreads to body	"Slapped cheeks" (erythema infectiosum/fifth disease: parvovirus B19)
Chorea, dementia, caudate degeneration	Huntington disease (autosomal dominant CAG repeat expansion)
Chorioretinitis, hydrocephalus, intracranial calcifications	Congenital toxoplasmosis

CLINICAL PRESENTATION	DIAGNOSIS/DISEASE
Chronic exercise intolerance with myalgia, fatigue, painful cramps, myoglobinuria	McArdle disease (skeletal muscle glycogen phosphorylase deficiency)
Cold intolerance	Hypothyroidism
Conjugate horizontal gaze palsy, horizontal diplopia	Internuclear ophthalmoplegia (damage to MLF; may be unilateral or bilateral)
Continuous "machine-like" heart murmur	PDA (close with indomethacin; open or maintain with PGE analogs)
Cutaneous/dermal edema due to connective tissue deposition	Myxedema (caused by hypothyroidism, Graves disease [pretibial])
Cutaneous flushing, diarrhea, bronchospasm	Carcinoid syndrome (right-sided cardiac valvular lesions, ↑ 5-HIAA)
Dark purple skin/mouth nodules in a patient with AIDS	Kaposi sarcoma, associated with HHV-8
Deep, labored breathing/hyperventilation	Kussmaul respirations (diabetic ketoacidosis)
Dermatitis, dementia, diarrhea	Pellagra (niacin [vitamin B_3] deficiency)
Dilated cardiomyopathy, edema, alcoholism or malnutrition	Wet beriberi (thiamine [vitamin B_1] deficiency)
Dog or cat bite resulting in infection	*Pasteurella multocida* (cellulitis at inoculation site)
Dry eyes, dry mouth, arthritis	Sjögren syndrome (autoimmune destruction of exocrine glands)
Dysphagia (esophageal webs), glossitis, iron deficiency anemia	Plummer-Vinson syndrome (may progress to esophageal squamous cell carcinoma)
Elastic skin, hypermobility of joints, ↑ bleeding tendency	Ehlers-Danlos syndrome (type V collagen defect, type III collagen defect seen in vascular subtype of ED)
Enlarged, hard left supraclavicular node	Virchow node (abdominal metastasis)
Episodic vertigo, tinnitus, hearing loss	Meniere disease
Erythroderma, lymphadenopathy, hepatosplenomegaly, atypical T cells	Mycosis fungoides (cutaneous T-cell lymphoma) or Sézary syndrome (mycosis fungoides + malignant T cells in blood)
Facial muscle spasm upon tapping	Chvostek sign (hypocalcemia)
Fat, female, forty, and fertile	Cholelithiasis (gallstones)
Fever, chills, headache, myalgia following antibiotic treatment for syphilis	Jarisch-Herxheimer reaction (rapid lysis of spirochetes results in endotoxin release)
Fever, cough, conjunctivitis, coryza, diffuse rash	Measles
Fever, night sweats, weight loss	B symptoms (staging) of lymphoma
Fibrous plaques in soft tissue of penis with abnormal curvature	Peyronie disease (connective tissue disorder)
Golden brown rings around peripheral cornea	Kayser-Fleischer rings (copper accumulation from Wilson disease)
Gout, intellectual disability, self-mutilating behavior in a boy	Lesch-Nyhan syndrome (HGPRT deficiency, X-linked recessive)
Hamartomatous GI polyps, hyperpigmentation of mouth/feet/hands/genitalia	Peutz-Jeghers syndrome (inherited, benign polyposis can cause bowel obstruction; ↑ cancer risk, mainly GI)
Hepatosplenomegaly, pancytopenia, osteoporosis, aseptic necrosis of femur, bone crises	Gaucher disease (glucocerebrosidase deficiency)

CLINICAL PRESENTATION	DIAGNOSIS/DISEASE
Hereditary nephritis, sensorineural hearing loss, cataracts	Alport syndrome (mutation in collagen IV)
Hyperphagia, hypersexuality, hyperorality, hyperdocility	Klüver-Bucy syndrome (bilateral amygdala lesion)
Hyperreflexia, hypertonia, Babinski sign present	UMN damage
Hyporeflexia, hypotonia, atrophy, fasciculations	LMN damage
Hypoxemia, polycythemia, hypercapnia	"Blue bloater" (chronic bronchitis: hyperplasia of mucous cells)
Indurated, ulcerated genital lesion	Nonpainful: chancre (1° syphilis, *Treponema pallidum*) Painful, with exudate: chancroid (*Haemophilus ducreyi*)
Infant with "cherry-red" spot on macula, hepatosplenomegaly, and neurodegeneration	Niemann-Pick disease (genetic sphingomyelinase deficiency)
Infant with cleft lip/palate, microcephaly or holoprosencephaly, polydactyly, cutis aplasia	Patau syndrome (trisomy 13)
Infant with hypoglycemia, hepatomegaly	Cori disease (debranching enzyme deficiency) or Von Gierke disease (glucose-6-phosphatase deficiency, more severe)
Infant with microcephaly, rocker-bottom feet, clenched hands, and structural heart defect	Edwards syndrome (trisomy 18)
Jaundice, palpable distended non-tender gallbladder	Courvoisier sign (distal obstruction of biliary tree)
Large rash with bull's-eye appearance	Erythema chronicum migrans from *Ixodes* tick bite (Lyme disease: *Borrelia*)
Lucid interval after traumatic brain injury	Epidural hematoma (middle meningeal artery rupture)
Male child, recurrent infections, no mature B cells	Bruton disease (X-linked agammaglobulinemia)
Mucosal bleeding and prolonged bleeding time	Glanzmann thrombasthenia (defect in platelet aggregation due to lack of GpIIb/IIIa)
Muffled heart sounds, distended neck veins, hypotension	Beck triad of cardiac tamponade
Multiple colon polyps, osteomas/soft tissue tumors, impacted/supernumerary teeth	Gardner syndrome (subtype of FAP)
Myopathy (infantile hypertrophic cardiomyopathy), exercise intolerance	Pompe disease (lysosomal α-1,4-glucosidase deficiency)
Neonate with arm paralysis following difficult birth	Erb-Duchenne palsy (superior trunk [C5–C6] brachial plexus injury: "waiter's tip")
No lactation postpartum, absent menstruation, cold intolerance	Sheehan syndrome (pituitary infarction)
Nystagmus, intention tremor, scanning speech, bilateral internuclear ophthalmoplegia	Multiple sclerosis
Painful blue fingers/toes, hemolytic anemia	Cold agglutinin disease (autoimmune hemolytic anemia caused by *Mycoplasma pneumoniae*, infectious mononucleosis, CLL)
Painful fingers/toes changing color from blue to white to red with cold or stress	Raynaud phenomenon (vasospasm in extremities)
Painful, raised red lesions on pads of fingers/toes	Osler nodes (infective endocarditis, immune complex deposition)

CLINICAL PRESENTATION	DIAGNOSIS/DISEASE
Painless erythematous lesions on palms and soles	Janeway lesions (infective endocarditis, septic emboli/microabscesses)
Painless jaundice	Cancer of the pancreatic head obstructing bile duct
Palpable purpura on buttocks/legs, joint pain, abdominal pain (child), hematuria	Henoch-Schönlein purpura (IgA vasculitis affecting skin and kidneys)
Pancreatic, pituitary, parathyroid tumors	MEN 1 (autosomal dominant)
Periorbital and/or peripheral edema, proteinuria, hypoalbuminemia, hypercholesterolemia	Nephrotic syndrome
Pink complexion, dyspnea, hyperventilation	"Pink puffer" (emphysema: centriacinar [smoking], panacinar [α_1-antitrypsin deficiency])
Polyuria, renal tubular acidosis type II, growth failure, electrolyte imbalances, hypophosphatemic rickets	Fanconi syndrome (multiple combined dysfunction of the proximal convoluted tubule)
Pruritic, purple, polygonal planar papules and plaques (6 P's)	Lichen planus
Ptosis, miosis, anhidrosis	Horner syndrome (sympathetic chain lesion)
Pupil accommodates but doesn't react	Argyll Robertson pupil (neurosyphilis)
Rapidly progressive limb weakness that ascends following GI/upper respiratory infection	Guillain-Barré syndrome (acute inflammatory demyelinating polyradiculopathy subtype)
Rash on palms and soles	Coxsackie A, 2° syphilis, Rocky Mountain spotted fever
Recurrent cold (noninflamed) abscesses, unusual eczema, high serum IgE	Hyper-IgE syndrome (Job syndrome: neutrophil chemotaxis abnormality)
Red "currant jelly" sputum in alcoholic or diabetic patients	*Klebsiella pneumoniae* pneumonia
Red "currant jelly" stools	Acute mesenteric ischemia (adults), intussusception (children)
Red, itchy, swollen rash of nipple/areola	Paget disease of the breast (sign of underlying neoplasm)
Red urine in the morning, fragile RBCs	Paroxysmal nocturnal hemoglobinuria
Renal cell carcinoma (bilateral), hemangioblastomas, angiomatosis, pheochromocytoma	von Hippel-Lindau disease (dominant tumor suppressor gene mutation)
Resting tremor, rigidity, akinesia, postural instability, shuffling gait	Parkinson disease (loss of dopaminergic neurons in substantia nigra pars compacta)
Retinal hemorrhages with pale centers	Roth spots (bacterial endocarditis)
Severe jaundice in neonate	Crigler-Najjar syndrome (congenital unconjugated hyperbilirubinemia)
Severe RLQ pain with palpation of LLQ	Rovsing sign (acute appendicitis)
Severe RLQ pain with rebound tenderness	McBurney sign (acute appendicitis)
Short stature, café au lait spots, thumb/radial defects, ↑ incidence of tumors/leukemia, aplastic anemia	Fanconi anemia (genetic loss of DNA crosslink repair; often progresses to AML)
Single palmar crease	Down syndrome
Situs inversus, chronic sinusitis, bronchiectasis, infertility	Kartagener syndrome (dynein arm defect affecting cilia)
Skin hyperpigmentation, hypotension, fatigue	1° adrenocortical insufficiency (e.g., Addison disease) causes ↑ ACTH and ↑ α-MSH production)
Slow, progressive muscle weakness in boys	Becker muscular dystrophy (X-linked missense mutation in dystrophin; less severe than Duchenne)

CLINICAL PRESENTATION	DIAGNOSIS/DISEASE
Small, irregular red spots on buccal/lingual mucosa with blue-white centers	Koplik spots (measles; rubeola virus)
Smooth, moist, painless, wart-like white lesions on genitals	Condylomata lata (2° syphilis)
Splinter hemorrhages in fingernails	Bacterial endocarditis
"Strawberry tongue"	Scarlet fever, Kawasaki disease
Streak ovaries, congenital heart disease, horseshoe kidney, cystic hygroma at birth, short stature, webbed neck, lymphedema	Turner syndrome (45,XO)
Sudden swollen/painful big toe joint, tophi	Gout/podagra (hyperuricemia)
Swollen gums, mucosal bleeding, poor wound healing, petechiae	Scurvy (vitamin C deficiency: can't hydroxylate proline/lysine for collagen synthesis)
Swollen, hard, painful finger joints	Osteoarthritis (osteophytes on PIP [Bouchard nodes], DIP [Heberden nodes])
Systolic ejection murmur (crescendo-decrescendo)	Aortic stenosis
Telangiectasias, recurrent epistaxis, skin discoloration, arteriovenous malformations, GI bleeding, hematuria	Osler-Weber-Rendu syndrome
Thyroid and parathyroid tumors, pheochromocytoma	MEN 2A (autosomal dominant *RET* mutation)
Thyroid tumors, pheochromocytoma, ganglioneuromatosis	MEN 2B (autosomal dominant *RET* mutation)
Toe extension/fanning upon plantar scrape	Babinski sign (UMN lesion)
Unilateral facial drooping involving forehead	LMN facial nerve (CN VII) palsy; UMN lesions spare the forehead
Urethritis, conjunctivitis, arthritis in a male	Reactive arthritis associated with HLA-B27
Vascular birthmark (port-wine stain) of the face	Nevus flammeus (benign, but associated with Sturge-Weber syndrome)
Vomiting blood following gastroesophageal lacerations	Mallory-Weiss syndrome (alcoholic and bulimic patients)
Weight loss, diarrhea, arthritis, fever, adenopathy	Whipple disease (*Tropheryma whipplei*)
"Worst headache of my life"	Subarachnoid hemorrhage

▶ CLASSIC LABS/FINDINGS

LAB/DIAGNOSTIC FINDING	DIAGNOSIS/DISEASE
Anticentromere antibodies	Scleroderma (CREST)
Anti-desmoglein (epithelial) antibodies	Pemphigus vulgaris (blistering)
Anti–glomerular basement membrane antibodies	Goodpasture syndrome (glomerulonephritis and hemoptysis)
Antihistone antibodies	Drug-induced SLE (e.g., hydralazine, isoniazid, phenytoin, procainamide)
Anti-IgG antibodies	Rheumatoid arthritis (systemic inflammation, joint pannus, boutonnière deformity)
Antimitochondrial antibodies (AMAs)	1° biliary cirrhosis (female, cholestasis, portal hypertension)
Antineutrophil cytoplasmic antibodies (ANCAs)	Microscopic polyangiitis and eosinophilic granulomatosis with polyangiitis (Churg-Strauss syndrome) (MPO-ANCA/ p-ANCA); granulomatosis with polyangiitis (Wegener; PR3-ANCA/c-ANCA)

LAB/DIAGNOSTIC FINDING	DIAGNOSIS/DISEASE
Antinuclear antibodies (ANAs: anti-Smith and anti-dsDNA)	SLE (type III hypersensitivity)
Antiplatelet antibodies	Idiopathic thrombocytopenic purpura
Anti-topoisomerase antibodies	Diffuse systemic scleroderma
Anti-transglutaminase/anti-gliadin/anti-endomysial antibodies	Celiac disease (diarrhea, weight loss)
"Apple core" lesion on barium enema x-ray	Colorectal cancer (usually left-sided)
Atypical lymphocytes	EBV
Azurophilic peroxidase ⊕ granular inclusions in granulocytes and myeloblasts	Auer rods (AML, especially the promyelocytic [M3] type)
Bacitracin response	Sensitive: *S. pyogenes* (group A); resistant: *S. agalactiae* (group B)
"Bamboo spine" on x-ray	Ankylosing spondylitis (chronic inflammatory arthritis: HLA-B27)
Basophilic nuclear remnants in RBCs	Howell-Jolly bodies (due to splenectomy or nonfunctional spleen)
Basophilic stippling of RBCs	Lead poisoning or sideroblastic anemia
Bloody or yellow tap on lumbar puncture	Subarachnoid hemorrhage
"Boot-shaped" heart on x-ray	Tetralogy of Fallot (due to RVH)
Branching gram-positive rods with sulfur granules	*Actinomyces israelii*
Bronchogenic apical lung tumor on imaging	Pancoast tumor (can compress cervical sympathetic chain and cause Horner syndrome)
"Brown" tumor of bone	Hyperparathyroidism or osteitis fibrosa cystica (deposited hemosiderin from hemorrhage gives brown color)
Cardiomegaly with apical atrophy	Chagas disease (*Trypanosoma cruzi*)
Cellular crescents in Bowman capsule	Rapidly progressive crescentic glomerulonephritis
"Chocolate cyst" of ovary	Endometriosis (frequently involves both ovaries)
Circular grouping of dark tumor cells surrounding pale neurofibrils	Homer-Wright rosettes (neuroblastoma, medulloblastoma)
Colonies of mucoid *Pseudomonas* in lungs	Cystic fibrosis (autosomal recessive mutation in *CFTR* gene → fat-soluble vitamin deficiency and mucous plugs)
↓ AFP in amniotic fluid/maternal serum	Down syndrome or other chromosomal abnormalities
Degeneration of dorsal column fibers	Tabes dorsalis (3° syphilis), subacute combined degeneration (dorsal columns, lateral corticospinal, spinocerebellar tracts affected)
"Delta wave" on EKG, short PR interval, supraventricular tachycardia	Wolf-Parkinson-White syndrome (Bundle of Kent bypasses AV node)
Depigmentation of neurons in substantia nigra	Parkinson disease (basal ganglia disorder: rigidity, resting tremor, bradykinesia)
Desquamated epithelium casts in sputum	Curschmann spirals (bronchial asthma; can result in whorled mucous plugs)
Disarrayed granulosa cells arranged around collections of eosinophilic fluid	Call-Exner bodies (granulosa cell tumor of the ovary)
Dysplastic squamous cervical cells with "raisinoid" nuclei and hyperchromasia	Koilocytes (HPV: predisposes to cervical cancer)

LAB/DIAGNOSTIC FINDING	DIAGNOSIS/DISEASE
Electrical alternans (alternating amplitude on EKG)	Pericardial tamponade
Enlarged cells with intranuclear inclusion bodies	"Owl eye" appearance of CMV
Enlarged thyroid cells with ground-glass nuclei with central clearing	"Orphan Annie" eyes nuclei (papillary carcinoma of the thyroid)
Eosinophilic cytoplasmic inclusion in liver cell	Mallory body (alcoholic liver disease)
Eosinophilic cytoplasmic inclusion in nerve cell	Lewy body (Parkinson disease)
Eosinophilic globule in liver	Councilman body (viral hepatitis, yellow fever), represents hepatocyte undergoing apoptosis
Eosinophilic inclusion bodies in cytoplasm of hippocampal and cerebellar neurons	Negri bodies of rabies
Extracellular amyloid deposition in gray matter of brain	Senile plaques (Alzheimer disease)
Giant B cells with bilobed nuclei with prominent inclusions ("owl's eye")	Reed-Sternberg cells (Hodgkin lymphoma)
Glomerulus-like structure surrounding vessel in germ cells	Schiller-Duval bodies (yolk sac tumor)
"Hair on end" ("Crew-cut") appearance on x-ray	β-thalassemia, sickle cell disease (marrow expansion)
hCG elevated	Choriocarcinoma, hydatidiform mole (occurs with and without embryo, and multiple pregnancy)
Heart nodules (granulomatous)	Aschoff bodies (rheumatic fever)
Heterophile antibodies	Infectious mononucleosis (EBV)
Hexagonal, double-pointed, needle-like crystals in bronchial secretions	Bronchial asthma (Charcot-Leyden crystals: eosinophilic granules)
High level of D-dimers	DVT, PE, DIC
Hilar lymphadenopathy, peripheral granulomatous lesion in middle or lower lung lobes (can calcify)	Ghon complex (1° TB: *Mycobacterium* bacilli)
"Honeycomb lung" on x-ray or CT	Interstitial pulmonary fibrosis
Hypercoagulability (leading to migrating DVTs and vasculitis)	Trousseau syndrome (adenocarcinoma of pancreas or lung)
Hypersegmented neutrophils	Megaloblastic anemia (B_{12} deficiency: neurologic symptoms; folate deficiency: no neurologic symptoms)
Hypertension, hypokalemia, metabolic alkalosis	Conn syndrome (primary hyperaldosteronism)
Hypochromic, microcytic anemia	Iron deficiency anemia, lead poisoning, thalassemia (fetal hemoglobin sometimes present)
Increased AFP in amniotic fluid/maternal serum	Dating error, anencephaly, spina bifida (neural tube defects)
Increased uric acid levels	Gout, Lesch-Nyhan syndrome, tumor lysis syndrome, loop and thiazide diuretics
Intranuclear eosinophilic droplet-like bodies	Cowdry type A bodies (HSV or VZV)
Iron-containing nodules in alveolar septum	Ferruginous bodies (asbestosis: ↑ chance of mesothelioma)
Keratin pearls on a skin biopsy	Squamous cell carcinoma
Large granules in phagocytes, immunodeficiency	Chédiak-Higashi disease (congenital failure of phagolysosome formation)
"Lead pipe" appearance of colon on abdominal imaging	Ulcerative colitis (loss of haustra)
Linear appearance of IgG deposition on glomerular and alveolar basement membranes	Goodpasture syndrome

LAB/DIAGNOSTIC FINDING	DIAGNOSIS/DISEASE
Low serum ceruloplasmin	Wilson disease (hepatolenticular degeneration)
"Lumpy bumpy" appearance of glomeruli on immunofluorescence	Poststreptococcal glomerulonephritis (due to deposition of IgG, IgM, and C3)
Lytic ("punched-out") bone lesions on x-ray	Multiple myeloma
Mammary gland ("blue domed") cyst	Fibrocystic change of the breast
Monoclonal antibody spike	<ul><li>Multiple myeloma (usually IgG or IgA)</li><li>Monoclonal gammopathy of undetermined significance (MGUS consequence of aging)</li><li>Waldenström (M protein = IgM) macroglobulinemia</li><li>Primary amyloidosis</li></ul>
Mucin-filled cell with peripheral nucleus	"Signet ring" (gastric carcinoma)
Narrowing of bowel lumen on barium x-ray	"String sign" (Crohn disease)
Necrotizing vasculitis (lungs) and necrotizing glomerulonephritis	Granulomatosis with polyangiitis (Wegener; PR3-ANCA/c-ANCA) and Goodpasture syndrome (anti–basement membrane antibodies)
Needle-shaped, negatively birefringent crystals	Gout (monosodium urate crystals)
Nodular hyaline deposits in glomeruli	Kimmelstiel-Wilson nodules (diabetic nephropathy)
Novobiocin response	Sensitive: *S. epidermidis*; resistant: *S. saprophyticus*
"Nutmeg" appearance of liver	Chronic passive congestion of liver due to right heart failure or Budd-Chiari syndrome
"Onion skin" periosteal reaction	Ewing sarcoma (malignant small blue cell tumor)
Optochin response	Sensitive: *S. pneumoniae*; resistant: viridans streptococci (*S. mutans, S. sanguis*)
Periosteum raised from bone, creating triangular area	Codman triangle on x-ray, Ewing sarcoma, pyogenic osteomyelitis)
Podocyte fusion or "effacement" on electron microscopy	Minimal change disease (child with nephrotic syndrome)
Polished, "ivory-like" appearance of bone at cartilage erosion	Eburnation (osteoarthritis resulting in bony sclerosis)
Protein aggregates in neurons from hyperphosphorylation of tau protein	Neurofibrillary tangles (Alzheimer disease) and Pick bodies (Pick disease)
Psammoma bodies	Meningiomas, papillary thyroid carcinoma, mesothelioma, papillary serous carcinoma of the endometrium and ovary
Pseudopalisading tumor cells on brain biopsy	Glioblastoma multiforme
RBC casts in urine	Glomerulonephritis
Rectangular, crystal-like, cytoplasmic inclusions in Leydig cells	Reinke crystals (Leydig cell tumor)
Recurrent infections, eczema, thrombocytopenia	Wiskott-Aldrich syndrome
Renal epithelial casts in urine	Intrinsic renal failure (e.g., ischemia or toxic injury)
Rhomboid crystals, positively birefringent	Pseudogout (calcium pyrophosphate dihydrate crystals)
Rib notching	Coarctation of the aorta
Ring-enhancing brain lesion in AIDS	*Toxoplasma gondii*, CNS lymphoma
Sheets of medium-sized lymphoid cells with scattered pale, tingible body–laden macrophages ("starry sky" histology)	Burkitt lymphoma (t[8:14] c-*myc* activation, associated with EBV; "starry sky" made up of malignant cells)
Silver-staining spherical aggregation of tau proteins in neurons	Pick bodies (Pick disease: progressive dementia, changes in personality)

LAB/DIAGNOSTIC FINDING	DIAGNOSIS/DISEASE
"Soap bubble" in femur or tibia on x-ray	Giant cell tumor of bone (generally benign)
"Spikes" on basement membrane, "dome-like" subepithelial deposits	Membranous nephropathy (nephrotic syndrome)
Stacks of RBCs	Rouleaux formation (high ESR, multiple myeloma)
"Steeple" sign on CXR	Croup (parainfluenza virus)
Stippled vaginal epithelial cells	"Clue cells" (*Gardnerella vaginalis*)
Streptococcus bovis bacteremia	Colon cancer
"Tennis racket"-shaped cytoplasmic organelles (EM) in Langerhans cells	Birbeck granules (Langerhans cell histiocytosis)
Thousands of polyps on colonoscopy	Familial adenomatous polyposis (autosomal dominant, mutation of APC gene)
Thrombi made of white/red layers	Lines of Zahn (arterial thrombus, layers of platelets/RBCs)
"Thumb sign" on lateral neck x-ray	Epiglottitis (*Haemophilus influenzae*)
Thyroid-like appearance of kidney	Chronic pyelonephritis (usually due to recurrent infections)
"Tram-track" appearance of capillary loops of glomerular basement membranes on light microscopy	Membranoproliferative glomerulonephritis
Triglyceride accumulation in liver cell vacuoles	Fatty liver disease (alcoholic or metabolic syndrome)
"Waxy" casts with very low urine flow	Chronic end-stage renal disease
WBC casts in urine	Acute pyelonephritis
WBCs that look "smudged"	CLL (almost always B cell)
"Wire loop" glomerular capillary appearance on light microscopy	Diffuse proliferative glomerulonephritis (usually seen with lupus)
Yellowish CSF	Xanthochromia (e.g., due to subarachnoid hemorrhage)

▶ CLASSIC/RELEVANT TREATMENTS

CONDITION	COMMON TREATMENT(S)
Absence seizures	Ethosuximide
Acute gout attack	NSAIDs, colchicine, glucocorticoids
Acute promyelocytic leukemia (M3)	All-*trans* retinoic acid
ADHD	Methylphenidate, CBT, atomoxetine
Alcoholism	Disulfiram, acamprosate, naltrexone, supportive care
Alcohol withdrawal	Long-acting benzodiazepines
Anorexia	Nutrition, psychotherapy, mirtazapine
Anticoagulation during pregnancy	Heparin
Arrhythmia in damaged cardiac tissue	Class IB antiarrhythmic (lidocaine, mexiletine)
B_{12} deficiency	Vitamin B_{12} supplementation (work up cause with Schilling test)
Benign prostatic hyperplasia	α_1-antagonists, 5α-reductase inhibitors, PDE-5 inhibitors

CONDITION	COMMON TREATMENT(S)
Bipolar disorder	Mood stabilizers (e.g., lithium, valproic acid, carbamazepine), atypical antipsychotics
Breast cancer in postmenopausal woman	Aromatase inhibitor (anastrozole)
Buerger disease	Smoking cessation
Bulimia nervosa	SSRIs
Candida albicans	Topical azoles (vaginitis); nystatin, fluconazole, caspofungin (oral/esophageal); fluconazole, caspofungin, amphotericin B (systemic)
Carcinoid syndrome	Octreotide
Chlamydia trachomatis	Doxycycline (+ ceftriaxone for gonorrhea coinfection), erythromycin eye drops (prophylaxis in infants)
Chronic gout	Xanthine oxidase inhibitors (e.g., allopurinol, febuxostat)
Chronic hepatitis B or C	IFN-α (HBV and HCV); ribavirin, simeprevir, sofosbuvir (HCV)
Chronic myelogenous leukemia	Imatinib
Clostridium botulinum	Antitoxin
Clostridium difficile	Oral metronidazole; if refractory, oral vancomycin
Clostridium tetani	Antitoxin
CMV	Ganciclovir, foscarnet, cidofovir
Crohn disease	Corticosteroids, infliximab, azathioprine
Cryptococcus neoformans	Fluconazole (in AIDS patients)
Cyclophosphamide-induced hemorrhagic cystitis	Mesna
Depression	SSRIs (first-line)
Diabetes insipidus	Desmopressin (central); hydrochlorothiazide, indomethacin, amiloride (nephrogenic)
Diabetes mellitus type 1	Dietary intervention (low carbohydrate) + insulin replacement
Diabetes mellitus type 2	Dietary intervention, oral hypoglycemics, and insulin (if refractory)
Diabetic ketoacidosis	Fluids, insulin, K^+
Enterococci	Vancomycin, aminopenicillins/cephalosporins
Erectile dysfunction	Sildenafil, tadalafil, vardenafil
ER ⊕ breast cancer	Tamoxifen
Ethylene glycol/methanol intoxication	Fomepizole (alcohol dehydrogenase inhibitor)
Haemophilus influenzae (B)	Rifampin (prophylaxis)
Generalized anxiety disorder	SSRIs, SNRIs (first line); buspirone (second line)
Granulomatosis with polyangiitis (Wegener)	Cyclophosphamide, corticosteroids
Heparin reversal	Protamine sulfate
HER2/neu ⊕ breast cancer	Trastuzumab
Hyperaldosteronism	Spironolactone

CONDITION	COMMON TREATMENT(S)
Hypercholesterolemia	Statin (first-line)
Hypertriglyceridemia	Fibrate
Immediate anticoagulation	Heparin
Infertility	Leuprolide, GnRH (pulsatile), clomiphene
Influenza	Oseltamivir, zanamivir
Kawasaki disease	IVIG, high-dose aspirin
Legionella pneumophila	Macrolides (e.g., azithromycin)
Long-term anticoagulation	Warfarin, dabigatran, rivaroxaban and apixaban
Malaria	Chloroquine, mefloquine, atovaquone/proguanil (for blood schizont), primaquine (for liver hypnozoite)
Malignant hyperthermia	Dantrolene
Medical abortion	Mifepristone
Migraine	Abortive therapies (e.g., sumatriptan, NSAIDs); prophylaxis (e.g., propranolol, topiramate, CCBs, amitriptyline)
Multiple sclerosis	Disease-modifying therapies (e.g., β-interferon, natalizumab); for acute flares, use IV steroids
Mycobacterium tuberculosis	RIPE (rifampin, isoniazid, pyrazinamide, ethambutol)
Neisseria gonorrhoeae	Ceftriaxone (add doxycycline to cover likely concurrent *C. trachomatis*)
Neisseria meningitidis	Penicillin/ceftriaxone, rifampin (prophylaxis)
Neural tube defect prevention	Prenatal folic acid
Osteomalacia/rickets	Vitamin D supplementation
Osteoporosis	Calcium/vitamin D supplementation (prophylaxis); bisphosphonates, PTH analogs, SERMs, calcitonin, denosumab (treatment)
Patent ductus arteriosus	Close with indomethacin; open or maintain with PGE analogs
Pheochromocytoma	α-antagonists (e.g., phenoxybenzamine)
Pneumocystis jirovecii	TMP-SMX (prophylaxis in AIDS patient)
Prolactinoma	Cabergoline/bromocriptine (dopamine agonists)
Prostate adenocarcinoma/uterine fibroids	Leuprolide, GnRH (continuous)
Prostate adenocarcinoma	Flutamide
Pseudomonas aeruginosa	Antipseudomonal penicillins, aminoglycosides, carbapenems
Pulmonary arterial hypertension (idiopathic)	Sildenafil, bosentan, epoprostenol
Rickettsia rickettsii	Doxycycline, chloramphenicol
Schizophrenia (negative symptoms)	Atypical antipsychotics
Schizophrenia (positive symptoms)	Typical and atypical antipsychotics
SIADH	Fluid restriction, IV hypertonic saline, conivaptan/tolvaptan, demeclocycline

CONDITION	COMMON TREATMENT(S)
Sickle cell disease	Hydroxyurea (↑ fetal hemoglobin)
Sporothrix schenckii	Itraconazole, oral potassium iodide
Stable angina	Sublingual nitroglycerin
Staphylococcus aureus	MSSA: nafcillin, oxacillin, dicloxacillin (antistaphylococcal penicillins); MRSA: vancomycin, daptomycin, linezolid, ceftaroline
Streptococcus bovis	Penicillin prophylaxis; evaluation for colon cancer if linked to endocarditis
Streptococcus pneumoniae	Penicillin/cephalosporin (systemic infection, pneumonia), vancomycin (meningitis)
Streptococcus pyogenes	Penicillin prophylaxis
Temporal arteritis	High-dose steroids
Tonic-clonic seizures	Levetiracetam, phenytoin, valproate, carbamazepine
Toxoplasma gondii	Sulfadiazine + pyrimethamine
Treponema pallidum	Penicillin
Trichomonas vaginalis	Metronidazole (patient and partner)
Trigeminal neuralgia (tic douloureux)	Carbamazepine
Ulcerative colitis	5-ASA preparations (e.g., mesalamine), 6-mercaptopurine, infliximab, colectomy
UTI prophylaxis	TMP-SMX
Warfarin reversal	Fresh frozen plasma (acute), vitamin K (chronic)

▶ KEY ASSOCIATIONS

DISEASE/FINDING	MOST COMMON/IMPORTANT ASSOCIATIONS
Actinic (solar) keratosis	Precursor to squamous cell carcinoma
Acute gastric ulcer associated with CNS injury	Cushing ulcer (↑ intracranial pressure stimulates vagal gastric H^+ secretion)
Acute gastric ulcer associated with severe burns	Curling ulcer (greatly reduced plasma volume results in sloughing of gastric mucosa)
Alternating areas of transmural inflammation and normal colon	Skip lesions (Crohn disease)
Aortic aneurysm, abdominal	Atherosclerosis
Aortic aneurysm, ascending or arch	3° syphilis (syphilitic aortitis), vasa vasorum destruction
Aortic aneurysm, thoracic	Marfan syndrome (idiopathic cystic medial degeneration)
Aortic dissection	Hypertension
Atrophy of the mammillary bodies	Wernicke encephalopathy (thiamine deficiency causing ataxia, ophthalmoplegia, and confusion)
Autosplenectomy (fibrosis and shrinkage)	Sickle cell disease (hemoglobin S)

DISEASE/FINDING	MOST COMMON/IMPORTANT ASSOCIATIONS
Bacteria associated with gastritis, peptic ulcer disease, and stomach cancer	*H. pylori*
Bacterial meningitis (adults and elderly)	*S. pneumoniae*
Bacterial meningitis (newborns and kids)	Group B streptococcus/*E.coli* (newborns), *S. pneumoniae*/*N. meningitidis* (kids/teens)
Bilateral ovarian metastases from gastric carcinoma	Krukenberg tumor (mucin-secreting signet ring cells)
Bleeding disorder with GpIb deficiency	Bernard-Soulier syndrome (defect in platelet adhesion to von Willebrand factor)
Brain tumor (adults)	Supratentorial: metastasis, astrocytoma (including glioblastoma multiforme), meningioma, schwannoma
Brain tumor (kids)	Infratentorial: medulloblastoma (cerebellum) or supratentorial: craniopharyngioma
Breast cancer	Invasive ductal carcinoma
Breast mass	Fibrocystic change, carcinoma (in postmenopausal women)
Breast tumor (benign)	Fibroadenoma
Cardiac 1° tumor (kids)	Rhabdomyoma, often seen in tuberous sclerosis
Cardiac manifestation of lupus	Marantic/thrombotic endocarditis (nonbacterial)
Cardiac tumor (adults)	Metastasis, myxoma (90% in left atrium; "ball and valve")
Cerebellar tonsillar herniation	Chiari II malformation
Chronic arrhythmia	Atrial fibrillation (associated with high risk of emboli)
Chronic atrophic gastritis (autoimmune)	Predisposition to gastric carcinoma (can also cause pernicious anemia)
Clear cell adenocarcinoma of the vagina	DES exposure in utero
Congenital adrenal hyperplasia, hypotension	21-hydroxylase deficiency
Congenital cardiac anomaly	VSD
Congenital conjugated hyperbilirubinemia (black liver)	Dubin-Johnson syndrome (inability of hepatocytes to secrete conjugated bilirubin into bile)
Constrictive pericarditis	TB (developing world); idiopathic, viral illness (developed world)
Coronary artery involved in thrombosis	LAD > RCA > circumflex
Cretinism	Iodine deficit/congenital hypothyroidism
Cushing syndrome	▪ Iatrogenic (from corticosteroid therapy) ▪ Adrenocortical adenoma (secretes excess cortisol) ▪ ACTH-secreting pituitary adenoma (Cushing disease) ▪ Paraneoplastic (due to ACTH secretion by tumors)
Cyanosis (early; less common)	Tetralogy of Fallot, transposition of great vessels, truncus arteriosus
Cyanosis (late; more common)	VSD, ASD, PDA
Death in CML	Blast crisis
Death in SLE	Lupus nephropathy

DISEASE/FINDING	MOST COMMON/IMPORTANT ASSOCIATIONS
Dementia	Alzheimer disease, multiple infarcts (vascular dementia)
Demyelinating disease in young women	Multiple sclerosis
DIC	Severe sepsis, obstetric complications, cancer, burns, trauma, major surgery
Dietary deficit	Iron
Diverticulum in pharynx	Zenker diverticulum (diagnosed by barium swallow)
Ejection click	Aortic stenosis
Esophageal cancer	Squamous cell carcinoma (worldwide); adenocarcinoma (U.S.)
Food poisoning (exotoxin mediated)	S. aureus, B. cereus
Glomerulonephritis (adults)	Berger disease (IgA nephropathy)
Gynecologic malignancy	Endometrial carcinoma (most common in U.S.); cervical carcinoma (most common worldwide)
Heart murmur, congenital	Mitral valve prolapse
Heart valve in bacterial endocarditis	Mitral > aortic (rheumatic fever), tricuspid (IV drug abuse)
Helminth infection (U.S.)	*Enterobius vermicularis, Ascaris lumbricoides*
Hematoma—epidural	Rupture of middle meningeal artery (trauma; lentiform shaped)
Hematoma—subdural	Rupture of bridging veins (crescent shaped)
Hemochromatosis	Multiple blood transfusions or hereditary *HFE* mutation (can result in heart failure, "bronze diabetes," and ↑ risk of hepatocellular carcinoma)
Hepatocellular carcinoma	Cirrhotic liver (associated with hepatitis B and C and with alcoholism)
Hereditary bleeding disorder	von Willebrand disease
Hereditary harmless jaundice	Gilbert syndrome (benign congenital unconjugated hyperbilirubinemia)
HLA-B27	Ankylosing spondylitis, reactive arthritis, ulcerative colitis, psoriatic arthritis
HLA-DR3	Diabetes mellitus type 1, SLE, Graves disease, Hashimoto thyroiditis
HLA-DR4	Diabetes mellitus type 1, rheumatoid arthritis
Holosystolic murmur	VSD, tricuspid regurgitation, mitral regurgitation
Hypercoagulability, endothelial damage, blood stasis	Virchow triad (↑ risk of thrombosis)
Hypertension, 2°	Renal disease
Hypoparathyroidism	Accidental excision during thyroidectomy
Hypopituitarism	Pituitary adenoma (usually benign tumor)
Infection 2° to blood transfusion	Hepatitis C
Infections in chronic granulomatous disease	S. aureus, E. coli, Aspergillus (catalase ⊕)
Intellectual disability	Down syndrome, fragile X syndrome

DISEASE/FINDING	MOST COMMON/IMPORTANT ASSOCIATIONS
Kidney stones	▪ Calcium = radiopaque ▪ Struvite (ammonium) = radiopaque (formed by urease ⊕ organisms such as *Klebsiella*, *Proteus* species, and *S. saprophyticus*) ▪ Uric acid = radiolucent
Late cyanotic shunt (uncorrected left to right becomes right to left)	Eisenmenger syndrome (caused by ASD, VSD, PDA; results in pulmonary hypertension/polycythemia)
Liver disease	Alcoholic cirrhosis
Lysosomal storage disease	Gaucher disease
Male cancer	Prostatic carcinoma
Malignancy associated with noninfectious fever	Hodgkin lymphoma
Malignancy (kids)	ALL, medulloblastoma (cerebellum)
Metastases to bone	Prostate, breast > lung > thyroid
Metastases to brain	Lung > breast > genitourinary > melanoma > GI
Metastases to liver	Colon >> stomach, pancreas
Mitochondrial inheritance	Disease occurs in both males and females, inherited through females only
Mitral valve stenosis	Rheumatic heart disease
Mixed (UMN and LMN) motor neuron disease	Amyotrophic lateral sclerosis
Myocarditis	Coxsackie B
Nephrotic syndrome (adults)	Focal segmental glomerulosclerosis
Nephrotic syndrome (kids)	Minimal change disease
Neuron migration failure	Kallmann syndrome (hypogonadotropic hypogonadism and anosmia)
Nosocomial pneumonia	*S. aureus*, *Pseudomonas*, other enteric gram-negative rods
Obstruction of male urinary tract	BPH
Opening snap	Mitral stenosis
Opportunistic infection in AIDS	*Pneumocystis jirovecii* pneumonia
Osteomyelitis	*S. aureus* (most common overall)
Osteomyelitis in sickle cell disease	*Salmonella*
Osteomyelitis with IV drug use	*Pseudomonas*, *Candida*, *S. aureus*
Ovarian tumor (benign, bilateral)	Serous cystadenoma
Ovarian tumor (malignant)	Serous cystadenocarcinoma
Pancreatitis (acute)	Gallstones, alcohol
Pancreatitis (chronic)	Alcohol (adults), cystic fibrosis (kids)
Patient with ALL /CLL /AML /CML	ALL: child, CLL: adult > 60, AML: adult ~ 65, CML: adult 45–85
Pelvic inflammatory disease	*C. trachomatis*, *N. gonorrhoeae*
Philadelphia chromosome t(9;22) (*BCR-ABL*)	CML (may sometimes be associated with ALL/AML)
Pituitary tumor	Prolactinoma, somatotropic adenoma
1° amenorrhea	Turner syndrome (45,XO)

DISEASE/FINDING	MOST COMMON/IMPORTANT ASSOCIATIONS
1° bone tumor (adults)	Multiple myeloma
1° hyperaldosteronism	Adenoma of adrenal cortex
1° hyperparathyroidism	Adenomas, hyperplasia, carcinoma
1° liver cancer	Hepatocellular carcinoma (chronic hepatitis, cirrhosis, hemochromatosis, α_1-antitrypsin deficiency, Wilson disease)
Pulmonary hypertension	COPD
Recurrent inflammation/thrombosis of small/medium vessels in extremities	Buerger disease (strongly associated with tobacco)
Renal tumor	Renal cell carcinoma: associated with von Hippel-Lindau and cigarette smoking; paraneoplastic syndromes (EPO, renin, PTHrP, ACTH)
Right heart failure due to a pulmonary cause	Cor pulmonale
S3 heart sound	↑ ventricular filling pressure (e.g., mitral regurgitation, HF), common in dilated ventricles
S4 heart sound	Stiff/hypertrophic ventricle (aortic stenosis, restrictive cardiomyopathy)
2° hyperparathyroidism	Hypocalcemia of chronic kidney disease
Sexually transmitted disease	*C. trachomatis* (usually coinfected with *N. gonorrhoeae*)
SIADH	Small cell carcinoma of the lung
Site of diverticula	Sigmoid colon
Sites of atherosclerosis	Abdominal aorta > coronary artery > popliteal artery > carotid artery
Stomach cancer	Adenocarcinoma
Stomach ulcerations and high gastrin levels	Zollinger-Ellison syndrome (gastrinoma of duodenum or pancreas)
t(14;18)	Follicular lymphomas (*BCL-2* activation, anti-apoptotic oncogene)
t(8;14)	Burkitt lymphoma (c-*myc* fusion, transcription factor oncogene)
t(9;22)	Philadelphia chromosome, CML (*BCR-ABL* activation, tyrosine kinase oncogene)
Temporal arteritis	Risk of ipsilateral blindness due to occlusion of ophthalmic artery; polymyalgia rheumatica
Testicular tumor	Seminoma (malignant, radiosensitive)
Thyroid cancer	Papillary carcinoma
Tumor in women	Leiomyoma (estrogen dependent, not precancerous)
Tumor of infancy	Strawberry hemangioma (usually regresses spontaneously by childhood)
Tumor of the adrenal medulla (adults)	Pheochromocytoma (usually benign)
Tumor of the adrenal medulla (kids)	Neuroblastoma (malignant)
Type of Hodgkin lymphoma	Nodular sclerosing (vs. mixed cellularity, lymphocytic predominance, lymphocytic depletion)
Type of non-Hodgkin lymphoma	Diffuse large B-cell lymphoma

DISEASE/FINDING	MOST COMMON/IMPORTANT ASSOCIATIONS
UTI	*E. coli*, *Staphylococcus saprophyticus* (young women)
Vertebral compression fracture	Osteoporosis (type I: postmenopausal woman; type II: elderly man or woman)
Viral encephalitis affecting temporal lobe	HSV-1
Vitamin deficiency (U.S.)	Folate (pregnant women are at high risk; body stores only 3- to 4-month supply; prevents neural tube defects)

▶ EQUATION REVIEW

TOPIC	EQUATION	PAGE
Sensitivity	$\text{Sensitivity} = TP / (TP + FN)$	49
Specificity	$\text{Specificity} = TN / (TN + FP)$	49
Positive predictive value	$PPV = TP / (TP + FP)$	49
Negative predictive value	$NPV = TN / (FN + TN)$	49
Odds ratio (for case-control studies)	$OR = \dfrac{a/c}{b/d} = \dfrac{ad}{bc}$	50
Relative risk	$RR = \dfrac{a/(a+b)}{c/(c+d)}$	50
Attributable risk	$AR = \dfrac{a}{a+b} - \dfrac{c}{c+d}$	50
Relative risk reduction	$RRR = 1 - RR$	50
Absolute risk reduction	$ARR = \dfrac{c}{c+d} - \dfrac{a}{a+b}$	50
Number needed to treat	$NNT = 1/\text{absolute risk reduction}$	50
Number needed to harm	$NNH = 1/\text{attributable risk}$	50
Hardy-Weinberg equilibrium	$p^2 + 2pq + q^2 = 1$ $p + q = 1$	81
Volume of distribution	$V_d = \dfrac{\text{amount of drug in the body}}{\text{plasma drug concentration}}$	243
Half-life	$t_{1/2} = \dfrac{0.693 \times V_d}{CL}$	243
Drug clearance	$CL = \dfrac{\text{rate of elimination of drug}}{\text{plasma drug concentration}} = V_d \times K_e \text{ (elimination constant)}$	243
Loading dose	$LD = \dfrac{C_p \times V_d}{F}$	243
Maintenance dose	$D = \dfrac{C_p \times CL \times \tau}{F}$	243

TOPIC	EQUATION	PAGE
Cardiac output	$$CO = \frac{\text{rate of } O_2 \text{ consumption}}{\text{arterial } O_2 \text{ content} - \text{venous } O_2 \text{ content}}$$	272
	$CO = \text{stroke volume} \times \text{heart rate}$	272
Mean arterial pressure	$MAP = \text{cardiac output} \times \text{total peripheral resistance}$	272
	$MAP = \frac{2}{3} \text{ diastolic} + \frac{1}{3} \text{ systolic}$	272
Stroke volume	$SV = EDV - ESV$	272
Ejection fraction	$$EF = \frac{SV}{EDV} = \frac{EDV - ESV}{EDV}$$	273
Resistance	$$\text{Resistance} = \frac{\text{driving pressure } (\Delta P)}{\text{flow } (Q)} = \frac{8\eta \text{ (viscosity)} \times \text{length}}{\pi r^4}$$	274
Capillary fluid exchange	$J_v = \text{net fluid flow} = K_f[(P_c - P_i) - \varsigma(\pi_c - \pi_i)]$	287
Renal clearance	$C_x = U_x V / P_x$	529
Glomerular filtration rate	$GFR = U_{inulin} \times V / P_{inulin} = C_{inulin}$	529
	$GFR = K_f [(P_{GC} - P_{BS}) - (\pi_{GC} - \pi_{BS})]$	
Effective renal plasma flow	$$eRPF = U_{PAH} \times \frac{V}{P_{PAH}} = C_{PAH}$$	530
Renal blood flow	$$RBF = \frac{RPF}{1 - Hct}$$	530
Filtration fraction	$$FF = \frac{GFR}{RPF}$$	530
Henderson-Hasselbalch equation (for extracellular pH)	$$pH = 6.1 + \log \frac{[HCO_3^-]}{0.03 \, P_{CO_2}}$$	538
Winters formula	$P_{CO_2} = 1.5 \, [HCO_3^-] + 8 \pm 2$	538
Physiologic dead space	$$V_D = V_T \times \frac{Pa_{CO_2} - Pe_{CO_2}}{Pa_{CO_2}}$$	602
Pulmonary vascular resistance	$$PVR = \frac{P_{\text{pulm artery}} - P_{\text{L atrium}}}{\text{cardiac output}}$$	606
Alveolar gas equation	$$Pa_{O_2} = Pi_{O_2} - \frac{Pa_{CO_2}}{R}$$	606

▶ NOTES

Top-Rated Review Resources

"Some books are to be tasted, others to be swallowed, and some few to be chewed and digested."

—Sir Francis Bacon

"Always read something that will make you look good if you die in the middle of it."

—P.J. O'Rourke

"So many books, so little time."

—Frank Zappa

"If one cannot enjoy reading a book over and over again, there is no use in reading it at all."

—Oscar Wilde

▶ HOW TO USE THE DATABASE

This section is an abbreviated database of top-rated basic science review books, sample examination books, software, Web sites, and apps that have been marketed to medical students studying for the USMLE Step 1. For each recommended resource, we list (where applicable) the **Title**, the **First Author** (or editor), the **Current Publisher**, the **Copyright Year**, the **Number of Pages**, the **Approximate List Price**, the **Format** of the resource, and the **Number of Test Questions**. Finally, each recommended resource receives a **Rating**. Within each section, resources are arranged first by Rating and then alphabetically by the first author within each Rating group.

For a complete list of resources, including summaries that describe their overall style and utility, go to **www.firstaidteam.com/bonus**.

A letter rating scale with six different grades reflects the detailed student evaluations for **Rated Resources**. Each rated resource receives a rating as follows:

A+	Excellent for boards review.
A A–	Very good for boards review; choose among the group.
B+ B	Good, but use only after exhausting better sources.
B–	Fair, but there are many better books in the discipline; or low-yield subject material.

The Rating is meant to reflect the overall usefulness of the resource in helping medical students prepare for the USMLE Step 1. This is based on a number of factors, including:

- The cost
- The readability of the text
- The appropriateness and accuracy of the material
- The quality and number of sample questions
- The quality of written answers to sample questions
- The quality and appropriateness of the illustrations (e.g., graphs, diagrams, photographs)
- The length of the text (longer is not necessarily better)
- The quality and number of other resources available in the same discipline
- The importance of the discipline for the USMLE Step 1

Please note that ratings do not reflect the quality of the resources for purposes other than reviewing for the USMLE Step 1. Many books with lower ratings are well written and informative but are not ideal for boards preparation. We have not listed or commented on general textbooks available in the basic sciences.

Evaluations are based on the cumulative results of formal and informal surveys of thousands of medical students at many medical schools across the country. The ratings represent a consensus opinion, but there may have been a broad range of opinion or limited student feedback on any particular resource.

Please note that the data listed are subject to change in that:

- Publishers' prices change frequently.
- Bookstores often charge an additional markup.
- New editions come out frequently, and the quality of updating varies.
- The same book may be reissued through another publisher.

We actively encourage medical students and faculty to submit their opinions and ratings of these basic science review materials so that we may update our database. (See p. xix, How to Contribute.) In addition, we ask that publishers and authors submit for evaluation review copies of basic science review books, including new editions and books not included in our database. We also solicit reviews of new books or suggestions for alternate modes of study that may be useful in preparing for the examination, such as flash cards, computer software, commercial review courses, apps, and Web sites.

Disclaimer/Conflict of Interest Statement

No material in this book, including the ratings, reflects the opinion or influence of the publisher. All errors and omissions will gladly be corrected if brought to the attention of the authors through our blog at www.firstaidteam.com. Please note that USMLE-Rx and the entire *First Aid for the USMLE* series are publications by the senior authors of this book; their ratings are based solely on recommendations from the student authors of this book as well as data from the student survey and feedback forms.

▶ TOP-RATED REVIEW RESOURCES

Question Banks

		AUTHOR	PUBLISHER	TYPE	PRICE
A⁺	*USMLEWorld Qbank*	USMLEWorld	www.usmleworld.com	Test/2200 q	$125–$399
A	*USMLE-Rx Qmax*	MedIQ Learning	www.usmle-rx.com	Test/2500 q	$99–$249
A⁻	*Kaplan Qbank*	Kaplan	www.kaplanmedical.com	Test/2200 q	$99–$299
B⁺	*USMLE Consult*	Elsevier	www.usmleconsult.com	Test/2500 q	$75–$395

Question Books

		AUTHOR	PUBLISHER	TYPE	PRICE
A	*First Aid Q&A for the USMLE Step 1*	Le	McGraw-Hill, 2012, 765 pp	Test/1000 q	$46
B⁺	*Kaplan USMLE Step 1 Qbook*	Kaplan	Kaplan, 2013, 456 pp	Test/850 q	$45
B⁺	*PreTest Clinical Vignettes for the USMLE Step 1*	McGraw-Hill	McGraw-Hill, 2010, 318 pp	Test/322 q	$37
B	*Lange Q&A: USMLE Step 1*	King	McGraw-Hill, 2008, 528 pp	Test/1200 q	$54

Internet Sites

		AUTHOR	PUBLISHER	TYPE	PRICE
A⁻	*First Aid Step 1 Express*		www.usmle-rx.com	Review/Test	$99–$249
B⁺	*Blue Histology*		www.lab.anhb.uwa.edu.au/mb140	Review/Test	Free
B⁺	*Firecracker*	Firecracker Inc.	www.firecracker.me	Review/Test/1500 q	$39/month
B⁺	*Radiopaedia.org*		www.radiopaedia.org	Cases/Test	Free
B⁺	*SketchyMicro*		www.sketchymicro.com	Review	$40–$70
B⁺	*WebPath: The Internet Pathology Laboratory*		library.med.utah.edu/WebPath/	Review/Test/1300 q	Free
B	*Dr. Najeeb Lectures*		http://www.drnajeeblectures.com/	Review	$399/year
B	*Medical School Pathology*	Minarcik		Review	Free
B	*The Pathology Guy*	Friedlander	www.pathguy.com	Review	Free
B	*Picmonic*		http://www.picmonic.com	Review	$29–$499
B	*The Whole Brain Atlas*	Johnson	www.med.harvard.edu/aanlib/	Review	Free
B⁻	*Digital Anatomist Interactive Atlases*	University of Washington	www9.biostr.washington.edu/da.html	Review	Free

Mobile Apps

		AUTHOR	PUBLISHER	TYPE	PRICE
A⁻	*Anki*		http://ankisrs.net	Flash cards	Free/ $25
B	*Cram Fighter*		www.cramfighter.com	Study plan	Variable
B	*Osmosis*		www.osmosis.org	Test	Variable

Comprehensive

		AUTHOR	PUBLISHER	TYPE	PRICE
A	*USMLE Step 1 Secrets*	Brown	Elsevier, 2012, 880 pp	Review	$43
A	*First Aid Cases for the USMLE Step 1*	Le	McGraw-Hill, 2012, 411 pp	Cases	$46
A⁻	*First Aid for the Basic Sciences: General Principles*	Le	McGraw-Hill, 2011, 560 pp	Review	$72
A⁻	*First Aid for the Basic Sciences: Organ Systems*	Le	McGraw-Hill, 2011, 858 pp	Review	$93
A⁻	*medEssentials for the USMLE Step 1*	Manley	Kaplan, 2012, 588 pp	Review	$55
B⁺	*Cases & Concepts Step 1: Basic Science Review*	Caughey	Lippincott Williams & Wilkins, 2012, 400 pp	Cases	$44
B⁺	*Step-Up to USMLE Step 1*	Jenkins	Lippincott Williams & Wilkins, 2014, 512 pp	Review	$52
B⁺	*Cracking the USMLE Step 1*	Princeton Review	Princeton Review, 2013, 832 pp	Review	$45
B⁺	*USMLE Images for the Boards: A Comprehensive Image-Based Review*	Tully	Elsevier, 2012, 296 pp	Review	$43
B	*Déjà Review: USMLE Step 1*	Naheedy	McGraw-Hill, 2010, 412 pp	Review	$23
B⁻	*USMLE Step 1 Made Ridiculously Simple*	Carl	MedMaster, 2014, 400 pp	Review/Test 100 q	$30

Anatomy, Embryology, and Neuroscience

		AUTHOR	PUBLISHER	TYPE	PRICE
A⁻	*High-Yield Embryology*	Dudek	Lippincott Williams & Wilkins, 2013, 176 pp	Review	$38
A⁻	*High-Yield Neuroanatomy*	Fix	Lippincott Williams & Wilkins, 2008, 160 pp	Review/ Test/50 q	$36
A⁻	*Anatomy—An Essential Textbook*	Gilroy	Thieme, 2013, 504 pp	Text/ Test/400 q	$45
A⁻	*Atlas of Anatomy*	Gilroy	Thieme, 2012, 704 pp	Text	$80
B⁺	*High-Yield Gross Anatomy*	Dudek	Lippincott Williams & Wilkins, 2014, 320 pp	Review	$38
B⁺	*Clinical Anatomy Made Ridiculously Simple*	Goldberg	MedMaster, 2012, 175 pp	Review	$30
B⁺	*Rapid Review: Gross and Developmental Anatomy*	Moore	Elsevier, 2010, 304 pp	Review/ Test/450 q	$43

Anatomy, Embryology, and Neuroscience *(continued)*

		AUTHOR	PUBLISHER	TYPE	PRICE
B⁺	*PreTest Neuroscience*	Siegel	McGraw-Hill, 2013, 412 pp	Test/500 q	$35
B⁺	*Crash Course: Anatomy*	Sternhouse	Elsevier, 2012, 288 pp	Review	$45
B⁺	*Déjà Review: Neuroscience*	Tremblay	McGraw-Hill, 2010, 266 pp	Review	$23
B⁺	*USMLE Road Map: Neuroscience*	White	McGraw-Hill, 2008, 224 pp	Review/Test/300 q	$38
B	*BRS Embryology*	Dudek	Lippincott Williams & Wilkins, 2014, 336 pp	Review/Test/220 q	$50
B	*Anatomy Flash Cards*	Gilroy	Thieme, 2008, 376 flash cards	Flash cards	$38
B	*Clinical Neuroanatomy Made Ridiculously Simple*	Goldberg	MedMaster, 2014, 90 pp + CD-ROM	Review/Test/Few q	$26
B	*Case Files: Anatomy*	Toy	McGraw-Hill, 2014, 400 pp	Cases	$35
B	*Case Files: Neuroscience*	Toy	McGraw-Hill, 2014, 416 pp	Cases	$35
B⁻	*Gray's Anatomy for Students Flash Cards*	Drake	Elsevier, 2014, 350 flash cards	Flash cards	$40
B⁻	*Netter's Anatomy Flash Cards*	Hansen	Saunders, 2014, 674 flash cards	Flash cards	$40

Behavioral Science

		AUTHOR	PUBLISHER	TYPE	PRICE
A	*High-Yield Behavioral Science*	Fadem	Lippincott Williams & Wilkins, 2012, 144 pp	Review	$35
A⁻	*BRS Behavioral Science*	Fadem	Lippincott Williams & Wilkins, 2013, 336 pp	Review/Test/700 q	$48
A⁻	*High-Yield Biostatistics, Epidemiology, and Public Health*	Glaser	Lippincott Williams & Wilkins, 2013, 168 pp	Review	$40
A⁻	*Clinical Biostatistics and Epidemiology Made Ridiculously Simple*	Weaver	MedMaster, 2011, 104 pp	Review	$23
B⁺	*USMLE Medical Ethics*	Fischer	Kaplan, 2012, 216 pp	Cases	$43
B⁺	*Jekel's Epidemiology, Biostatistics, Preventive Medicine, and Public Health*	Katz	Saunders, 2013, 420 pp	Review/Test/477 q	$60
B	*Déjà Review: Behavioral Science*	Quinn	McGraw-Hill, 2010, 240 pp	Review	$23

Biochemistry

		AUTHOR	PUBLISHER	TYPE	PRICE
A	*Lange Flash Cards Biochemistry and Genetics*	Baron	McGraw-Hill, 2013, 184 flash cards	Flash cards	$36
A⁻	*Rapid Review: Biochemistry*	Pelley	Elsevier, 2010, 208 pp	Review/Test/350 q	$43
B⁺	*Lippincott's Illustrated Reviews: Biochemistry*	Ferrier	Lippincott Williams & Wilkins, 2012, 560 pp	Review/Test/500 q	$73
B⁺	*Déjà Review: Biochemistry*	Manzoul	McGraw-Hill, 2010, 206 pp	Review	$23

Biochemistry *(continued)*

		AUTHOR	PUBLISHER	TYPE	PRICE
B+	*Medical Biochemistry—An Illustrated Review*	Panini	Thieme, 2013, 441 pp	Review/ Test/400 q	$40
B+	*PreTest Biochemistry and Genetics*	Wilson	McGraw-Hill, 2013, 570 pp	Test/500 q	$35
B	*Clinical Biochemistry Made Ridiculously Simple*	Goldberg	MedMaster, 2010, 95 pp + foldout	Review	$25
B	*BRS Biochemistry, Molecular Biology, and Genetics*	Lieberman	Lippincott Williams & Wilkins, 2013, 432 pp	Review/Test	$49
B−	*Case Files: Biochemistry*	Toy	McGraw-Hill, 2008, 456 pp	Cases	$37
B−	*High-Yield Biochemistry*	Wilcox	Lippincott Williams & Wilkins, 2009, 128 pp	Review	$39

Cell Biology and Histology

		AUTHOR	PUBLISHER	TYPE	PRICE
A−	*High-Yield Cell and Molecular Biology*	Dudek	Lippincott Williams & Wilkins, 2010, 151 pp	Review	$36
B	*Elsevier's Integrated Review: Genetics*	Adkison	Elsevier, 2011, 272 pp	Review	$43
B	*High-Yield Genetics*	Dudek	Lippincott Williams & Wilkins, 2008, 134 pp	Review	$36
B	*BRS Cell Biology and Histology*	Gartner	Lippincott Williams & Wilkins, 2014, 432 pp	Review/ Test/320 q	$46
B	*PreTest Anatomy, Histology, and Cell Biology*	Klein	McGraw-Hill, 2010, 654 pp	Test/500 q	$35
B	*USMLE Road Map: Genetics*	Sack	McGraw-Hill, 2008, 224 pp	Review	$36
B	*Déjà Review: Histology and Cell Biology*	Song	McGraw-Hill, 2011, 300 pp	Review	$23
B	*Crash Course: Cell Biology and Genetics*	Stubbs	Elsevier, 2013, 216 pp	Review	$50
B−	*Wheater's Functional Histology*	Young	Elsevier, 2013, 464 pp	Text	$83

Microbiology and Immunology

		AUTHOR	PUBLISHER	TYPE	PRICE
A	*Déjà Review: Microbiology & Immunology*	Chen	McGraw-Hill, 2010, 424 pp	Review	$23
A	*Clinical Microbiology Made Ridiculously Simple*	Gladwin	MedMaster, 2014, 400 pp	Review	$37
A	*Lange Microbiology & Infectious Diseases Flash Cards*	Somers	McGraw-Hill, 2010, 189 flash cards	Flash cards	$41
A−	*Basic Immunology*	Abbas	Elsevier, 2012, 336 pp	Review	$72
A−	*The Big Picture: Medical Microbiology*	Chamberlain	McGraw-Hill, 2008, 456 pp	Review/ 100 q	$61
A−	*Microcards: Microbiology Flash Cards*	Harpavat	Lippincott Williams & Wilkins, 2011, 310 flash cards	Flash cards	$47

Microbiology and Immunology (continued)

		AUTHOR	PUBLISHER	TYPE	PRICE
A⁻	*Lange Review of Medical Microbiology and Immunology*	Levinson	McGraw-Hill, 2014, 800 pp	Text/Test/654 q	$55
A⁻	*Medical Microbiology and Immunology Flash Cards*	Rosenthal	Elsevier, 2008, 324 flash cards	Flash cards	$40
B⁺	*Elsevier's Integrated Immunology and Microbiology*	Actor	Elsevier, 2012, 192 pp	Review	$43
B⁺	*Lippincott's Illustrated Reviews: Immunology*	Doan	Lippincott Williams & Wilkins, 2012, 384 pp	Review/Test/Few q	$63
B⁺	*Lippincott's Illustrated Reviews: Microbiology*	Harvey	Lippincott Williams & Wilkins, 2012, 448 pp	Review/Test/Few q	$65
B⁺	*Review of Medical Microbiology and Immunology*	Levinson	McGraw-Hill, 2014, 800 pp	Review/Test/654 q	$55
B	*Case Studies in Immunology: Clinical Companion*	Geha	Garland Science, 2011, 363 pp	Cases	$59
B	*Pretest: Microbiology*	Kettering	McGraw-Hill, 2013, 462 pp	Test/500 q	$35
B	*Rapid Review: Microbiology and Immunology*	Rosenthal	Elsevier, 2010, 240 pp	Review/Test/400 q	$43
B	*Case Files: Microbiology*	Toy	McGraw-Hill, 2014, 400 pp	Cases	$35

Pathology

		AUTHOR	PUBLISHER	TYPE	PRICE
A⁺	*Rapid Review: Pathology*	Goljan	Elsevier, 2013, 784 pp	Review/Test/400 q	$56
A⁺	*Pathoma: Fundamentals of Pathology*	Sattar	Pathoma, 2011, 218 pp	Review/Lecture	$85
A⁻	*Lange Pathology Flash Cards*	Baron	McGraw-Hill, 2013, 300 flash cards	Flash cards	$38
A⁻	*Déjà Review: Pathology*	Davis	McGraw-Hill, 2010, 474 pp	Review	$23
A⁻	*Lippincott's Illustrated Q&A Review of Rubin's Pathology*	Fenderson	Lippincott Williams & Wilkins, 2010, 336 pp	Test/1000 q	$56
A⁻	*The Big Picture: Pathology*	Kemp	McGraw-Hill, 2007, 512 pp	Review/Test/130 q	$58
A⁻	*Robbins and Cotran Review of Pathology*	Klatt	Elsevier, 2014, 504 pp	Test/1100 q	$50
A⁻	*BRS Pathology*	Schneider	Lippincott Williams & Wilkins, 2013, 480 pp	Review/Test/450 q	$48
B⁺	*Cases & Concepts Step 1: Pathophysiology Review*	Caughey	Lippincott Williams & Wilkins, 2009, 376 pp	Cases	$49
B⁺	*Case Files: Pathology*	Toy	McGraw-Hill, 2008, 456 pp	Cases	$38
B⁺	*USMLE Road Map: Pathology*	Wettach	McGraw-Hill, 2009, 412 pp	Review/Test/500 q	$40

Pathology (continued)

		AUTHOR	PUBLISHER	TYPE	PRICE
B	*PreTest Pathology*	Brown	McGraw-Hill, 2010, 612 pp	Test/500 q	$35
B	*High-Yield Histopathology*	Dudek	Lippincott Williams & Wilkins, 2011, 328 pp	Review	$36
B	*Pathophysiology of Disease: Introduction to Clinical Medicine*	McPhee	McGraw-Hill, 2014, 784 pp	Text/Test/ Few q	$76
B	*Haematology at a Glance*	Mehta	Blackwell Science, 2014, 136 pp	Review	$45
B	*PreTest Pathophysiology*	Mufson	McGraw-Hill, 2010, 500 pp	Test/500 q	$35
B	*Color Atlas of Physiology*	Silbernagl	Thieme, 2009, 456 pp	Review	$50
B	*Crash Course: Pathology*	Xiu	Elsevier, 2012, 356 pp	Review	$45
B⁻	*Pocket Companion to Robbins and Cotran Pathologic Basis of Disease*	Mitchell	Elsevier, 2011, 800 pp	Review	$41

Pharmacology

		AUTHOR	PUBLISHER	TYPE	PRICE
A	*Déjà Review: Pharmacology*	Gleason	McGraw-Hill, 2010, 236 pp	Review	$23
A⁻	*Lange Pharmacology Flash Cards*	Baron	McGraw-Hill, 2013, 230 flash cards	Flash cards	$38
A⁻	*Kaplan Medical USMLE Pharmacology and Treatment Flashcards*	Fischer	Kaplan, 2011, 200 flash cards	Flash cards	$45
A⁻	*Lippincott's Illustrated Reviews: Pharmacology*	Harvey	Lippincott Williams & Wilkins, 2014, 680 pp	Review/ Test/380 q	$67
A⁻	*Pharm Cards: Review Cards for Medical Students*	Johannsen	Lippincott Williams & Wilkins, 2010, 240 flash cards	Flash cards	$45
B⁺	*Crash Course: Pharmacology*	Battista	Elsevier, 2012, 248 pp	Review	$45
B⁺	*Pharmacology Flash Cards*	Brenner	Elsevier, 2012, 200 flash cards	Flash cards	$40
B⁺	*Elsevier's Integrated Pharmacology*	Kester	Elsevier, 2011, 264 pp	Review	$43
B⁺	*Rapid Review: Pharmacology*	Pazdernik	Elsevier, 2010, 360 pp	Review/ Test/450 q	$43
B⁺	*BRS Pharmacology*	Rosenfeld	Lippincott Williams & Wilkins, 2013, 384 pp	Review/ Test/200 q	$49
B⁺	*Katzung & Trevor's Pharmacology: Examination and Board Review*	Trevor	McGraw-Hill, 2012, 640 pp	Review/ Test/1000 q	$54
B	*PreTest Pharmacology*	Shlafer	McGraw-Hill, 2013, 567 pp	Test/500 q	$35
B	*Case Files: Pharmacology*	Toy	McGraw-Hill, 2013, 453 pp	Cases	$35
B	*High-Yield Pharmacology*	Weiss	Lippincott Williams & Wilkins, 2009, 160 pp	Review	$36

Physiology

		AUTHOR	PUBLISHER	TYPE	PRICE
A	*BRS Physiology*	Costanzo	Lippincott Williams & Wilkins, 2014, 328 pp	Review/ Test/350 q	$50
A	*Acid-Base, Fluids, and Electrolytes Made Ridiculously Simple*	Preston	MedMaster, 2010, 156 pp	Review	$23
A⁻	*Physiology*	Costanzo	Saunders, 2013, 520 pp	Text	$63
A⁻	*The Big Picture: Medical Physiology*	Kibble	McGraw-Hill, 2009, 448 pp	Review/ Test/108 q	$55
B⁺	*BRS Physiology Cases and Problems*	Costanzo	Lippincott Williams & Wilkins, 2012, 368 pp	Cases	$49
B⁺	*Déjà Review: Physiology*	Gould	McGraw-Hill, 2010, 298 pp	Review	$23
B⁺	*PreTest Physiology*	Metting	McGraw-Hill, 2013, 505 pp	Test/500 q	$35
B	*Rapid Review: Physiology*	Brown	Elsevier, 2011, 288 pp	Test/350 q	$43
B	*Vander's Renal Physiology*	Eaton	McGraw-Hill, 2013, 240 pp	Text	$43
B	*Endocrine Physiology*	Molina	McGraw-Hill, 2013, 320 pp	Review	$46
B	*Netter's Physiology Flash Cards*	Mulroney	Saunders, 2009, 200+ flash cards	Flash cards	$40
B	*Case Files: Physiology*	Toy	McGraw-Hill, 2008, 456 pp	Cases	$37
B	*Pulmonary Pathophysiology: The Essentials*	West	Lippincott Williams & Wilkins, 2012, 208 pp	Review/ Test/50 q	$50
B⁻	*Clinical Physiology Made Ridiculously Simple*	Goldberg	MedMaster, 2010, 160 pp	Review	$25

Commercial Review Courses

▶ COMMERCIAL REVIEW COURSES

Commercial preparation courses can be helpful for some students, but such courses are expensive and may leave limited time for independent study. They are usually an effective tool for students who feel overwhelmed by the volume of material they must review in preparation for the boards. Also note that while some commercial courses are designed for first-time test takers, others are geared toward students who are repeating the examination. Still other courses have been created for IMGs who want to take all three Steps in a limited amount of time. Finally, student experience and satisfaction with review courses are highly variable, and course content and structure can evolve rapidly. We thus suggest that you discuss options with recent graduates of review courses you are considering. Some student opinions can be found in discussion groups on the Internet.

Becker Healthcare

Becker Healthcare provides intensive and comprehensive live, online, and self-study review courses for students preparing for the USMLE. The 7-week live Step 1 reviews are held throughout the year with high student involvement and instructor accessibility. Becker Healthcare uses an active learning system that focuses on comprehension, retention, and application of concepts. Online program components include:

- Over 275 hours of video lectures
- Lecture notes
- Interactive ebooks
- USMLEWorld QBank for 3 months
- Becker's Step 1 question bank for 6 months
- Clinical vignettes and case studies
- 2 NBME practice exams

Live programs are currently offered in Dallas, Chicago, Fort Lauderdale, and New York City. The fee range is $2799–$6499. The all-inclusive live review program includes all of the above plus:

- Lodging and local hotel shuttle service
- Breakfast and lunch
- Access to a tutor
- High-speed Internet service

Becker's Self-Study USMLE Step 1 Review Course includes:

- Diagnostic exam
- Streaming video lectures
- Interactive series of ebooks featuring Becker's new curriculum
- Dual-degree MD and/or PhD instructors
- Becker's Step 1 Qbank
- Optional full set of color textbooks
- 3-month USMLEWorld or 6-month USMLE Consult Qbank subscription

For more information, contact:

Becker Healthcare
3005 Highland Parkway
Downers Grove, IL 60515
Phone: (800) 683-8725
www.becker.com/health

Kaplan Medical

For more than 40 years, Kaplan Medical has helped medical students and physicians in the U.S. and across the world to prepare efficiently for their Boards and match into the residency program of their choice.

USMLE Step 1 Comprehensive Program Live Lectures. Kaplan's LivePrep offers a highly structured, interactive live lecture series led by all-star faculty and is available at Kaplan centers in major cities with 7-, 14-, and 16-week options. Includes a 7-volume, full-color set of lecture notes.

Live Online Lectures. Kaplan's Classroom Anywhere™ includes over 240 hours of live, interactive instruction delivered by expert faculty from wherever Internet access is available. Includes a 7-volume set of lecture notes.

Center Study. Kaplan's CenterPrep provides more than 200 hours of video lectures to study at your own pace at Kaplan centers. Available for 3-, 6-, or 9-month periods and includes a 7-volume set of lecture notes.

On-demand Lectures. Kaplan's OnlinePrep gives access to over 200 hours of video lectures delivered by expert faculty and is accessible at any time wherever Internet access is available.

USMLE Step 1 High-Yield Program. Utilize Kaplan's Master Faculty and these key features:

- Review 55 hours of core lectures organized by General Principle and Organ System (39 hours at 1.5× speed)
- Warm up with 28 basic science exercises to review your first year
- Make it stick with clinical correlates, heart sounds, and dynamic visuals throughout your core lectures
- Practice with over 2000 USMLE review exercises in your printed workbook and watch the video explanations
- Connect core lectures with page references to First Aid, Pathoma, and medEssentials
- Strengthen your skills with core lecture quizzes and watch the video explanations
- Prep on-the-go with USMLE Step 1 High Yield on your iPad®

Until Your Test®. Use a structured study guide to map out your schedule for up to 12 months.

USMLE Step 1 High-Yield Program. Includes Step 1 Qbank:

- Master your material with 3000 USMLE practice questions and 200 mini-lectures in Kaplan's Step 1 Qbank, including diagnostic and 2 simulated exams
- Turn downtime into a higher score with free Qbank mobile app for iPhone® and Android™

To learn more, call 1-800-KAP-TEST or visit www.kaplanmedical.com.

Med School Tutors

Since 2007, Med School Tutors has helped students prepare for Step 1 by working with them one-on-one. Instead of offering courses, lectures, or videos, MST's approach is tailored to each student's weaknesses and strengths, according to their learning styles and schedules, and is guided by a personal coach who has scored high on Step 1.

Med School Tutors are medical students and residents who have excelled in their medical studies and training. Their minimum credentials include:

- Training at top medical schools and residency programs
- Superior standardized test scores (e.g., Step 1 > 245)
- Significant and verifiable teaching experience
- Interviewing and training with MST's most experienced USMLE tutors

Med School Tutors assists students according to their needs. Comprehensive packages include:

- Personal day-by-day study schedule and plan
- Test-taking techniques and confidence-building exercises
- Assessment by question bank performance and NBME test analysis
- Selection and use of high-yield resources
- Integrated review of content with emphasis on student's weaknesses
- Emphasis on question/vignette-based learning
- Clinical reasoning skills training
- Holistic support throughout study period

Students start with a complimentary consultation and discussion of their needs and goals. This is followed by the tutor matching process and introduction to the tutor. Students then begin formal work with a trial session at half the cost. The trial session encompasses a review of a recent self-assessment (or question block), the first steps in creating a personal study plan, and Q&A. Nearly 80% of MST's students work with tutors seamlessly online via Web conferences. In-person tutoring is also offered in Manhattan near select universities and medical centers.

For more information, visit www.medschooltutors.com or call (212) 327-0098.

Northwestern Medical Review

Since 1986, Northwestern Medical Review (NMR) has been offering review courses in preparation for the USMLE Step 1 and COMLEX Level I examinations. The curriculum of Northwestern Review allows students to select a variety of live or online courses ranging in length from 5–18 days. The courses are developed in a high-yield and clinically oriented format and address concepts that are commonly tested on the exams. Courses are taught by the authors of the Northwestern Review Books and/or authors of best-selling books. The uniqueness of the NMR curriculum is the multimedia live-lecture TALLP™ instructional methodology that incorporates simulated test items, cartoons, animations, and uplifting mnemonics into the courses. Another feature of the courses is the built-in Adaptive-Flexi-Pass™ teaching methodology that progressively customizes live courses around the academic needs of the participating students. The format of the workbooks allows students to actively and effectively assimilate the presented concepts. In addition to organized lecture notes and review books for all subjects, students will receive access to more than 2500 Web-based question bank items, audio CDs, and a large pool of practice questions and simulated exams. All study plans are available in a customized and onsite format for groups of students. Additionally, public sessions are frequently offered in East Lansing, Philadelphia, Los Angeles, Chicago, New York City, and San Juan. Live courses are also globally available in certain countries. NMR offers a free retake option as well as a liberal cancellation policy.

For more information, contact:

Northwestern Medical Review
P.O. Box 22174
Lansing, MI 48909-2174
Phone: (866) MedPass
Fax: (517) 347-7005
E-mail: contactus@northwesternmedicalreview.com
www.northwesternmedicalreview.com

PASS Program

USMLE and COMLEX Review Program. The PASS Program offers a concept-based, clinically integrated curriculum to help students increase board scores, obtain residencies, and broaden their perspective of medicine. Helpful for a wide spectrum of students, including those trying to maximize scores on the first try and those struggling to stay in medical school. PASS accommodates all types of learners: auditory, visual, or kinesthetic, and, with the help of small class sizes, encourages students to interact and to ask questions.

Live Lectures. PASS offers 4-, 6-, 8-week, or extended-stay programs in Champaign, IL, and St. Augustine, FL. Facilities include computer labs, a state-of-the-art lecture hall, student lounges and study areas, and housing. Drill sessions and small study groups take place throughout the week. Tuition, which includes housing and security deposit, is $4050 for the 4-week course, $6850 for the 6-week course, and $7700 for the 8-week course.

One-on-One Tutoring. Included with tuition, students receive one-on-one tutoring from an MD each week they attend the program. Six-week students receive two sessions per week and 8-week students receive three sessions in weeks 1–5 of the program and five sessions in weeks 6–8.

Online Program. The online program includes new lectures on nearly 40 topics and the current edition of the Course Notes book. Also included are sample questions by topic with video explanations from Dr. Francis, two NBME exams, and a 1-year KISSPharm subscription (www.kisspharm.com). There are weekly drill sessions and a student discussion board, and the program is available for 6- or 12-month access.

For more information, contact:

PASS Program
2302 Moreland Blvd.
Champaign, IL 61822
Phone: (217) 378-8018
Fax: (217) 378-7809
www.passprogram.net

The Princeton Review

The Princeton Review offers two flexible preparation options for the USMLE Step 1: the USMLE Online Course and the USMLE Online Workout.

USMLE Online Courses. The USMLE Online Courses offer the following:

- 75 hours of online review, including lessons, vignettes, and drills
- Complete review of all USMLE Step 1 subjects
- Three full-length CBTs
- Seven 1-hour subject-based tests
- Complete set of print materials
- 24/7 access to technical support
- Three months of access to tests, drills, and lessons

More information can be found on The Princeton Review's Web site at www.princetonreview.com.

Youel's™ Prep, Inc.

Youel's Prep, Inc., has specialized in medical board preparation for 30 years. The company provides DVDs, audiotapes, videotapes, a CD (PowerPrep Quick Study), books, live lectures, and tutorials for small groups as well as for individuals (TutorialPrep™). All DVDs, videotapes, audiotapes, live lectures, and tutorials are correlated with a three-book set of Prep Notes consisting of two textbooks, *Youel's Jewels I* and *Youel's Jewels II* (984 pages), and *Case Studies*, a question-and-answer book (1854 questions, answers, and explanations).

The Comprehensive DVD program consists of 56 hours of lectures by the systems with a three-book set: *Youel's Jewels I and II* and *Case Studies.* Integrated with these programs are pre-tests and post-tests.

All Youel's Prep courses are taught and written by physicians, reflecting the clinical slant of the boards. All programs are systems based. In addition, all programs are updated continuously. Accordingly, books are not printed until the order is received.

Delivery in the United States or overseas is usually within 1 week. Optional express delivery is also available. Youel's Prep Home Study Program™ allows students to own their materials and to use them for repetitive study in the convenience of their homes. Purchasers of any of Youel's Prep materials, programs, or services are enrolled as members of the Youel's Prep Family of Students™, which affords them access to free telephone tutoring at (800) 645-3985. Students may call 24/7. Youel's Prep live lectures are held at select medical schools at the invitation of the school and students.

Programs are custom-designed for content, number of hours, and scheduling to fit students' needs. First-year students are urged to call early to arrange live-lecture programs at their schools for next year.

For more information, contact:

Youel's Prep, Inc.
P.O. Box 31479
Palm Beach Gardens, FL 33420
Phone: (800) 645-3985
Fax: (561) 622-4858
Email: info@youelsprep.com
www.youelsprep.net

Publisher Contacts

ASM Press
P.O. Box 605
Herndon, VA 20172
(800) 546-2416
Books@asmusa.org
www.asmscience.org

CRC Press
Taylor & Francis Group
6000 Broken Sound Parkway, NW, Suite 300
Boca Raton, FL 33487
(800) 272-7737
Fax: (800) 374-3401
orders@crcpress.com
www.crcpress.com

Elsevier, Inc.
3251 Riverport Lane
Maryland Heights, MO 63043
(800) 401-9962
Fax: (314) 447-8078
www.us.elsevierhealth.com

Exam Master
100 Lake Drive, Suite 6
Newark, DE 19702
(800) 572-3627
Fax: (302) 283-1222
customerservice@exammaster.com
www.exammaster.com

Garland Science
711 Third Avenue, 8th Floor
New York, NY 10017
(203) 281-4487
Fax: (212) 947-3027
science@garland.com
www.garlandscience.com

Gold Standard Board Prep
Apollo Audiobooks, LLC
2508 27th Street
Lubbock, TX 79410
(806) 773-3197
info@ApolloAudiobooks.com
www.boardprep.net

John Wiley & Sons
1 Wiley Drive
Somerset, NJ 08875-1272
(800) 225-5945
Fax: (732) 302-2300
custserv@wiley.com
www.wiley.com

Kaplan, Inc.
395 Hudson Street, 4th Floor
New York, NY 10014
(800) 527-8378
customer.care@kaplan.com

Lippincott Williams & Wilkins
16522 Hunters Green Parkway
Hagerstown, MD 21740
(800) 638-3030
Fax: (301) 223-2400
orders@lww.com
www.lww.com

McGraw-Hill Companies
Order Services
P.O. Box 182604
Columbus, OH 43272-3031
(800) 262-4729
Fax: (614) 759-3749
pbg_ecommerce_custserv@mheducation.com
www.mhprofessional.com

MedMaster, Inc.
P.O. Box 640028
Miami, FL 33164
(800) 335-3480
Fax: (954) 962-4508
mmbks@aol.com
www.medmaster.net

Princeton Review
2315 Broadway
New York, NY 10024
(888) 955-4600
www.princetonreview.com

Thieme Medical Publishers, Inc.
333 Seventh Avenue
New York, NY 10001
(800) 782-3488
Fax: (212) 947-0108
www.thieme.com
customerservice@thieme.com

▶ NOTES

SECTION IV

Abbreviations and Symbols

ABBREVIATION	MEANING
1°	primary
2°	secondary
3°	tertiary
A-a	alveolar-arterial [gradient]
AA	Alcoholics Anonymous, amyloid A
AAMC	Association of American Medical Colleges
Ab	antibody
ABP	androgen-binding protein
ACA	anterior cerebral artery
Acetyl-CoA	acetyl coenzyme A
ACD	anemia of chronic disease
ACE	angiotensin-converting enzyme
ACh	acetylcholine
AChE	acetylcholinesterase
ACL	anterior cruciate ligament
ACom	anterior communicating [artery]
ACTH	adrenocorticotropic hormone
ADA	adenosine deaminase, Americans with Disabilities Act
ADH	antidiuretic hormone
ADHD	attention-deficit hyperactivity disorder
ADP	adenosine diphosphate
ADPKD	autosomal-dominant polycystic kidney disease
AFP	α-fetoprotein
Ag	antigen, silver
AICA	anterior inferior cerebellar artery
AIDS	acquired immunodeficiency syndrome
AIHA	autoimmune hemolytic anemia
AL	amyloid light [chain]
ALA	aminolevulinic acid
ALL	acute lymphoblastic (lymphocytic) leukemia
ALP	alkaline phosphatase
α_1, α_2	sympathetic receptors
ALS	amyotrophic lateral sclerosis
ALT	alanine transaminase
AMA	American Medical Association, antimitochondrial antibody
AML	acute myelogenous (myeloid) leukemia
AMP	adenosine monophosphate
ANA	antinuclear antibody
ANCA	antineutrophil cytoplasmic antibody
ANOVA	analysis of variance
ANP	atrial natriuretic peptide
ANS	autonomic nervous system
anti-CCP	anti-cyclic citrullinated peptide
AOA	American Osteopathic Association

ABBREVIATION	MEANING
AP	action potential, A & P [ribosomal binding sites]
A & P	ribosomal binding sites
APC	antigen-presenting cell, activated protein C
APP	amyloid precursor protein
APRT	adenine phosphoribosyltransferase
APSAC	anistreplase
aPTT	activated partial thromboplastin time
Apo	apolipoprotein
AR	attributable risk, autosomal recessive, aortic regurgitation
ara-C	arabinofuranosyl cytidine (cytarabine)
ARB	angiotensin receptor blocker
ARDS	acute respiratory distress syndrome
Arg	arginine
ARMD	age-related macular degeneration
ARPKD	autosomal-recessive polycystic kidney disease
AS	aortic stenosis
ASA	anterior spinal artery
ASD	atrial septal defect
ASO	anti–streptolysin O
AST	aspartate transaminase
AT	angiotensin, antithrombin
ATCase	aspartate transcarbamoylase
ATN	acute tubular necrosis
ATP	adenosine triphosphate
ATPase	adenosine triphosphatase
ATTR	transthyretin-mediated amyloidosis
AV	atrioventricular
AZT	azidothymidine
β_1, β_2	sympathetic receptors
BAL	British anti-Lewisite [dimercaprol]
BCG	bacille Calmette-Guérin
BIMS	Biometric Identity Management System
BM	basement membrane
BMI	body-mass index
BMR	basal metabolic rate
BP	bisphosphate, blood pressure
BPG	bisphosphoglycerate
BPH	benign prostatic hyperplasia
BT	bleeding time
BUN	blood urea nitrogen
Ca^{2+}	calcium ion
CAD	coronary artery disease
CAF	common application form
CALLA	common acute lymphoblastic leukemia antigen
cAMP	cyclic adenosine monophosphate

ABBREVIATION	MEANING
CBG	corticosteroid-binding globulin
Cbl	cobalamin
CBSSA	Comprehensive Basic Science Self-Assessment
CBT	computer-based test, cognitive behavioral therapy
CCK	cholecystokinin
CCS	computer-based case simulation
CD	cluster of differentiation
CDK	cyclin-dependent kinase
cDNA	complementary deoxyribonucleic acid
CEA	carcinoembryonic antigen
CETP	cholesterol-ester transfer protein
CF	cystic fibrosis
CFTR	cystic fibrosis transmembrane conductance regulator
CFX	circumflex [artery]
CGD	chronic granulomatous disease
cGMP	cyclic guanosine monophosphate
CGN	cis-Golgi network
$C_H1–C_H3$	constant regions, heavy chain [antibody]
ChAT	choline acetyltransferase
χ^2	chi-squared
CI	confidence interval
CIN	candidate identification number, carcinoma in situ, cervical intraepithelial neoplasia
CIS	Communication and Interpersonal Skills
CK	clinical knowledge, creatine kinase
CK-MB	creatine kinase, MB fraction
C_L	constant region, light chain [antibody]
CL	clearance
Cl^-	chloride ion
CLL	chronic lymphocytic leukemia
CML	chronic myelogenous (myeloid) leukemia
CMV	cytomegalovirus
CN	cranial nerve
CN^-	cyanide ion
CNS	central nervous system
CNV	copy number variation
CO	carbon monoxide, cardiac output
CO_2	carbon dioxide
CoA	coenzyme A
COMLEX-USA	Comprehensive Osteopathic Medical Licensing Examination
COMSAE	Comprehensive Osteopathic Medical Self-Assessment Examination
COMT	catechol-O-methyltransferase
COOH	carboxyl group
COP	coat protein
COPD	chronic obstructive pulmonary disease
CoQ	coenzyme Q
COX	cyclooxygenase
C_p	plasma concentration
CPAP	continuous positive airway pressure
CPK	creatine phosphokinase
CPR	cardiopulmonary resuscitation
Cr	creatinine
CRC	colorectal cancer

ABBREVIATION	MEANING
CREST	calcinosis, Raynaud phenomenon, esophageal dysfunction, sclerosis, and telangiectasias [syndrome]
CRH	corticotropin-releasing hormone
CRP	C-reactive protein
CS	clinical skills
C-section	cesarean section
CSF	cerebrospinal fluid
CT	computed tomography
CTP	cytidine triphosphate
CVA	cerebrovascular accident
CVID	common variable immunodeficiency
CXR	chest x-ray
Cys	cysteine
DAF	decay-accelerating factor
DAG	diacylglycerol
dATP	deoxyadenosine triphosphate
DCIS	ductal carcinoma in situ
DCT	distal convoluted tubule
ddC	dideoxycytidine [zalcitabine]
ddI	didanosine
DES	diethylstilbestrol
DHAP	dihydroxyacetone phosphate
DHB	dihydrobiopterin
DHEA	dehydroepiandrosterone
DHF	dihydrofolic acid
DHS	Department of Homeland Security
DHT	dihydrotestosterone
DI	diabetes insipidus
DIC	disseminated intravascular coagulation
DIP	distal interphalangeal [joint]
DKA	diabetic ketoacidosis
DLCO	diffusing capacity for carbon monoxide
DM	diabetes mellitus
DNA	deoxyribonucleic acid
dNTP	deoxynucleotide triphosphate
DO	doctor of osteopathy
DPGN	diffuse proliferative glomerulonephritis
DPM	doctor of podiatric medicine
DPP-4	dipeptidyl peptidase-4
DS	double stranded
dsDNA	double-stranded deoxyribonucleic acid
dsRNA	double-stranded ribonucleic acid
d4T	didehydrodeoxythymidine [stavudine]
dTMP	deoxythymidine monophosphate
DTR	deep tendon reflex
DTs	delirium tremens
dUDP	deoxyuridine diphosphate
dUMP	deoxyuridine monophosphate
DVT	deep venous thrombosis
EBV	Epstein-Barr virus
EC	ejection click
ECF	extracellular fluid
ECFMG	Educational Commission for Foreign Medical Graduates
ECG	electrocardiogram
ECL	enterochromaffin-like [cell]

ABBREVIATION	MEANING
ECM	extracellular matrix
ECT	electroconvulsive therapy
ED_{50}	median effective dose
EDRF	endothelium-derived relaxing factor
EDTA	ethylenediamine tetra-acetic acid
EDV	end-diastolic volume
EEG	electroencephalogram
EF	ejection fraction
EGF	epidermal growth factor
EHEC	enterohemorrhagic *E. coli*
ELISA	enzyme-linked immunosorbent assay
EM	electron micrograph/microscopy
EMB	eosin–methylene blue
Epi	epinephrine
EPO	erythropoietin
EPS	extrapyramidal system
ER	endoplasmic reticulum, estrogen receptor
ERAS	Electronic Residency Application Service
ERCP	endoscopic retrograde cholangiopancreatography
ERP	effective refractory period
eRPF	effective renal plasma flow
ERT	estrogen replacement therapy
ERV	expiratory reserve volume
ESR	erythrocyte sedimentation rate
ESRD	end-stage renal disease
ESV	end-systolic volume
ETEC	enterotoxigenic *E. coli*
EtOH	ethyl alcohol
EV	esophageal vein
F	bioavailability
FA	fatty acid
Fab	fragment, antigen-binding
FAD	flavin adenine dinucleotide
FAD^+	oxidized flavin adenine dinucleotide
$FADH_2$	reduced flavin adenine dinucleotide
FAP	familial adenomatous polyposis
F1,6BP	fructose-1,6-bisphosphate
F2,6BP	fructose-2,6-bisphosphate
FBPase	fructose bisphosphatase
Fc	fragment, crystallizable
FcR	Fc receptor
5f-dUMP	5-fluorodeoxyuridine monophosphate
Fe^{2+}	ferrous ion
Fe^{3+}	ferric ion
FENa	excreted fraction of filtered sodium
FEV_1	forced expiratory volume in 1 second
FF	filtration fraction
FFA	free fatty acid
FGF	fibroblast growth factor
FGFR	fibroblast growth factor receptor
FISH	fluorescence in situ hybridization
FKBP	FK506 binding protein
FLAIR	fluid-attenuated inversion recovery
f-met	formylmethionine
FMG	foreign medical graduate

ABBREVIATION	MEANING
FMN	flavin mononucleotide
FN	false negative
FNHTR	febrile nonhemolytic transfusion reaction
FP	false positive
F1P	fructose-1-phosphate
F6P	fructose-6-phosphate
FRC	functional residual capacity
FSH	follicle-stimulating hormone
FSMB	Federation of State Medical Boards
FTA-ABS	fluorescent treponemal antibody—absorbed
5-FU	5-fluorouracil
FVC	forced vital capacity
GABA	γ-aminobutyric acid
Gal	galactose
GBM	glomerular basement membrane
GC	glomerular capillary
G-CSF	granulocyte colony-stimulating factor
GERD	gastroesophageal reflux disease
GFAP	glial fibrillary acid protein
GFR	glomerular filtration rate
GGT	γ-glutamyl transpeptidase
GH	growth hormone
GHB	γ-hydroxybutyrate
GHRH	growth hormone–releasing hormone
G_I	G protein, I polypeptide
GI	gastrointestinal
GIP	gastric inhibitory peptide
GIST	gastrointestinal stromal tumor
GLUT	glucose transporter
GM	granulocyte macrophage
GM-CSF	granulocyte-macrophage colony stimulating factor
GMP	guanosine monophosphate
GnRH	gonadotropin-releasing hormone
GP	glycoprotein
G3P	glucose-3-phosphate
G6P	glucose-6-phosphate
G6PD	glucose-6-phospate dehydrogenase
GPe	globus pallidus externa
GPi	globus pallidus interna
GPI	glycosyl phosphatidylinositol
GRP	gastrin-releasing peptide
G_S	G protein, S polypeptide
GS	glycogen synthase
GSH	reduced glutathione
GSSG	oxidized glutathione
GTP	guanosine triphosphate
GTPase	guanosine triphosphatase
GU	genitourinary
H^+	hydrogen ion
H_1, H_2	histamine receptors
HAART	highly active antiretroviral therapy
HAV	hepatitis A virus
HAVAb	hepatitis A antibody
Hb	hemoglobin
Hb^+	oxidized hemoglobin

ABBREVIATION	MEANING
Hb^-	ionized hemoglobin
HBcAb	hepatitis B core antibody
HBcAg	hepatitis B core antigen
HBeAb	hepatitis B early antibody
HBeAg	hepatitis B early antigen
HBsAb	hepatitis B surface antibody
HBsAg	hepatitis B surface antigen
$HbCO_2$	carbaminohemoglobin
HBV	hepatitis B virus
HCC	hepatocellular carcinoma
hCG	human chorionic gonadotropin
HCO_3^-	bicarbonate
Hct	hematocrit
HCTZ	hydrochlorothiazide
HCV	hepatitis C virus
HDL	high-density lipoprotein
HDV	hepatitis D virus
H&E	hematoxylin and eosin
HEV	hepatitis E virus
HF	heart failure
Hfr	high-frequency recombination [cell]
HGPRT	hypoxanthine-guanine phosphoribosyltransferase
HHb	human hemoglobin
HHV	human herpesvirus
5-HIAA	5-hydroxyindoleacetic acid
HIE	hypoxic ischemic encephalopathy
His	histidine
HIT	heparin-induced thrombocytopenia
HIV	human immunodeficiency virus
HL	hepatic lipase
HLA	human leukocyte antigen
HMG-CoA	hydroxymethylglutaryl-coenzyme A
HMP	hexose monophosphate
HMSN	hereditary motor and sensory neuropathy
HMWK	high-molecular-weight kininogen
hnRNA	heterogeneous nuclear ribonucleic acid
H_2O	water
H_2O_2	hydrogen peroxide
HPA	hypothalamic-pituitary-adrenal [axis]
HPO	hypothalamic-pituitary-ovarian [axis]
HPV	human papillomavirus
HR	heart rate
HRE	hormone receptor element
HSV	herpes simplex virus
5-HT	5-hydroxytryptamine (serotonin)
HTLV	human T-cell leukemia virus
HTN	hypertension
HTR	hemolytic transfusion reaction
HUS	hemolytic-uremic syndrome
HVA	homovanillic acid
HZV	herpes zoster virus
IBD	inflammatory bowel disease
IBS	irritable bowel syndrome
IC	inspiratory capacity, immune complex
I_{Ca}	calcium current [heart]

ABBREVIATION	MEANING
I_f	funny current [heart]
ICA	internal carotid artery
ICAM	intracellular adhesion molecule
ICD	implantable cardioverter defibrillator
ICE	Integrated Clinical Encounter
ICF	intracellular fluid
ICP	intracranial pressure
ID	identification
ID_{50}	dose at which pathogen produces infection in 50% of population
IDDM	insulin-dependent diabetes mellitus
IDL	intermediate-density lipoprotein
I/E	inspiratory/expiratory [ratio]
IF	immunofluorescence, initiation factor
IFN	interferon
Ig	immunoglobulin
IGF	insulin-like growth factor
I_K	potassium current [heart]
IL	interleukin
IM	intramuscular
IMA	inferior mesenteric artery
IMED	International Medical Education Directory
IMG	international medical graduate
IMP	inosine monophosphate
IMV	inferior mesenteric vein
I_{Na}	sodium current [heart]
INO	internuclear ophthalmoplegia
INR	International Normalized Ratio
IO	inferior oblique [muscle]
IOP	intraocular pressure
IP_3	inositol triphosphate
IPV	inactivated polio vaccine
IR	current × resistance [Ohm's law], inferior rectus [muscle]
IRV	inspiratory reserve volume
ITP	idiopathic thrombocytopenic purpura
IUD	intrauterine device
IUGR	intrauterine growth restriction
IV	intravenous
IVC	inferior vena cava
IVDU	intravenous drug use
IVIG	intravenous immunoglobulin
JAK/STAT	Janus kinase/signal transducer and activator of transcription [pathway]
JGA	juxtaglomerular apparatus
JVD	jugular venous distention
JVP	jugular venous pulse
K^+	potassium ion
KatG	catalase-peroxidase produced by *M. tuberculosis*
K_e	elimination constant
K_f	filtration constant
KG	ketoglutarate
K_m	Michaelis-Menten constant
KOH	potassium hydroxide
L	left
LA	left atrial, left atrium

ABBREVIATION	MEANING
LAD	left anterior descending [artery]
LAF	left anterior fascicle
LCA	left coronary artery
LCAT	lecithin-cholesterol acyltransferase
LCFA	long-chain fatty acid
LCL	lateral collateral ligament
LCME	Liaison Committee on Medical Education
LCMV	lymphocytic choriomeningitis virus
LCX	left circumflex artery
LD	loading dose
LD_{50}	median lethal dose
LDH	lactate dehydrogenase
LDL	low-density lipoprotein
LES	lower esophageal sphincter
LFA	leukocyte function–associated antigen
LFT	liver function test
LGN	lateral geniculate nucleus
LGV	left gastric vein
LH	luteinizing hormone
LLQ	left lower quadrant
LM	light microscopy
LMN	lower motor neuron
LP	lumbar puncture
LPL	lipoprotein lipase
LPS	lipopolysaccharide
LR	lateral rectus [muscle]
LT	labile toxin leukotriene
LV	left ventricle, left ventricular
Lys	lysine
M_1-M_5	muscarinic (parasympathetic) ACh receptors
MAC	membrane attack complex, minimal alveolar concentration
MALT	mucosa-associated lymphoid tissue
MAO	monoamine oxidase
MAOI	monoamine oxidase inhibitor
MAP	mean arterial pressure, mitogen-activated protein
MASP	mannose-binding lectin–associated serine protease
MBL	mannose-binding lectin
MC	midsystolic click
MCA	middle cerebral artery
MCAT	Medical College Admissions Test
MCHC	mean corpuscular hemoglobin concentration
MCL	medial collateral ligament
MCP	metacarpophalangeal [joint]
MCV	mean corpuscular volume
MD	maintenance dose
MEN	multiple endocrine neoplasia
Mg^{2+}	magnesium ion
MGN	medial geniculate nucleus
$MgSO_4$	magnesium sulfate
MGUS	monoclonal gammopathy of undetermined significance
MHC	major histocompatibility complex
MI	myocardial infarction
MIF	müllerian inhibiting factor
MLCK	myosin light-chain kinase
MLF	medial longitudinal fasciculus

ABBREVIATION	MEANING
MMC	migrating motor complex
MMR	measles, mumps, rubella [vaccine]
MOPP	mechlorethamine-vincristine (Oncovin)-prednisone-procarbazine [chemotherapy]
6-MP	6-mercaptopurine
MPGN	membranoproliferative glomerulonephritis
MPO	myeloperoxidase
MPO-ANCA/ p-ANCA	perinuclear antineutrophil cytoplasmic antibody
MR	medial rectus [muscle], mitral regurgitation
MRI	magnetic resonance imaging
mRNA	messenger ribonucleic acid
MRSA	methicillin-resistant S. aureus
MS	mitral stenosis, multiple sclerosis
MSH	melanocyte-stimulating hormone
MSM	men who have sex with men
mtDNA	mitochondrial DNA
mtRNA	mitochondrial RNA
mTOR	mammalian target of rapamycin
MTP	metatarsophalangeal [joint]
MTX	methotrexate
MUA/P	Medically Underserved Area and Population
MVO_2	myocardial oxygen consumption
MVP	mitral valve prolapse
N/A	not applicable
Na^+	sodium ion
NAD	nicotinamide adenine dinucleotide
NAD^+	oxidized nicotinamide adenine dinucleotide
NADH	reduced nicotinamide adenine dinucleotide
$NADP^+$	oxidized nicotinamide adenine dinucleotide phosphate
NADPH	reduced nicotinamide adenine dinucleotide phosphate
NBME	National Board of Medical Examiners
NBOME	National Board of Osteopathic Medical Examiners
NBPME	National Board of Podiatric Medical Examiners
NC	no change
NE	norepinephrine
NF	neurofibromatosis
NFAT	nuclear factor of activated T-cell
NH_3	ammonia
NH_4^+	ammonium
NIDDM	non-insulin-dependent diabetes mellitus
NK	natural killer [cells]
N_M	muscarinic ACh receptor in neuromuscular junction
NMDA	N-methyl-D-aspartate
NMJ	neuromuscular junction
NMS	neuroleptic malignant syndrome
N_N	nicotinic ACh receptor in autonomic ganglia
NRMP	National Residency Matching Program
NNRTI	non-nucleoside reverse transcriptase inhibitor
NO	nitric oxide
N_2O	nitrous oxide
NPH	neutral protamine Hagedorn, normal pressure hydrocephalus
NPV	negative predictive value
NRI	norepinephrine receptor inhibitor
NRTI	nucleoside reverse transcriptase inhibitor

ABBREVIATION	MEANING
NSAID	nonsteroidal anti-inflammatory drug
NSTEMI	non–ST-segment elevation myocardial infarction
OA`A	oxaloacetic acid
OCD	obsessive-compulsive disorder
OCP	oral contraceptive pill
OH	hydroxy
OH_2	dihydroxy
1,25-OH D_3	calcitriol (active form of vitamin D)
25-OH D_3	storage form of vitamin D
3′ OH	hydroxyl
OMT	osteopathic manipulative technique
OPV	oral polio vaccine
OR	odds ratio
OS	opening snap
OTC	ornithine transcarbamoylase
OVLT	organum vasculosum of the lamina terminalis
P-450	cytochrome P-450 family of enzymes
PA	posteroanterior
PABA	*para*-aminobenzoic acid
$Paco_2$	arterial Pco_2
$PAco_2$	alveolar Pco_2
PAH	*para*-aminohippuric acid
PAN	polyarteritis nodosa
Pao_2	partial pressure of oxygen in arterial blood
PAo_2	partial pressure of oxygen in alveolar blood
PAP	Papanicolaou [smear], prostatic acid phosphatase
PAS	periodic acid–Schiff
PC	plasma colloid osmotic pressure, platelet count, pyruvate carboxylase
PCA	posterior cerebral artery
PCL	posterior cruciate ligament
Pco_2	partial pressure of carbon dioxide
PCom	posterior communicating [artery]
PCOS	polycystic ovarian syndrome
PCP	phencyclidine hydrochloride, *Pneumocystis jirovecii* pneumonia
PCR	polymerase chain reaction
PCT	proximal convoluted tubule
PCWP	pulmonary capillary wedge pressure
PD	posterior descending [artery]
PDA	patent ductus arteriosus
PDC	pyruvate dehydrogenase complex
PDE	phosphodiesterase
PDGF	platelet-derived growth factor
PDH	pyruvate dehydrogenase
PE	pulmonary embolism
PECAM	platelet–endothelial cell adhesion molecule
$PEco_2$	expired air Pco_2
PEP	phosphoenolpyruvate
PF	platelet factor
PFK	phosphofructokinase
PFT	pulmonary function test
PG	phosphoglycerate
P_i	plasma interstitial osmotic pressure, inorganic phosphate
PICA	posterior inferior cerebellar artery
PID	pelvic inflammatory disease

ABBREVIATION	MEANING
PIo_2	Po_2 in inspired air
PIP	proximal interphalangeal [joint]
PIP_2	phosphatidylinositol 4,5-bisphosphate
PKD	polycystic kidney disease
PKR	interferon-α–induced protein kinase
PKU	phenylketonuria
PLP	pyridoxal phosphate
PLS	Personalized Learning System
PML	progressive multifocal leukoencephalopathy
PMN	polymorphonuclear [leukocyte]
P_{net}	net filtration pressure
PNET	primitive neuroectodermal tumor
PNS	peripheral nervous system
Po_2	partial pressure of oxygen
PO_4	salt of phosphoric acid
PO_4^{3-}	phosphate
PPAR	peroxisome proliferator-activated receptor
PPD	purified protein derivative
PPI	proton pump inhibitor
PPV	positive predictive value
PR3-ANCA/ c-ANCA	cytoplasmic antineutrophil cytoplasmic antibody
PrP	prion protein
PRPP	phosphoribosylpyrophosphate
PSA	prostate-specific antigen
PSS	progressive systemic sclerosis
PT	prothrombin time
PTH	parathyroid hormone
PTHrP	parathyroid hormone–related protein
PTSD	post-traumatic stress disorder
PTT	partial thromboplastin time
PV	plasma volume, venous pressure
PVC	polyvinyl chloride
PVR	pulmonary vascular resistance
R	correlation coefficient, right, R variable [group]
R_3	Registration, Ranking, & Results [system]
RA	right atrium
RAAS	renin-angiotensin-aldosterone system
RANK-L	receptor activator of nuclear factor-κ B ligand
RAS	reticular activating system
RBC	red blood cell
RBF	renal blood flow
RCA	right coronary artery
REM	rapid eye movement
RER	rough endoplasmic reticulum
Rh	*rhesus* antigen
RLQ	right lower quadrant
RNA	ribonucleic acid
RNP	ribonucleoprotein
ROS	reactive oxygen species
RPF	renal plasma flow
RPGN	rapidly progressive glomerulonephritis
RPR	rapid plasma reagin
RR	relative risk, respiratory rate
rRNA	ribosomal ribonucleic acid

ABBREVIATION	MEANING
RS	Reed-Sternberg [cells]
RSV	respiratory syncytial virus
RTA	renal tubular acidosis
RUQ	right upper quadrant
RV	residual volume, right ventricle, right ventricular
RVH	right ventricular hypertrophy
Rx	medical prescription
[S]	substrate concentration
SA	sinoatrial
SAA	serum amyloid–associated [protein]
SAM	S-adenosylmethionine
SARS	severe acute respiratory syndrome
SAT	Scholastic Aptitude Test
SC	subcutaneous
SCC	squamous cell carcinoma
SCD	sudden cardiac death
SCID	severe combined immunodeficiency disease
SCJ	squamocolumnar junction
SCM	sternocleidomastoid muscle
SCN	suprachiasmatic nucleus
SD	standard deviation
SEM	standard error of the mean
SEP	Spoken English Proficiency
SER	smooth endoplasmic reticulum
SERM	selective estrogen receptor modulator
SHBG	sex hormone–binding globulin
SIADH	syndrome of inappropriate [secretion of] antidiuretic hormone
SLE	systemic lupus erythematosus
SLL	small lymphocytic lymphoma
SLT	Shiga-like toxin
SMA	superior mesenteric artery
SMX	sulfamethoxazole
SNARE	soluble NSF attachment protein receptor
SNc	substantia nigra pars compacta
SNP	single nucleotide polymorphism
SNr	substantia nigra pars reticulata
SNRI	serotonin and norepinephrine receptor inhibitor
snRNP	small nuclear ribonucleoprotein
SO	superior oblique [muscle]
SOAP	Supplemental Offer and Acceptance Program
spp.	species
SR	superior rectus [muscle]
SS	single stranded
ssDNA	single-stranded deoxyribonucleic acid
SSPE	subacute sclerosing panencephalitis
SSRI	selective serotonin reuptake inhibitor
ssRNA	single-stranded ribonucleic acid
SSSS	staphylococcal scalded-skin syndrome
ST	Shiga toxin
STD	sexually transmitted disease
STEMI	ST-segment elevation myocardial infarction
STN	subthalamic nucleus
SV	splenic vein, stroke volume
SVC	superior vena cava

ABBREVIATION	MEANING
SVT	supraventricular tachycardia
$t_{1/2}$	half-life
T_3	triiodothyronine
T_4	thyroxine
TAPVR	total anomalous pulmonary venous return
TB	tuberculosis
TBG	thyroxine-binding globulin
3TC	dideoxythiacytidine [lamivudine]
TCA	tricarboxylic acid [cycle], tricyclic antidepressant
Tc cell	cytotoxic T cell
TCR	T-cell receptor
TDF	tenofovir disoproxil fumarate
TdT	terminal deoxynucleotidyl transferase
TFT	thyroid function test
TG	triglyceride
6-TG	6-thioguanine
TGA	*trans*-Golgi apparatus
TGF	transforming growth factor
TGN	*trans*-Golgi network
Th cell	helper T cell
THF	tetrahydrofolic acid
TI	therapeutic index
TIA	transient ischemic attack
TIBC	total iron-binding capacity
TIPS	transjugular intrahepatic portosystemic shunt
TLC	total lung capacity
T_m	maximum rate of transport
TMP	trimethoprim
TN	true negative
TNF	tumor necrosis factor
TNM	tumor, node, metastases [staging]
TOEFL	Test of English as a Foreign Language
ToRCHeS	*Toxoplasma gondii*, rubella, CMV, HIV, HSV-2, syphilis
TP	true positive
tPA	tissue plasminogen activator
TPP	thiamine pyrophosphate
TPR	total peripheral resistance
TR	tricuspid regurgitation
TRAP	tartrate-resistant acid phosphatase
TRH	thyrotropin-releasing hormone
tRNA	transfer ribonucleic acid
TSH	thyroid-stimulating hormone
TSS	toxic shock syndrome
TSST	toxic shock syndrome toxin
TTP	thrombotic thrombocytopenic purpura
TTR	transthyretin
TV	tidal volume
Tx	translation [factor]
TXA_2	thromboxane A_2
UCV	Underground Clinical Vignettes
UDP	uridine diphosphate
UMN	upper motor neuron
UMP	uridine monophosphate
UPD	uniparental disomy
URI	upper respiratory infection

ABBREVIATION	MEANING
USMLE	United States Medical Licensing Examination
UTI	urinary tract infection
UTP	uridine triphosphate
UV	ultraviolet
V_1, V_2	Vasopressin receptors
VA	Veterans Affairs
VC	vital capacity
V_d	volume of distribution
VD	physiologic dead space
V(D)J	heavy-chain hypervariable region [antibody]
VDRL	Venereal Disease Research Laboratory
VEGF	vascular endothelial growth factor
V_H	variable region, heavy chain [antibody]
VHL	von Hippel-Lindau [disease]
VIP	vasoactive intestinal peptide
VIPoma	vasoactive intestinal polypeptide-secreting tumor
VJ	light-chain hypervariable region [antibody]
VL	ventral lateral [nucleus]; variable region, light chain [antibody]

ABBREVIATION	MEANING
VLDL	very low density lipoprotein
VMA	vanillylmandelic acid
V_{max}	maximum velocity
VPL	ventral posterior nucleus, lateral
VPM	ventral posterior nucleus, medial
VPN	vancomycin, polymyxin, nystatin [media]
V/Q	ventilation/perfusion [ratio]
VRE	vancomycin-resistant enterococcus
VSD	ventricular septal defect
V_T	tidal volume
vWF	von Willebrand factor
VZV	varicella-zoster virus
WHOML	"worst headache of my life"
WBC	white blood cell
XR	X-linked recessive
XX	normal complement of sex chromosomes for female
XY	normal complement of sex chromosomes for male
ZDV	zidovudine [formerly AZT]

Image Acknowledgments

In this edition, in collaboration with McGraw-Hill, MedIQ Learning, LLC, and a variety of other partners, we are pleased to include the following clinical images and diagrams for the benefit of integrative student learning.

℞ Portions of this book identified with the symbol ℞ are copyright © USMLE-Rx.com (MedIQ Learning, LLC).

RU Portions of this book identified with the symbol RU are copyright © Dr. Richard Usatine and are provided under license through MedIQ Learning, LLC.

✳ Portions of this book identified with the symbol ✳ are listed below by page number.

This symbol refers to material that is available in the public domain.

This symbol refers to the Creative Commons Attribution license, full text at: *http://creativecommons.org/licenses/by/3.0/legalcode.*

This symbol refers to the Creative Commons Attribution-Share Alike license, full text at: *http://creativecommons.org/.*

Biochemistry

74 Cilia structure. Courtesy of Louisa Howard and Michael Binder. The image may have been modified by cropping, labeling, and/or captions. All rights to this adaptation by MedIQ Learning, LLC are reserved.

76 Osteogenesis imperfecta: Image A. Skeletal deformities in child. This image is a derivative work, adapted from the following source, available under . Courtesy of Vanakker OM, Hemelsoet D, De Paepe. Hereditary connective tissue diseases in young adult stroke: a comprehensive synthesis. Stroke Res Treat 2011;712903. doi 10.4061/2011/712903. The image may have been modified by cropping, labeling, and/or captions. MedIQ Learning, LLC makes this image available under .

76 Osteogenesis imperfecta: Image B. Blue sclera. This image is a derivative work, adapted from the following source, available under . Courtesy of Fred H, van Dijk H. Images of memorable cases: cases 40, 41 & 42. Connexions Web site. December 3, 2008. Available at: *http://cnx.org/content/m15020/1.3/.*

77 Ehlers-Danlos syndrome. Finger hypermobility. This image is a derivative work, adapted from the following source, available under . Courtesy of Piotr Dołżonek.

95 Muscular dystrophies. Fibrofatty replacement of muscle. Courtesy of the U.S. Department of Health and Human Services and Dr. Edwin P. Ewing, Jr. The image may have been modified by cropping, labeling, and/or captions. All rights to this adaptation by MedIQ Learning, LLC are reserved.

90 Vitamin A. Pellagra. This image is a derivative work, adapted from the following source, available under . van Dijk HA, Fred H. Images of memorable cases: case 2. Connexions Web site. Dec 4, 2008. Available at: *http://cnx.org/contents/3d3dcb2e-8e98-496f-91c2-fe94e93428a1@3@3/.*

93 Vitamin D. Rickets. This image is a derivative work, adapted from the following source, available under . Courtesy of Dr. Michael L. Richardson.

94 Malnutrition. Child with kwashiorkor. Courtesy of the U.S. Department of Health and Human Services and Dr. Lyle Conrad.

108 Alkaptonuria (ochronosis). Pigment granules on dorsum of hand. This image is a derivative work, adapted from the following source, available under . Vasudevan B, Sawhney MPS, Radhakrishnan S. Alkaptonuria associated with degenerative collagenous palmar plaques. *Indian J Dermatol* 2009;54:299-301. doi 10.4103/0019-5154.55650.

108 Cystinuria. Hexagonal stones in cystinuria. This image is a derivative work, adapted from the following source, available under . Courtesy of Cayla Devine.

111 Lysosomal storage diseases: Image A. Gaucher cells in Gaucher disease. This image is a derivative work, adapted from the following source, available under . Sokołowska B, Skomra D, Czartoryska B. et al. Gaucher disease diagnosed after bone marrow trephine biopsy—a report of two cases. Folia Histochemica et Cytobiologica 2011;49:352-356. doi 10.5603/FHC.2011.0048. The image may have been modified by cropping, labeling, and/or captions. All rights to this adaptation by MedIQ Learning, LLC are reserved.

111 Lysosomal storage diseases: Image B. Foam cells in Niemann-Pick disease. This image is a derivative work, adapted from the following source, available under . Hypercholesterolemia boosts joint destruction in chronic arthritis. An experimental model aggravated by foam macrophage infiltration. Prieto-Potin I, Roamn-Blas JA, Martinez-Calatrava MJ, et al. *Arthritis Res Ther* 2013;15:R81. doi 10.1186/ar4261. The image may have been modified by cropping, labeling, and/or captions. All rights to this adaptation by MedIQ Learning, LLC are reserved.

111 Lysosomal storage diseases: Image C. "Cherry-red" spot on macula in Tay-Sachs disease. This image is a derivative work, adapted from the following source, available under . Courtesy of Dr. Jonathan Trobe.

Microbiology

122   Catalase-positive organisms. Oxygen bubbles released during catalase reaction. This image is a derivative work, adapted from the following source, available under [cc] BY-SA. Courtesy of Stefano Nase.

125   Endotoxin. Functions of endotoxin. Adapted, with permission, from Levinson W. *Review of medical microbiology and immunology*, 12th ed. New York: McGraw-Hill, 2012: Fig. 7-4.

128   α-hemolytic bacteria. α-hemolysis. This image is a derivative work, adapted from the following source, available under [cc] BY-SA. Courtesy of Y. Tambe.

128   β-hemolytic bacteria. β-hemolysis. This image is a derivative work, adapted from the following source, available under [cc] BY-SA. Courtesy of Y. Tambe.

128   *Staphylococcus aureus*. Gram stain. [public domain] Courtesy of the U.S. Department of Health and Human Services and Dr. Richard Facklam.

129   *Streptococcus pyogenes* (group A streptococci). Gram stain. This image is a derivative work, adapted from the following source, available under [cc] BY-SA. Courtesy of Y. Tambe.

130   *Corynebacterium diphtheriae*. Pseudomembranous pharyngitis. This image is a derivative work, adapted from the following source, available under [cc] BY-SA. Courtesy of Wikimedia Commons. The image may have been modified by cropping, labeling, and/or captions. MedIQ Learning, LLC makes this image available under [cc] BY-SA.

131   Clostridia (with exotoxins): Image A. Gas gangrene due to *Clostridium perfringens* infection. This image is a derivative work, adapted from the following source, available under [cc] 0. Courtesy of Engelbert Schröpfer, Stephan Rauthe, and Thomas Meyer.

131   Clostridia (with exotoxins): Image B. Pseudomembranous enterocolitis on colonoscopy. This image is a derivative work, adapted from the following source, available under [cc] 0. Courtesy of Klinikum Dritter Orden für die Überlassung des Bildes zur Veröffentlichu. The image may have been modified by cropping, labeling, and/or captions. MedIQ Learning, LLC makes this image available under [cc] BY-SA.

131   Clostridia (with exotoxins): Image C. CT of thickened bowel walls in *C. difficile* infection. This image is a derivative work, adapted from the following source, available under [cc] 0. Bowel wall thickening at CT: simplifying the diagnosis. Teresa Fernandes, Maria I. Oliveira, Ricardo Castro, et al. Insights Imaging 2014;5:195–208. doi 10.1007/s13244-013-0308-y. The image may have been modified by cropping, labeling, and/or captions. All rights to this adaptation by MedIQ Learning, LLC are reserved.

132   Anthrax: Image A. Gram-positive rods of *Bacillus anthracis*. [public domain] Courtesy of the U.S. Department of Health and Human Services.

132   Anthrax: Image B. Ulcer with black eschar. [public domain] Courtesy of the U.S. Department of Health and Human Services and James H. Steele.

132   *Listeria monocytogenes*. Actin rockets. This image is a derivative work, adapted from the following source, available under [cc] 0. Schuppler M, Loessner MJ. The opportunistic pathogen *Listeria monocytogenes*: pathogenicity and interaction with the mucosal immune system. *Int J Inflamm* 2010;2010:704321. doi 10.4061/2010/704321.

133   *Actinomyces* vs. *Nocardia*: Image A. *Actinomyces israelii* on Gram stain. [public domain] Courtesy of the U.S. Department of Health and Human Services.

133   *Actinomyces* vs. *Nocardia*: Image B. *Nocardia* on acid-fast stain. This image is a derivative work, adapted from the following source, available under [cc] 0. Leli C, Moretti A, Guercini F, et al. Fatal *Nocardia farcinica* bacteremia diagnosed by matrix-assisted laser desorption-ionization time of flight mass spectrometry in a patient with myelodysplastic syndrome treated with corticosteroids. *Case Rep Med* 2013;2013:368637. doi 10.1155/2013/368637.

134   Mycobacteria. Acid-fast stain. [public domain] Courtesy of the U.S. Department of Health and Human Services and Dr. Roger Feldman.

134   Leprosy (Hansen disease): Image B. "Glove and stocking" distribution. This image is a derivative work, adapted from the following source, available under [cc] BY-SA. Courtesy of Bruno Jehle. The image may have been modified by cropping, labeling, and/or captions. MedIQ Learning, LLC makes this image available under [cc] BY-SA.

136   Neisseria: Image A. Photomicrograph. [public domain] Courtesy of the U.S. Department of Health and Human Services and Dr. Mike Miller.

136   Haemophilus influenzae: Image A. Epiglottitis. This image is a derivative work, adapted from the following source, available under [cc] BY-SA. Courtesy of Wikimedia Commons. The image may have been modified by cropping, labeling, and/or captions. MedIQ Learning, LLC makes this image available under [cc] BY-SA.

137   Legionella pneumophila. [public domain] Courtesy of Grottola A, Forghieri F, Meacci M, et al. Severe pneumonia caused by *Legionella pneumophila* serogroup 11, Italy. *Emerg Infect Dis* 2012. doi 10.3201/eid1811.120216. The image may have been modified by cropping, labeling, and/or captions. All rights to this adaptation by MedIQ Learning, LLC are reserved.

137   Pseudomonas aeruginosa: Image A. Blue-green pigment. This image is a derivative work, adapted from the following source, available under [cc] BY-SA. Courtesy of Hansen. The image may have been modified by cropping, labeling, and/or captions. MedIQ Learning, LLC makes this image available under [cc] BY-SA.

137   Pseudomonas aeruginosa: Image B. Ecthyma gangrenosum. This image is a derivative work, adapted from the following source, available under [cc] 0. Gencer S, Ozer S, Gul AE, et al. Ecthyma gangrenosum without bacteremia in a previously healthy man: a case report. *J Med Case Rep* 2008;2:14. doi 10.1186/1752-1947-2-14. The image may have been modified by cropping, labeling, and/or captions. MedIQ Learning, LLC makes this image available under [cc] BY-SA.

139 **Vibrio cholerae.** This image is a derivative work, adapted from the following source, available under [CC]. Phetsouvanh R, Nakatsu M, Arakawa E, et al. Fatal bacteremia due to immotile *Vibrio cholerae* serogroup O21 in Vientiane, Laos—a case report. *Ann Clin Microbiol Antimicrob* 2008;7:10. doi 10.1186/1476-0711-7-10.

140 *Helicobacter pylori.* [PD] Courtesy of the U.S. Department of Health and Human Services, Dr. Patricia Fields, and Dr. Collette Fitzgerald.

140 **Spirochetes.** This image is a derivative work, adapted from the following source, available under [CC]. Larsson C, Berström. A novel and simple method for laboratory diagnosis of relapsing fever borreliosis. *Open Microbiol J* 2008;2:10–12. doi 10.2174/1874285800802010010.

140 **Lyme disease: Image A.** *Ixodes* tick. [PD] Courtesy of the U.S. Department of Health and Human Services and Dr. Michael L. Levin.

140 **Lyme disease: Image B.** Erythema chronicum migrans. [PD] Courtesy of the U.S. Department of Health and Human Services and James Gathany.

141 **Syphilis: Image A.** Painless cancer. [PD] Courtesy of the U.S. Department of Health and Human Services and M. Rein.

141 **Syphilis: Image B.** Treponeme on dark-field microscopy. [PD] Courtesy of the U.S. Department of Health and Human Services and Renelle Woodall.

141 **Syphilis: Image D.** Rash on palms in 2° syphilis. [PD] Courtesy of the U.S. Department of Health and Human Services and Robert Sumpter.

141 **Syphilis: Image E.** Condyloma lata. [PD] Courtesy of the U.S. Department of Health and Human Services and Susan Lindsley.

141 **Syphilis: Image F.** Gumma. This image is a derivative work, adapted from the following source, available under [CC]. Chakir K, Benchikhi H. Granulome centro-facial révélant une syphilis tertiaire. *Pan Afr Med J* 2013;15:82. doi 10.11604/pamj.2013.15.82.3011.

141 **Syphilis: Image G.** Congenital syphilis. [PD] Courtesy of the U.S. Department of Health and Human Services and Dr. Norman Cole.

141 **Syphilis: Image H.** Hutchinson teeth. [PD] Courtesy of the U.S. Department of Health and Human Services and Susan Lindsley.

142 *Gardnerella vaginalis.* [PD] Courtesy of the U.S. Department of Health and Human Services and M. Rein.

143 **Rickettsial diseases and vector-borne illness: Image A.** Rash of Rocky Mountain spotted fever. [PD] Courtesy of the U.S. Department of Health and Human Services.

143 **Rickettsial diseases and vector-borne illnesses: Image B.** *Ehrlichia* morulae. This image is a derivative work, adapted from the following source, available under [CC]. Dantas-Torres F. Canine vector-borne diseases in Brazil. *Parasit Vectors* 2008;1:25. doi 10.1186/1756-3305-1-25. The image may have been modified by cropping, labeling, and/or captions. MedIQ Learning, LLC makes this image available under [CC BY-SA].

144 *Mycoplasma pneumoniae.* This image is a derivative work, adapted from the following source, available under [CC]. Rottem S, Kosower NS, Kornspan JD. Contamination of tissue cultures by *Mycoplasma*. In: Ceccherini-Nelli L, ed: *Biomedical tissue culture*. doi 10.5772/51518.

145 **Systemic mycoses: Image A.** *Histoplasma.* [PD] Courtesy of the U.S. Department of Health and Human Services and Dr. D.T. McClenan.

145 **Systemic mycoses: Image B.** *Blastomyces.* This image is a derivative work, adapted from the following source, available under [CC BY-SA]. Courtesy of Joel Mills. The image may have been modified by cropping, labeling, and/or captions. MedIQ Learning, LLC makes this image available under [CC BY-SA].

145 **Systemic mycoses: Image D.** *Paracoccidioides.* [PD] Courtesy of the U.S. Department of Health and Human Services and Dr. Lucille K. Georg.

146 **Cutaneous mycoses: Image G.** Tinea versicolor. This image is a derivative work, adapted from the following source, available under [CC BY-SA]. Courtesy of Sarah (Rosenau) Korf. The image may have been modified by cropping, labeling, and/or captions. MedIQ Learning, LLC makes this image available under [CC BY-SA].

147 **Opportunistic fungal infections: Image A, left.** Budding yeast of *Candida albicans.* This image is a derivative work, adapted from the following source, available under [CC BY-SA]. Courtesy of Y. Tambe. The image may have been modified by cropping, labeling, and/or captions. MedIQ Learning, LLC makes this image available under [CC BY-SA].

147 **Opportunistic fungal infections: Image A, right.** Germ tubes of *Candida albicans.* This image is a derivative work, adapted from the following source, available under [CC BY-SA]. Courtesy of Y. Tambe. The image may have been modified by cropping, labeling, and/or captions. MedIQ Learning, LLC makes this image available under [CC BY-SA].

147 **Opportunistic fungal infections: Image B.** Oral thrush. [PD] Courtesy of the U.S. Department of Health and Human Services and Dr. Sol Silverman, Jr.

147 **Opportunistic fungal infections: Image C, right.** Conidiophores of *Aspergillus fumigatus.* [PD] Courtesy of the U.S. Department of Health and Human Services.

147 **Opportunistic fungal infections: Image D.** *Cryptococcus neoformans.* [PD] Courtesy of the U.S. Department of Health and Human Services and Dr. Leanor Haley.

147 **Opportunistic fungal infections: Image E.** *Mucor.* [PD] Courtesy of the U.S. Department of Health and Human Services and Dr. Libero Ajello.

148 *Pneumocystis jirovecii:* **Image A.** *Pneumocystis* pneumonia (PCP). This image is a derivative work, adapted from the following source, available under [CC]. Cho J-Y, Kim D-M, Kwon YE, et al. Newly formed cystic lesions for the development of pneumomediastinum in *Pneumocystis jirovecii* pneumonia. *BMC Infect Dis* 2009;9:171. doi 10.1186/1471-2334-9-171. The image may have been modified by cropping, labeling, and/or captions. All rights to this adaptation by MedIQ Learning, LLC are reserved.

149 Protozoa—GI infections: Image B. *Giardia lamblia* cyst. ▣ Courtesy of the U.S. Department of Health and Human Services.

149 Protozoa—GI infections: Image C. *Entamoeba histolytica* trophozoites. ▣ Courtesy of the U.S. Department of Health and Human Services.

149 Protozoa—GI infections: Image D. *Entamoeba histolytica* cyst. ▣ Courtesy of the U.S. Department of Health and Human Services.

149 Protozoa—GI infections: Image E. *Cryptosporidium* oocysts. ▣ Courtesy of the U.S. Department of Health and Human Services.

150 Protozoa—CNS infections: Image A. Cerebral toxoplasmosis. This image is a derivative work, adapted from the following source, available under ▣. Adurthi S, Mahadevan A, Bantwal R, et al. Utility of molecular and serodiagnostic tools in cerebral toxoplasmosis with and without tuberculous meningitis in AIDS patients: a study from South India. *Ann Indian Acad Neurol* 2010;13:263–270. doi 10.4103/0972-2327.74197. The image may have been modified by cropping, labeling, and/or captions. All rights to this adaptation by MedIQ Learning, LLC are reserved.

150 Protozoa—CNS infections: Image B. *Toxoplasma gondii* tachyzoite. ▣ Courtesy of the U.S. Department of Health and Human Services and Dr. L.L. Moore, Jr.

150 Protozoa—CNS infections: Image C. *Naegleria fowleri* amoebas. ▣ Courtesy of the U.S. Department of Health and Human Services.

150 Protozoa—CNS infections: Image D. *Trypanosoma brucei gambiense.* ▣ Courtesy of the U.S. Department of Health and Human Services and Dr. Mae Melvin.

151 Protozoa—Hematologic infections: Image A. *Plasmodium* trophozoite ring form. ▣ Courtesy of the U.S. Department of Health and Human Services.

151 Protozoa—Hematologic infections: Image B. *Plasmodium* schizont containing merozoites. ▣ Courtesy of the U.S. Department of Health and Human Services and Steven Glenn.

151 Protozoa—Hematologic infections: Image C. *Babesia.* ▣ Courtesy of the U.S. Department of Health and Human Services.

152 Protozoa—Others: Image A. *Trypanosoma cruzi.* ▣ Courtesy of the U.S. Department of Health and Human Services and Dr. Mae Melvin.

152 Protozoa—Others: Image B. *Leishmania donovani.* ▣ Courtesy of the U.S. Department of Health and Human Services and Dr. Francis W. Chandler. The image may have been modified by cropping, labeling, and/or captions. All rights to this adaptation by MedIQ Learning, LLC are reserved.

152 Protozoa—Others: Image C. *Trichomonas vaginalis.* ▣ Courtesy of the U.S. Department of Health and Human Services.

153 Nematodes (roundworms): Image A. *Enterobius vermicularis* eggs. ▣ Courtesy of the U.S. Department of Health and Human Services, B.G. Partin, and Dr. Moore.

153 Nematodes (roundworms): Image B. *Ascaris lumbricoides* egg. ▣ Courtesy of the U.S. Department of Health and Human Services.

153 Nematodes (roundworms): Image C. Elephantiasis. ▣ Courtesy of the U.S. Department of Health and Human Services.

154 Cestodes (tapeworms): Image A. *Taenia solium* scolex. This image is a derivative work, adapted from the following source, available under ▣ BY-SA. Courtesy of Robert J. Galindo. The image may have been modified by cropping, labeling, and/or captions. MedIQ Learning, LLC makes this image available under ▣ BY-SA.

154 Cestodes (tapeworms): Image B. Neurocysticercosis. This image is a derivative work, adapted from the following source, available under ▣. Coyle CM, Tanowitz HB. Diagnosis and treatment of neurocysticercosis. *Interdiscip Perspect Infect Dis* 2009;2009:180742. doi 10.1155/2009/180742. The image may have been modified by cropping, labeling, and/or captions. All rights to this adaptation by MedIQ Learning, LLC are reserved.

154 Cestodes (tapeworms): Image C. *Echinococcus granulosus* scolex. ▣ Courtesy of the U.S. Department of Health and Human Services and Dr. L.A.A. Moore, Jr.

154 Cestodes (tapeworms): Image D. Gross hyatid cyst of *Echinococcus granulosus.* ▣ Courtesy of the U.S. Department of Health and Human Services and Dr. I. Kagan.

154 Cestodes (tapeworms): Image E. *Echinococcus granulosus* cyst in liver. This image is a derivative work, adapted from the following source, available under ▣. Ma Z, Yang W, Yao Y, et al. The adventitia resection in treatment of liver hydatid cyst: a case report of a 15-year-old boy. *Case Rep Surg* 2014;2014:123149. doi 10.1155/2014/123149.

155 Trematodes (flukes): Image A. *Schistosoma mansoni* egg with terminal spine. ▣ Courtesy of the U.S. Department of Health and Human Services.

155 Trematodes (flukes): Image B. *Schistosoma mansoni* egg with lateral spine. ▣ Courtesy of the U.S. Department of Health and Human Services.

159 Herpesviruses: Image A. Keratoconjunctivitis in HSV-1 infection. This image is a derivative work, adapted from the following source, available under ▣. Yang HK, Han YK, Wee WR, et al. Bilateral herpetic keratitis presenting with unilateral neurotrophic keratitis in pemphigus foliaceus: a case report. *J Med Case Rep* 2011;5:328. doi 10.1186/1752-1947-5-328.

159 Herpesviruses: Image B. Herpes labialis. ▣ Courtesy of the U.S. Department of Health and Human Services and Dr. Herrmann.

159 Herpesviruses: Image E. Varicella-zoster virus. This image is a derivative work, adapted from the following source, available under ▣ BY-SA. Courtesy of Fisle. The image may have been modified by cropping, labeling, and/or captions. MedIQ Learning, LLC makes this image available under ▣ BY-SA.

159 Herpesviruses: Image F. Lymphadenopathy in VZV infection. This image is a derivative work, adapted from the following source, available under ▣ BY-SA. Courtesy of Dr. James Heilman.

159 Herpesviruses: Image G. Atypical lymphocytes in Epstein-Barr virus infection. This image is a derivative work, adapted from the following source, available under ▣ BY-SA. Courtesy of Dr. Ed Uthman. The image may have been modified by cropping, labeling, and/or captions. MedIQ Learning, LLC makes this image available under ▣ BY-SA.

159 Herpesviruses: Image I. Roseola. ▣ Courtesy of Emiliano Burzagli.

159 Herpesvirus: Image J. Kaposi sarcoma. ▣ Courtesy of the U.S. Department of Health and Human Services.

160 HSV identification. Positive Tzank smear in HSV-2 infection. This image is a derivative work, adapted from the following source, available under ▣. Courtesy of Yale Rosen. The image may have been modified by cropping, labeling, and/or captions. MedIQ Learning, LLC makes this image available under ▣.

162 Yellow fever virus. *Aedes aegypti* mosquito. ▣ Courtesy of the U.S. Department of Health and Human Services and James Gathany.

162 Rotavirus. ▣ Courtesy of the U.S. Department of Health and Human Services and Erskine Palmer.

163 Rubella virus: Image A. Rubella rash. ▣ Courtesy of the U.S. Department of Health and Human Services.

163 Rubella virus: Image B. Congenital rubella virus infection. ▣ Courtesy of the U.S. Department of Health and Human Services and Dr. Andre J. Lebrun.

164 Croup (acute laryngotracheobronchitis). Steeple sign. Reproduced, with permission, from Dr. Frank Gaillard and *www.radiopaedia.org.*

164 Measles (rubeola) virus: Image A. Koplik spots. ▣ Courtesy of the U.S. Department of Health and Human Services the U.S. Department of Health and Human Services. The image may have been modified by cropping, labeling, and/or captions. All rights to this adaptation by MedIQ Learning, LLC are reserved.

164 Measles (rubeola) virus: Image B. Rash of measles. ▣ Courtesy of the U.S. Department of Health and Human Services.

165 Mumps virus. Swollen neck and parotid glands. ▣ Courtesy of the U.S. Department of Health and Human Services.

165 Rabies virus: Image A. Transmission electron micrograph. ▣ Courtesy of the U.S. Department of Health and Human Services Dr. Fred Murphy, and Sylvia Whitfield.

165 Rabies virus: Image B. Negri bodies. ▣ Courtesy of the U.S. Department of Health and Human Services and Dr. Daniel P. Perl.

165 Ebola virus. ▣ Courtesy of the U.S. Department of Health and Human Services and Cynthia Goldsmith.

171 Prions. Spongiform changes in Creutzfeld-Jacob disease. This image is a derivative work, adapted from the following source, available under ▣. Courtesy of DRdoubleB. The image may have been modified by cropping, labeling, and/or captions. MedIQ Learning, LLC makes this image available under ▣.

173 Osteomyelitis: Images A and B. This image is a derivative work, adapted from the following source, available under ▣. Pandey V, Rao SP, Rao S, et al. *Burkholderia pseudomallei* musculoskeletal infections (melioidosis) in India. *Indian J Orthop* 2010;44:216-220. doi 10.4103/0019-5413.61829.

174 Common vaginal infections: Image C. *Candida* vulvovaginitis. ▣ Courtesy of Mikael Häggström.

178 Pelvic inflammatory disease: Image A. Purulent cervical discharge. This image is a derivative work, adapted from the following source, available under ▣. Courtesy of SOS-AIDS Amsterdam The image may have been modified by cropping, labeling, and/or captions. MedIQ Learning, LLC makes this image available under ▣.

178 Pelvic inflammatory disease: Image B. Adhesions in Fitz-Hugh–Curtis syndrome. ▣ Courtesy of Hic et nunc.

Immunology

199 Sinusoids of spleen. Red and white pulp. This image is a derivative work, adapted from the following source, available under ▣. Heinrichs S, Conover LF, Bueso-Ramos CE, et al. *MYBL2* is a sub-haploinsufficient tumor suppressor gene in myeloid malignancy. *eLife* 2013;2:e00825. doi 10.7554/eLife.00825. The image may have been modified by cropping, labeling, and/or captions. All rights to this adaptation by MedIQ Learning, LLC are reserved.

215 Immunodeficiencies. Giant granules in granulocytes in Chédiak-Higashi syndrome. This image is a derivative work, adapted from the following source, available under ▣. Bharti S, Bhatia P, Bansal D, et al. The accelerated phase of Chediak-Higashi syndrome: the importance of hematological evaluation. *Turk J Haematol* 2013;30:85-87. doi 10.4274/tjh.2012.0027. The image may have been modified by cropping, labeling, and/or captions. All rights to this adaptation by MedIQ Learning, LLC are reserved.

Pathology

223 Necrosis: Image A. Coagulative necrosis. ▣ Courtesy of the U.S. Department of Health and Human Services and Dr. Steven Rosenberg.

223 Necrosis: Image B. Liquefactive necrosis. ▣ Courtesy of Daftblogger.

223 Necrosis: Image C. Caseous necrosis. This image is a derivative work, adapted from the following source, available under ▣. Courtesy of Dr. Yale Rosen. The image may have been modified by cropping, labeling, and/or captions. MedIQ Learning, LLC makes this image available under ▣.

223 Necrosis: Image D. Fat necrosis. This image is a derivative work, adapted from the following source, available under ▣. Courtesy of Patho. The image may have been modified by cropping, labeling, and/or captions. MedIQ Learning, LLC makes this image available under ▣.

223 Necrosis: Image E. Fibrinoid necrosis. This image is a derivative work, adapted from the following source, available under ▣. Courtesy of Dr. Yale Rosen. The image may have been modified by cropping, labeling, and/or captions. MedIQ Learning, LLC makes this image available under ▣.

223 Necrosis: Image F. Acral gangrene. ▣ Courtesy of the U.S. Department of Health and Human Services and William Archibald.

224 Infarcts: red vs. pale: Image A, right. Pale infarct. ▣ Courtesy of the U.S. Department of Health and Human Services and Armed Forces Institute of Pathology.

240   **Common metastases: Image E.** Renal cell carcinoma metastases to bone. This image is a derivative work, adapted from the following source, available under [cc BY-SA]. Courtesy of Hellerhoff. The image may have been modified by cropping, labeling, and/or captions. MedIQ Learning, LLC makes this image available under [cc BY-SA].

240   **Common metastases: Image F.** Bone metastases. This image is a derivative work, adapted from the following source, available under [cc 0]. M. Emmanuel.

Pharmacology

244   **Elimination of drugs.** Adapted, with permission, from Katzung BG, Trevor AJ. *Pharmacology: examination & board review*, 5th ed. Stamford, CT: Appleton & Lange, 1998:5.

246   **Receptor binding: Images A and B.** Adapted, with permission, from Trevor AJ et al: *Katzung & Trevor's pharmacology: examination & board review*, 8th ed. New York: McGraw-Hill, 2008:14.

246   **Receptor binding: Image C.** Adapted, with permission, from Katzung BG. *Basic and clinical pharmacology*, 7th ed. Stamford, CT: Appleton & Lange, 1997:13.

247   **Central and peripheral nervous system.** Adapted, with permission, from Katzung BG. *Basic and clinical pharmacology*, 10th ed. New York: McGraw-Hill, 2007:76.

254   **Norepinephrine vs. isoproterenol.** Adapted, with permission, from Katzung BG, Trevor AJ. *Pharmacology: examination & board review*, 5th ed. Stamford, CT: Appleton & Lange, 1998:72.

255   **α-blockers.** Adapted, with permission, from Katzung BG, Trevor AJ. *Pharmacology: examination & board review*, 5th ed. Stamford, CT: Appleton & Lange, 1998:80.

Cardiovascular

288   **Congenital heart diseases: Image A.** Tetralogy of Fallot. This image is a derivative work, adapted from the following source, available under [cc 0]. Rashid AKM: Heart diseases in Down syndrome. In: Dey S, ed: Down syndrome. doi 10.5772/46009. The image may have been modified by cropping, labeling, and/or captions. All rights to this adaptation by MedIQ Learning, LLC are reserved.

288   **Congenital heart diseases: Image B.** Atrial septal defect. This image is a derivative work, adapted from the following source, available under [cc 0]. Teo KSL, Disney PJ, Dundon BK, et al. Assessment of atrial septal defects in adults comparing cardiovascular magnetic resonance with transesophageal echocardiography. *J Cardiovasc Magnet Resonance* 2010;12:44. doi 10.1186/1532-429X-12-44.

288   **Congenital heart diseases: Image C.** Clubbing of fingers in Eisenmenger syndrome. [cc] Courtesy of Ann McGrath.

290   **Hypertension: Image A.** "String of beads" appearance in fibromuscular dysplasia. This image is a derivative work, adapted from the following source, available under [cc 0]. Plouin PF, Perdu J, LaBatide-Alanore A, et al. Fibromuscular dysplasia. *Orphanet J Rare Dis* 2007;7:28. doi 10.1186/1750-1172-2-28. The image may have been modified by cropping, labeling, and/or captions. All rights to this adaptation by MedIQ Learning, LLC are reserved.

290   **Hypertension: Image B.** Hypertensive nephropathy. This image is a derivative work, adapted from the following source, available under [cc BY-SA]. Courtesy of Nephron. The image may have been modified by cropping, labeling, and/or captions. MedIQ Learning, LLC makes this image available under [cc BY-SA].

291   **Hyperlipidemia signs: Image C.** Tendinous xanthoma. This image is a derivative work, adapted from the following source, available under [cc BY-SA]. Courtesy of Min.neel. The image may have been modified by cropping, labeling, and/or captions. MedIQ Learning, LLC makes this image available under [cc BY-SA].

291   **Atherosclerosis: Image A.** Hyaline type. This image is a derivative work, adapted from the following source, available under [cc BY-SA]. Courtesy of Nephron. The image may have been modified by cropping, labeling, and/or captions. MedIQ Learning, LLC makes this image available under [cc BY-SA].

291   **Atherosclerosis: Image B.** Hyperplastic type. This image is a derivative work, adapted from the following source, available under [cc BY-SA]. Courtesy of Paco Larosa. The image may have been modified by cropping, labeling, and/or captions. MedIQ Learning, LLC makes this image available under [cc BY-SA].

291   **Arteriosclerosis: Image C.** Monckeberg medial calcific sclerosis. This image is a derivative work, adapted from the following source, available under [cc BY-SA]. Courtesy of C.E. Couri, G.A. da Silva, J.A. Martinez, F.A. Pereira, and F. de Paula. The image may have been modified by cropping, labeling, and/or captions. All rights to this adaptation by MedIQ Learning, LLC are reserved.

292   **Atherosclerosis: Image B.** Carotid plaque. This image is a derivative work, adapted from the following source, available under [cc BY-SA]. Courtesy of Dr. Ed Uthman. The image may have been modified by cropping, labeling, and/or captions. MedIQ Learning, LLC makes this image available under [cc BY-SA].

293   **Aortic dissection.** This image is a derivative work, adapted from the following source, available under [cc 0]. Apostolakis EE, Baikoussis NG, Katsanos K, et al. Postoperative peri-axillary seroma following axillary artery cannulation for surgical treatment of acute type A aortic dissection: case report. *J Cardiothor Surg* 2010;5:43. doi 0.1186/1749-8090-5-43.

294   **Evolution of MI.** LV free wall rupture. This image is a derivative work, adapted from the following source, available under [cc 0]. Zacarias ML, da Trindade H, Tsutsu J, et al. Left ventricular free wall impeding rupture in post-myocardial infarction period diagnosed by myocardial contrast echocardiography: case report. *Cardiovasc Ultrasound* 2006;4:7. doi 10.1186/1476-7120-4-7.

295   **MI complications.** Papillary muscle rupture. This image is a derivative work, adapted from the following source, available under [cc 0]. Routy B, Huynh T, Fraser R, et al. Vascular endothelial cell function in catastrophic antiphospholipid syndrome: a case report and review of the literature. *Case Rep Hematol* 2013;2013:710365. doi 10.1155/2013/710365.

296   **Cardiomyopathies: Image A.** Dilated cardiomyopathy. This image is a derivative work, adapted from the following source, available under [cc 0]. Gho JMIH, van Es R, Stathonikos N, et al. High resolution systematic digital histological quantification of cardiac fibrosis and adipose tissue in phospholamban p.Arg14del mutation associated cardiomyopathy. *PLoS One* 2014;9:e94820. doi 10.1371/journal.pone.0094820.

297 Heart failure. Pedal edema. This image is a derivative work, adapted from the following source, available under [CC BY-SA]. Courtesy of Dr. James Heilman. The image may have been modified by cropping, labeling, and/or captions. MedIQ Learning, LLC makes this image available under [CC BY-SA].

298 Bacterial endocarditis: Image A. Janeway lesions on foot. This image is a derivative work, adapted from the following source, available under [CC 0]. DeNanneke.

299 Rheumatic fever. Aschoff body and Anitschkow cells. This image is a derivative work, adapted from the following source, available under [CC BY-SA]. Courtesy of Dr. Ed Uthman. The image may have been modified by cropping, labeling, and/or captions. MedIQ Learning, LLC makes this image available under [CC BY-SA].

299 Cardiac tamponade. This image is a derivative work, adapted from the following source, available under [CC 0]. Jana M, Gamanagatti SR, Kumar A. Case series: CT scan in cardiac arrest and imminent cardiogenic shock: case series. *Indian J Radiol Imaging* 2010;20:150–153. doi 10.4103/0971-3026.63037.

301 Vascular tumors: Image A. Bacillary angiomatosis. This image is a derivative work, adapted from the following source, available under [CC 0]. Fulchini R, Bloemberg G, Boggian K. Bacillary angiomatosis and bacteremia due to *Bartonella quintana* in a patient with chronic lymphocytic leukemia. *Case Rep Infect Dis* 2013;2013:694765. doi 10.1155/2013/694765.

301 Vascular tumors: Image C. Cystic hygroma. This image is a derivative work, adapted from the following source, available under [CC 0]. Sannoh S, Quezada E, Merer DM, et al. Cystic hygroma and potential airway obstruction in a newborn: a case report and review of the literature. *Cases J* 2009;2:48. doi 10.1186/1757-1626-2-48. The image may have been modified by cropping, labeling, and/or captions. All rights to this adaptation by MedIQ Learning, LLC are reserved.

301 Vascular tumors: Image D. Pyogenic granuloma. This image is a derivative work, adapted from the following source, available under [CC BY-SA]. Courtesy of L. Wozniak and K.W. Zielinski. The image may have been modified by cropping, labeling, and/or captions. MedIQ Learning, LLC makes this image available under [CC BY-SA].

301 Raynaud phenomenon. This image is a derivative work, adapted from the following source, available under [CC BY-SA]. Courtesy of Jamclaassen. The image may have been modified by cropping, labeling, and/or captions. MedIQ Learning, LLC makes this image available under [CC BY-SA].

303 Vasculitides: Image A. Temporal arteritis histology. This image is a derivative work, adapted from the following source, available under [CC BY-SA]. Courtesy of Marvin. The image may have been modified by cropping, labeling, and/or captions. MedIQ Learning, LLC makes this image available under [CC BY-SA].

303 Vasculitides: Image B. Takayasu arteritis angiography. [CC PUBLIC] Courtesy of the U.S. Department of Health and Human Services and Justin Ly.

303 Vasculitides: Image C. Microaneurysms in polyarteritis nodosa. Reproduced, with permission, from Dr. Frank Gaillard and *www.radiopaedia.org*.

303 Vasculitides: Image D. Kawasaki disease and strawberry tongue. This image is a derivative work, adapted from the following source, available under [CC BY-SA]. Courtesy of Natr.

303 Vasculitides: Image E. Kawasaki disease and coronary artery aneurysm. This image is a derivative work, adapted from the following source, available under [CC 0]. Wikimedia Commons. The image may have been modified by cropping, labeling, and/or captions. All rights to this adaptation by MedIQ Learning, LLC are reserved.

303 Vasculitides: Image F. Buerger disease. This image is a derivative work, adapted from the following source, available under [CC 0]. Afsjarfard A, Mozaffar M, Malekpour F, et al. The wound healing effects of iloprost in patients with Buerger's disease: claudication and prevention of major amputations. *Iran Red Crescent Med J* 2011;13:420-423. PMCID PMC3371931.

303 Vasculitides: Image G. Granulomatosis with polyangiitis (Wegener) and PR3-ANCA/c-ANCA. [CC PUBLIC] Courtesy of the U.S. Department of Health and Human Services. M.A. Little.

303 Vasculitis: Image H. Microscopic polyangiitis and MPO-ANCA/p-ANCA. [CC PUBLIC] Courtesy of the U.S. Department of Health and Human Services. M.A. Little.

303 Vasculitis: Image I. Churg-Strauss syndrome histology. This image is a derivative work, adapted from the following source, available under [CC BY-SA]. Courtesy of Nephron. The image may have been modified by cropping, labeling, and/or captions. MedIQ Learning, LLC makes this image available under [CC BY-SA].

303 Vasculitis: Image J. Henoch-Schönlein purpura. [CC PUBLIC] Courtesy of the U.S. Department of Health and Human Services. Okwikikim.

306 Lipid-lowering agents. Adapted, with permission, from Katzung BG, Trevor AJ. *USMLE road map: pharmacology.* New York: McGraw-Hill, 2003:56.

Endocrine

312 Thyroid development. Thyroglossal duct cyst. This image is a derivative work, adapted from the following source, available under [CC 0]. Karlatti PD, Nagvekar S, Lekshmi TP, Kothari As. Migratory intralaryngeal thyroglossal duct cyst. *Indian J Radiol Imaging* 2010;20: 115-117. doi 10.4103/0971-3026.63053. The image may have been modified by cropping, labeling, and/or captions. All rights to this adaptation by MedIQ Learning, LLC are reserved.

312 Adrenal cortex and medulla. [CC PUBLIC] Courtesy of Wikimedia Commons. The image may have been modified by cropping, labeling, and/or captions. All rights to this adaptation by MedIQ Learning, LLC are reserved.

320 Parathyroid hormone. Adapted, with permission, from Chandrosoma P et al. *Concise pathology*, 3rd ed. Stamford, CT: Appleton & Lange, 1998.

323 Cushing syndrome. Abdominal striae. An image that belongs to this book.

324 Adrenal insufficiency. Mucosal hyperpigmentation in 1° adrenal insufficiency. [CC PUBLIC] Courtesy of the U.S. Department of Health and Human Services. FlatOut. The image may have been modified by cropping, labeling, and/or captions. All rights to this adaptation by MedIQ Learning, LLC are reserved.

325 **Neuroblastoma: Image B.** This image is a derivative work, adapted from the following source, available under CC BY. Koumarianou A, Oikonomopoulou P, Baka M, et al. Implications of the incidental finding of a MYCN amplified adrenal tumor: a case report and update of a pediatric disease diagnosed in adults. *Case Rep Oncol Med* 2013;2013:393128. doi 10.1155/2013/393128.

326 **Pheochromocytoma: Image A.** Pheochromocytoma involving adrenal medulla. This image is a derivative work, adapted from the following source, available under CC BY. Dr. Michael Feldman.

326 **Pheochromocytoma: Image B.** Chromaffin cells. This image is a derivative work, adapted from the following source, available under CC BY-SA. Courtesy of KGH. The image may have been modified by cropping, labeling, and/or captions. MedIQ Learning, LLC makes this image available under CC BY-SA.

328 **Hypothyroidism: Image B.** Congenital hypothyroidism. This image is a derivative work, adapted from the following source, available under CC BY-SA. Courtesy of Sadasiv Swain. The image may have been modified by cropping, labeling, and/or captions. MedIQ Learning, LLC makes this image available under CC BY-SA.

328 **Hypothyroidism: Image C: Before and after treatment of congenital hypothyroidism.** CC PUBLIC DOMAIN Courtesy of the U.S. Department of Health and Human Services.

332 **Hyperparathyroidism.** Multiple lytic lesions. This image is a derivative work, adapted from the following source, available under CC BY. Khaoula BA, Kaouther BA, Ines C, et al. An unusual presentation of primary hyperparathyroidism: pathological fracture. *Case Rep Orthop* 2011;2011:521578. doi 10.1155/2011/521578.

332 **Pituitary adenoma.** Reproduced, with permission, from Dr. Frank Gaillard and *www.radiopaedia.org*.

336 **Carcinoid syndrome.** Carcinoid tumor histology. CC PUBLIC DOMAIN Courtesy of the U.S. Department of Health and Human Services and Armed Forces Institute of Pathology.

Gastrointestinal

340 **Pancreas and spleen embryology.** Annular pancreas. This image is a derivative work, adapted from the following source, available under CC BY. Mahdi B, Selim S, Hassen T, et al. A rare cause of proximal intestinal obstruction in adults—annular pancreas: a case report. *Pan Afr Med J* 2011;10:56. PMCID PMC3290886.

349 **Liver anatomy.** Kupffer cells. This image is a derivative work, adapted from the following source, available under CC BY-SA. Courtesy of Nephron. The image may have been modified by cropping, labeling, and/or captions. MedIQ Learning, LLC makes this image available under CC BY-SA.

350 **Biliary structures.** Gallstones. This image is a derivative work, adapted from the following source, available under CC BY-SA. Courtesy of J. Guntau. The image may have been modified by cropping, labeling, and/or captions. MedIQ Learning, LLC makes this image available under CC BY-SA.

356 **Peyer patches.** This image is a derivative work, adapted from the following source, available under CC BY-SA. Courtesy of Plainpaper. The image may have been modified by cropping, labeling, and/or captions. MedIQ Learning, LLC makes this image available under CC BY-SA.

357 **Salivary gland tumors.** Pleomorphic adenoma. This image is a derivative work, adapted from the following source, available under CC BY-SA. Courtesy of Wikimedia Commons. The image may have been modified by cropping, labeling, and/or captions. MedIQ Learning, LLC makes this image available under CC BY-SA.

357 **Achalasia.** This image is a derivative work, adapted from the following source, available under CC BY-SA. Courtesy of Farnoosh Farrokhi and Michael F. Vaezi. The image may have been modified by cropping, labeling, and/or captions. MedIQ Learning, LLC makes this image available under CC BY-SA.

358 **Esophageal pathologies: Image A.** Pneumomediastinum in Boerhaave syndrome. This image is a derivative work, adapted from the following source, available under CC BY-SA. Courtesy of Wikimedia Commons. The image may have been modified by cropping, labeling, and/or captions. MedIQ Learning, LLC makes this image available under CC BY-SA.

358 **Esophageal pathologies: Image B.** Esophageal varices on endoscopy. This image is a derivative work, adapted from the following source, available under CC BY. Costaguta A, Alvarez F. Etiology and management of hemorrhagic complications of portal hypertension in children. *Int J Hepatol* 2012;2012:879163. doi 10.1155/2012/879163.

358 **Esophageal pathologies: Image C.** Esophageal varices on CT. This image is a derivative work, adapted from the following source, available under CC BY-SA. Courtesy of Hellerhoff. The image may have been modified by cropping, labeling, and/or captions. MedIQ Learning, LLC makes this image available under CC BY-SA.

358 **Barrett esophagus.** This image is a derivative work, adapted from the following source, available under CC BY-SA. Courtesy of Nephron. The image may have been modified by cropping, labeling, and/or captions. MedIQ Learning, LLC makes this image available under CC BY-SA.

359 **Esophageal cancer.** This image is a derivative work, adapted from the following source, available under CC BY. Brooks PJ, Enoch M-A, Goldman D, et al. The alcohol flushing response: an unrecognized risk factor for esophageal cancer from alcohol consumption. *PLOS Med* 2009;6:e1000050. doi 10.1371/journal.pmed.1000050.

359 **Ménétrier disease.** This image is a derivative work, adapted from the following source, available under CC BY-SA. Courtesy of Hellerhoff. The image may have been modified by cropping, labeling, and/or captions. MedIQ Learning, LLC makes this image available under CC BY-SA.

360 **Ulcer complications.** Reproduced, with permission, from Dr. Frank Gaillard and *www.radiopaedia.org*.

361 **Malabsorption syndromes: Image B.** Whipple disease. This image is a derivative work, adapted from the following source, available under CC BY-SA. Courtesy of Nephron.

378 **Acid suppression therapy.** Adapted, with permission, from Katzung BG, Trevor AJ. *USMLE road map: pharmacology*. New York: McGraw-Hill, 2003:159.

Hematology and Oncology

382 **Erythrocyte.** Courtesy of the U.S. Department of Health and Human Services and Drs. Noguchi, Rodgers, and Schechter.

382 **Thrombocyte (platelet).** Reproduced, with permission, from Mescher AL. *Junquiera's basic histology: text and atlas*, 12th ed. New York: McGraw-Hill, 2010: Fig. 12-13A.

382 **Neutrophil.** Courtesy of the U.S. Department of Health and Human Services. B. Lennert.

383 **Monocyte.** This image is a derivative work, adapted from the following source, available under BY-SA. Courtesy of Dr. Graham Beards.

383 **Macrophage.** Courtesy of the U.S. Department of Health and Human Services.

383 **Eosinophil.** This image is a derivative work, adapted from the following source, available under 0. Dr. Ed Uthman.

383 **Basophil.** This image is a derivative work, adapted from the following source, available under BY-SA. Courtesy of Dr. Erhabor Osaro. The image may have been modified by cropping, labeling, and/or captions. MedIQ Learning, LLC makes this image available under BY-SA.

383 **Mast cell.** Courtesy of the U.S. Department of Health and Human Services. Wikimedia Commons.

384 **Dendritic cell.** This image is a derivative work, adapted from the following source, available under 0. Behnsen J, Narang P, Hasenberg M, et al. Environmental dimensionality controls the interaction of phagocytes with the pathogenic fungi Aspergillus fumigatus and *Candida albicans*. *PLoS Pathogens* 2007;3:e13. doi10.1371/journal.ppat.0030013.

384 **Lymphocyte.** This image is a derivative work, adapted from the following source, available under BY-SA. Courtesy of Wikimedia Commons.

385 **Plasma cell.** This image is a derivative work, adapted from the following source, available under 0. Sharma A, Kaushal M, Chaturvedi N, et al. Cytodiagnosis of multiple myeloma presenting as orbital involvement: a case report. *Cytojournal* 2006;3:19. doi 10.1186/1742-6413-3-19.

388 **Pathologic RBC forms: Image A.** Acanthocyte. This image is a derivative work, adapted from the following source, available under BY-SA. Courtesy of Dr. Ed Uthman.

388 **Pathologic RBC forms: Image B.** Basophilic stippling. This image is a derivative work, adapted from the following source, available under 0. van Dijk HA, Fred HL. Images of memorable cases: case 81. Connexions Web site. December 3, 2008. Available at *http://cnx.org/contents/3196bf3e-1e1e-4c4d-a1ac-d4fc9ab65443@4@4*.

388 **Pathologic RBC forms: Image C.** Degmacyte. This image is a derivative work, adapted from the following source, available under BY-SA. Courtesy of Wikidocs.

388 **Pathologic RBC forms: Image D.** Elliptocyte. Courtesy of Wikimedia Commons.

388 **Pathologic RBC forms: Image E.** Macro-ovalocyte. This image is a derivative work, adapted from the following source, available under BY-SA. Courtesy of Dr. Graham Beards.

388 **Pathologic RBC forms: Image F.** Ringed sideroblast. This image is a derivative work, adapted from the following source, available under BY-SA. Courtesy of Paulo Henrique Orlandi Mourao.

388 **Pathologic RBC forms: Image G.** Schistocyte. Courtesy of Dr. Ed Uthman.

389 **Pathologic RBC forms: Image H.** Sickle cell. Courtesy of the U.S. Department of Health and Human Services. The Sickle Cell Foundation of Georgia, Jackie George, and Beverly Sinclair.

389 **Pathologic RBC forms: Image J.** Dacrocyte. This image is a derivative work, adapted from the following source, available under BY-SA. Courtesy of Paulo Henrique Orlandi Mourao.

389 **Other RBC pathologies: Image A.** Heinz bodies. Reproduced, with permission, from Lichtman MA et al. *Lichtman's atlas of hematology*. New York: McGraw-Hill, 2007: Fig. I.B.2.

389 **Other RBC pathologies: Image B.** Howell-Jolly body. This image is a derivative work, adapted from the following source, available under BY-SA. Courtesy of Paulo Henrique Orlandi Mourao and Mikael Häggström. The image may have been modified by cropping, labeling, and/or captions. MedIQ Learning, LLC makes this image available under BY-SA.

391 **Microcytic, hypochromic anemia: Image D.** Lead poisoning. Reproduced, with permission, from Dr. Frank Gaillard and *www.radiopaedia.org*.

391 **Microcytic, hypochromic anemia: Image E.** Sideroblastic anemia. This image is a derivative work, adapted from the following source, available under 0. Courtesy of Paulo Henrique Orlandi Moura.

392 **Macrocytic anemia.** This image is a derivative work, adapted from the following source, available under BY-SA. Courtesy of Dr. Ed Uthman.

396 **Heme synthesis, porphyrias, and lead poisoning.** Basophilic stippling in lead poisoning. This image is a derivative work, adapted from the following source, available under 0. van Dijk HA, Fred HL. Images of memorable cases: case 81. Connexions Web site. December 3, 2008. Available at *http://cnx.org/contents/3196bf3e-1e1e-4c4d-a1ac-d4fc9ab65443@4@4*.

397 **Coagulation disorders.** Hemarthrosis. This image is a derivative work, adapted from the following source, available under 0. Rodriguez-Merchan EC. Prevention of the musculoskeletal complications of hemophilia. *Adv Prev Med* 2012;2012:201271. doi 10.1155/2012/201271.

401 **Multiple myeloma: Image B.** RBCs in rouleaux formation. This image is a derivative work, adapted from the following source, available under 0. Michail Charakidis and David Joseph Russell.

401 **Multiple myeloma: Image C.** Plasma cells. This image is a derivative work, adapted from the following source, available under 0. Sharma A, Kaushal M, Chaturvedi NK, et al. Cytodiagnosis of multiple myeloma presenting as orbital involvement: a case report. *Cytojournal* 2006;3:19. doi 10.1186/1742-6413-3-19.

403 **Langerhans cell histiocytosis: Image A.** Lytic bone lesion. This image is a derivative work, adapted from the following source, available under ⊛ⓘ. Dehkordi NR, Rajabi P, Naimi A, et al. Langerhans cell histiocytosis following Hodgkin lymphoma: a case report from Iran. *J Res Med Sci* 2010;15:58-61. PMCID PMC3082786.

403 **Langerhans cell histiocytosis: Image B.** Birbeck granules. This image is a derivative work, adapted from the following source, available under ⓒ BY-SA. Courtesy of Dr. Yale Rosen. The image may have been modified by cropping, labeling, and/or captions. MedIQ Learning, LLC makes this image available under ⓒ BY-SA.

403 **Langerhans cell histiocytosis: Image A.** Erythromelalgia in polycythemia vera. This image is a derivative work, adapted from the following source, available under ⊛ⓘ. Fred H, van Dijk H. Images of memorable cases: case 151. Connexions Web site. December 4, 2008. Available at *http://cnx.org/content/ m14932/1.3/*.

403 **Chronic myeloproliferative disorders: Image B.** Enlarged megakaryocytes in essential thrombocytosis. This image is a derivative work, adapted from the following source, available under ⓒ BY-SA. Courtesy of Simon Caulton.

403 **Chronic myeloproliferative disorders: Image C.** Myelofibrosis. This image is a derivative work, adapted from the following source, available under ⓒ BY-SA. Courtesy of Dr. Ed Uthman.

405 **Warfarin.** Toxic effect. This image is a derivative work, adapted from the following source, available under ⊛ⓘ. Fred H, van Dijk H. Images of memorable cases: cases 84 and 85. Connexions Web site. December 2, 2008. Available at *http://cnx. org/content/m14932/1.3/*.

Musculoskeletal, Skin, and Connective Tissue

416 **Common knee conditions: Image A, left (prepatellar bursitis) and right (Baker cyst).** This image is a derivative work, adapted from the following source, available under ⊛ⓘ. Hirji Z, Hunhun JS, Choudur HN. Imaging of the bursae. *J Clin Imaging Sci* 2011;1:22. doi 10.4103/2156-7514.80374.

417 **Wrist bones.** Adapted, with permission, from Brunicardi FC et al. *Schwartz' principles of surgery*, 9th ed. New York: McGraw-Hill, 2009: Fig. 44-2B.

418 **Upper extremity nerves.** Adapted, with permission, from White JS. *USMLE road map: gross anatomy*, 2nd ed. New York: McGraw-Hill, 2005: 145-147.

423 **Muscle conduction to contraction.** Human skeletal muscle. ⊛ⓘ Courtesy of Louisa Howard. The image may have been modified by cropping, labeling, and/or captions. All rights to this adaptation by MedIQ Learning, LLC are reserved.

425 **Osteopetrosis.** This image is a derivative work, adapted from the following source, available under ⊛ⓘ. Kant P, Sharda N, Bhowate RR. Clinical and radiological findings of autosomal dominant osteopetrosis type II: a case report. *Case Rep Dent* 2013;2013:707343. doi 10.1155/2013/707343.

426 **Paget disease of bone: Image A.** Histology. This image is a derivative work, adapted from the following source, available under ⓒ BY-SA. Courtesy of Nephron.

426 **Paget disease of bone: Image B.** Thickened calvarium. This image is a derivative work, adapted from the following source, available under ⊛ⓘ. Dawes L. Paget's disease. [Radiology Picture of the Day Website]. Published June 21, 2007. Available at *http://www.radpod.org/2007/06/21/pagets-disease/*.

426 **Osteonecrosis (avascular necrosis).** This image is a derivative work, adapted from the following source, available under ⊛ⓘ. Ding H, Chen S-B, Lin S, et al. The effect of postoperative corticosteroid administration on free vascularized fibular grafting for treating osteonecrosis of the femoral head. *Sci World J* 2013;2013:708014. doi 10.1155/2013/708014.

428 **Primary bone tumors: Image A.** Giant cell tumor. Reproduced, with permission, from Dr. Frank Gaillard and *www.radiopaedia. org*.

428 **Primary bone tumors: Image B.** Osteochondroma. This image is a derivative work, adapted from the following source, available under ⓒ BY-SA. Courtesy of Lucien Monfils. The image may have been modified by cropping, labeling, and/or captions. MedIQ Learning, LLC makes this image available under ⓒ BY-SA.

428 **Primary bone tumors: Image C.** Osteosarcoma. Reproduced, with permission, from Dr. Frank Gaillard and *www.radiopaedia.org*.

430 **Sjögren syndrome.** Lymphocytic infiltration. ⊛ PUBLIC Courtesy of the U.S. Department of Health and Human Services.

430 **Gout: Image B.** Uric acid crystals under polarized light. This image is a derivative work, adapted from the following source, available under ⓒ BY-SA. Courtesy of Robert J. Galindo

430 **Gout: Image C.** Podagra. This image is a derivative work, adapted from the following source, available under ⊛ⓘ. Roddy E. Revisiting the pathogenesis of podagra: why does gout target the foot? *J Foot Ankle Res* 2011;4:13. doi 10.1186/1757-1146-4-13.

431 **Pseudogout.** Calcium phosphate crystals. ⊛ PUBLIC Courtesy of the U.S. Department of Health and Human Services.

432 **Infectious arthritis.** Joint effusion. This image is a derivative work, adapted from the following source, available under ⓒ BY-SA. Courtesy of Dr. James Heilman. The image may have been modified by cropping, labeling, and/or captions. All rights to this adaptation by MedIQ Learning, LLC are reserved.

432 **Seronegative spondyloarthropathies: Image C, left.** Bamboo spine. This image is a derivative work, adapted from the following source, available under ⓒ BY-SA. Courtesy of Stevenfruitsmaak. The image may have been modified by cropping, labeling, and/ or captions. MedIQ Learning, LLC makes this image available under ⓒ BY-SA.

432 **Seronegative spondyloarthropathies: Image C, right.** Bamboo spine. ⊛ PUBLIC Courtesy of the U.S. Department of Health and Human Services. Heather Hawker.

434 **Sarcoidosis: Image B (X-ray of the chest) and Image C (CT of the chest).** This image is a derivative work, adapted from the following source, available under ⊛ⓘ. Lønborg J, Ward M, Gill A, et al. Utility of cardiac magnetic resonance in assessing right-sided heart failure in sarcoidosis. *BMC Med Imaging* 2013;13:2. doi 10.1186/1471-2342-13-2.

Neurology

479 Normal eye. This image is a derivative work, adapted from the following source, available under (cc) BY-SA. Courtesy of Jan Kaláb. The image may have been modified by cropping, labeling, and/or captions. MedIQ Learning, LLC makes this image available under (cc) BY-SA.

479 Aqueous humor pathway. Adapted, with permission, from Riordan-Eva P, Whitcher JP. *Vaughan & Asbury's general ophthalmology*, 17th ed. New York: McGraw-Hill, 2008.

480 Cataract: Image A, left. Cataract associated with aging. Courtesy of EyeRounds.

480 Cataract: Image A, right. Juvenile cataract. This image is a derivative work, adapted from the following source, available under (cc) O. Roshan M, Vijaya PH, Lavanya GR, et al. A novel human *CRYGD* mutation in a juvenile autosomal dominant cataract. *Mol Vis* 2010;16:887-896. PMCID PMC2875257.

480 Glaucoma: Image A (normal optic cup) and Image B (optic cup in glaucoma). Courtesy of EyeRounds.

480 Glaucoma: Image C. Closed/narrow angle glaucoma. This image is a derivative work, adapted from the following source, available under (cc) O. Low S, Davidson AE, Holder GE, et al. Autosomal dominant Best disease with an unusual electrooculographic light rise and risk of angle-closure glaucoma: a clinical and molecular genetic study. *Mol Vis* 2011;17:2272-2282. PMCID PMC3171497.

480 Glaucoma: Image D. Acute angle closure glaucoma. This image is a derivative work, adapted from the following source, available under (cc) O. Courtesy of Dr. Jonathan Trobe.

480 Uveitis. Courtesy of EyeRounds.

481 Age-related macular degeneration. (PD) Courtesy of the U.S. Department of Health and Human Services.

481 Diabetic retinopathy. Courtesy of EyeRounds.

481 Retinal vein occlusion. This image is a derivative work, adapted from the following source, available under (cc) O. Alasil T, Rauser ME. Intravitreal bevacizumab in the treatment of neovascular glaucoma secondary to central retinal vein occlusion: a case report. *Cases J* 2009;2:176. doi 10.1186/1757-1626-2-176.

481 Retinal detachment. This image is a derivative work, adapted from the following source, available under (cc) O. Hirano Y, Yasukawa T, Ogura Y. Bilateral serous retinal detachments associated with accelerated hypertensive choroidopathy. *Int J Hypertens* 2010;2010:964513. doi 10.4061/2010/964513.

482 Retinitis pigmentosa. Courtesy of EyeRounds.

482 Retinitis. (PD) Courtesy of the U.S. Department of Health and Human Services.

483 Pupillary control. Pupillary light reflex. Adapted, with permission, from Simon RP, et al. *Clinical neurology*, 7th ed. New York: McGraw-Hill, 2009: Fig. 4-12.

484 Ocular motility. Anatomy. Reproduced, with permission, from Morton D et al. *The big picture: gross anatomy*. New York: McGraw-Hill, 2011: Fig. 18-3C.

484 Ocular motility. Testing ocular muscles. This image is a derivative work, adapted from the following source, available under (cc) BY-SA. Courtesy of Au.yousef.

485 Cranial nerve III, IV, VI palsies: Image A. Cranial nerve III damage. This image is a derivative work, adapted from the following source, available under (cc) O. Hakim W, Sherman R, Rezk T, et al. An acute case of herpes zoster ophthalmicus with ophthalmoplegia. *Case Rep Ophthalmol Med* 2012;2012:953910. doi 10.1155/2012/953910.

485 Cranial nerve III, IV, VI palsies: Image B. Cranial nerve IV damage. This image is a derivative work, adapted from the following source, available under (cc) O. Mendez JA, Arias CR, Sanchez D, et al. Painful ophthalmoplegia of the left eye in a 19-year-old female, with an emphasis in Tolosa-Hunt syndrome: a case report. *Cases J* 2009; 2: 8271. doi 10.4076/1757-1626-2-8271.

485 Cranial nerve III, IV, VI palsies: Image C. Cranial nerve VI damage. This image is a derivative work, adapted from the following source, available under (cc) BY-SA. Courtesy of Jordi March i Nogué.

487 Dementia: Image B. Pick bodies in frontotemporal dementia. This image is a derivative work, adapted from the following source, available under (cc) O. Niedowicz DM, Nelson PT, Murphy MP. Alzheimer's disease: pathological mechanisms and recent insights. *Curr Neuropharmacol* 2011;9:674-684. doi 10.2174/157015911798376181.

488 Multiple sclerosis. Periventricular plaques. This image is a derivative work, adapted from the following source, available under (cc) O. Buzzard KA, Broadley SA, Butzkueven H. What do effective treatments for multiple sclerosis tell us about the molecular mechanisms involved in pathogenesis? *Int J Mol Sci* 2012;13:12665-12709. doi 10.3390/ijms131012665.

491 Neurocutaneous disorders: Image A. Sturge-Weber syndrome and port wine stain. This image is a derivative work, adapted from the following source, available under (cc) BY-SA. Courtesy of Babaji P, Bansal A, Krishna G, et al. Sturge-Weber syndrome with osteohypertrophy of maxilla. *Case Rep Pediatr* 2013. doi 10.1155/2013/964596.

491 Neurocutaneous disorders: Image B. Leptomeningeal angioma in Sturge-Weber syndrome. Reproduced, with permission, from Dr. Frank Gaillard and *www.radiopaedia.org*.

491 Neurocutaneous disorders: Image C. Tuberous sclerosis. This image is a derivative work, adapted from the following source, available under (cc) O. Fred H, van Dijk H. Images of memorable cases: case 143. Connexions Web site. December 4, 2008. Available at: *http://cnx.org/content/m14923/1.3/*.

491 Neurocutaneous disorders: Image D. Ash leaf spots in tuberous sclerosis. This image is a derivative work, adapted from the following source, available under (cc) O. Tonekaboni SH, Tousi P, Ebrahimi A, et al. Clinical and para clinical manifestations of tuberous sclerosis: a cross sectional study on 81 pediatric patients. *Iran J Child Neurol* 2012;6:25-31. PMCID PMC3943027.

491 Neurocutaneous disorders: Image E. Angiomyolipoma in tuberous sclerosis. This image is a derivative work, adapted from the following source, available under (cc) O. KGH.

491 Neurocutaneous disorders: Image F. Café-au-lait spots in neurofibromatosis. This image is a derivative work, adapted from the following source, available under (cc) BY-SA. Courtesy of Wikimedia Commons.

491 Neurocutaneous disorders: Image G. Lisch nodules in neurofibromatosis. Courtesy of the U.S. Department of Health and Human Services.

491 Neurocutaneous disorders: Image H. Cutaneous neurofibromas. This image is a derivative work, adapted from the following source, available under . Kim BK, Choi YS, Gwoo S, et al. Neurofibromatosis type 1 associated with papillary thyroid carcinoma incidentally detected by thyroid ultrasonography: a case report. *J Med Case Rep* 2012;6:179. doi 10.1186/1752-1947-6-179.

491 Neurocutaneous disorders: Image I. Cerebellar hemangioblastomas histology. This image is a derivative work, adapted from the following source, available under . Courtesy of Nephron.

491 Neurocutaneous disorders: Image H. Cerebellar hemangioblastomas imaging. This image is a derivative work, adapted from the following source, available under . Park DM, Zhuang Z, Chen L, et al. von Hippel-Lindau disease-associated hemangioblastomas are derived from embryologic multipotent cells. *PLOS Medicine* Feb. 13, 2007. doi 10.1371/journal.pmed.0040060.

492 Adult primary brain tumors: Image A. Glioblastoma multiforme at autopsy. Courtesy of the U.S. Department of Health and Human Services and Armed Forces Institute of Pathology.

492 Adult primary brain tumors: Image B. Glioblastoma multiforme histology. This image is a derivative work, adapted from the following source, available under . Courtesy of Wikimedia Commons. The image may have been modified by cropping, labeling, and/or captions. MedIQ Learning, LLC makes this image available under .

492 Adult primary brain tumors: Image C. Dural tail in meningioma. Courtesy of the U.S. Department of Health and Human Services and Armed Forces Institute of Pathology.

492 Adult primary brain tumors: Image D. Meningioma histology. This image is a derivative work, adapted from the following source, available under . Courtesy of Nephron. The image may have been modified by cropping, labeling, and/or captions. MedIQ Learning, LLC makes this image available under .

492 Adult primary brain tumors: Image E. MRI of hemangioblastoma. This image is a derivative work, adapted from the following source, available under . Park DM, Zhuang Z, Chen L, et al. von Hippel-Lindau disease-associated hemangioblastomas are derived from embryologic multipotent cells. PLoS Med 2007;4:e60. doi 10.1371/journal.pmed.0040060.

492 Adult primary brain tumors: Image F. Hemangioblastoma histology. This image is a derivative work, adapted from the following source, available under . Courtesy of Wikimedia Commons.

492 Adult primary brain tumors: Image G. MRI of schwannoma. Courtesy of the U.S. Department of Health and Human Services. Wikimedia Commons.

492 Adult primary brain tumors: Image H. Schwannoma histology. This image is a derivative work, adapted from the following source, available under . Courtesy of Nephron.

492 Adult primary brain tumors: Image I. MRI of oligodendroglioma. This image is a derivative work, adapted from the following source, available under . Celzo FG, Venstermans C, De Belder F, et al. Brain stones revisited—between a rock and a hard place. *Insights Imaging* 2013;4:625-635. doi 10.1007/s13244-013-0279-z.

492 Adult primary brain tumors: Image J. Oligodendroglioma histology. This image is a derivative work, adapted from the following source, available under . Courtesy of Nephron.

492 Adult primary brain tumors: Image K. MRI of prolactinoma. Reproduced, with permission, from Dr. Frank Gaillard and *www.radiopaedia.org.*

492 Adult primary brain tumors: Image L. Field of vision in bitemporal hemianopia. This image is a derivative work, adapted from the following source, available under . Courtesy of Wikimedia Commons.

493 Childhood primary brain tumors: Image A. MRI of pilocytic astrocytoma. This image is a derivative work, adapted from the following source, available under . Hafez RFA. Stereotaxic gamma knife surgery in treatment of critically located pilocytic astrocytoma: preliminary result. *World J Surg Oncol* 2007;5:39. doi 10.1186/1477-7819-5-39.

493 Childhood primary brain tumors: Image C. CT of medulloblastoma. Courtesy of the U.S. Department of Health and Human Services and Armed Forces Institute of Pathology.

493 Childhood primary brain tumors: Image D. Medulloblastoma histology. This image is a derivative work, adapted from the following source, available under . Courtesy of KGH.

493 Childhood primary brain tumors: Image E. MRI of ependymoma. This image is a derivative work, adapted from the following source, available under . Courtesy of Hellerhoff.

493 Childhood primary brain tumors: Image F: Ependymoma histology. This image is a derivative work, adapted from the following source, available under . Courtesy of Nephron.

493 Childhood primary brain tumors: Image G. CT of craniopharyngioma. This image is a derivative work, adapted from the following source, available under . Garnet MR, Puget S, Grill J, et al. Craniopharyngioma. *Orphanet J Rare Dis* 2007;2:18. doi 10.1186/1750-1172-2-18.

493 Childhood primary brain tumor: Image H. Craniopharyngioma histology. This image is a derivative work, adapted from the following source, available under . Courtesy of Nephron.

Renal

526 Potter sequence (syndrome). Courtesy of the U.S. Department of Health and Human Services and Armed Forces Institute of Pathology.

528 Ureters: course. This image is a derivative work, adapted from the following source, available under . Courtesy of Wikimedia Commons.

533 Relative concentrations along proximal convoluted tubule. Adapted, with permission, from Ganong WF. *Review of medical physiology*, 22nd ed. New York: McGraw-Hill, 2005.

570   **Female reproductive epithelial histology.** Transformation zone. This image is a derivative work, adapted from the following source, available under [cc][BY-SA]. Courtesy of Dr. Ed Uthman. The image may have been modified by cropping, labeling, and/ or captions. MedIQ Learning, LLC makes this image available under [cc][BY-SA].

572   **Seminiferous tubules.** This image is a derivative work, adapted from the following source, available under [cc][BY-SA]. Courtesy of Dr. Anlt Rao.

583   **Pregnancy complications.** Ectopic pregnancy. This image is a derivative work, adapted from the following source, available under [cc][BY-SA]. Courtesy of Dr. Ed Uthman.

585   **Polycystic ovarian syndrome.** This image is a derivative work, adapted from the following source, available under [cc][0]. Lujan ME, Chizen DR, Peppin AK, et al. Improving inter-observer variability in the evaluation of ultrasonographic features of polycystic ovaries. *Reprod Biol Endocrinol* 2008;6:30. doi 10.1186/1477-7827-6-30.

586   **Ovarian neoplasms: Image C.** Mature cystic teratoma. This image is a derivative work, adapted from the following source, available under [cc][BY-SA]. Courtesy of Nephron.

587   **Ovarian neoplasms: Image F.** Yolk sac tumor. This image is a derivative work, adapted from the following source, available under [cc][BY-SA]. Courtesy of Jensflorian. The image may have been modified by cropping, labeling, and/or captions. MedIQ Learning, LLC makes this image available under [cc][BY-SA].

588   **Endometrial conditions: Image A.** Leiomyoma (fibroid), gross specimen. This image is a derivative work, adapted from the following source, available under [cc][BY-SA]. Courtesy of Hic et nunc. The image may have been modified by cropping, labeling, and/or captions. MedIQ Learning, LLC makes this image available under [cc][BY-SA].

588   **Endometrial conditions: Image B.** Leiomyoma (fibroid) histology. This image is a derivative work, adapted from the following source, available under [cc][BY-SA]. Courtesy of KGH.

588   **Endometrial conditions: Image D.** Endometritis. This image is a derivative work, adapted from the following source, available under [cc][BY-SA]. Courtesy of Nephron.

588   **Endometrial conditions: Image E (endometrial hyperplasia) and image F (endometrial carcinoma).** This image is a derivative work, adapted from the following source, available under [cc][0]. Izadi-Mood N, Yarmohammadi M, Ahmadi SA, et al. Reproducibility determination of WHO classification of endometrial hyperplasia/well differentiated adenocarcinoma and comparison with computerized morphometric data in curettage specimens in Iran. *Diagn Pathol* 2009;4:10. doi 10.1186/1746-1596-4-10.

591   **Common breast conditions: Image B.** Comedocarcinoma. Reproduced, with permission, from Schroge JO et al. *Williams gynecology.* New York: McGraw-Hill, 2008: Fig. 12-11.

591   **Common breast conditions: Image C.** Paget disease of breast. Muttarak M, Siriya B, Kongmebhol P, et al. Paget's disease of the breast: clinical, imaging and pathologic findings: a review of 16 patients. *Biomed Imaging Interv J* 2011;7:e16. doi 10.2349/biij.7.2.e16.

591   **Common breast conditions: Image D.** Invasive ductal carcinoma. This image is a derivative work, adapted from the following source, available under [cc][0]. Zhou X-C, Zhou, Ye Y-H, et al. Invasive ductal breast cancer metastatic to the sigmoid colon. *World J Surg Oncol* 2012;10:256. doi 10.1186/1477-7819-10-256.

591   **Common breast conditions: Image E.** Invasive lobular carcinoma. This image is a derivative work, adapted from the following source, available under [cc][0]. Franceschini G, Manno A, Mule A, et al. Gastro-intestinal symptoms as clinical manifestation of peritoneal and retroperitoneal spread of an invasive lobular breast cancer: report of a case and review of the literature. *BMC Cancer* 2006;6:193. doi 10.1186/1471-2407-6-193.

591   **Common breast conditions: Image F.** Peau d'orange of inflammatory breast cancer. [public domain] Courtesy of the U.S. Department of Health and Human Services.

Respiratory

600   **Pneumocytes.** Type II pneumocyte. This image is a derivative work, adapted from the following source, available under [cc][0]. Courtesy of Dr. Thomas Caceci.

608   **Rhinosinusitis.** This image is a derivative work, adapted from the following source, available under [cc][0]. Smith KD, Edwards PC, Saini TS, et al. The prevalence of concha bullosa and nasal septal deviation and their relationship to maxillary sinusitis by volumetric tomography. *Int J Dent* 2010;2010:2404982. doi 10.1155/2010/404982.

608   **Deep venous thrombosis.** This image is a derivative work, adapted from the following source, available under [cc][BY-SA]. Courtesy of Dr. James Heilman.

609   **Pulmonary embolism: Image C.** This image is a derivative work, adapted from the following source, available under [cc][BY-SA]. Courtesy of Dr. Carl Chartrand-Lefebvre.

610   **Obstructive lung diseases: Image A.** Emphysema histology. This image is a derivative work, adapted from the following source, available under [cc][BY-SA]. Courtesy of Nephron.

610   **Obstructive lung disease: Image B.** Centriacinar emphysema, gross specimen. [public domain] Courtesy of the U.S. Department of Health and Human Services and Dr. Edwin P. Ewing, Jr.

610   **Obstructive lung disease: Image C.** CT of centriacinar emphysema. This image is a derivative work, adapted from the following source, available under [cc][0]. Oikonomou A, Prassopoulo P. Mimics in chest disease: interstitial opacities. *Insights Imaging* 2013;4:9-27. doi 10.1007/s13244-012-0207-7.

610   **Obstructive lung disease: Image D.** Barrel-shaped chest in emphysema. This image is a derivative work, adapted from the following source, available under [cc][BY-SA]. Courtesy of Dr. James Heilman.

610   **Obstructive lung disease: Image E.** Curschmann spirals. [public domain] Courtesy of Dr. James Heilman.

610   **Obstructive lung disease: Image F.** Mucus plugs in asthma. This image is a derivative work, adapted from the following source, available under [cc][BY-SA]. Courtesy of Dr. Yale Rosen.

610   **Obstructive lung disease: Image F.** Bronchiectasis in cystic fibrosis. This image is a derivative work, adapted from the following source, available under [cc][BY-SA]. Courtesy of Dr. Yale Rosen.

611 Restrictive lung disease. This image is a derivative work, adapted from the following source, available under ![BY-SA]. Courtesy of IPFeditor.

612 Hypersensitivity pneumonitis: Image A. Pleural plaques in asbestosis. This image is a derivative work, adapted from the following source, available under ![BY-SA]. Courtesy of Dr. Yale Rosen.

612 Hypersensitivity pneumonitis: Image B. CT scan of asbestosis. This image is a derivative work, adapted from the following source, available under ![0]. Miles SE, Sandrini A, Johnson AR, et al. Clinical consequences of asbestos-related diffuse pleural thickening: a review. *J Occup Med Toxicol* 2008;3:20. doi 10.1186/1745-6673-3-20.

612 Hypersensitivity pneumonitis: Image C. Ferruginous bodies in asbestosis. This image is a derivative work, adapted from the following source, available under ![BY-SA]. Courtesy of Nephron.

613 Neonatal respiratory distress syndrome. This image is a derivative work, adapted from the following source, available under ![0]. Alorainy IA, Balas NB, Al-Boukai AA. Pictorial essay: infants of diabetic mothers. *Indian J Radiol Imaging* 2010;20:174-181. doi 10.4103/0971-3026.69349.

613 Acute respiratory distress syndrome. This image is a derivative work, adapted from the following source, available under ![BY-SA]. Courtesy of Samir.

615 Pleural effusions: Images A and B. This image is a derivative work, adapted from the following source, available under ![BY-SA]. Courtesy of Toshikazu A, Takeoka H, Nishioka K, et al. Successful management of refractory pleural effusion due to systemic immunoglobulin light chain amyloidosis by vincristine adriamycin dexamethasone chemotherapy: a case report. *Med Case Rep* 2010;4:322. doi 10.1186/1752-1947-4-322.

616 Pneumonia: Image B. Lobar pneumonia, gross specimen. This image is a derivative work, adapted from the following source, available under ![BY-SA]. Courtesy of Dr. Yale Rosen.

616 Pneumonia: Image C. Acute inflammatory infiltrates in bronchopneumonia. This image is a derivative work, adapted from the following source, available under ![BY-SA]. Courtesy of Dr. Yale Rosen.

616 Pneumonia: Image D. Bronchopneumonia, gross specimen. This image is a derivative work, adapted from the following source, available under ![BY-SA]. Courtesy of Dr. Yale Rosen.

617 Lung abscess: Image A. Gross specimen. This image is a derivative work, adapted from the following source, available under ![BY-SA]. Courtesy of Dr. Yale Rosen.

617 Lung abscess: Image B. X-ray. This image is a derivative work, adapted from the following source, available under ![BY-SA]. Courtesy of Dr. Yale Rosen.

617 Pancoast tumor. This image is a derivative work, adapted from the following source, available under ![0]. Manenti G, Raguso M, D'Onofrio S, et al. Pancoast tumor: the role of magnetic resonance imaging. *Case Rep Radiol* 2013;2013:479120. doi 10.1155/2013/479120.

618 Superior vena cava syndrome: Image A (blanching of skin with pressure) and image B (CT of chest). This image is a derivative work, adapted from the following source, available under ![0]. Shaikh I, Berg K, Kman N. Thrombogenic catheter-associated superior vena cava syndrome. *Case Rep Emerg Med* 2013; 2013: 793054. doi 10.1155/2013/793054.

619 Lung cancer: Image B. Adenocarcinoma histology. ![PUBLIC] Courtesy of the U.S. Department of Health and Human Services and Armed Forces Institute of Pathology.

619 Lung cancer: Image C. Squamous cell carcinoma. This image is a derivative work, adapted from the following source, available under ![BY-SA]. Courtesy of Dr. James Heilman.

Index

T

Tabes dorsalis
  lab/diagnostic findings, 629
  spinal cord lesions in, 471
Tachyarrhythmia, in thyroid
    storm, 329
Tachycardia
  alcohol withdrawal as cause, 519
  in female sexual response, 571
  levothyroxine/triiodothyronine as
    cause, 339
  tricyclic antidepressants as
    cause, 523
Tachypnea, in asthma, 610
Tacrine, 502
Tacrolimus, 218
Tacrolimus (FK-506), 258
Tactile hallucinations, 509
Tadalafil, 598
Taenia solium, 154
Takayasu arteritis, 302
Tamoxifen, **412**, 596
  for breast cancer, 633
  reactions to, 258
Tamponade. *See* Cardiac tamponade
Tamsulosin, 594, **598**, 632
Tanner stages of sexual
    development, **574**
Tapeworms (cestodes), 154
TAPVR (total anomalous pulmonary
    venous return), 288
Tarasoff decision, 57
Tardive dyskinesia, 521
  as drug reaction, 259
Target cells, 389
  in β-thalassemia, 391
  postsplenectomy, 199
Tarsal tunnel syndrome, 421
Tartrate-resistant acid phosphatase
    as hairy cell leukemia test, 402
Taut form of hemoglobin, 603
Taxols, 411
Tay-Sachs disease, 111
  clinical presentation of, 624
Tazobactam, 181
TBG (thyroxine-binding
    globulin), 322
TCA cycle, **97**
  rate-determining enzymes, 96
T-cell lymphomas, and celiac
    sprue, 361
T-cell receptor (TCR), 209
T cells, 384. *See also* Killer T cells
  activation of, **203**
  adaptive immunity and, 200
  anergy, 209
  bacterial toxin effect on, 209
  cytokines secreted by, 207
  cytokines stimulating
      differentiation of, **202**, 207
  cytotoxic, 202, 209
  deficiencies, infections caused
      by, 216
  in delayed (type IV)
      hypersensitivity, 211
  differentiation and maturation, 199
  disorders of, 214–215

helper T cells, 202, 209
  in HIV infection, 169
  location of, in lymph node, 198
  major functions of, **201**
  neoplasms of, 400
  polyclonal activation with
      TSST, 128
  positive and negative selection, 202
  regulatory, 209
  regulatory T cells, **202**
  in spleen, 199
  surface proteins, 209, 384
Teardrop cells, 389
  in myelofibrosis, 404
Teeth
  bacterial flora on, 171
  discolored, from tetracyclines, 259,
      560
  Hutchinson's, in congenital
      syphilis, 141, 175
  impacted/supernumerary, in
      Gardner syndrome, 626
  in Sjögren syndrome, 430
TEF. *See* Tracheoesophageal fistula
Telangiectasias
  in basal cell carcinoma, 443
  in CREST syndrome, 436
  Osler-Weber-Rendu syndrome as
      cause, 628
Telencephalon, 448
Telomerase, 65
Telophase, 72
Temazepam, 497
Temporal arteritis, 302
  associations, common/
      important, 639
  common treatments for, 635
  polymyalgia rheumatica and, 434
Temporal fracture, 466
Temporalis muscle, 478, 565
Temporal lobe, 460
  aphasia and, 460
  stroke effects, 464
Tendinous xanthomas, 291
Tendonitis
  as drug reaction, 259
  fluoroquinolones as cause, 187
Tendons, 75
Tenecteplase, 406
Teniposide, **411**
Tennis elbow, 417
Tenofovir
  Fanconi syndrome caused by, 533
Tenofovir (TDF), 194
Tenosynovitis, 432
Tension headaches, 490
Tension pneumothorax, 614, 615
Tensor tympani muscle, 565
Tensor veli patini muscle, 565
Teratogens, **560**. *See also* Pregnancy
  ACE inhibitors as, 555
  aminoglycosides, 184
  carbamazepine as, 496
  in fetal development, 558
  fluoroquinolones, 187
  griseofulvin, 191, 195
  isoretinoin as, 89

lithium as, 522
  methimazole, 339
  methotrexate as, 409
  phenytoin as, 496
  retinol as, 89
  ribavirin, 195
  tetracyclines, 185
  warfarin as, 405
Teratomas, 593
  immature, 587
Terazosin, 255, 594
Terbinafine, 190, **191**
Terbutaline, 597
  for priapism, 592
Teres minor muscle, 417
Teriparatide, 445
Terminal duct, 589
Terminal ileum
  angiodysplasia in, 365
Tertiary disease prevention, 55
Tesamorelin, 315
Testes
  cryptorchidism, 592
  descent of, 569
  diagram of, 571
  drainage of, 569
  embryonic development of, 559
  progesterone production by, 573
  reproductive hormones and, 595
Testicular arteries, 346
Testicular atrophy
  alcohol use as cause, 519
  cirrhosis as cause, 368
  hemochromatosis as cause, 373
  Klinefelter syndrome as cause, 578
Testicular cancer
  bleomycin for, 410
  drug therapy for, 411
Testicular feminization, 579
Testicular lymphoma, 593
Testicular tumors, **593**
  associations, common/
      important, 639
  gynecomastia caused by, 590
Testis-determining factor, 567
Testosterone, 577
  in cryptorchidism, 592
  secretion of, 572, 595
  in sex chromosome disorders, 579
  in sex development disorders, 579
  SHBG, effect on, 321
  signaling pathway for, 321
  synthesis of, 318
Testosterone (exogenous), **597**
Testosterone-secreting tumors, 579
Tetanospasmin, 124, 131
Tetanus, 131. *See also* Clostridium
    tetani
  bacterial spores causing, 130
Tetanus toxin, 210
Tetany, in hypoparathyroidism, 331
Tetrabenazine, 502
Tetracaine, 499
Tetracyclines, **185**
  expired, reactions to, 259
  mechanism of action, 180
  as protein synthesis inhibitors, 184

reactions to, 259
  as teratogen, 195, 560
Tetralogy of Fallot, 269, 288
  22q11 syndromes and, 290
  cyanosis and, 636
  lab/diagnostic findings, 629
Tetrodotoxin, 252
TGF-β (transforming growth
    factor β), 229
Thalamus, **456**
  central post-stroke pain syndrome
      and, 465
  development of, 448
Thalassemia
  anemia caused by, 390
  labs/diagnostic findings, 630
  target cells in, 389
Thalidomide, 560
Theca-lutein cysts, 585
Thecomas, 586
Thenar eminence, 420
Thenar muscles, 420
  brachial plexus lesions
      affecting, 419
Theophylline, 621
  therapeutic index (TI) value, 246
Therapeutic antibodies, 220
Therapeutic index, **246**
Therapeutic privilege, 56
Thiamine. *See* Vitamin B₁
Thiazide diuretics, 532
  labs/diagnostic findings, 630
Thiazides, 554
  electrolytes, effect on, 554
  gout, effect on, 430
  for heart failure, 297
  for kidney stones, 544
  reactions to, 259
  site of action, 552
  as sulfa drug, 260
Thiazolidinediones, 338
Thick ascending loop of Henle, 532,
    533
Thin descending loop of Henle, 532
Thiopental, 497, 498
Thioridazine, 521
Thiosulfate
  as antidote, 257
Thoracic aortic aneurysms, 272, 292
Thoracic artery, 422
Thoracic duct, 198
  diaphragm and, 601
Thoracic nerve lesions, 419
Thoracic outlet syndrome, 419
Threonine, 104
Throat cancer
  oncogenic microbes, 237
Thrombi
  as atherosclerosis complication, 292
  calcification and, 226
  lines of Zahn, 632
Thrombin, 386
  heparin, effect on, 405
Thromboangiitis obliterans, 302
Thromboangiitis obliterans (Buerger
    disease), 541
Thrombocytes, 382

About the Authors

Tao Le, MD, MHS

Tao developed a passion for medical education as a medical student. He currently edits more than 15 titles in the *First Aid* series. In addition, he is the founder and editor of the *USMLE-Rx* test bank and online video series as well as a cofounder of the *Underground Clinical Vignettes* series. As a medical student, he was editor-in-chief of the University of California, San Francisco (UCSF) *Synapse,* a university newspaper with a weekly circulation of 9000. Tao earned his medical degree from UCSF in 1996 and completed his residency training in internal medicine at Yale University and fellowship training at Johns Hopkins University. Tao subsequently went on to cofound Medsn, a medical education technology venture, and served as its chief medical officer. He is currently conducting research in asthma education at the University of Louisville.

Vikas Bhushan, MD

Vikas is a writer, editor, entrepreneur, and teleradiologist on sabbatical. In 1990 he conceived and authored the original *First Aid for the USMLE Step 1*. His entrepreneurial endeavors include a student-focused medical publisher (S2S), an e-learning company (medschool.com/Medsn), and an ER teleradiology practice (24/7 Radiology). Firmly anchored to the Left Coast, Vikas completed a bachelor's degree at the University of California Berkeley; an MD with thesis at UCSF; and a diagnostic radiology residency at UCLA. His eclectic interests include technology, information design, photography, South Asian diasporic culture, and avoiding a day job. Always finding the long shortcut, Vikas is an adventurer, knowledge seeker, and occasional innovator. He enjoys novice status as a kiteboarder and single father, and strives to raise his children as global citizens.

Matthew Sochat, MD

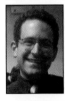

Matthew began residency training in neurology at New York University in 2014. He earned his medical degree from Brown University in 2013 and completed his undergraduate studies at the University of Massachusetts-Amherst, graduating in 2008 with degrees in biochemistry and the classics. In his (limited) spare time, Matthew enjoys skiing, cooking/baking, traveling, the company of friends/loved ones, and computer/video gaming. Be warned: he also loves to come up with corny jokes at (in)opportune moments.

Michael Mehlman

Michael is in his sixth and final year of medical school and research at the University of Queensland, Australia. Prior to medical school, he completed an undergraduate degree at Boston University and a research internship at University of Sydney. Michael would be most fortunate for a transitional/preliminary year in order to gain a greater diversity of experience and perspective before committing to any field for the long term. In his (lack of) spare time, he teaches students across the world preparation tactics for the USMLE Step 1 and is an avid member of the Student Doctor Network. Outside of medicine, Michael is interested in chess, artisanal hot sauce, and lexicology.

Patrick Sylvester

Patrick is a fourth-year student at the Ohio State University College of Medicine. Originally from Illinois, he completed his undergraduate studies at the University of Illinois at Urbana-Champaign. Recently married, Patrick enjoys spending his free time with his infinitely patient wife, Julie, and their dog, Chief.

Kimberly Kallianos, MD

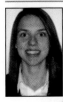

Originally from Atlanta, Kimberly graduated from the University of North Carolina at Chapel Hill in 2006 and from Harvard Medical School in 2011. She is currently a third-year radiology resident at the University of California, San Francisco.

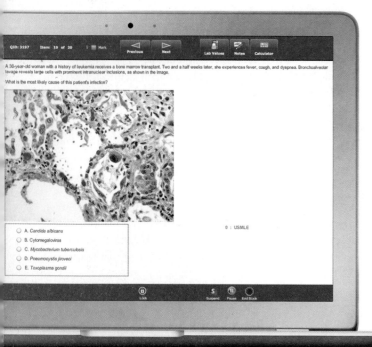
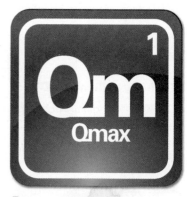